Vertebrate hormones	Molecular weight
Lysine vasopressin (LVP)	1,056
Lysylbradykinin	1,188
Melanin-concentrating hormone (MCH)	2,387
α-Melanocyte-stimulating hormone (α-MSH); α-melanotropin	1,665
Melatonin (*N*-acetyl-5-methoxytryptamine)	232
Mesotocin	1,007
Methionine enkephalin (Met-enkephalin)	574
Motilin	2,670
MSH release-inhibiting factor (MIF)	
Müllerian regression factor (MRF, anti-Müllerian hormone, AMH)	
Nerve growth factor (NGF)	
NPY	4,272
	1,673
	103
Oxytocin	1,007
Pancreatic polypeptide (PP)	4,221 (b)
Parathormone (PTH)	
Platelet-derived growth factor (PDGF)	
Progesterone	314
Prostacyclin I_2 (PGI_2)	353
Prostaglandin E_2 (PGE_2)	352
Prostaglandin $F_{2\alpha}$ ($PGF_{2\alpha}$)	355
Relaxin	
Secretin	3,055 (p)
Serotonin (5-hydroxytryptamine, 5-HT)	176
Serum thymic factor (STF)	876
Somatostatin (SST)	1,639
Substance P (SP)	1,347 (b)
Testosterone	288
Thromboxane A_2 (TXA_2)	
Thymopoietin	
Thymosin$_{\alpha 1}$	
Thymosin$_{\alpha 4}$	
Thyrotropin; thyroid-stimulating hormone (TSH)	
Thyrotropin-releasing hormone (TRH)	362
Thyroxine (T_4)	777
Transforming growth factor (TGF)	
Triiodothyronine (T_3)	651
Vasoactive intestinal peptide (VIP)	3,326 (p)
Vasotocin	1,050
Vitamin D_3(1α,25-dihydroxycholecalciferol) (1α,25(OH)$_2$D$_3$) (calcitriol)	417

[a]All hormones are of human origin unless otherwise noted (p, procine; b, bovine; f, frog). The molecular weights (MW) are derived from the constituent amino acids of the peptides. It should be noted that commercially available or synthetically prepared peptides may contain a number of counter ions (e.g., acetate, Na$^+$, etc.) depending on the final purification and isolation procedures. This should be carefully considered when using the dry weight of the lyophilized powder to prepare molar concentrations of peptides.

Endocrinology

Sixth Edition

Mac E. Hadley

Department of Cell Biology & Anatomy
The University of Arizona
Tucson, Arizona

Jon E. Levine

Department of Neurobiology and Physiology
Northwestern University
Evanston, Illinois

PEARSON

Prentice
Hall

Upper Saddle River, NJ 07458

Library of Congress Cataloging-in-Publication Data

Hadley, Mac E.
    Endocrinology / Mac E. Hadley, Jon E. Levine.—6th ed.
        p. cm.
    Includes bibliographical references and index.
    ISBN 0-13-187606-6
    1. Endocrinology.   I. Levine, Jon E.   II. Title
    [DNLM: 1. Endocrine System.   2. Hormones.   WK 100 H131e 2006]
    QP187.H17 2006
    573.4—dc22

                                      2006026786

Executive Editor: Gary Carlson
Editor-in-Chief, Science: Dan Kaveney
Executive Managing Editor: Kathleen Schiaparelli
Assistant Managing Editor: Beth Sweeten
Media Editor: Patrick Shriner
Senior Managing Editor, Science and Math Media:
    Nicole M. Jackson
Assistant Managing Editor, Science Supplements:
    Karen Bosch
Manufacturing Manager: Alexis Heydt-Long
Manufacturing Buyer: Alan Fischer
Director of Creative Services: Paul Belfanti
Creative Director: Juan R. López
Art Director: Maureen Eide
Interior Design: Koala Bear

Cover Design: Michael Fruibeis
Senior Managing Editor, AV Production and Management:
    Patricia Burns
Manager, Production Technologies: Matthew Haas
Managing Editor, Art Management: Abigail Bass
Art Development Editor: Jay McElroy
AV Production Editor: Connie Long
Manager, Art Production: Sean Hogan
Assistant Manager, Art Production: Ronda Whitson
Illustrations: Artworks, Adam Steinberg
Editorial Assistant: Jessica Neumann
Cover Image: Photomicrographs courtesy of
    Gloria Hoffman, Ph.D., Department of Anatomy &
    Neurobiology, University of Maryland School of Medicine,
    Baltimore MD.

© 2007, 2000, 1996, 1992, 1988, 1982 by Pearson Education, Inc.
Pearson Prentice Hall
Pearson Education, Inc.
Upper Saddle River, New Jersey 07458

Pearson Prentice Hall™ is a trademark of Pearson Education, Inc.

Printed in the United States of America
10 9 8 7 6 5 4 3 2 1

ISBN 0-13-187606-6

Pearson Education Ltd., *London*
Pearson Education Australia Pty., Limited, *Sydney*
Pearson Education Singapore, Pte. Ltd
Pearson Education North Asia Ltd., *Hong Kong*
Pearson Education Canada, Ltd., *Toronto*
Pearson Educación de Mexico, S.A. de C.V.
Pearson Education—Japan, *Tokyo*
Pearson Education Malaysia, Pte. Ltd.

CONTENTS

2   *The Vertebrate Endocrine System*   *17*

3   *General Mechanisms of Hormone Action*   39

4   *Endocrine Methodologies*   67

11 *Pancreatic Hormones and Metabolic Regulation   237*

12 *Growth Hormones*   264

15 *Adrenal Steroid Hormones   337*

18 *Hormones and Female Reproductive Physiology   408*

PREFACE

As the new co-author this sixth edition of ***Endocrinology***, I am by no means a stranger to the book. It has been a smart and dependable friend – one that has helped me to teach my course, *Vertebrate Endocrinology*, to both undergraduates and graduate students at Northwestern University for the past ten years. Knowing firsthand the heuristic value of this textbook, I have endeavored to update and revise it, without changing its basic organization and flow. I have also attempted to match, to the extent possible, Mac Hadley's lucid and authoritative writing style. New to this edition is an expanded treatment of the basic concepts and research methodologies in endocrinology in Chapters 1–4. Moreover, Chapters 3 and 4 in the previous edition have been swapped in this edition, so as to complete discussions of fundamentals and basic principles before delving into modern and classic research methods. In each of the succeeding chapters, specific endocrine systems are described and analyzed according to the same general format used in previous editions of Hadley's ***Endocrinology***.

Chapters 5–20 have been updated and revised, each to the extent dictated by research advances in the study of each endocrine system. For example, new sections have been added to Chapter 11 on the adipocytokines, leptin and adiponectin, and their roles in feeding and energy homeostasis. Similarly, the multiple functions of the recently characterized gut hormone, ghrelin, are included in Chapters 10, 11, and 12. Discussions of estrogen receptors and estrogen actions have also been revised in several chapters, based on advances made using molecular biology and gene targeting approaches. In this edition, we have also opted to move much of the material contained within the previous Chapter 21, "Neurohormones," to other appropriate places within the book. Opioid peptides, for example, are discussed in Chapter 8 of this edition.

This edition of ***Endocrinology*** has two additional features that we hope will enhance its usefulness in the classroom. Throughout the book, subheadings now consist of declarative statements, each succinctly summarizing the major concept discussed in the text that follows it. Students are thus given notice as to the point of the ensuing text, and are better prepared to digest and understand the information and arguments that support it. For instructors, these subheadings will also provide a logically ordered series of major concepts to be addressed during lectures. The second new feature of ***Endocrinology*** is a section at the end of each chapter entitled "Think, Analyze and Discuss." These contain challenging questions that can be used as provocative starting points for in-class discussions or group study sessions.

The science of endocrinology is remarkably fast-moving, and encompasses a myriad of today's "hot issues." Indeed, the student of endocrinology may be surprised to find that endocrine science intersects with so many contemporary concerns. Body weight regulation and obesity, hormone replacement therapy in menopause, "doping" by competitive athletes, responses to stress, sex partner preference, effects of environmental pollutants on wildlife—all of these ostensibly unrelated topics have, at their core, an endocrine basis. We hope that this textbook will continue to enlighten and inform readers, and provide them with the firm grounding in current endocrine science needed to intelligently consider issues such as these.

Jon E. Levine
Northwestern University
Department of Neurobiology and Physiology
Evanston, IL 60208
Tel: (847) 491-7180
Fax: (847) 491-5211
Email: jlevine@northwestern.edu

The central theme of this text is the role of chemical messengers, or hormones, whether they are of endocrine or neural origin, in the control of physiological processes. Although endocrine physiology has been separated from neurophysiology in the past, it is now amply documented that hormones may originate from either endocrine or neural tissue. Thus has emerged the field of neuroendocrinology. Several eminent endocrinologists have been awarded Nobel Prizes in Physiology/Medicine for their monumental efforts leading to the discovery and elucidation of the chemical structure of several brain neuropeptides (neurohormones); this clearly emphasizes the importance of the concept of neuroendocrine physiology. It is now also realized that the so-called "classical" hormones are produced in many sites throughout the body and may be released directly into the blood, into neuronal synapses, or into the immediate intercellular space to affect adjacent cellular activity. This more inclusive definition of "hormone," therefore, has been employed, as suggested by Nobel laureate Roger Guillemin. The important point emphasized in this definition is that it is both the method of delivery as well as the source of the hormone that is of greatest physiological significance.

In **Introduction to Endocrinology**, a short chronology of endocrine research is presented. The concept of homeostasis is then discussed with special reference given to the roles of chemical messengers in the control of homeostatic systems. The reader is then provided with a general description of **The Vertebrate Endocrine System**, wherein an initial working vocabulary is established. Included here is a discussion of the general classes of chemical messengers and other cellular regulators (steroid and peptide hormones, neurohormones, chalones, growth factors, eicosanoids, pheromones); the cellular synthesis of chemical messengers and their secretion, delivery, and metabolism; and a general overview of the physiological role of hormones. It was considered important to provide, early in the book, a discussion of **General Mechanisms of Hormone Action**, because these concepts are a necessary component of each of the following chapters. Included within this chapter is a discussion of cellular receptors, cyclic nucleotides as second messengers, prostaglandins (and prostacyclins, thromboxanes, and leukotrienes), stimulus-response coupling, calmodulin (a cellular calcium receptor), and phosphorylated proteins as physiological effectors. In consideration of the various methodologies used in present-day endocrine research, it was also considered necessary to add a chapter on **Endocrine Methodologies** early in the text. Classical surgical and histological techniques are discussed, as are more recent methods including radioimmunoassay, radioreceptor assay, radioisotope enzyme assay, autoradiography, reverse-transcriptase polymerase chain reaction (RT-PCR), recombinant-DNA methodologies, transgenesis, and gene targeting. The source, synthesis, chemistry, and general role of the **Pituitary Hormones** in the control of endocrine physiology are discussed next, because the pituitary gland is a major source of hormones regulating many other endocrine glands. More specific details of the roles and actions of these hormones are provided in subsequent chapters. Because the secretion of each of the pituitary hormones is controlled by hypophysiotropic hormones of hypothalamic origin, a chapter on the role of **The Endocrine Hypothalamus** is provided. The evidence supporting the neurovascular hypothesis is emphasized.

Chapter 7, **Neurohypophysial Hormones**, provides a complete coverage of the source, synthesis, chemistry, secretion, metabolism, biological actions, and mechanisms of action of the posterior pituitary hormones, oxytocin and vasopressin. The evolution of hormone structure is emphasized under the comparative endocrinology of neurohypophysial hormones. Chapter 8, **The Opiomelanotropic Hormones**, emphasizes the recent discovery that proopiomelanocortin is the precursor protein of α-melanotropin, adrenocorticotropin, and humans' own analgesic hormones, the endorphins (opiate-like peptides). The author (MEH) has done considerable research in the field of melanotropins and vertebrate pigmentation, particularly in relationship to the control of melanocyte-stimulating hormone secretion and the mechanisms of action of the melanotropins. Because the secretion and actions of almost all hormones involve the calcium ion, the roles of parathormone, calcitonin, and vitamin D in the **Hormonal Control of Calcium Homeostasis** are discussed early in the book (Chap. 9).

The next six chapters are grouped together because they all relate to aspects of metabolic endocrinology. The **Gastrointestinal Hormones** play important roles in the control of food-stuff movement through the gastrointestinal tract and its transport through the intestinal mucosa and into the general circulation. The chapter on **Pancreatic Hormones and Metabolic Endocrinology** discusses the roles of the endocrine pancreas in the storage and utilization of metabolic substrates. The contrasting roles of insulin and glucagon are explored, as are the possible roles of the newer pancreatic hormones, somatostatin and pancreatic polypeptide. In a chapter on **Growth Hormones**, the varied roles of the somatomedins and other peptide-growth hormones, such as nerve growth factor, epidermal growth factor, erythropoietin, and the thymic growth factors, as well as growth inhibitory factors (chalones) are discussed, in addition to an in-depth coverage of pituitary somatotropin (growth hormone).

In the chapter on **Thyroid Hormones**, evidence is marshaled demonstrating that triiodothyronine is the physiologically relevant thyroid hormone at the cellular level. An up-to-date review of a model of thyroid hormone action is provided. A discussion of the integrated functional aspects of **Catecholamines and the Sympathoadrenal System** provides recent data on the developmental biology of catecholamine biosynthesis within adrenal chromaffin tissue and sympathetic neurons. The physiological roles of catecholamines as mediated through adrenergic receptors (adrenoceptors) is discussed, and the pharmacology of the autonomic nervous system, particularly the sympathoadrenal system, is reviewed. The chapter on the **Adrenal Steroid Hormones** completes the general discussion of the roles and actions of hormones in the control of metabolic homeostasis. Steroid hormone structure and nomenclature are reviewed. The roles of cortisol, a glucocorticoid, and aldosterone, a mineralocorticoid, are discussed in detail. The pathophysiology of adrenocortical dysfunction provides an in-depth view of the etiological bases for endocrine pathophysiology.

The next five chapters deal with the endocrinology of vertebrate reproductive systems, mostly mammalian systems. In the **Endocrinology of Sex Differentiation and Development**, the role of the Sry/SRY gene and its product, the testes-determining factor, in the regulation of gonadal differentiation is discussed. The early organizational roles of gonadal steroids in the development of neural centers (e.g., dimorphic nucleus) within the central nervous system, and the activation roles of steroids in CNS function in the adult animal are reviewed. In **Hormones and Male Reproductive Physiology**, as in **Hormones and Female Reproductive Physiology**, the origin, synthesis, chemistry, secretion, metabolism, biological roles, and mechanisms of actions of the male and female reproductive hormones are reviewed. A discussion of the pathophysiology of reproductive function in the human male and female provides an insight into the many genetic and congenital defects that affect normal growth and development of the human reproductive systems. In **Endocrinology of Pregnancy, Parturition, and Lactation**, the roles of hormones in the fertile period of the female are reviewed. Next is included a chapter on the **Endocrine Role of the Pineal Gland**, which reviews its putative role in reproductive physiology. This chapter is long overdue; the pineal gland is clearly an endocrine organ.

Generally, each chapter is subdivided as follows: (1) Introduction (which provides a historical perspective to the particular topic), (2) Source, (3) Synthesis, (4) Chemistry, (5) Secretion, (6) Metabolism, (7) Physiological Roles, (8) Mechanism of Action, (9) Pathophysiology (of endocrine dysfunction), and (10) Comparative Endocrinology. Due to space limitations and other considerations the coverage of neuroendocrine physiology generally has been restricted to vertebrates, mainly mammals, particularly the human. Therefore, this book should be of special appeal to preprofessional students in medicine, dentistry, pharmacology, nutrition, nursing, and other related medical or animal sciences. Within each chapter, however, where appropriate, is included a short coverage of comparative endocrinology.

References are provided with each chapter, but, because space limitations place a premium on those selected, the most recently available are used. These references will provide the reader with most of the important earlier studies related to a particular topic. The author therefore acknowledges the unreferenced contributions of many investigators in the field of neuroendocrine physiology.

Individuals interested in the topic of endocrinology mainly fall into the following general categories: (1) teachers and their students interested in a general (comprehensive) coverage of the topic, (2) teachers and their students with preprofessional interests (premedical, predental, other health-related sciences), (3) teachers and students interested in comparative endocrinology, and (4) professional scientists in research and health-related professions. Since time is limited and the coverage of endocrinology is extensive, some teachers of general or comparative endocrinology may desire to omit (not cover) the last section of each chapter dealing with *Pathophysiology*.

The authors appreciate the very informative figures that have been provided for this sixth edition by leading authorities in the field of endocrine physiology. I am particularly grateful to my past students, both in the classroom and the research laboratory, who provided me with an opportunity to develop the thoughts that are now presented in this textbook of endocrinology.

Helpful criticisms, corrections, or other comments are most welcome and may be addressed to the authors.

Mac E. Hadley
University of Arizona
College of Medicine
Department of Cell Biology & Anatomy
Tucson, AZ 85724
Tel: (520) 626-0966
Fax: (520) 626-6354
E mail: erectide@aol.com

Introduction to Endocrinology

Development of a multicellular organism commences on fertilization and subsequent division of the egg. Further development is then dependent on continued cell proliferation, growth, and differentiation, including the formation of tissues and organs. The integration of these developmental events, as well as the coordination of such physiological processes as metabolism, respiration, excretion, movement, reproduction, and sensory perception, are dependent on chemical cues, substances synthesized and secreted by cells within the animal. The role of these **chemical messengers** in the growth and regulation of cellular and organ function in the vertebrate is the topic of this book.

Endocrinology is a subdiscipline of the broader field, physiology, and is concerned with the study of **hormones**, which are chemical messengers secreted by cells of endocrine glands (ductless glands) and tissues that regulate the activity of other cells in the body. Besides the obvious study of the physiological roles of hormones, endocrinologists also study the cellular source, biosynthesis, chemistry and storage of hormones, the factors and mechanisms controlling hormonal secretion, the cellular mechanisms of hormone action, and the pathophysiology of endocrine system dysfunction. The comparative endocrinologist is particularly interested in the study of the endocrine systems of non-human vertebrate as well as invertebrate species [3].

Endocrine Systems

In evolutionary history, Metazoa appeared as the earliest multicellular organisms in which different cell groups assumed specific functions. The emergence of these animals coincided with the development of systems that allowed for communication and functional integration among the specialized cell groups. Two types of intercellular communication systems evolved—one endocrine and the other nervous—to assume these important physiological roles. Both endocrine and nervous systems acquired the same basic components of cell–cell signaling: "sender" cells that produce and release chemical messengers into the extracellular environment, and "target" cells that receive, transduce, and respond to the chemical signal.

In a nervous system, communication between neurons, or from neurons to peripheral tissues, is mediated by electrochemical signals; excitation of the sender or presynaptic cell leads to release of a *neurotransmitter* into a synapse (microscopic cleft between the sender and target cell). The neurotransmitter diffuses across the synaptic cleft and binds to specific molecules called *receptors*, located on the target cell, which in turn activate a cascade of signals to the interior of the target cell. In *endocrine systems*, by contrast, the sender cells typically produce and secrete *hormones* into the bloodstream to exert their actions via receptors on cells in distant target tissues. Many hormones are specifically produced by ductless organs or tissues called *glands*, such as the pituitary gland, thyroid gland, parathyroid glands, and endocrine pancreas. Other hormones are produced and secreted into the bloodstream by certain cells within the brain, kidney, gonads, bones, heart, and other tissues with additional major non-endocrine functions. Neurons in the brain that produce hormones are referred to as *neuroendocrine* cells, and the process of release from these cells into the bloodstream is called *neurosecretion*; the hormones released by neurons are accordingly known as *neurohormones*.

Each specific hormone, together with its cells of origin and target tissues, constitutes a specific endocrine system. As described in several chapters in this book, however, virtually none of the specific endocrine systems operate in isolation from other endocrine systems. Thus, in a more general sense, "endocrine system" is also used to describe a set of endocrine tissues, hormones, and target tissues that operate as a functionally integrated unit. In some cases, multiple hormones may be produced by the same organ or different organs to control a particular physiological variable. Blood glucose levels, for example, are regulated in a reciprocal manner by two pancreatic hormones, insulin and glucagon, as well as by hormones of the pituitary and adrenal glands. In other endocrine systems, one endocrine organ may regulate another, which may then reciprocally regulate the first, or even regulate a third organ. The control of gonadal function, for example, is exerted in a hierarchical manner: neurosecretion of a neurohormone called gonadotropin-releasing hormone (GnRH) directs the secretion of gonadotropic hormones from the pituitary gland, which in turn stimulate production of gonadal steroid hormones and regulate gonadal function. How does one go about gaining an understanding of endocrine systems such as these? For the student of endocrinology, it is most instructive to first understand the scientific processes that were used to acquire the basic knowledge of these systems, as presented below.

Historical Perspective

Endocrinology is a relatively infant science that began with the first recorded endocrine experiment published by Berthold (1849) [5]. No other truly significant discoveries were made until about 50 years later (1889–1902). The pace quickened after 1910, and the outlines of vertebrate and invertebrate endocrine systems were generally complete by 1950. From then on, chemistry and physiology played most important roles in the development of the science and many advances in the field were made. Molecular biology and genetics are now advancing the field at an ever more rapid pace. The elucidation of the gene structure for hormones and their receptors is providing important insights into the evolutionary history of endocrine systems.

The Science of Endocrinology Progressed from Simple Observations to Complex Experimentation

Early medical writings described the general symptoms of many endocrine dysfunctions long before the pathophysiology of any of the now well-characterized *endocrinopathies* was understood. In the age of the great European microscopists of the nineteenth century, most tissues and organs of the vertebrate body were described in great detail, but the functional significance of what we now refer to as endocrine glands was not evident. Clinical correlations between tissue or organ abnormalities, such as atrophy or enlargement, and a change in a particular physiological state were occasionally noted. This led to the study of the possible effects of tissue or organ removal from animals and subsequent alteration in physiological function. The use of organ transplants or extracts in replacement therapy for the absent tissue or organ then followed. Successful replacement therapy led to the purification of these physiologically active extracts and ultimately to the identification of the hormonal substances concerned.

Berthold's Experiments in Roosters Lead to the Discovery of Testosterone

Berthold, a French scientist, in the earliest endocrinological study on record, noted that if he castrated roosters they failed to develop their comb and wattles, and they also failed to exhibit male behavior [5]. Transplant of the testes (one or both) back into the abdominal cavity of the same or another castrated bird resulted in normal development of the comb and wattles, and the birds exhibited male behavior, which involved an interest in hens and aggressive action toward other males. The transplanted testes were functional, yet they were not dependent on any direct nervous innervation for their activity. Berthold also observed

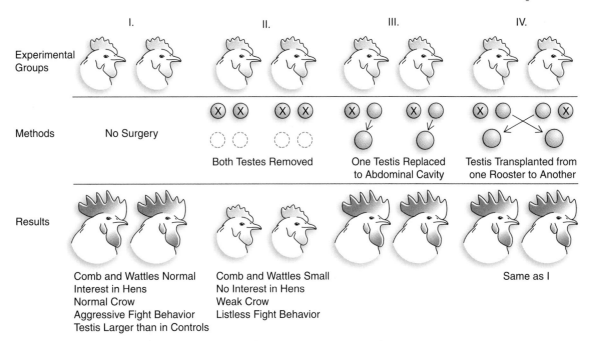

I.   II.   III.   IV.

Experimental Groups

Methods   No Surgery   Both Testes Removed   One Testis Replaced to Abdominal Cavity   Testis Transplanted from one Rooster to Another

Results

Comb and Wattles Normal
Interest in Hens
Normal Crow
Aggressive Fight Behavior
Testis Larger than in Controls

Comb and Wattles Small
No Interest in Hens
Weak Crow
Listless Fight Behavior

Same as I

Figure 1.1   Berthold's experiment: the first endocrine experiment.

that a transplanted single testis was larger than either testis of the host when both were present together in the bird. Thus he discovered, but may not have appreciated, what is now referred to as *compensatory hypertrophy*, an increase in the size of an organ to compensate functionally for the activity of the other lost organ. His results also demonstrated that an organ from one (donor) animal could be transplanted to another (host) animal where it can become functional (Fig. 1.1).

Berthold concluded that the testes secreted something that conditioned the blood, and he speculated that the blood then acted on the body of the cockerel to cause the development of male characteristics. Actually, these experiments only demonstrated the need for the presence of the testes to maintain male characteristics. The testes could maintain such behavioral and physiological functions by a number of possible means: (1) activation or transformation of one or more constituents of the blood into active agents, hormones, (2) removal of an inhibitory substance from the blood or, as is now known, (3) release of a hormone into the circulation. That the testes produce a substance that is released into the blood to affect masculine features and behavior was not proven until many years later when it was shown that extracts of the testes could functionally replace the testes of a castrated animal. The hormone of the testes, *testosterone*, was finally obtained in pure crystalline form in 1935 and shown to be the active substance.

Secretin is Discovered by Bayliss and Starling

In 1902, the first critical experiment, the *experimentum cruces*, demonstrating the existence of a hormone was reported [2]. Bayliss and Starling, British physiologists, discovered that a substance was liberated by the mucosa of the small intestine that stimulates the flow of pancreatic juice. It was known that the acid present in chyme (partially digested food) stimulated pancreatic secretion after it entered into the small intestine from the stomach. Introduction of acid into an isolated (denervated) but vascularized section of the jejunum (portion of the small intestine) caused a similar flow of pancreatic juice. This observation supported the view that the control of pancreatic enzyme secretion was mediated by humoral (bloodborne) rather than nervous stimulation. Extracts of jejunal epithelium produced similar effects on pancreatic secretion. The active substance was given the name *secretin* and was further shown to be localized only to those regions of the small intestine that could be stimulated by acid to induce pancreatic fluid flow. Starling (1905) [26] introduced the term *hormone* (from the Greek for "I arouse to activity" or "I excite") for this humoral factor.

Insulin is Determined to be a Pancreatic Hormone that Regulates Blood Glucose

In 1889, Von Mering and Minkowski showed by surgical methods that removal of the pancreas from dogs led to symptoms similar to those characteristics of human *diabetes mellitus*. In these dogs, as in diabetic humans, blood sugar levels were remarkably elevated; this suggested that diabetes mellitus might result from a defect of carbohydrate metabolism due to lack of pancreatic function. Banting and Best [1], Canadian physiologists, concluded from other investigations that the islets of Langerhans, rather than the pancreatic acini, which make up the bulk of the pancreas, are essential in the control of carbohydrate metabolism. They suggested that the pancreatic islets regulate blood glucose levels by producing an internal secretion, rather than by modifying the blood. In 1922, they successfully obtained extracts of the pancreatic islets and showed that these preparations caused a dramatic drop in blood glucose levels when administered to diabetic dogs [6]. This hormone of the pancreas was given the name *insulin* as originally proposed by Schaefer in 1912. In 1953, Frank Sanger established the amino acid sequence of this protein hormone [22]. For this crucial work in the characterization of hormone structure, he received a Nobel Prize. The structures of many of the other major protein hormones were subsequently elucidated using Sanger's methods.

The Nervous System is Shown to Release Neurotransmitters

Hormones are released from cells into the general circulation to mediate their effects on distant target cells, while neurotransmitters are released from neurons into close proximity to the effector cells that they regulate. Some neurotransmitters can function in both capacities depending upon the source of the neurochemical. The catecholamines, norepinephrine and epinephrine, for example, function as neurotransmitters at synaptic junctions, and they are also released from adrenal medullary cells into the systemic circulation to act as hormones. As neurotransmitters, these chemical messengers of neural origin play important roles in both the *central nervous system* (CNS) and the *autonomic nervous system* (ANS) function. Walter Cannon was the first physiologist to stress the role of the ANS in the "self-regulation of physiological processes" [7]. As is described in Chapter 14, the ANS regulates the activity of such so-called "autonomic" activities as gastrointestinal (GI) smooth muscle contraction and relaxation; GI secretions (including hormone secretions from the stomach and gut), cardiovascular muscle contraction and relaxation, and adipose tissue metabolism.

That nerves release neurotransmitters to control effector cell activity was first demonstrated in 1921 by Otto Loewi [16]. A frog heart with its attached vagus nerve was incubated in physiological saline solution, and after residing therein for a period of time, the solution was removed and used to bathe a second heart. There was no effect of the solution on the *inotropic* (amplitude of beat) or *chronotropic* (rate of beat) characteristics of the incubated heart. If, on the other hand, the vagus nerve innervating an incubated heart was electrically stimulated a number of times and the saline solution then transferred to another beaker containing another frog heart, a decreased (negative) inotropic and chronotropic activity was noted. These diminished myotropic responses could be blocked by addition of the drug atropine, which was known to be inhibitory to vagal nerve-induced relaxation of the heart. The atropinized heart preparations did, however, respond to saline solution taken from vagus nerve-stimulated hearts by an increased rate and strength of contraction. These experiments demonstrated that the vagus nerve released substances that affect the relaxation and contraction of cardiac muscle. For this work, Loewi received a Nobel Prize. The "vagustuff" (vagal substance) was identified as *acetylcholine* and the accelerator substance as *norepinephrine*. These two neurotransmitters play very important roles in endocrine physiology (Chap. 14).

Vincent du Vigneaud carried out the first laboratory syntheses of peptide hormones by synthesizing the neurohormones oxytocin and a vasopressin. For this work he, too, received a Nobel Prize. Most interestingly, he also synthesized a related structure (analog) of oxytocin, which turned out to be a hormone found in the pituitaries of most vertebrates. Thus, he synthesized the structure of a hormone (vasotocin) before it was actually discovered (Chap. 7).

Sutherland and Colleagues Discover Cyclic AMP

How do hormones exert their biological effects in cells? In early endocrine research, this question was of particular importance for those hormones that were known to not pass freely through cell plasma membrane, but instead were suspected to act on the exterior

Figure 1.2 Structure of cyclic AMP, a second messenger of hormone action.

surfaces of cells. In 1962, Earl Sutherland and his colleagues presented a number of papers describing the presence of adenosine 3′,5′-monophosphate (*cyclic AMP, cAMP*) in biological materials. These papers also dealt with adenylate cyclase, the enzyme responsible for the cellular production of this cyclic nucleotide. Sutherland and his co-workers had previously demonstrated that hormones could stimulate broken cell membrane preparations to activate liver phosphorylase, the enzyme responsible for the normal breakdown of liver glycogen (the principal carbohydrate reserve). These workers established that when certain hormones were incubated with a particulate (cell membrane) fraction of liver cells, a factor was produced that could, in turn, activate the phosphorylase enzyme present in the supernatant fraction of the tissue homogenate. This substance was identified by Sutherland as cAMP (Fig. 1.2).

For this monumental discovery, Sutherland received the Nobel Prize in Physiology/Medicine in 1971 [27]. Cyclic AMP, the so-called *second messenger* of hormone action, is now implicated in the actions of many hormones and other stimuli on cellular physiological processes. The importance of this cyclic nucleotide to biochemistry, pharmacology, physiology, and medicine is enormous. Much of this book is, in fact, a discussion of the role of cAMP in hormone action and in normal and abnormal cellular function. Many more second messengers have since been discovered and are discussed in the context of hormone signal transduction pathways throughout this textbook.

Discovery of Hypothalamic Releasing Factors Starts a "Race to Stockholm"

Another crucial breakthrough was the demonstration that the pituitary gland, the so-called "master gland" of the body, was controlled by the brain, specifically the area known as the *hypothalamus* [13, 14]. Geoffrey Harris, an English endocrinologist, had provided data suggesting that the release of the pituitary hormones was controlled by humoral factors, probably of hypothalamic origin [12]. A number of workers then showed that extracts of the hypothalamus contained substances that affected the release of pituitary hormones [23]. The "race to Stockholm" for a Nobel Prize was then on [17, 30]. Andrew Schally and Roger Guillemin, working independently of each other, began purification of hypothalamic extracts from pig and sheep tissue sources. After the extraction of about 250,000 pig hypothalami, Schally and colleagues were able to provide the structure of the factor that stimulates the release of thyroid-stimulating hormone (TSH) from the pituitary gland. The structure of this thyrotropin-releasing hormone (TRH) (Fig. 1.3) was similar to that of the same factor isolated from sheep brains by Guillemin and reported at about the same time. This work was followed by the isolation and structural identification of several other hypothalamic hormones that control the secretion of pituitary hormones [13, 14, 17, 18].

Andrew Schally and his collaborators were also able to provide the chemical structure of porcine GnRH, which controls the release of the gonadotropins from the pituitary. Guillemin and colleagues then revealed that sheep GnRH was identical in structure. Understanding the structure of GnRH was of immense importance [19]. With this knowledge, it became possible to control fertility in humans and domestic animals with synthetic GnRH. It also became possible to modify the structure of the natural GnRH to provide analogs that enhance gonadotropin secretion from the pituitary, which can enhance the probability of conception. On the other hand, antihormone analogs (antagonists) have also been synthesized, which can be used as contraceptive agents.

Guillemin and colleagues were the first to discover and report the structure of a hypothalamic peptide, somatostatin, that was inhibitory to pituitary growth hormone (GH) secretion. Somatostatin, also found in other regions of the brain as well as in the pancreas, inhibits a number of hormone secretions, including the pancreatic hormones glucagon and insulin.

Figure 1.3 Structure of thyrotropin-releasing hormone, a neuro-hormone.

Somatostatin and related analogs have also been found to possess anti-proliferative properties. Thus, the clinical importance of somatostatin and its related analogs has been vast, ranging from the diagnosis and treatment of growth disorders and pituitary tumors to its potential use in cancer chemotherapies.

For their contribution to the isolation and determination of the structures of the hypothalamic regulatory peptides, Guillemin and Schally received the Nobel Prize in Physiology/Medicine in 1978 [10, 23]. Certainly, the pioneering work of Geoffrey Harris and many others provided the great impetus for the important accomplishments of Schally and Guillemin, as they have acknowledged. Many other chemists and endocrinologists provided important discoveries that contributed to the determination of the structures and roles of hypothalamic peptide hormones. Understanding the structures and functions of these hypothalamic regulatory hormones has been of the greatest importance for the welfare of humanity. As discussed later, many hypothalamic factors have been discovered and their roles in endocrine physiology explained (Chap. 6).

Development of Immunoassays Permits Hormone Measurements at Physiological Concentrations

The ability to chemically characterize and quantitate the hypothalamic (hypophysiotropic) factors, as well as most peripheral hormones, was revolutionized by the development of the radioimmunoassay (RIA). This method makes use of antibodies that specifically recognize and bind to the hormone of interest, which in turn provides the means to detect and quantify the amount of hormone present in a sample of blood or other bodily fluid. By the use of RIAs, it became possible to detect the presence of hormones in the blood or in tissues at most physiological concentrations. Possibilities for uses of immunoassays in basic science research and clinical diagnostics have proven to be virtually limitless [31]. For the development of the RIA, Rosalyn Yalow received the Nobel Prize in Physiology/Medicine in 1978, along with Schally and Guillemin.

Boundaries of Endocrinology are Broadened with the Discovery of Growth Factors

The development of refined immunometric and biological assays led to the discovery of chemical messengers that regulate cell growth and development. In contrast to the classical hormones that circulate in plasma, many of these growth factors are released into the local extracellular spaces and exert their actions on cells adjacent to their site of synthesis, or in some cases on the same cells in which they are produced. The Nobel Prize for Physiology/Medicine was awarded to Rita Levi-Montalcini and Stanley Cohen for their discoveries of several of these cell growth factors [18]. Levi-Montalcini discovered *nerve growth factor* (NGF, Chap. 12), a peptide hormone required for the growth, development, and maintenance of certain nerve cells of the peripheral nervous system, as well as in the brain. Cohen discovered *epidermal growth factor* (EGF), a peptide hormone that stimulates differentiation and growth of a variety of epithelial and other cells (Chap. 12). These discoveries opened up a vast field of research on NGF and EGF, as well as numerous other growth factors. The biological actions of these peptide hormones are providing important insights for an understanding of normal and abnormal cell growth.

Advances in Molecular Biology and Genetics Spawn a New Era in Endocrine Research

With the advent of recombinant DNA technologies, the science of endocrinology was propelled into an unparalleled era of progress. Among the earliest milestones in molecular endocrinology was the characterization, cloning, and expression of genes encoding pituitary (GH), by Philip Seeburg and his colleagues in 1977 [25]. This accomplishment was followed by a flood of investigations of hormone gene structure and regulation. Soon after these pioneering studies, many of the hormone receptor genes were similarly characterized. The primary structure and expression of the gene encoding the receptor for the adrenal glucocorticoid hormones (Chap. 15), for example, was first reported by Evans and colleagues in 1985 [8]. Early in the same decade, Palmiter and colleagues were among the first to develop transgenic animal models, viz. animals expressing embryonically introduced transgenes, for endocrine research. In these studies they engineered mice that overexpressed a transgene encoding GH and hence, grew to "giant" proportions [21]. The use of gene targeting approaches to produce gene "knockout" animals was similarly pioneered by several laboratories in the early 1990s, when advances in genetics first permitted development of mice bearing targeted deletions of hormone receptor genes. The use of embryonic stem cells and homologous recombination techniques (Chap. 4) to disrupt the gene encoding receptors for the gonadal hormone estrogen [15] represents one of the earliest of these remarkable achievements. Continued advances in molecular genetics have since permitted widespread use of a virtually limitless repertoire of in vitro and in vivo approaches to study molecular, cellular, physiological, and behavioral aspects of hormone expression and action.

The Science of Endocrinology

Endocrine glands secrete their hormones into the immediate extracellular space; from here, the hormones enter the circulatory system. These ductless glands differ from *exocrine glands* (e.g., salivary glands) whose products are released into ducts that lead to the digestive tract and then to the exterior of the body. Endocrinology is, therefore, the study of the ductless glands or tissues and their hormonal products. Hormones were originally considered to be synthesized only within specific endocrine organs and then secreted into the bloodstream to act on specific target tissues some distance away to evoke a specific physiological response. These definitions of endocrine glands and their hormones, while they accurately describe the secretory tissues such as the pituitary, thyroid, adrenal, and other glands, are too restrictive as they do not include other tissues that secrete hormones but have other major physiological functions. For example, Bayliss and Starling clearly demonstrated that secretin is released from the jejunum of the small intestine, a tissue that was not originally suspected to be of importance in endocrine function. Secretin is actually produced and secreted by individual cells distributed individually throughout the epithelial lining of the jejunum. Thus, the GI tract, which is also the source of other hormones, could well be considered the largest endocrine organ of the body.

The definition of endocrine glands and hormones has additionally been complicated by the finding that a single chemical messenger can be produced in multiple tissues, and even in different cell types within a single tissue, to mediate several different physiological activities. For example, the GI-derived hormone cholecystokinin (CCK) travels by way of the blood to act on the pancreas to induce pancreatic secretions; however, CCK and other "gut" peptides are also released from specific nerve cells within the brain to act as neurotransmitters on adjacent or nearby neurons. In the latter case the chemical messenger, functioning as a neurotransmitter, does not travel from its source of origin to its site of action by way of the bloodstream.

The Importance of Comparative Endocrinology is Multidimensional

Much of what is known about the endocrine physiology of humans derives from data obtained from patients manifesting signs of endocrine dysfunction. Research on other animals, particularly the rat and the mouse, has also provided a wealth of information on the endocrine system of mammals, including that of humans. In *comparative endocrinology*, researchers investigate the specific adaptations of basic endocrine systems in various animal species, as well as the similarities that they share with these same systems in humans. It is arguable that the great majority of clinical advances in endocrinology have depended upon information obtained in basic science research with animals, or with cells and tissues derived from animals. The "bench to bedside" translation of basic scientific knowledge to clinical practice remains a bedrock strategy of sponsored biomedical research in endocrinology.

One should also appreciate, however, the contributions that comparative endocrinology has provided for a broader evolutionary view of the endocrine system [3, 9]. Although the chemical structures of most human hormones have been elucidated, this information obviously does not provide an understanding of the evolution of these hormones. Once the structures of the related hormones of other vertebrates are determined, however, it becomes possible to trace the changes in the structure of the hormones that have evolved over time. In comparing the amino acid sequences of similar peptide structures from primitive and more recent vertebrates, one can determine the approximate rates of evolutionary change in hormones and when particular chemical changes probably occurred in earth history. The structures and phylogenetic distribution of the neurohypophysial hormones have been particularly well documented (see Table 7.1).

Knowledge of how hormones work owes much to early studies on the large chromosomes from salivary glands of such dipteran flies as *Drosophila* and *Chironomus*. The actions of hormones on genes were first visualized using the large chromosomes from these glands. Certain insect hormones were found to cause so-called "puffs" in the chromosome structure that represent areas where DNA is exposed and RNA synthesis is increased (see Fig. 3.4). One could follow the sequential puffing patterns of these large chromosomes during the larval development of the insects. Therefore, the genomic actions of hormones that relate to the temporal aspects of developmental changes could be precisely delineated. Since these classic studies, a variety of invertebrate and vertebrate animals have been utilized to delineate common signaling mechanisms among different animal species, as well as species-specific adaptations in signaling pathways, that mediate hormone action and endocrine function. Knowledge of invertebrate hormone structure and mechanisms of action has also proven to be of great commercial value, as it can provide a potent tool in the fight against disease-carrying or crop-damaging insects. Moreover, understanding the endocrine system of other vertebrate and invertebrate species provides important information that may be essential to animal husbandry and to the culture and raising of species such as shrimp and other edible crustaceans or mollusks [3, 9].

Clinical Endocrinologists Address a Multitude of Important Health Issues

Endocrine research has revealed a wealth of information on the biology and pathophysiology of endocrine systems. Consequently, major advances have been made in the diagnosis and treatment of a variety of human disease states, each of which is addressed in the appropriate chapters of this book. Obesity, diabetes, osteoporosis, infertility, hypertension, certain mental illnesses, and growth disorders are just a few of the major medical concerns that have a substantial endocrine basis. Understanding hormone and receptor structure and function has permitted development of a modern endocrine pharmacology for the treatment of many of these conditions. Particularly noteworthy has been the development of methods to synthesize structural analogs of hormone molecules with predicted biological activity. This is important because some hormones are not available in large enough quantities to supply the medicinal needs of humans. For example, a lack of GH results in a failure of growth in humans. GH is commercially available and normal growth and body stature can be attained following continued administration of the hormone. Introduction of the human GH gene into bacteria by recombinant DNA techniques provides a means for the large-scale production of the hormone (Chap. 4) [28]. The discovery and elucidation of the hypothalamic GH-releasing hormone (GHRH) structure has also allowed production of this peptide for the stimulation of pituitary GH secretion.

The Concept of Homeostasis

Claude Bernard, a nineteenth-century French physiologist, first formulated the concept of homeostasis [4, 11]. He pointed out that an individual lives within two environments: the exterior environment that surrounds us, and, more important, a *milieu interieur*. This internal environment is the fluid compartment within which the cells of our body are bathed. Bernard noted that this fluid is produced and controlled by the organism. He believed that organisms become more independent of changes in the outer world by maintaining constant their own internal environment. He emphasized that "it is the fixity of the milieu interieur which is the condition of free and independent life" and that "all the vital mechanisms, however varied they may be, have only one objective, that of preserving constant the conditions of life in the internal environment" [4].

This internal fluid environment bathes the cells with nutrients and inorganic and organic ions of critical importance to normal cell functioning [26]. The blood carries important metabolites to all the cells in the body: metabolic substrates, such as sugars, fatty acids, and amino acids; cofactors, such as the vitamins needed for enzyme function; and electrolytes, such as calcium, sodium, and potassium ions, which are necessary for stability of the electrical properties of cells.

Walter Cannon [7] later stated that "the coordinated physiological processes which maintain most of the steady states in the organism are so complex and so peculiar to living beings—involving, as they may, the brain and nerves, the heart, lungs, kidneys and spleen, all working cooperatively that I have suggested a specific designation for these states, homeostasis." Mammals, for example, maintain a very stringent control over the concentration of glucose, Ca^{2+}, and Na^+, and other constituents of the body fluids. Only small fluctuations in these important fluid components are tolerated or the animal will suffer immediate and often fatal consequences. Homeostatic settings, however, are not invariant; they depend on the time of day, time of year, stage of development, age, and reproductive status of an animal. It is the ability to maintain a constant internal environment in the face of adverse environmental conditions that has undoubtedly favored the wide distribution of mammals to all types of environmental habitats. Many poikilothermic ("cold-blooded") vertebrates, on the other hand, are restricted to narrow environmental niches. The price that homeotherms ("warm-blooded") animals must pay for maintenance of the homeostatic state is a need for a constant food supply. Many poikilotherms hibernate or estivate (remain in a torpid, or relatively quiescent state) until more favorable climatic conditions occur, when they become active again. They are, nevertheless, successful in their particular niches as they need not always depend on a continuous supply of metabolic substrates.

Homeostatic Systems Use Negative Feedback Control Mechanisms

How does the body maintain precise control over the concentrations of such fluid components as glucose, and calcium and sodium ions? Certain sensory and endocrine cells in the body, either individually or functioning as a unit, seem to possess a definite set point (like a thermostat) for monitoring the concentrations of these substances. If the plasma concentration of a metabolite is diminished, for example, by loss through the urine or by perspiration, these receptive cells respond by releasing a substance, in this context a hormone, which then acts on other cells to release their stores of the needed metabolite or to prevent its loss from the body. These responses to hormonal stimulation elevate the levels of such factors as Na^+ or glucose in the blood to a point where, for example, the cellular osmostat or glucostat, respectively, shuts off release of its chemical messenger. Increased metabolite availability therefore functions as a *negative feedback* stimulus (Fig. 1.4).

Virtually all endocrine systems within the vertebrate body have been found to operate under the control of one or more negative feedback mechanisms. Specific mechanisms controlling each of the major hormone systems are addressed in corresponding chapters in this textbook. For a very few physiological circumstances, however, there also exist examples of *positive feedback*. This occurs when rising concentrations of a hormone cause another gland to release a second hormone, which is then stimulatory to an increased output of the first hormone (Fig. 1.4). A positive feedback system must have some mechanism of shutting off release of the first hormone or the system would increase continuously in amplitude. In the primate, estradiol, a gonadal estrogen, increases the release of pituitary gonadotropic hormones, which, in turn, stimulate ovarian estrogen production. Consequently, estrogen levels as well as the pituitary gonadotropic hormone levels increase concomitantly. The monthly demise of the ovarian follicle, the source of estradiol, results in a subsequent fall in plasma estrogen and gonadotropin levels (Chap. 18). Presently, there are only a few recognized examples of positive feedback.

In a number of feedback systems, an increase in the plasma levels of one hormone may be stimulatory to the release of a metabolite (e.g., glucose) from a target tissue. Elevated plasma levels of the metabolite may then be stimulatory to the release of a second hormone, which has an inhibitory effect on the release of the metabolite from the target tissue. The lowered level of the metabolite would, in turn, be the stimulus to the release of the first hormone (Fig. 1.5). Some specific examples of the roles of hormones in plasma metabolite homeostasis will now be discussed.

Figure 1.4 General scheme of negative and positive feedback systems.

many other more subtle cellular functions. In most mammals, the concentration of Ca^{2+} in the blood is maintained within very narrow limits. Any deviation from this set point will cause homeostatic mechanisms to bring the concentration of Ca^{2+} back to this level. If Ca^{2+} levels fall, this is perceived by cells in the parathyroid glands and they secrete parathormone (also called parathyroid hormone, Chap. 9). This hormone then (1) acts on bone to release stored Ca^{2+}, (2) stimulates Ca^{2+} absorption from the gut, and (3) enhances resorption of Ca^{2+} from the urine by the kidney. All these actions tend to bring the concentration of the cation back to normal. Lack of parathormone, on the other hand, leads to a lowering of serum Ca^{2+}, which may lead to tetanic convulsions and death.

If serum Ca^{2+} becomes elevated, as it may after a meal, then other cells release a hormone, calcitonin, which lowers the level of circulating Ca^{2+}. In mammals, this hormone is released from parafollicular cells within the thyroid gland (Chap. 9). Somehow, these cells are capable of detecting elevated levels of Ca^{2+} (see Fig. 9.13). Calcitonin causes deposition of Ca^{2+} into bone, and it may have other actions on the gut and kidney to prevent Ca^{2+} uptake and resorption. The hormonal homeostatic mechanisms controlling serum Ca^{2+} levels are shown in Fig. 1.7.

Example 3: Sodium Homeostasis is Controlled by the Renin-Angiotensin System and Atriopeptin

Although the sodium ion (Na^+) is the major electrolyte in body fluids, Na^+ is continuously being lost from the body in urine and sweat. Specialized cells in the walls of certain blood vessels within the kidney can act as *osmoreceptors* and continuously monitor the Na^+ concentration of the blood. If a drop in Na^+ concentration and hence blood osmolarity is noted, these cells release a substance, renin, which, acting as an enzyme, is able to split a plasma protein into a smaller peptide. This peptide is then acted on by yet another enzyme to release a still smaller peptide, angiotensin II, a hormone. Angiotensin II then stimulates certain cells of the adrenal cortex to release aldosterone, another hormone. This hormone then acts on certain collecting tubules of the kidney to cause resorption of Na^+ from the urine. Thus a complex set of hormonal actions are brought into play to maintain the proper levels of blood Na^+ (see Fig. 15.10).

Atrial distension due to blood volume expansion is a stimulus to renal salt and water diuresis (excretion in urine). In the past, it was generally held that the cardiac atria served to sense the fullness of the vascular fluid compartment. The resulting "reflex" diuresis resulting from atrial stretch receptors was thought to result from activation of neural stretch receptors located within the innermost layers of the atrium. The pioneering work of de Bold [29] revealed that saline extracts of atria, but not of ventricles, provoked a marked increase in urinary salt and water excretion when injected into rats. An *atrial natriuretic peptide* (ANP)

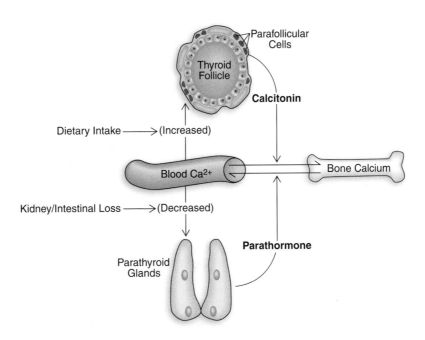

Figure 1.7 Hormonal control of calcium homeostasis.

extracted from atria is a polypeptide whose structure has been elucidated, synthesized, and biologically characterized [29]. This cardiac hormone (*atriopeptin*) may be a major regulator of the physiological responses to volume overload. The homeostatic regulation of ANP release and volume regulation is depicted in Fig. 15.15. The therapeutic potential of this newly discovered hormone is of obvious clinical importance, as will be discussed.

Neuroendocrine Integration in Homeostasis

A variety of stimuli of both *extrinsic* (external/environmental) and *intrinsic* (within the body) origin affect physiological processes within an animal. The body must interpret changes in environmental temperature and day length. The recognition of specific odors (*pheromones*) produced by members of the opposite sex may be important in the control of reproductive behavior. Changes in fluid electrolyte levels or metabolic substrate levels must be monitored. Pain stimuli, whether of extrinsic or intrinsic origin, must be perceived. The recognition of these factors is accomplished by cellular sensory elements (receptors), which may be referred to as mechanoreceptors, chemoreceptors, osmoreceptors, or baroreceptors, depending on which modality is monitored. These sensory elements may be cellular components of glands, such as the pancreas, or they may be neural elements of the eye, nasal (olfactory) epithelium, or other tissues. These sensory cells respond to sensory cues by releasing a hormone directly into the blood or by transmitting a nerve impulse to other neurons or cellular elements that then release one or more chemical messengers. After the stomach contents (chyme) are released into the small intestine, hydrogen ions (protons from hydrochloric acid) interact with specific cells of the gut epithelium, which results in the release of the hormone secretin. Secretin then enters the bloodstream and interacts with cells of the pancreas to release a fluid secretion that neutralizes the acid within the small intestine. This is the classical example of a hormone, as first described by Bayliss and Starling [2], and a further example of a homeostatic mechanism (see Fig. 10.6).

The release of most hormones is not as simple as that seen in the example of secretin. Sensory cues are often transmitted from one neuron to one or more other neurons, which may ultimately result in the release of a hormone. Therefore, the nervous system, working through the endocrine system, plays an important role in the homeostasis of a number of such physiological processes as water balance, temperature regulation, and even feeding behavior. The following examples of neuroendocrine integration are discussed in more detail in several succeeding chapters.

Example 1: Neuroendocrine Regulation of Fluid Homeostasis is Mediated by Vasopressin

If water is lost and not replaced, dehydration results. The hyperosmolality (increase in fluid Na^+ concentration) and hypovolemia (decrease in fluid volume) are detected by *osmoreceptors* and *baroreceptors*, sensory cells that monitor changes in Na^+ concentration or volume (pressure), respectively, of the blood. Baroreceptor neurons, located within the carotid sinus, for example, relay information to specific sites within the brain. Integration of this information within the hypothalamus results in the release of a hormone, vasopressin, from neurons that are components of the posterior pituitary gland. This hormone, also referred to as antidiuretic hormone (ADH) (or, more specifically, arginine vasopressin (AVP), is released into the blood and acts on certain cells of kidney collecting tubules to cause water reabsorption. Vasopressin also causes contraction of certain smooth muscles of the vasculature, which results in partial restoration of blood pressure. In addition, sensory neurons within the brain may also monitor fluid osmolarity, and, under dehydrating conditions, neurotransmitters are released to act within the brain to initiate drinking (*dipsogenic*) behavior. The complexity of this neuroendocrine control of water balance is discussed more fully in Chap. 7.

Example 2: Neuroendocrine Control of Body Temperature is Regulated by Thyroid Hormones and Autonomic Activity

The temperature of the body, at least that of humans, is maintained at a precise level, although it does exhibit a circadian (daily) variation. Hormones and neuronal mechanisms are crucial in temperature regulation. Alterations in body temperature are monitored by sensory neurons within the brain. These neurons release neurotransmitter substances that stimulate other neurons to initiate physiological processes that lead to warming or cooling of the body back to the normal state. Under cooling conditions when body heat is lost, neurons within the brain release one or more neurohormones that increase metabolic activity and heat production within the body. Specifically, a hormone released from neuroendocrine cells within the hypothalamus of the brain stimulates the release of a thyroid-stimulating hormone (TSH) from the pituitary (Fig. 1.3). This hormone released into the circulation stimulates cells of the thyroid gland to release one or more thyroid hormones, thyroxine and triiodothyronine, which then stimulate metabolism within various cells of the body with resulting heat production. In addition, neurohormones released within the brain also activate the *sympathetic nervous system* and the adrenal gland to release hormones that also affect metabolic processes by causing the release of glucose from the liver; this can then be utilized as a metabolic substrate for heat production. The sympathetic nervous system will also release neurotransmitters that cause vasoconstriction, which will result in decreased heat loss from the skin. These are only a few of the neuroendocrine mechanisms involved in the complex physiological processes that maintain body temperature.

Example 3: Neuroendocrine Control of Energy Homeostasis is Mediated by Neuropeptides and Peripheral Feedback Signals

Body weight is generally controlled within narrow limits by neuroendocrine homeostatic control mechanisms. While these control mechanisms have long been known to exist, neuroendocrine studies have only recently revealed some of their major cellular and hormonal components. Neurons located in the basal portion of the hypothalamus have been identified as critically important regulators of energy homeostasis, as they control both the intake of food and the rate of energy utilization. Many of these cells produce neuropeptide neurotransmitters that are either orexigenic (stimulate food intake) or anorexigenic (inhibit food intake). The relative activities of these cell groups appear to manifest the prevailing motivational state, i.e., satiety or hunger. These cell groups are influenced, in turn, by neural and hormonal signals that convey information about the availability of metabolic energy substrates. Some of these signals arise from the gut and provide short-term cues about the absence or presence of food in the stomach. Others are hormonal signals that represent the levels of metabolic substrates in blood and stored in fat cells and other tissues. The adipocyte-derived hormone, leptin, is one such hormonal regulator that has been shown to suppress food intake and increase energy utilization. Insulin appears to exert similar feedback effects. Not surprisingly, the targets of leptin and insulin feedback effects on food intake and energy utilization are the same basal hypothalamic neuropeptidergic neurons that appear to be crucial in inducing or inhibiting feeding behavior and energy utilization. The long-term, homeostatic regulation of body weight thus appears to be controlled by a "feedforward" neuroendocrine mechanism that controls energy intake and utilization, and a negative feedback regulation of these same neuronal groups by leptin, insulin, and other factors that are raised as a consequence of energy intake and storage. How the hypothetical set point for body weight regulation may be established, and how it may be altered in morbidly obese individuals, remains the subject of intense study.

Hormones and Behavior

Besides the behaviors associated with water and food intake to maintain volume and nutrient homeostasis, hormones regulate many other behaviors necessary for survival.

Gonadal Hormones Regulate Reproductive Behaviors

Hormones regulate courtship, mating, and maternal behaviors that are necessary for reproductive success and perpetuation of the species. Libido in the human male is critically dependent on hormones (androgens) produced by the gonads, which then manifest themselves through actions on the brain. Libido in the human female may be "encephalized" and less dependent on a hormonal directive. In other mammals, however, female behavior is acutely affected and directed by the hormonal milieu of the animal. Gonadal steroids have also been found to exert effects in the brain that impact mood, learning, and memory (Chap. 18).

Fetal Hormones can "Program" Behavior

The fetal and neonatal brain is subject to the trophic (growth-inducing) influences of several hormones during specific "critical periods" of development. The best characterized of these organizational effects of hormones are those induced by testicular androgen secretions in the male fetus. The presence of a testosterone surge in the male directs the development of circuitries that later support male-typical behaviors. On the other hand, the absence of testosterone during prenatal or perinatal (shortly before or after birth) life is permissive for development of the female neuroanatomy and subsequent female-type behaviors. The degree to which prenatal hormone exposures may "program" the behavioral tendencies of an animal in adulthood is likely species-specific. Whether such programming may or may not pertain to human behavior is not well known, and remains a hotly debated issue. For example, to what extent, if any, are hormones responsible for sexual behaviors that might be considered by some to differ from the norm? If there is a biological (hormonal) basis for these anomalous sexual behaviors, then how can such actions be viewed as "deviant"? Some evidence suggests that the anatomy of the brain of some homosexual males may be somewhere between the male and female anatomical construct. If true, then we may have to accept that certain sexual activities may therefore be biologically driven and not due to some societal directive (Chap. 17).

Other behaviors may similarly be programmed by early exposure to hormones. Animal studies suggest that pre- or postnatal stress can influence brain development and subsequent responses to stress in adulthood. Glucocorticoid hormones produced by the adrenal glands certainly may play an important role in this regard (Chap. 15).

Hormones, Growth Regulation, and Cancer

Just as hormones regulate glucose, Ca^{2+}, and Na^+ balance, a number of hormones also control the growth of the cellular components of tissues and organs. The growth factors are now known to be involved in homeostasis of body growth and function. A major discovery in cancer research is the finding of a relationship between normal growth regulation by hormones and growth factors and by *oncogenes*, proto-oncogenes that acquire cancerous (oncogenic) characteristics. Proto-oncogenes, which are postulated to control normal cellular growth, particularly in early development, may themselves become uncontrolled (mutated) and produce growth factors or growth factor receptors that activate cellular mechanisms leading to uncontrolled (abnormal) cell growth, or cancer. In some tissues, hormones such as estrogen and progesterone may normally exert their growth effects by regulating growth factor production and actions. Cancers of the breast and uterus, normal target organs of these gonadal hormones, may thus develop as hormone-dependent neoplasms. These hormone-like growth factor peptides may even be products of cancer-causing viruses and may be responsible for tumor formation (Chap. 12).

REVIEW EXERCISES

Compare and contrast each of the following terms. How are they related? How do they differ?

baroreceptor/osmoreceptor
estivation/hibernation
endocrine gland/exocrine gland
   homeotherm/poikilotherm
intrinsic stimulus/extrinsic stimulus
endocrinology/neuroendocrinology
inotropic/chronotropic (activities of the heart)
negative feedback/positive feedback
first messenger/second messenger (of hormone action)

Define or otherwise characterize each of the following terms:

hypothalamus
pheromone
homeostasis
diabetes mellitus

oncogene
hypophysotropic factor
Vagustuff
Second messenger

Think, analyze and discuss:

1. Berthold's experiments demonstrated that removal of the testes from rooster results in failure of development of the wattles and combs, and an absence of male-typical

behaviors in these animals. Replacement of the testes in the abdominal cavity reversed all of these effects.

   a. One explanation for these results is that the testes produce a hormone that normally stimulates the development of the wattle and comb, as well as sexual and aggressive behavior. Describe an experiment that would demonstrate the existence of a testes-derived hormone (testosterone) that exerts these effects in roosters.

   b. In Berthold's experiments, he noted that transplantation of a single testis in the abdomen of a castrated rooster resulted in the growth of that testis to an abnormally large size. What is the name of this phenomenon?

   c. Pituitary hormones normally stimulate testosterone release from the testes and promote their growth and development. Testosterone can exert negative feedback on pituitary cells to restrain pituitary hormone release. Considering this negative feedback control mechanism, construct a reasonable hypothesis as to why the single transplanted testis may have become enlarged in Berthold's roosters.

2. Otto Loewi demonstrated the existence of substances released by the vagus nerve that decrease (acetylcholine) and increase (norepinephrine) the inotropic and chronotropic characteristics of the incubated frog heart. He stimulated the vagus nerve attached to one heart, and applied the surrounding *conditioned medium* to a second heart and observed the effects on its activity.

   a. Suppose that this experiment were performed several times, and in each trial a high, medium, or low intensity of electrical stimulation was applied to the vagus nerve. In each case, the magnitude of the change in heartbeats per minute (increased or decreased) was recorded. Make a histogram plot of the data that would likely be obtained in this experiment, demonstrating the relationship between the change in beats per minute and the intensity of the vagal nerve stimulation.

   b. Make a plot of the expected results from an experiment performed as in (a), except that the drug atropine is added to the incubation solution of the second heart.

3. Which of the following chemical messengers are primarily released into the bloodstream to act on distant organs and tissues? Which would be expected to act within the tissue of origin or adjacent tissues? Why?

   a. insulin
   b. testosterone
   c. vasopressin
   d. NGF
   e. GH
   f. EGF

4. Homeostatic mechanisms exert tight control over concentrations of vital constituents of body fluids. Endocrine glands and their hormones usually assume central roles in these regulatory systems. Some homeostatic mechanisms involve two or more hormones that may act in parallel or opposite manners to maintain a metabolic or mineral constituent within a narrow physiological range of values. For the three homeostatic systems controlling serum glucose, Ca^+, and Na^+, respectively, construct schematic diagrams of the systems, and include in each the following system components:

   a. stimulatory hormone, and the gland that produces it
   b. inhibitory hormone, and the gland that produces it
   c. target tissues of the stimulatory and inhibitory hormone
   d. feedback mechanism

For all three variables, consider and predict the sequence of events that would follow an increase in the level of the variable (e.g., elevated blood glucose after a meal), and those that would ensue following a drop in the level of the variable (e.g., reduced blood glucose with strenuous exercise).

5. Neuroendocrine systems affect homeostatic control of fluid balance, body temperature, and food intake. Construct schematic diagrams of the systems controlling these three physiological variables, and include in them the hormone(s) that mediate control over the level of the variable, the glands and/or cell groups that produce the hormone(s), the target tissues of the hormone(s), and the feedback mechanisms that operate within the system. As for question 4, above, consider and predict the sequence of events that would follow an increase in the level of the variable (e.g., elevated body temperature) and those that would ensue following a drop in the level of the variable (e.g., reduced body temperature).

References

[1] Banting, F. G., and G. H. Best. 1922. The internal secretion of the pancreas. *J. Lab. Clin. Med.* 7:241–66.

[2] Bayliss, W. M., and E. H. Starling. 1902. Mechanisms of pancreatic secretion. *J. Physiol.* 28:325–53.

[3] Bern, H. A. 1990. The "new" endocrinology: Its scope and its impact. *Am. Zool.* 30:877–85.

[4] Bernard, C. 1865. *Introduction à l'étude de la médicine expérimentale.* Paris: J. B. Baillière et Fils.

[5] Berthold, A. A. 1849. Transplantation der Hoden. *Arch. Anat. Physiol. Wiss. Med.* 16:42–6.

[6] Bliss, M. 1989. J. J. R. Macleod and the discovery of insulin. *Q. J. Exp. Physiol.* 74:87–96.

[7] Cannon, W. B. 1960. *The wisdom of the body.* New York: W. W. Norton.

[8] Evans, R. M. 1988. The steroid and thyroid hormone receptor superfamily. *Science* 240:889–95.

[9] Gorbman, A., et al. 1983. *Comparative endocrinology.* New York: John Wiley.

[10] Guillemin, R. 1978. Peptides in the brain: The new endocrinology of the neuron. *Science* 202:390–402.

[11] Guillemin, R., and L. Guillemin (Trans.) 1974. Claude Bernard. *Lectures on the phenomena of life common to animals and plants.* Springfield: Charles Thomas.

[12] Harris, G. W. 1955. *Neural control of the pituitary gland.* London: Edward Arnold.

[13] Klavdieva, M. M. 1995. The history of neuropeptides I. *Front. Neuroendocrinol.* 16:293–321.

[14] Klavdieva, M. M. 1996. The history of neuropeptides II. *Front. Neuroendocrinol.* 17:126–53.

[15] Korach, K. S., et al. 1996. Estrogen receptor gene disruption: molecular characterization and experimental and clinical phenotypes. *Recent Prog. Horm. Res.* 51:159–86.

[16] Loewi, O. 1921. Uebertragbarkeit der Herznervenwirkung. *Pflüger's Arch. Ges. Physiol.* 189:239–42.

[17] Marx, J. L. 1986. The 1986 Nobel Prize for physiology or medicine. *Science* 234:543–4.

[18] Marx, J. L. 1988. The 1988 Nobel Prize for physiology or medicine: Three researchers are honored for developing drugs that combat some of mankind's most common diseases. *Science* 242:516–17.

[19] Martini, L., et al. 1997. LHRF, LHRH, GnRH: What controls the secretion of this hormone? *Mol. Psychiat.* 2:373–5.

[20] O'Malley, B. W. 1995. Thirty years of steroid hormone action: Personal recollections of an investigator. *Steroids* 60:490.

[21] Palmiter R. D., et al. 1982. Dramatic growth of mice that develop from eggs microinjected with metallothionein-growth hormone fusion genes. *Nature* 300:611–15.

[22] Sanger, F. 1959. Chemistry of insulin. *Science* 129:1340–4.

[23] Schally, A. V. 1978. Aspects of hypothalamic regulation of the pituitary gland. *Science* 202:18–28.

[24] Schultz, S. G. 1996. Homeostasis, Humpty Dumpty, and integrative biology. *News Physiol. Sci.* 11:238–46.

[25] Seeburg P. H., et al. 1977. Nucleotide sequence and amplification in bacteria of structural gene for rat growth hormone. *Nature* 270:486–94.

[26] Starling, E. H. 1905. The chemical correlation of the functions of the body. *Lancet* i:340–1.

[27] Sutherland, E. 1972. Studies on the mechanisms of hormone action. *Science* 177:401–8.

[28] Tattersall, R. 1996. A history of growth hormone. *Horm. Res.* 46:236–47.

[29] Vesely, D. L. 1991. *The atrial peptides.* Prentice Hall Endocrinology Series. Englewood Cliffs, NJ: Prentice Hall.

[30] Wade, N. 1978. Guillemin and Schally. *Science* 200:279–82; 411–14; 510–13.

[31] Yalow, R. S. 1978. Radioimmunoassay: A probe for the fine structure of biologic systems. *Science* 200:1236–45.

The Vertebrate Endocrine System

*A*fter fertilization of the vertebrate egg, a number of inductive processes ensue that cause the zygote to divide and develop into an embryo. The chemical messengers regulating early embryonic differentiation and development are being clarified. The fetus will grow, develop, use metabolic substrates, respire, move, and excrete various waste products. The extent to which these physiological processes are regulated by hormones of fetal or maternal origin is also poorly understood. Whether the embryo will develop in a male or female direction is, however, determined by early endocrine influences (Chap. 16). The fetus will be liberated from the environment of the womb at parturition; the infant will continue to grow and develop, and new physiological functions and morphological changes will occur during growth and development of the young animal. The adolescent will develop into an adult and the adult may bear offspring of its own. A large number of hormones are required to control and coordinate these various physiological activities. Some hormones may only function during specific developmental stages, and their physiological roles may even change over time. Growth hormone and thyroid hormones, for example, are necessary for normal bone growth in the young animal; these same hormones assume new or additional functions in the adult.

Some hormones cause rapid responses after being secreted, such as milk release and uterine contraction in response to oxytocin. Epinephrine, a hormone of the adrenal medulla, causes an almost instantaneous change in the rate and force of the heartbeat. Other hormones, such as gonadal steroids, initiate a slower response, for instance, protein synthesis within muscle and other tissues. Testosterone or one of its metabolites affects the development of the brain at an early developmental period, but these effects may not become manifest until the animal approaches sexual maturity. In some animals, this may occur many years later. Some hormones, for example adrenocorticotropin (ACTH), may only control a few physiological functions; others, like testosterone, may affect physiological processes in many target tissues. A large and diverse number of hormones are required for coordinating the complex physiological events associated with reproductive processes, especially in the female. These may include differentiation of the gonads, germ cell maturation, development of secondary sexual characteristics, milk production, labor at parturition, and sexual behavior.

In this chapter, the general characteristics of the vertebrate endocrine system are considered. Each endocrine gland or tissue and its hormones will be discussed in greater detail later in the text.

Endocrine Glands and their Hormones

Tissues are composed of one functional cell type, and a number of tissues usually function together to form an organ. An endocrine gland, for example, is composed of a prominent mass (parenchyma) of secretory cells, as well as connective tissue, blood vessels, and nerves. Endocrine glands (ductless glands) secrete their products directly into the bloodstream. This is in contrast to exocrine glands (e.g., salivary glands), which release their products into ducts leading into the lumen of other organs, such as the intestine, or to the outside of the animal. The hormones of the adrenal steroidogenic tissue are synthesized within a compact mass of tissue, but some hormones are secreted by individual cells or groups of cells found distributed within other nonendocrine tissue. The pancreatic islets, for example, which are the source of insulin and glucagon, are found embedded within the much larger exocrine pancreas. Gastrointestinal hormones are produced by individual isolated cells, distributed diffusely throughout the endothelial lining of the stomach and gut [17]. A few endocrine glands are transient in nature. For example, hormones are produced by the placenta during pregnancy; the placenta and its endocrine tissue are lost during parturition but return, de novo, during a subsequent pregnancy. Endocrine glands usually secrete more than one hormone, but the parathyroids may be an example where an endocrine organ secretes only one hormone.

The pituitary gland is the source of a large number of hormones. The anterior lobe, or pars distalis, contains at least six well-characterized hormones and a number of other hormonal candidates (Chap. 5). The pars intermedia (the intermediate lobe of the pituitary) contains one or more hormones, and the posterior lobe, or neurohypophysis, contains at least two hormones. Although the pituitary gland was once considered the master gland of the body, its function is subservient to the brain, in particular, the hypothalamus (Chap. 6). The secretion of the pituitary principles of the pars distalis and pars intermedia is under the control of hypothalamic releasing and inhibiting hormones. Some of these hypothalamic factors have not yet been chemically characterized and are only considered as candidate hormones; they are often referred to as factors rather than hormones (e.g., prolactin-releasing factor, PRF). Numerous other hormones are also present within the hypothalamus and other parts of the brain; the brain is one of the richest sources of hormones. The hormones of the hypothalamus and pituitary (Table 2.1), as well as hormones from other sources (Table 2.2), are listed with a brief statement of their functions.

Hormones Defined

Bayliss and Starling discovered that the small intestine is the source of a substance released into the bloodstream that acts on cells of the exocrine pancreas, causing the fluid (bicarbonate) secretion necessary to neutralize the acid present within the chyme [2]. This substance, secretin, was subsequently referred to as a hormone. Hormones are generally considered to be chemical messengers that are released from cells into the bloodstream to exert their action on target cells some distance away. These bloodborne messengers of the endocrine system originally were distinguished from *neurotransmitters*, the chemical messengers released from neurons into a synapse between the nerve and its *effector cells*, such as secretory cells, muscle cells, or other neurons. It was discovered that the posterior pituitary gland mainly consisted of axonal endings of neurons that stored the hormones oxytocin and vasopressin. These hormones are released on appropriate stimulation into the bloodstream to regulate target tissues of the mammary gland, uterus, and kidney. These peptide hormones of neural origin were referred to as *neurohormones* to distinguish them from such neurotransmitter substances as acetylcholine, norepinephrine, and serotonin [21].

Many peptide hormones, such as somatostatin (SST), cholecystokinin (CCK), and others, which function in the classical sense as bloodborne hormones, are also synthesized within specific neurons in the central and peripheral nervous system. Some of these peptide hormones may function as neurotransmitters within the nervous system. On the other hand, dopamine, which has always been considered a classic example of a neurotransmitter, is released from nerves within the brain (hypothalamus) into the specialized hypophysial portal

TABLE 2.1 Vertebrate hypothalamic and pituitary hormones

Source of Hormone			Major Physiological Roles[a]
Hypothalamus			
Gonadotropin-releasing hormone	GnRH	↑	FSH and LH secretion
Thyrotropin-releasing hormone	TRH	↑	TSH secretion
Corticotropin-releasing hormone	CRH	↑	ACTH secretion
Dopamine	DA	↓	Prolactin secretion
Melanocyte-stimulating hormone (MSH) release inhibiting factor	MIF[b]	↓	MSH secretion
Somatostatin	SST	↓	GH secretion
Growth hormone-releasing hormone	GHRH	↑	GH secretion
Pituitary gland			
Posterior lobe (pars nervosa):[c]			
Oxytocin	OT	↑	Milk secretion; uterine contraction
Vasopressin (arginine vasopressin) (antidiuretic hormone)	AVP ADH	↑	Renal water absorption; vasoconstriction
Melanin-concentrating hormone	MCH	↑	Melanosome aggregation (teleost fishes)
Intermediate lobe (pars intermedia):			
Melanocyte-stimulating hormone	MSH	↑	Integumental melanogenesis; melanosome dispersion
Anterior lobe (pars distalis):			
Follicle-stimulating hormone (follitropin)	FSH	↑	Female: ovarian follicle growth; estradiol synthesis
		↑	Male: spermatogenesis
Luteinizing hormone (lutropin)	LH	↑	Female: ovulation; ovarian estradiol and progesterone synthesis
		↑	Male: testicular androgen synthesis
Prolactin	PRL	↑	Milk synthesis; corpus luteum progesterone synthesis in some species
Thyrotropin (thyroid-stimulating hormone)	TSH	↑	Thyroid hormone (T_4 and T_3) synthesis and secretion
Adrenocorticotropin (adrenal cortical stimulating hormone)	ACTH	↑	Adrenal steroidogenesis
Growth hormone	GH	↑	Hepatic somatomedin (IGF-I, II) biosynthesis

[a]The effect of each hormone on either an increased or stimulated (↑) or a decreased or inhibited (↓) physiological response is indicated.
[b]There is some evidence for putative PRL- and MSH-releasing factors.
[c]See Chap. 7 for other vertebrate neurohypophysial hormones.

vasculature and carried to the pituitary gland where it functions in the control of prolactin and melanocyte-stimulating hormone (α-MSH) secretion. Here, then, is an example of a neurotransmitter functioning as a neurohormone. One can no longer separate the endocrine and nervous system into unrelated physiological systems. The hypothalamus, for example, is the richest source of chemical messengers and should be considered the "endocrine hypothalamus" (Chap. 6).

Based simply on anatomical considerations, hormones derived from nerve cells may be called neurohormones, a specific subclass of hormones; they may be *neuropeptides* or nonpeptidergic in nature (e.g., dopamine). Although peptide neurohormones may be secreted into the bloodstream, the same molecules may also regulate neuronal function within the nervous system as neurotransmitters or as *neuromodulators*. In contrast to the rapid actions of neurotransmitters, neuromodulatory substances are considered to exert slower, but more sustained actions on neurons. Their actions are believed to enhance or inhibit (and therefore modulate) the response of neurons to neurotransmitters. Neuromodulatory hormones may also originate from non-neuronal sources. For example, adrenocortical steroids, such as cortisol, or androgens and estrogens of gonadal origin may modulate central nervous system activity and therefore play an important role in sexual and other behaviors (Chaps 16–18).

TABLE 2.2 Some other vertebrate hormones

Source of Hormone			Major Physiological Roles[a]
Thyroid			
Thyroxine	T_4	↑	Growth; differentiation; calorigenesis (↑ metabolic rate and oxygen consumption)
Triiodothyronine	T_3		Same as for thyroxine
Adrenal steroidogenic tissue (adrenal cortex)			
Cortisol		↑	Carbohydrate metabolism; sympathetic function
Corticosterone		↑	Carbohydrate metabolism; sympathetic function
Aldosterone		↑	Sodium retention
Adrenal chromaffin tissue (adrenal medulla)			
Epinephrine	E		Multiple ↑ and ↓ effects on nerves, muscles, cellular secretions, and metabolism
Norepinephrine	NE		Generally same physiological roles as epinephrine
Ovary (preluteal follicle)			
Estradiol	E_2	↑	Female sexual development and behavior
Ovary (corpus luteum)			
Progesterone		↑	Uterine and mammary gland growth; maternal behavior
Relaxin		↑	Relaxation of pubic symphysis and dilation of uterine cervix
Placenta			
Chorionic gonadotropin (choriogonadotropin)	CG	↑	Corpus luteum progesterone synthesis
Placental lactogen	PL	↑	Possibly fetal growth and development, mammary gland development in the mother
Testes (Leydig cells)			
Testosterone		↑	Male sexual development and behavior
Testes (Sertoli cells)			
Inhibin		↓	Pituitary FSH secretion
Anti-Müllerian Hormone	AMH		Müllerian duct regression (atrophy)
Pineal (epiphysis)			
Melatonin		↓	Gonadal development (antigonadotropic action)
Thymus gland			
Thymic hormones		↑	Proliferation and differentiation of lymphocytes
Pancreatic islets			
Insulin		↓	Blood glucose; ↑ protein, glycogen, and fat synthesis
Glucagon		↑	Blood glucose; gluconeogenesis; glycogenolysis
Somatostatin	SST	↓	Secretion of other pancreatic islet hormones
Pancreatic polypeptide	PP	↑↓	Secretion of other pancreatic islet hormones
Gastrointestinal (GI) tract			
Gastrin		↑	HCL secretion
Secretin		↑	Pancreatic acinar cell fluid (bicarbonate) secretion
Cholecystokinin	CCK	↑	Pancreatic acinar cell enzyme secretion; gall bladder contraction
Gastric inhibitory peptide	GIP	↓ ↑	Gastric acid (HCL) secretion, Insulin secretion
Vasoactive intestinal peptide	VIP	↑	Intestinal secretion of electrolytes; smooth muscle relaxation
Glucagon-like peptide-1	GLP-1	↑	Insulin secretion
Motilin		↑	Gastric acid secretion; villous motility
Neurotensin	NT		Enteric neurotransmitter
Substance P	SP		Enteric neurotransmitter
Gastrin-releasing peptide	GRP	↑	Gastrin secretion; gastric acid secretion
Parathyroid glands			
Parathormone	PTH	↑ ↓	Blood calcium (Ca^{2+}) Blood phosphate (PO_4^{-3})
Thyroid parafollicular cells (or ultimobranchial glands)			
Calcitonin	CT	↓	Blood Ca^{2+}

TABLE 2.2 Continued

Source of Hormone			Major Physiological Roles
Skin, liver, kidney vitamin D$_3$		↑	Blood Ca^{2+}; intestinal Ca^{2+} absorption, renal Ca^{2+} reabsorption
Plasma angiotensinogen Angiotensin II	All	↑	Vasoconstriction; aldosterone secretion; thirst (dipsogenic behavior)
Kidney Erythropoietin	EP	↑	Erythropoiesis
Most all tissues Prostaglandins (PGs)	PGE$_2$	↑	Second messenger formation
	PGF$_{2\alpha}$	↑	Second messenger formation
Prostacyclins	PGI$_2$	↑	Second messenger formation
Thromboxanes	TXA$_2$	↑	Second messenger formation
Leukotrienes	LTE$_4$	↑↓	Second messenger formation
Various tissues Epidermal growth factor	EGF	↑	Epithelial cell proliferation
Fibroblast growth factor	FGF	↑	Fibroblast proliferation
Nerve growth factor	NGF	↑	Neurite development
Somatomedins	IGF-I, II	↑	Cellular growth and proliferation
Endorphins (e.g., enkephalins)		↑	Opiate-like activity
Heart Atrial natriuretic factor (atriopeptin)	ANF	↓↑	Renal salt and water diuresis

[a]The major effect of each putative chemical messenger on either an increased or stimulated (↑) or a decreased or inhibited (↓) physiological response is indicated.

Some cells within the gastrointestinal epithelium and other tissues of the body secrete peptide hormones and neurotransmitter substances (e.g., serotonin) locally to regulate adjacent cells. Here are examples of neurotransmitter substances acting nonsynaptically and hormones acting locally rather than by a bloodborne route. Growth inhibitory substances, *chalones*, may represent other examples of local hormones [7]. Some chemical messengers are released to the exterior of animals where by air convection or water dispersal they interact with cells (e.g., nasal olfactory epithelium) of other members of the same species to evoke a response; these substances are referred to as *pheromones* [22, 24].

In consideration of the multiple sources of peptide hormones, within glandular cells or within neurons, and the observation that classical neurotransmitters may function as a local hormone, neurotransmitter, or neuromodulatory substance, some have proposed that a broader definition of a hormone be adopted. Guillemin suggested that a hormone be defined as "any substance released by a cell and which acts on another cell near or far, regardless of the singularity or ubiquity of the source and regardless of the means of conveyance, blood stream, axoplasmic flow, or immediate intercellular space" [14]. In this book, however, the term hormone will be used in its more standard context, referring to any chemical messenger that is released from a cell and conveyed through the bloodstream to act on a distant target tissue. Neurohormone may be used to indicate specific examples of hormones that undergo neurosecretion from central or peripheral neurons; neurotransmitter may be used to describe many of the same messengers when they function at synaptic junctions (Table 2.3). Endocrinology is, by this definition, the study of hormones derived from the classical endocrine glands (e.g., pituitary, thyroid, adrenal, gonads) or from other cells or tissues such as the brain or gastrointestinal tract (GI).

TABLE 2.3   Hormone terminology

Chemical messenger:	Any substance produced by a cell of endogenous or exogenous origin that plays a physiological role in the control of the activity of another cell
Hormone:	The general circulation or a specialized vascular system, to regulate another cell. May be delivered by an endocrine or neuroendocrine, route
Neurohormone:	A hormone produced by a nerve cell
Neuropeptide:	A peptidergic neurohormone or neurotransmitter (e.g., substance P)
Non-peptidergic neurotransmitter:	Any non-peptidergic neurotransmitter, such as acetylcholine, histamine, norepinephrine, and serotonin
Neurotransmitter:	A neurochemical that acts trans-synaptically
Neuromodulator:	A neurochemical that modulates the response of a neuron to a neurotransmitter or hormone
Pheromones:	Chemical messengers released to the exterior of one animal to stimulate a response in another member of the same species
Lumones:	Chemical messengers released into the lumen of the gastrointestinal tract
Chalones:	Putative cellular mitotic inhibitors
Growth factors:	Mitogenic peptides, most often acting locally within tissues.

One problem arising from the recognition of the varied distribution of hormones relates to the physiological roles of a hormone. If one wants to know the functional role of a specific hormone, it is necessary to inquire as to which source of the hormone is being discussed. For example, the peptide hormone somatostatin (SST) is released from specific neurons in the brain to regulate the release of growth hormone (GH) and possibly other hormones from the pituitary gland (Chap. 6). SST is also present in other neurons within the central nervous system (CNS) where it may function as a neurotransmitter or a neuromodulator. SST is also found within the gut epithelium and the pancreas, and it undoubtedly functions in these sites by a local mechanism to regulate gastrin, glucagon, and insulin secretion (Chap. 11). Portal plasma levels of SST are elevated after a meal; the peptide may function in this example as a bloodborne chemical messenger (hormone in the classical sense), as it does in the regulation of pituitary GH secretion. SST eventually may be shown to have as many functions as the particular neurons or cells within which it is localized. Like the neurotransmitter dopamine, which is distributed widely within the brain and which subserves many functions, the localization of peptide hormones to specific neurons suggests that they, too, probably regulate a diverse number of functions.

General Classes of Chemical Messengers

Although there are many vertebrate hormones, they may be conveniently categorized into groups that bear structural and/or functional similarities. Generally, these groupings also imply some major differences in cellular source and synthesis of the particular chemical messengers that comprise the group.

Protein Hormones Comprise the Most Diverse Family of Chemical Messengers

As implied by the subgroup classification, these hormones are composed of amino acids. There may be as few as three amino acids (as in thyrotropin-releasing hormone, TRH, see Fig. 1.3) or as many as 180 or more in the pituitary gonadotropins. Although the individual hormones could be referred to as peptide, polypeptide, or protein in nature, depending on their specific chain length, for the sake of brevity here they are referred to as *peptide* hormones. Peptide hormones may be composed of a linear chain, as in α-MSH or angiotensin II, or may contain a ring structure due to bridge formation through disulfide bonds, as in the *neurohypophysial hormones* oxytocin and vasopressin (see Fig. 7.2) or SST (see Fig. 6.7). Some of the larger protein hormones are composed of two chains, as in insulin (see Fig. 11.5), thyrotropin (TSH), and the gonadotropins (follicle-stimulating hormone, FSH, and luteinizing hormone, LH). Dimeric hormones may be synthesized as the combination of two portions of the same gene product, such as in the case of insulin (Chap. 11). They may also arise from the post-translational dimerization of two protein subunits encoded by two different genes, as is true for the gonadotropins (Chap. 5). The dimeric (quaternary) structure of insulin is held together by interchain disulfide bonds. Intrachain disulfide bonds are also present in insulin and in prolactin (PRL), GH, and in some other hormones. These covalent bonds may be important for establishing the tertiary structure (conformation) necessary for producing the active site within these peptides or, in some instances, for protecting the hormones from enzymatic degradation [3].

Other special features of peptide hormones can also be important in determining their biological activity. In some peptide hormones, tyrosine is sulfated (e.g., gastrin; see Fig. 10.1), and the glutamic acid moiety may be cyclized into a pyrrole structure (as in TRH; see Fig. 1.3). Some of the larger peptides (FSH, LH, TSH, and human chorionic gonadotropin (hCG) are *glycoproteins*, that is, they are conjugated to one or more carbohydrate residues. Because peptide hormones are composed of a linear sequence of amino acids, there is usually an amino (NH_2)- or N-terminal and a carboxy (COOH)- or C-terminal group present in the structure. In some peptides the C-terminal end may be amidated (to a carboxamide) and the N-terminal group may be acetylated (as in α-MSH; see Fig. 8.1).

The amino acid sequence (primary sequence) of a hormone may differ between species (e.g., ACTH and calcitonin; see Figs 5.8 and 9.4, respectively). Two or more *isoforms* of a peptide hormone may be present within a single species of animal. Isoforms of hormones can arise from differential splicing of mRNA, as products of separate genes or as post-transcriptional or post-translational modifications (sulfation, glycosylation, etc.) of the peptide. Knowledge of such species differences in primary sequence provides information on the evolution of the hormone. Single amino acid substitutions may even lead to the evolution of new hormone structures within an individual species [8]. Although oxytocin and vasopressin are closely related structurally and presumably evolutionarily, they play entirely different physiological roles within an individual animal. Based on similarity of structure, one can group hormones into families of peptides that undoubtedly are derived from a common evolutionary precursor. The insulin family of peptides includes nerve growth factor (NGF), relaxin, and one or more of the somatomedins. The melanocortin family of peptides includes ACTH, α-MSH, and possibly other melanotropins (see Fig. 8.1). Invariant sequences of amino acids within the primary structure of a peptide may suggest that such sequences are components of the active site of the hormone (see Fig. 8.1).

The amino acid structure of peptide hormones generally renders them hydrophilic, and as such they do not passively permeate cells by diffusion through the plasma membrane. It is thus not surprising that virtually all peptide hormones exert their actions by activating specific receptor molecules present in the plasma membrane, which are in turn coupled to the activation of intracellular second and tertiary (third) messenger signal transduction pathways. The molecular and functional properties of these peptide hormone receptors are discussed in the next chapter.

The Thyroid Gland Produces Iodine-Containing Hormones, Thyroxine and Triiodothyronine (T_3)

The thyroid gland synthesizes two hormones, thyroxine and triiodothyronine (T_3), from the precursor amino acid tyrosine (see Fig. 13.1). These two iodinated hormones have a diverse number of functions within and between members of the different vertebrate classes. Thyroxine and T_3 are unique in that an inorganic ion, iodine, is incorporated into their structures and is required for their biological activity. These hormones are indispensable for normal growth and development. In their absence, somatic and mental growth is severely retarded. In contrast to the protein hormones, yet similar to steroid hormones (see below), the thyroid hormones exert their actions through receptors that are located in the nuclei of target cells.

Cortisol

Corticosterone

Aldosterone

Figure 2.1 Examples of adrenal steroid hormones.

Testosterone

Estradiol

Progesterone

Figure 2.2 Examples of gonadal steroid hormones.

Steroid Hormones are Produced Primarily by the Adrenal Cortex and Gonads

Steroid hormones are produced from their common precursor, cholesterol, by steroidogenic cells of the adrenal cortex and gonads (testes and ovaries). The adrenal steroidogenic tissue produces two types of corticosteroids: *glucocorticoids* (e.g., cortisol, corticosterone, and cortisone) and *mineralocorticoids* (e.g., aldosterone). These *corticosteroids* play important roles in carbohydrate metabolism and electrolyte balance, respectively. The pathway of steroid biosynthesis is complex, and many steroid precursors are formed in the synthetic pathway of any particular steroid hormone (e.g., see Fig. 15.3). Under abnormal conditions of biosynthesis, the production of these metabolites may increase and exert undesirable physiological effects. Figure 2.1 shows the structures of the major adrenal steroid hormones.

The steroidogenic tissue of the gonads produces a number of sex (gonadal) steroids: *androgens* (masculinizing), *estrogens* (feminizing), and *progestins* (related to pregnancy, gestation). The testes produce testosterone; in the ovary estradiol and progesterone are the main steroids synthesized and secreted. During pregnancy the placenta is an additional source of estrogens and progestins (progestogens). Under certain developmental conditions, the adrenal steroidogenic tissue may be an important additional source of androgens and estrogens. Figure 2.2 shows the structure of three important gonadal steroid hormones. As derivatives of cholesterol, most steroid hormones possess lipophilic properties that permit the passive diffusion of these molecules through the plasma and nuclear membranes. Likely as a consequence of these properties, the receptor molecules that bind steroids and then mediate their actions have evolved as linear protein molecules that are primarily contained within the nucleus and cytoplasm of cells. Structures and functions of members of the superfamily of steroid receptor molecules are addressed in more detail in Chap. 3.

Many Neurotransmitters are Enzymatically Modified Amino Acids

Neurotransmitters are synthesized by neurons and are usually released into a specialized structure, the synaptic cleft, adjacent to the cell to be regulated (effector/target cell). These neural messengers regulate another nerve cell, a muscle cell, or a secretory cell (e.g., salivary gland cell). The common neurotransmitters are acetylcholine, norepinephrine, dopamine, serotonin (5-hydroxytryptamine, 5-HT), gamma-aminobutyric acid (GABA), and glutamate, but there are a number of other putative neurotransmitters (Chaps 6, 21) [9, 10]. Dopamine released from hypothalamic neurons of the brain may also function as a bloodborne hormone to regulate pituitary hormone secretion. Figure 2.3 shows the structures of three important neurotransmitters. Other biogenic amines (see Figs 6.13, 6.14) themselves, also function as neurotransmitters within the central and peripheral nervous systems [5]. All of these neurotransmitter molecules, with the exception of acetylcholine, are enzymatically processed from amino acid precursors or they are themselves neurochemically active amino acids (e.g., glutamate). Upon release and diffusion across a synaptic cleft, virtually all of the neurotransmitters exert their actions by activating specific receptor molecules present on postsynaptic membranes.

Neuropeptides can Function as Neurohormones, Neurotransmitters, and Neuromodulators

Some neuropeptides (e.g., vasopressin and oxytocin) were first characterized as hormones secreted into the peripheral circulation from nerve terminals in the posterior pituitary gland. Other neuropeptides were identified as hypothalamic releasing factors (e.g., GnRH, CRH, GHRH) or inhibiting factors (e.g., SST) that are released into a specialized pituitary portal vasculature (Chap. 6) as neurohormones that direct secretion of anterior pituitary hormones. Almost all of these neuropeptides, however, as well as many more that do not regulate pituitary function, have been found throughout the central and peripheral nervous systems where they are synthesized by specific neurons and localized to specific nerve tracts [21]. Such a discrete localization within the brain is entirely consistent with the function of these neuropeptides as neurotransmitters and/or neuromodulators. As neurotransmitters they may conduct information synaptically between neurons, and as neuromodulators they may affect the response of a neuron to other neurotransmitters released from the same or other neurons. Indeed, some neuropeptides are distributed quite widely throughout the central nervous system. The *endorphins*, for example, are

Figure 2.3 Examples of neurotransmitters.

expressed at many levels of the neuroaxis and act as neuroregulators via so-called opiate receptors and, in humans at least, function as analgesic (pain-relieving) hormones. Methionine enkephalin, leucine enkephalin, and β-endorphin are examples of opioid peptides.

Growth Factors are a Diverse Group of Locally Acting Peptide Messengers

A number of peptides of diverse origin possessing cellular growth-regulating activity have been identified. In some cases, the structural characteristics of the molecules have been partially or fully determined. The thymus may produce one or more thymosins, which are believed to induce maturation of white blood cells that then function in the immune response. Nerve growth factor (NGF) is responsible for neuron maturation in developing systems. The NGF polypeptide is a member of a larger family of trophic (growth-promoting) factors called the neurotrophins, which also includes brain-derived neurotrophic factor (BDNF) and neurotrophin-3 (NT-3). A superfamily of growth factors has also been identified that are structurally related to transforming growth factor β (TGFβ). The TGFβ itself has pronounced antiproliferative effects on cells, and loss of TGFβ signaling is associated with abnormal cell proliferation and development of certain human malignancies. Endogenous mitotic inhibitors such as TGFβ are referred to as *chalones*. Other members of the TGFβ family are primarily positive regulators of cell division and growth during development; the bone morphogenetic proteins (BMPs), for example, are important in inducing bone growth, while the inhibins and activins are TGFβ superfamily members that regulate early development of the reproductive tract. The inhibins and activins also function as important reproductive hormones in adulthood (Chaps 17, 18). These and other growth-stimulating peptides, such as erythropoietin (erythrocyte-stimulating factor) epidermal growth factor (EGF), fibroblast growth factor (FGF), and the somatomedins (insulin-like growth factors) will be discussed in Chap. 12, along with the membrane receptors that mediate their actions.

Eicosanoids are Fatty Acid Derivatives that Include Prostaglandins, Thromboxanes, and Leukotrienes

Prostaglandins are one class of chemical messengers known as eicosanoids. They are ubiquitous and affect the activity of many physiological processes. Prostaglandins are synthesized from fatty acid substrates (e.g., arachidonic acid) within the membranes of cells, and they are generally thought to act locally, within the same tissues in which they are produced. Their generic name was derived from the fact they were first discovered within seminal fluid. They are composed of a 20-membered fatty acid carbon skeleton folded into a hairpin-like structure by incorporating a 5-membered ring at the bend of the molecule. The thromboxanes, prostacyclins, and leukotrienes are related chemical messengers that play significant roles in physiological processes (Chap. 4) as diverse as contractions of the uterus, ovulatory cyclicity, inflammation, and fever. Figure 2.4 shows the structure of two important prostaglandins. Other classes of eicosanoid hormones are discussed in Chap. 4.

Figure 2.4 Examples of two common prostaglandins.

Figure 2.5 Examples of vertebrate and invertebrate pheromones.

Pheromones are a Diverse Group of Chemical Messengers that Mediate Signaling between Individuals

Most hormones act on cells within the animal in which they are produced. Chemical signals are also used for transmitting information between individuals of the same species [11, 22, 24]. The term pheromone denotes a chemical substance that is liberated by one animal and that causes a relatively specific behavior modification in a recipient animal following its chemoreception [22]. This chemical communication is implied to function within a species. Pheromones are classified into two types, a *signaler* (or *releaser*) pheromone, which brings about a prompt behavioral reaction, and a *primer* pheromone, which causes a slower effect, such as an alteration of the endocrine and reproductive systems. These effects are produced through neuroendocrine mechanisms for which the primary stimulus is chemosensory, mediated in most species by an accessory olfactory system, and not the main olfactory pathways. Pheromones play important roles in insects and other invertebrates. Pheromones are generally aliphatic, thus facilitating their volatilization and subsequent transport by air. The structure of the vertebrate pheromone civetone (from the civet) and the invertebrate pheromone bombykol (from the silkworm moth) are shown (Fig. 2.5). Pheromones may also be delivered (dispersed) within an aquatic environment. The structures of these pheromones are therefore hydrophilic in nature.

Electrolytes and Metabolites can also Convey Physiological Signals

Besides the well-recognized classes of hormones, other substances play important roles as chemical messengers controlling cellular function. The simplest such messenger is the hydrogen (H^+) ion (proton). Hydrochloric acid present within chyme is responsible for stimulating secretin release from cells of the duodenal epithelium (see Fig. 10.6). Because other acids will similarly stimulate secretin release, it is presumed that interaction of the hydrogen ion with specific cellular components of secretin-producing cells elicits release of this hormone. Osmoreceptors also monitor sodium ion (Na^+) levels within the plasma. These chemoreceptor cells undoubtedly have special recognition sites for this monovalent cation (Chap. 15). The divalent calcium (Ca^{2+}) ion is an important regulator of parathormone and calcitonin secretion from the parathyroid glands and parafollicular cells, respectively. These cells have specific recognition sites (Ca^{2+}-sensing receptors) for this important cation (Chap. 9, Fig. 9.13).

Glucose is a specific stimulus for insulin secretion from the beta (β) cells of the pancreatic islets. Glucose is also inhibitory to glucagon secretion from the alpha (α) cells of the pancreatic islets. Glucose is bound and transported into the pancreatic α and β cells by plasmalemmal structural elements referred to as glucose transporters (Chap. 11). This process also takes place in special glucose-sensitive neurons in the brain, where glucose uptake and metabolism can directly alter the electrophysiological activity of specific neurons. It is believed that some of these glucose-responsive neurons function as "glucostats," as they appear to detect significant alterations in plasma glucose concentrations and if necessary, they can activate protective neurophysiological responses to dangerously low blood sugar levels [16].

Certain amino acids (e.g., arginine) may function as specific stimulants of insulin secretion from the pancreatic islets. Certain neurons within the hypothalamus also monitor the levels of certain circulating amino acids; these sensory elements may then regulate the release of pituitary growth hormone. Glutamate, a derivative of glutamic acid, functions as a major stimulatory neurotransmitter throughout the CNS. The simplest amino acid, glycine, probably functions in a similar manner. Other as yet unrecognized metabolic substrates or end products may also play important roles in cellular regulation.

Hormone Synthesis

Because of the diversity of hormone structures, a number of interesting synthetic processes are involved in hormone biosynthesis. The simplest of hormones or neurotransmitters are amino acids themselves or derivatives thereof (see Fig. 6.14). For example, glycine and glutamic acid (glutamate) are certainly implicated as neurotransmitters within the brain. The amino acids phenylalanine and tyrosine (a derivative of phenylalanine) are precursors for the synthesis of dopamine, norepinephrine, and epinephrine, which function as neurotransmitters or as bloodborne hormones. Tyrosine is also the substrate for biosynthesis of the thyroid hormones, triiodothyronine and thyroxine (see Fig. 13.1). The amino acid tryptophan is the precursor for the formation of serotonin, a CNS neurotransmitter, and melatonin, a pineal hormone (see Fig. 20.2).

Protein Hormone Synthesis Involves DNA Transcription, mRNA Translation, and Prohormone Processing

Most vertebrate hormones are peptide in nature and are therefore composed of amino acids. Like other proteins, they are synthesized on ribosomes where their specific amino acid sequence is determined (*translated*) from a specific mRNA sequence (codon). The nucleotide sequences of the mRNA are dictated (*transcribed*) from specific nucleotide sequences (genes) in the DNA of chromosomes. The nascent proteins are then released and transported into the cisternae (microscopic cavity) of the rough endoplasmic reticulum (ER). Most often, this process of *hormone gene expression*—the transcription of a protein hormone gene and translation of the corresponding mRNA—culminates in the ribosomal synthesis of a *prepro-hormone* protein that is longer, but inclusive of the specific hormone amino acid sequence itself. In part, this preprohormone is longer because it additionally contains an amino terminal, hydrophobic *signal peptide* sequence that functions to permit movement of the protein across the ER membrane into the Golgi apparatus. There it undergoes further enzymatic modifications, prior to packaging into secretory granules. The removal of the signal sequence, which yields the *prohormone*, is typically followed by the actions of proteolytic processing enzymes that additionally attack dibasic amino acid cleavage sites. These processing enzymes thereby release the *mature hormone* protein sequence from the remaining prohormone precursor molecule. Other peptide sequences with known biological activity, or without any known biological functions, i.e., *cryptic peptides*, may also be produced by these enzymatic cleavages. Within the Golgi elements the hormone may additionally be altered by processing enzymes that conjugate carbohydrate, or other specific chemical moieties (functional groups) to the molecule. In the synthesis of some protein hormones, processing enzymes direct the covalent linkage of two different sulfur-containing cysteine residues within the same hormone molecule. This creates the "disulfide bridge" that often endows the molecule with secondary and tertiary structures required for its biological activity.

Vesicles containing the mature protein hormone and possibly other products (e.g., proteolytic enzymes) are then pinched off the terminal cisternae of the Golgi apparatus. These secretory vesicles are then distributed within the cytoplasm in patterns generally characteristic of the cell type involved. Release of the hormone from the cell thereafter occurs through *exocytosis*, a process that involves fusion of the secretory granule with the plasma membrane and diffusion of its contents into the extracellular space, as discussed later in this chapter.

Steroid Hormones are Derived from Cholesterol

In contrast to peptide hormones, steroid hormones are not synthesized through expression of specific genes. Instead, steroid hormones are synthesized from the enzymatic processing of their common precursor molecule, cholesterol, which in turn is primarily available from fats ingested in the diet. Cholesterol is conveyed to cells via the bloodstream, transported into the cytoplasm and delivered to the mitochondria. Sequential modifications of cholesterol are made by steroidogenic enzymes present in both the mitochondria and cytoplasm, leading to the formation of specific steroid hormone molecules, such as estradiol, cortisol, or aldosterone. The relative abundance and activity of specific steroidogenic enzymes in a given steroidogenic cell determines the relative amounts of each intermediate and end product that are produced. The enzymatic activities present in the steroidogenic cells of the gonads, for example, preferentially direct steroid synthesis along the metabolic pathways leading to production of the gonadal steroids (estradiol, progesterone, and testosterone), while the steroidogenic enzymes present in the outermost layer of steroidogenic cells in the adrenal cortex produce much higher levels of the mineralocorticoid hormone aldosterone. Specific steroidogenic pathways are discussed in detail in subsequent chapters, as they relate to adrenocortical (Chap. 15) and gonadal hormone (Chaps 16–18) synthesis. Because of the great number of enzymes involved in the biosynthesis of any one steroid hormone, mutations leading to faulty enzymes may result in one or a number of pathophysiological states, and these are also discussed in relevant chapters (Chaps 15–18).

Thyroid Hormone Synthesis Requires a Unique Series of Biochemical Processes in Follicular Cells

The synthesis of the thyroid hormones, thyroxine and T_3, involves the addition of iodine moieties on tyrosine residues contained within the proteinaceous substrate, thyroglobulin. Pairs of the resulting iodotyrosines are joined by an ether linkage and released from the thyroglobulin protein, yielding active hormones containing either three (T_3) or four (thyroxine) iodine moieties. The synthesis of these iodine-containing hormones occurs on the extracellular (luminal) surface of the follicular cells of the thyroid. They are then taken up by endocytosis and transported through the follicular cells where they are enzymatically released from the carrier protein prior to secretion (Chap. 13).

Non-Peptide Neurotransmitters are Synthesized in Nerve Endings

Non-peptidergic neurotransmitters, such as acetylcholine and the biogenic amines (dopamine, norepinephrine, epinephrine, serotonin), are synthesized via enzymatic modification of precursors within the axonal endings of neurons (Chap. 14). The enzymes needed for the many neurotransmitter production steps are, however, synthesized on ribosomes in the perikarya (cell bodies) of neurons and are subsequently transported by axoplasmic flow to the neuron terminals. The secreted neurotransmitter may then be taken back up into axon terminals for further use (see Fig. 14.5). Acetylcholine is inactivated by enzymatic cleavage after secretion, but the constituent moieties (acetate and choline) are then taken up for resynthesis of the hormone.

Gases can Function as Chemical Messengers

Some neurons and cells of a variety of peripheral tissues produce gases, such as *nitric oxide* (NO) and *carbon monoxide* (CO), that function as neurotransmitters and locally acting hormones [10]. In endothelial (vascular) cells, for example, the formation of NO from oxygen and the amino acid arginine is catalyzed by the enzyme nitric oxide synthase (NOS). The NO diffuses locally to bind and activate NO receptors in adjacent smooth muscle cells; activation of the NO receptor is coupled to the generation of the second messenger, cyclic guanylyl monophosphate (cGMP), which in turn activates subsequent signals leading to relaxation of the smooth muscle cell and vasodilation. A neuronal isoform of NOS similarly catalyzes the formation of NO in brain, where NO can function as a neurotransmitter.

Peptide Neurohormones and Neurotransmitters are Synthesized in the Same Manner as Protein Hormones

The peptide neurohormones (e.g., oxytocin and vasopressin) are synthesized in neuronal perikarya and are transported within vesicles for long distances for storage in the axon terminals (see Fig. 7.1). Numerous other neuropeptides are synthesized within discrete neurons in the brain by genomic mechanisms of transcription and translation.

Some Peptide and Steroid Hormones are Derived from Prohormones after Secretion

Some peptide hormones are composed of only a small number of amino acids. Oxytocin and other neurohypophysial hormones, for example, contain only nine amino acids (nonapeptides). These hormones are synthesized in the same manner as described for the larger protein hormones: Protein sequences of about 100 amino acids and longer (e.g., neurophysins) are initially synthesized (Chap. 7), and these proteins are then packaged within secretory vesicles along with proteolytic enzymes. These enzymes (endopeptidases) then cleave the protein into one or more smaller peptides, in some cases, the definitive hormone. A number of cleavage events may take place during post-translational processing before the definitive hormone is produced. Thus, most peptide hormones are derived indirectly by way of a prohormone that is processed in the secretory cell, prior to secretion. In other cases, however, prohormone molecules may be secreted themselves, and then processed to yield a mature hormone in the blood or even in a target tissue. Some large plasma proteins, such as angiotensinogen, serve as prohormones for hormone production. Renin, an enzyme released from the juxtaglomerular cells of the kidneys, acts on angiotensinogen, a substrate protein produced by the liver, to convert it to a smaller fragment. This fragment, angiotensin I, is then converted by another enzyme to the active hormone, angiotensin II. Large precursor plasma proteins, kininogens, are converted by certain serine proteases, referred to as kallikreins, to kinins, such as bradykinin, an important hormone in regulating blood flow in certain vascular beds (Chap. 15). Bradykinin and angiotensin II are examples of hormones that are released from liver cells as larger prohormones to be converted into active hormonal peptides within the blood.

Certain steroids serve as prohormones in the production of other definitive steroid hormones. For example, certain cells possess the enzyme 5α-reductase that converts testosterone to dihydrotestosterone, the effector molecule for activating these cells (see Fig. 16.8). Within the brain, testosterone is also aromatized within certain neurons to estradiol, which is the biologically active steroid structure required for activation of these cells (see Fig. 6.10). A steroid hormone produced locally in the brain from its precursor is referred to as a *neurosteroid*.

Control of Hormone Secretion

Hormones are synthesized within cells and, except for the thyroid and steroid hormones, are packaged within secretory vesicles until released. Stimuli of both an intrinsic (internal) or extrinsic (light, sound, smell, temperature, etc.) nature can affect hormone secretion.

Hormone Secretion can be a Regulated or Constitutive Process

In most protein hormone-secreting cells, chemical or electrical stimulation results in an elevation of intracellular Ca^{2+} levels, which prompts vesicular fusion with the plasma membrane and *exocytosis* of the granule contents. This Ca^{2+}-*dependent, exocytotic* process is the basic secretion mechanism of the *regulated release* pathway. In this type of release mechanism, hormone-containing granules are stored within the cell and a proportion of them form a *readily releasable pool* of hormone, which can be rapidly exocytosed upon receipt of a stimulatory signal. By contrast, hormones that undergo *constitutive release*, such as the steroid and thyroid hormones, are minimally stored within fat droplets within the cells. They are released as a consequence of passive diffusion along their concentration gradients, out of the cell. In these constitutive release pathways the rate of hormone release is dependent upon the rate of synthesis, which in turn depends upon the relative activities of the enzymes that control their synthesis; that is, the amount released is proportional to the amount produced. Control over the constitutively released hormone is thus governed by stimuli that regulate the level of activities of these synthetic enzymes.

Secretion of One Hormone is often Controlled by the Actions of Another

Hormones often stimulate hormone secretion from other endocrine glands. For example, pituitary hormones, such as TSH, LH, and ACTH, stimulate target tissue cells of the thyroid, gonads, and adrenal gland, respectively, to secrete their own respective hormones: thyroxine, gonadal steroids, and adrenal glucocorticoids (see Fig. 6.16). Hormone-secreting cells of the neurohypophysis, the adrenal medulla (*chromaffin tissue*), and the pineal gland are regulated by direct neural innervation. Stimulation of hormone secretion by nerves is referred to as *neuroendocrine transduction.* Metabolic substrates (glucose, amino acids, free fatty acids) and inorganic ions also provide a selective stimulus to hormone secretion by some cells.

Secretions of Some Hormones are Controlled by the Ionic, Metabolic or Hormonal Factors they Regulate

Calcium ion levels are monitored directly by parathormone- and calcitonin-secreting cells. Thus, the hormone-secreting cells that regulate Ca^{2+} levels do so by sensing the extracellular Ca^{2+} concentration [6]. Glucose concentration is monitored by the glucagon- and insulin-secreting cells of the pancreatic islets. These cells regulate blood glucose levels by sensing the circulating glucose concentration. Growth hormone stimulates tissue uptake of amino acids, and the amino acids that are present in the blood at increased levels after a meal provide cues to growth hormone secretion.

The pituitary hormones, FSH, LH, TSH, and ACTH, stimulate hormone secretion from the gonads, thyroid, and adrenal, respectively, and are controlled through negative feedback mechanisms. Target organ hormones, gonadal steroids, and thyroxine or adrenal glucocorticoids feed back to the hypothalamus and pituitary to inhibit further secretion of pituitary hormones (see Fig. 6.16). Some hormones may exert a negative feedback on the cells within which they are synthesized by a so-called *autoinhibition.*

The factors that stimulate cellular secretion, whether they are hormones or metabolites, interact with cellular receptors of the secretory cells. For example, epinephrine, a blood-borne hormone, or norepinephrine, a neurotransmitter, interacts with cell membrane adrenergic receptors (Chap. 14). Hormone interaction with some membrane receptors results in membrane *depolarization.* This stimulates the movement of Ca^{2+} into the cells, which then results in secretory vesicle exocytosis (so-called *stimulus-secretion coupling*). Some chemical messengers are inhibitory to cellular secretion, and their effects are mediated by cell membrane *hyperpolarization.* Changes in cellular secretion are generally correlated with changes in levels of intracellular cyclic nucleotides or other second messengers (e.g., Ca^{2+}). Secretion is often correlated with elevation of intracellular cyclic adenosine monophosphate (cAMP) levels.

Most hormone-secreting cells only exhibit minimal (basal) secretion in the absence of stimulatory cues. Prolactin- and MSH-secreting cells of some species are unique as hormone-secreting cells, in that they spontaneously secrete their hormones when placed in vitro or when the pituitary gland is transplanted to an ectopic site in the animal. These cells are normally under tonic inhibition by the brain, and they spontaneously depolarize and secrete their hormones in the absence of such inhibitory input (Chaps 5, 8).

The temporal pattern of hormone secretions can be of critical importance. Secretion of the adrenal hormone cortisol, for example, occurs in a well-characterized *circadian* (24-h) rhythmic pattern. Cortisol secretions reach their apex prior to awakening, and thus may prepare for the energetic demands of daily activity. The molecular mechanisms that comprise the biological clock controlling 24-h rhythms, including the rhythmic stimulation of cortisol secretion, have recently been delineated (Chaps 6, 20) [25]. Many hormones are also secreted in rhythmic patterns that vary with *ultradian* (shorter than 24-h) periodicities. The frequency and amplitude of these fluctuations in secretion may be physiologically modulated to elicit different responses from target tissues under different physiological circumstances. The neurohormone gonadotropin-releasing hormone (GnRH), for example, is released as a train of pulses into the hypophysial portal vessels to stimulate release of the gonadotropic hormones from the anterior pituitary gland. The frequency and amplitude of this *pulsatile release* pattern—and not just the total amount of GnRH itself—have been shown to be critically important variables that determine the magnitude of the gonadotropin secretory responses. An increase in the frequency of pulsatile GnRH release, for example, is believed to be the primary neural signal that stimulates pubertal maturation. This knowledge has been of importance in the design of effective pulsatile hormone replacement therapies for certain infertility syndromes, such as those that result from an absence of GnRH release.

Endocrine

Neuroendocrine

Paracrine

Neurocrine

Autocrine

Figure 2.6 Methods of hormone delivery. Modified from [12].

Hormone Delivery

Chemical messengers are delivered from the cell of origin to their target cells by one of several routes [11, 14, 27]: (1) *endocrine*, where the messenger substance is bloodborne (the classical definition of a hormone); (2) *neuroendocrine*, where the hormone released by a nerve is bloodborne; and (3) *paracrine*, where the released hormone diffuses to its adjacent target cells through the immediate extracellular space; (4) *neurocrine*, where a neuron contacts its target cells by axonal extensions and then releases the hormone into a synaptic cleft between the two cells; or even (5) *lumonal*, where the hormone is released into the lumen of the gut. Chemical messengers may also be released into the environment by a pheromonal route [22, 24]. Following the release of a hormone, it may also feed back on the cell of origin by a so-called *autocrine* mechanism [15] (Fig. 2.6). Somatostatin is an example of a hormone that may be delivered to its target tissue by all these routes. It is delivered to the pituitary by way of the hypophysial portal system (neuroendocrine route) to regulate GH secretion. SST is localized within other specific neurons of the CNS and controls target tissue neurons by a neurocrine (synaptic) mechanism. SST regulates pancreatic islet function by a local paracrine mechanism, and in the gut, the peptide may also function as a local hormone and control gastrin secretion by a paracrine mechanism. Portal blood SST levels are increased after a meal, suggesting an additional endocrine method of delivery to undetermined target sites.

Hormones achieve selectivity of target cell activation by several means. Neurotransmitters may be delivered (by a neurocrine mechanism) only to those target cells being innervated. Some selectivity of hormone action is achieved by delivery through specialized circulatory routes, such as the hypophysial portal system linking the hypothalamus to the pituitary. The specificity of target tissue receptors also assures that these cells will respond only to certain hormones. Under certain pathological states, overproduction of a hormone and its excessive release results in undesirable target tissue responses due to excess amounts of the hormone. Most neurons in the brain are protected from systemic endocrine influences by a *blood–brain barrier* (BBB); this is a continuous layer of endothelial cells connected by tight junctions, which function to oppose passage of some ions and most high-molecular weight compounds from blood to brain. Hormone analogs can, however, be synthesized which are permeable to the BBB.

Hormone Circulation and Metabolism

Hormones are secreted from endocrine cells to initiate immediate target tissue responses or to set in motion more long-term effects. In either case, hormones must be continuously inactivated or the cellular response would be continuously activated. Both intracellular and extracellular mechanisms function in the cessation of hormone-mediated responses.

Peptide Hormones Have Short Half-Lives in the Circulation

The half-life of a hormone or other active agent is defined as the amount of time required for half the molecules to become inactivated or cleared from the circulation. Shorter peptides usually have particularly short half-lives (possibly 2 to 30 min). The large protein hormone TSH is reported to have a half-life of about 60 min, and this may be one example of a long half-life. Peptidases, enzymes responsible for metabolizing peptides, play an essential role in biological regulation because of the close involvement of peptide messengers in the maintenance of homeostasis. Proteolytic enzymes are intimately concerned with all stages in the life of a biologically active peptide, from synthesis in the ribosomes to ultimate hydrolysis to individual amino acids. The initial proteolytic events occur within the secretory cell in a highly organized and compartmentalized manner and involve conversion of large gene products to smaller secretory forms of the peptide. Once secreted from a nerve ending or an endocrine cell, a peptide will encounter peptidases either associated with cellular membranes or soluble in tissue fluids. The postsecretory metabolism of peptides may inactivate the peptide (Fig. 2.7) or even convert it to forms with different biological activities.

Figure 2.7 General scheme for hormone production from a precursor peptide.

Enzymes inactivate peptide hormones by splitting the molecules at specific peptide bonds. *Exopeptidases*, both *carboxypeptidases* and *aminopeptidases*, cleave off the C-terminal or N-terminal amino acids, respectively. Peptide hormones may also be inactivated by simple deamination at either the N- or C-terminal (if amidated) ends of the molecule. *Endopeptidases* split the molecule at other specific peptide bonds within the molecule. The sites of internal cleavage are quite specific, for example, often between repeating sequences of certain basic amino acids, such as Lys-Lys, Arg-Lys, Lys-Arg, Arg-Arg, as found in β-LPH (see Figs 6.6 and 8.4). The clinical use of some peptides has been limited because of their short half-lives. Understanding biodegradation mechanisms may facilitate the preparation of appropriate peptide hormone analogs with longer lasting actions.

Insulin is composed of two chains held together by a pair of disulfide bonds. The hormone is inactivated by a so-called insulinase, an enzyme complex that inactivates the hormone by reduction of the interchain disulfide bonds, thus splitting the hormone into two individual inactive chains. A hypothetical model for the action of various proteolytic enzymes on hormone degradation is shown (Fig. 2.8).

Steroid and Thyroid Hormone are Bound by Globulins that Increase their Half-Lives

Most steroid hormones are bound to plasma proteins that are accordingly referred to as steroid hormone binding globulins. The half-life of steroid hormones is apparently enhanced by their ability to be bound to these plasma proteins. Aldosterone, a steroid that is not readily bound, has a shorter half-life than other steroid hormones with specific carrier (transport) proteins. In the liver, both adrenal and gonadal steroids usually are conjugated to glucuronic acid or they are sulfated (Fig. 2.9). These structural modifications may render them inactive and more soluble so they can be more readily excreted in the urine. Some of the glucuronide salts are secreted with the bile salts and may be reabsorbed into the blood. Thyroxine and triiodothyronine are deiodinated in many tissues. These hormones are also conjugated in the liver to form sulfates and glucuronides that enter the bile to pass into the intestine where they are reabsorbed or eliminated from the bowel.

Figure 2.8 Model of peptide degradation by proteolytic enzymes.

Figure 2.9 Steroid
hormone sulfation and
glucuronide formation.

Steroid Sulphates

Steroid Glucuronides

Adrenal Catecholamines and Neurotransmitters are Enzymatically Inactivated in Liver and Brain, Respectively

The metabolism of circulating catecholamines occurs mainly in the liver by orthomethylation and oxidative deamination by catechol *O*-methyltransferase (COMT) and monoamine oxidase (MAO), respectively (see Fig. 14.4). Neurotransmitter action within synapses is terminated rapidly by a number of enzymatic or other processes. Norepinephrine and dopamine are inactivated in the synapse by COMT. These neurotransmitters are also taken back into the presynaptic axon to be used again or to be inactivated by MAO. Acetylcholine liberated into the synapse from cholinergic neurons is split into choline and acetate by the enzyme acetylcholinesterase. The reaction products, choline and acetate, are also taken back into the presynaptic axon to be resynthesized into acetylcholine.

Physiological Roles of Hormones

Hormones control the activity of virtually all cells in the body. The vast number of effects produced by hormones can, however, be reduced to a few general processes.

1. Hormones affect cellular **synthesis and secretion** of other biologically active molecules, such as other hormones within other endocrine glands or neurotransmitters in neurons. Hormones affect the secretion of digestive tract products, such as enzymes, hydrochloric acid, and bile salts. They also affect epithelial mucus and milk synthesis and secretion, as well as integumental sebum and sweat production and release. Hormones also affect the production and secretion of pheromones and probably other odoriferous substances [22, 24].

2. Hormones affect **metabolic processes**, both *anabolic* and *catabolic*, in most cells. The synthesis and degradation of carbohydrates, lipids, and proteins are controlled by hormones to meet the specific energy or growth needs of the individual.

3. Hormones affect **contraction, relaxation**, and **metabolism of muscle**. They cause contraction and relaxation of vascular and gastrointestinal smooth muscle, as well as genital tract musculature such as the uterus and oviducts. Hormones also affect cardiac and skeletal muscle contractile properties. Some steroid hormones profoundly affect anabolic and catabolic processes within muscle.

4. Hormones control **reproductive processes**, such as gonadal differentiation, maturation, and gametogenesis.

5. Hormones stimulate or inhibit **cellular proliferation**, thus affecting growth. Hormones also play regulatory roles in the earliest aspects of cell division and differentiation of the fertilized egg.

6. The **excretion and reabsorption of inorganic cations and anions** from the kidney is regulated by hormones. Sodium, potassium, calcium, and phosphate ions are particularly affected.

7. Hormones have **permissive actions** on the effects of other hormones: the effectiveness of certain hormones is often considerably enhanced by the action of another hormone. The permissive hormone may be without any noticeable effect of its own, but it may be an absolute requirement for the actions of the other hormone.

8. Hormones play important roles in **animal behavior**. Sexual and aggressive behaviors are affected by hormones, particularly during certain phases of the reproductive cycle. Maternal behavior is controlled by gonadal hormones and by pituitary hormones. Group behavior may even be affected by the release of pheromones into the environment [22].

Hormones may control certain physiological functions at one stage in life and certain others at a later developmental stage. Some hormones are secreted on an off-and-on basis to control fluctuations in serum constituents, such as glucose and calcium. Hormones may be secreted spasmodically to meet particular needs; oxytocin, for example, is generally secreted at parturition and during suckling of the breast. Adrenal catecholamines, on the other hand, are usually secreted under conditions of stress. The continuous secretion of hormones (e.g., cortisol) under prolonged stress may, because of their catabolic actions, debilitate an organism [23]. Some hormones are not secreted in large amounts until a later stage in development. The gonadotropic hormones, for example, increase in secretion after puberty to stimulate the gonads and subsequent growth and development of the secondary sex characteristics.

Some hormones may come into existence only a few times in the life of an individual. Human chorionic gonadotropin and other peptide hormones are made by the placenta and therefore are only produced during pregnancy. Some hormones lose their function with time; after menopause, for example, FSH secretion is enhanced, but the ovary no longer responds to the hormone. Thyroid hormone secretion and/or effectiveness is diminished with age, and this results in a decreased capacity for thermogenesis (as noted in the elderly).

General Mechanisms of Hormone Action

The physiological processes regulated by hormones result from interaction of the hormone with specific constituents of the cell, referred to as *receptors*. All peptide hormones, as well as most non-peptidergic neurotransmitters, act on membrane receptors. The major families of membrane receptor molecules include the G-protein-coupled receptors, cytokine receptors, receptor tyrosine kinases, and receptor serine/threonine kinases. The structures and functions of these receptors, and the coupling of receptor activation to signal transduction in cells, are discussed in detail in the following chapters. Stimulation of many membrane receptors leads to activation of cyclizing enzymes, which initiate the production of a cyclic nucleotide, either cAMP or cGMP. Other membrane receptors are coupled to phosphoinostol hydrolysis, which results in the production of diacylglycerol and inositol triphosphate (IP_3). These and other so-called second messengers of hormone action generally activate one or more specific protein phosphorylation events within the cell. Addition of a phosphate group to a protein, an enzyme, for example, by a phosphoprotein kinase may result in its activation. Phosphorylation of another protein might enhance its contractile activity. Protein substrate phosphorylation, in contrast, may also inactivate an enzyme. Phosphoprotein phosphatases, on the other hand, remove phosphate groups from proteins, and this can result in either inactivation or activation of the particular protein (see Fig. 7.13).

Steroid hormones, unlike most other chemical messengers, interact with intracellular receptors. These receptors within the nucleus interact with the chromatin (DNA) of specific chromosomes, which initiates mRNA synthesis (transcription) and protein synthesis (translation; see Figs 4.13 and 9.11). Thyroid hormones also interact with intracellular receptors to activate protein synthetic processes (see Fig. 13.10).

The cellular response to membrane receptor activation may be instantaneous as in nerve–nerve or nerve–muscle communication. The ultimate physiological response of cells to steroid or thyroid hormones is obviously much slower as the genomic and synthetic events require more time to be consummated.

Endocrine Pathophysiology

Endocrine glands release their hormones in response to bodily needs. The released hormones exert their effects on target tissues and are rapidly degraded and excreted. Failure of a gland or tissue to secrete enough hormone can lead to fatal consequences. For example, in the absence of insulin, elevated blood glucose (hyperglycemia) occurs and adversely affects other physiological processes. Individuals with diabetes mellitus may go into coma and die, or they may ultimately succumb to destructive alterations of other physiological processes. Lack of parathormone leads to hypocalcemia and this results in tetanic convulsions and death. Failure to secrete vasopressin results in severe water loss (*diabetes insipidus*) and dehydration.

Failure to secrete enough hormone may result from destruction of the endocrine gland, as can happen to the adrenal cortex due to tuberculosis. Failure to secrete cortisol (*Addison's disease*) may result from destruction of the adrenal cortex or failure of the pituitary to secrete ACTH, which is responsible for stimulation of adrenal cortisol formation. Failure to secrete ACTH can result from pituitary gland dysfunction or failure of the hypothalamus to secrete corticotropin-releasing hormone (CRH). Diabetes insipidus may result from a lack of vasopressin, but, if the kidney fails to respond to the hormone, this also results in *nephrogenic diabetes insipidus*.

Overproduction of hormone secretion, on the other hand, can also lead to pathophysiological states and possible death. Excess cortisol secretion (*Cushing's syndrome*) can cause altered carbohydrate, fat, and protein metabolism. This usually leads to hyperglycemia and pancreatic beta cell exhaustion resulting in diabetes mellitus. Oversecretion of aldosterone may lead to severe hypertension because of the hypervolemia (increased blood volume) caused by the hypernatremia (increased blood Na^+) characteristic of *hyperaldosteronism (aldosteronism)*.

Many endocrinopathies of excess hormone secretion result from neoplasms where the tumor produces an excess of a hormone. Adrenal cortical tumors may secrete tremendous amounts of cortisol (Cushing's syndrome). Insulinomas secrete excessive amounts of insulin, which results in lowered blood glucose levels. The resulting hypoglycemia may cause rapid coma and death since nerve cells must have a constant supply of glucose to function.

Endocrine disorders can result from a number of events related to hormone–target cell interaction. For example, the structure of a peptide hormone may be altered due to a mutation (nucleotide base change) in the gene coding for the hormone, as in one form of familial hyperinsulinemia. In the *testicular feminizing syndrome*, target tissues lack receptors for testosterone, and the body may then differentiate along the direction of the female phenotype [19]. In pseudohypoparathyroidism, although blood Ca^{2+} levels are low, there is an excess of parathormone [13]. The target tissue of the hormone, the kidney, apparently lacks functional receptors responsible for the production of cAMP; therefore, the cells fail to respond to the hormone. Other examples of endocrine dysfunction are discussed in Table 2.4 and in more detail within the following chapters [6, 18].

Comparative Endocrinology

Most information on the vertebrate endocrine system is derived from experiments on mammals, particularly rats and mice. Endocrine dysfunction in humans has, of course, contributed immensely to understanding the role of hormones in normal physiological processes. Primates, the closest relatives of humans, provide important experimental model systems for understanding the roles of hormones.

Much less is known about the endocrinology of nonmammalian forms. Studies on these vertebrates have, however, provided particularly interesting insights into the specialized aspects of endocrine regulation. Thyroid hormones, for example, are required for the metamorphic change necessary for the emergence of some amphibians (e.g., frogs, toads, salamanders) from the aquatic to the terrestrial environment [26]. The hormonal form of vitamin D, because of its crucial role in Ca^{2+} homeostasis, is of special importance to egg laying in the bird. Prolactin is necessary for successful transition of certain species of fishes from the saline (marine) to the freshwater environment. Prolactin is required for broodpatch development in some birds. Melanocyte-stimulating hormone plays an important role in regulating color changes of the integument of many vertebrates (Chap. 8). Understanding the diverse roles of each of the vertebrate hormones provides interesting insights into the evolution of hormone structure and function.

TABLE 2.4 Some examples of endocrinopathies

Disease	Etiology	Symptoms
Diabetes mellitus	Lack of insulin	Hyperglycemia, glucosuria (excretion of glucose in urine)
Diabetes insipidus:		
Pituitary	Lack of AVP (ADH)	Water loss, hypovolemia (low blood volume), dehydration
Nephrogenic	Renal unresponsiveness to AVP (ADH)	Water loss, hypovolemia, dehydration
Addison's disease:		
Primary	Adrenal cortical destruction (lack of all adrenal steroids)	Altered carbohydrate metabolism, salt-losing syndrome
Secondary	Lack of ACTH secretion	Altered carbohydrate metabolism
Cushing's syndrome:		
Primary	Adrenal tumor (excess cortisol secretion)	Protein catabolism, hyperglycemia
Secondary	Pituitary adenoma (excess ACTH and cortisol secretion)	Protein catabolism, hyperglycemia
Cretinism (infantile hypothyroidism)	Lack of T_4–T_3 secretion	Lowered basal metabolic rate (BMR), decreased mentation, growth failure
Myxedema (adult hypothyroidism)	Lack of T_4–T_3 secretion	Lowered BMR, decreased mentation
Hyperthyroidism (thyrotoxicosis)	Excess T_4–T_3 secretion	Enhanced BMR, hyperexcitability
Hypoparathyroidism	Parathyroid gland destruction	Lowered blood Ca^{2+} levels
Hyperparathyroidism	Parathyroid gland tumor or hypertrophy (increased PTH secretion)	Elevated blood Ca^{2+} levels
Pseudohypoparathyroidism	Lack of renal response to PTH	Lowered blood Ca^{2+} levels
Testicular feminizing syndrome	Absent or defective androgen receptors	Genital tract feminization in the male
Hyperaldosteronism (Conn's disease)	Adrenocortical tumor (excess aldosterone secretion)	Sodium retention (hypernatremia), hypervolemia, hypertension

REVIEW EXERCISES

Compare and contrast each of the following terms:

mineralocorticoid/
  glucocorticoid
androgen/estrogen
endocrine/neuroendocrine
  (delivery of a hormone)
translation/
  transcription (in peptide
  hormone synthesis)
endopeptidase/exopeptidase

oxytocin/vasopressin
neurohormone/
  neuropeptide
adrenal chromaffin/
  adrenal steroid (tissue)
endorphin/opiate
endocytosis/exocytosis

Define or otherwise characterize each of the follwing terms:

hypovolemia
isohormone
arachidonic acid
adenohypophysis

pheromone
chemoreceptor
autoinhibition
glucoronide formation

Match the glandular tissues in column A with the hormone(s) that they produce in column B:

(A)	(B)
Ovary	LH, FSH, GH, ACTH, PRL, TSH
Pancreas	GnRH, TRH, SST, GHRH, DA, CRH
Anterior pituitary gland	Testosterone, inhibin
Adrenal cortex	Atriopeptin
Heart	Calcitonin
Posterior pituitary gland	Insulin, glucagon
Thyroid gland	T_3, thyroxine
Testis	cortisol, aldosterone, testosterone
Hypothalamus	estrogen, progesterone, inhibin
Parathyroid gland	vasopressin, oxytocin

Think, analyze and discuss:

1. The neurohormone GnRH was the first of the hypophysiotropic releasing factors to be chemically characterized. It is synthesized in hypothalamic neurons, released into the hypophysial portal vessels, and conveyed to the anterior pituitary gland, where it stimulates LH and FSH secretion.
   a. GnRH belongs to which major structural class of hormones?
   b. What is the precursor to the GnRH molecule? Is it encoded by a gene? Describe the molecular processes by which GnRH synthesis takes place in GnRH neurons.
   c. Is it likely that GnRH is secreted into the portal vessel blood by a regulated or constitutive release mechanism?
   d. Do you think that GnRH has a long or short half-life in blood? Is it likely bound to a carrier molecule in blood?
   e. Would you expect that receptors for GnRH are located on the plasma membrane or in the cytoplasm or nucleus of the gonadotrope cells of the anterior pituitary gland?

2. Estrogen is a hormone that is produced in greatest amounts by the ovaries. It has numerous functions within the reproductive tract, brain, and many non-reproductive tissues and organs.
   a. Estrogen belongs to which major structural class of hormones?
   b. What is the initial substrate in the metabolic pathway leading to estrogen synthesis? Is it encoded by a gene? Describe the biochemical processes by which estrogen is synthesized in ovarian thecal cells.
   c. Is it likely that estrogen is secreted into the circulation by a regulated or a constitutive release mechanism?
   d. Do you think that estrogen has a long or short-half life in blood? Is it likely bound to a carrier molecule in blood?
   e. Would you expect that receptors for estrogen would be located on the plasma membrane, or in the cytoplasm or nucleus in cells of its target tissues?

3. Dopamine is a neurotransmitter and neurohormone that is produced by several different groups of neurons in the brain. One of these dopaminergic cell groups releases dopamine into the hypophysial portal vessels, where it is conveyed to the anterior pituitary gland to function as a prolactin-inhibiting hormone.
   a. Dopamine belongs to which major structural class of hormones?
   b. What is the initial biochemical substrate in the metabolic pathway leading to dopamine synthesis? Is it encoded by a gene? Describe the biochemical process by which dopamine is synthesized in dopaminergic neurons.
   c. Is it likely that dopamine is secreted into the portal vessel blood by a regulated or constitutive release mechanism?
   d. Would you expect that receptors for dopamine would be located on the plasma membrane, or in the cytoplasm or nucleus of lactotrope cells in the anterior pituitary gland?

4. Hormone secretions are regulated by a variety of physiological signals, as well as by feedback mechanisms. Often the secretion of a hormone is subject to regulation by the very same physiological variable that it, in turn, regulates. What are the major input signals that regulate secretion of insulin, glucagon, parathyroid hormone, and calcitonin, respectively? For each, predict whether they would stimulate or inhibit secretion of the hormone.

5. Name an example of one or more hormones that are produced and secreted . . .
   a. . . . only during a specific physiological circumstance, such as in pregnancy.
   b . . . in response to specific physiological stimulation, such as suckling by an infant.
   c. . . . in a pulsatile pattern.
   d. . . . with a circadian rhythmicity.
   e. . . . in response to a physical or behavioral stress.
   f. . . . at higher levels during pubertal maturation.

References

[1] Aoki, E., I. K. Takeuchi, and R. Shoji. 1995. Nitric oxide: An attractive signaling molecule. *Acta Histochem. Cytochem.* 28:97–106.

[2] Bayliss, W. M., and E. H. Starling. 1902. The mechanism of pancreatic secretion. *J. Physiol.* 28:325–53.

[3] Beebe, J. S., et al. 1990. Role of disulfide bond formation in the folding of human chorionic gonadotropin beta subunit into an alpha beta dimer assembly-competent form. *J. Biol. Chem.* 265:312–17.

[4] Boekhoff, I., et al. 1993. Pheromone-induced second-messenger signaling in insect antennae. *Insect Biochem. Mol. Biol.* 23:757–62.

[5] Brann, D. W., and V. B. Mahesh. 1997. Excitatory amino acids: Evidence for a role in the control of reproduction and anterior pituitary hormone secretion. *Endocr. Rev.* 18:678–700.

[6] Brown, E. M., et al. 1993. Cloning and characterization of an extracellular Ca^{2+}-sensing receptor from bovine parathyroid. *Nature Lond.* 366:575–80.

[7] Bullough, W. S. 1975. Mitotic control in adult mammalian tissue. *Biol. Rev.* 50:99–127.

[8] Castrucci, A. M. L., et al. 1989. Melanocyte stimulating hormone (MSH) and melanin concentrating hormone (MCH) may be structurally and evolutionarily related. *Reg. Pept.* 24:27–35

[9] Civelli, O., et al. 2001, Novel neurotransmitters as natural ligands of orphan G-protein-coupled receptors. *Trends Neurosci.* 24:230–7.

[10] Costa, A., et al. 1996. Gaseous transmitters as new agents in neuroendocrine regulation. *J. Endocrinol.* 149:199–207.

[11] Cutler, W. B., et al. 1986. Human axillary secretions influence women's menstrual cycles: The role of donor extract from men. *Horm. Behav.* 20:463–73.

[12] Dockray, G. J. 1979. Evolutionary relationship of the gut hormones. *Fed. Proc.* 38:2295–301.

[13] Farfel, Z., et al. 1996. Pseudohypoparathyroidism, a novel mutation in the βγ-contact region of $G_s\alpha$ impairs receptor stimulation. *J. Biol. Chem.* 271:19653–5.

[14] Guillemin, R. 1977. The expanding significance of hypothalamic peptides, or, is endocrinology a branch of neuroendocrinology. *Recent Prog. Horm. Res.* 33:1–28.

[15] Karlson, P. 1982. Was sind Hormone? Der Hormonbegriff in Geschichte und Gegenwart. *Naturwissenschaften* 69:3–14.

[16] Levin B. E., et al. 2004. Neuronal glucosensing: what do we know after 50 years? Diabetes 53:2521–8.

[17] Makhlouf, G. M. 1990. Neural and hormonal regulation of function in the gut. *Hosp. Pract.* 25:79–98.

[18] O'Riordan, J. L. H. 1997. Rickets, from history to molecular biology, from monkeys to YACS. *J. Endocrinol.* 154:S3–13.

[19] Quigley, C. A., et al. 1995. Androgen receptor defects: Historical, clinical, and molecular perspectives. *Endocr. Rev.* 16:271–321.

[20] Rosbash, M., and J. C. Hall. 1989. The molecular biology of circadian rhythms. *Neuron* 3:387–98.

[21] Scharrer, B. 1987. Neurosecretion: Beginnings and new directions in neuropeptide research. *Annu. Rev. Neurosci.* 10:1–17.

[22] Schneider, D. 1992. 100 years of pheromone research. *Naturwissenschaften* 79:241–50.

[23] Selye, H. 1976. *The stress of life.* New York: McGraw-Hill.

[24] Stowers, L., and T. F. Marton. 2005. What is a pheromone? Mammalian pheromones reconsidered. *Neuron* 46:699–702.

[25] Takahashi, J. S. 2004. Finding new clock components: past and future. *J. Biol. Rhythms* 19:339–47.

[26] Tata, J. R. 1996. Amphibian metamorphosis: an exquisite model for hormonal regulation of postembryonic development in vertebrates. *Develop. Growth Differ.* 38:223–31.

[27] Zimmerman, G. A., et al. 1993. Juxtacrine intercellular signalling: Another way to do it. *Am. J. Respir. Cell Mol. Biol.* 9:573–7.

General Mechanisms of Hormone Action

All hormones exert their effects by interacting with **receptors**. These are protein molecules that bind hormone with a high degree of specificity, and are activated as a consequence of this binding process. Activation of a receptor by a hormone results in the initiation of a sequence of molecular events that produce a change in some activity of the cell. These sequences of molecular events are referred to as **signal transduction pathways**, and a surprisingly limited number of them mediate the great majority of hormone signals in target cells. In general, hormone-induced intracellular signals can produce changes in the activity of existing protein molecules in the cell, changes in the amounts of certain proteins that are produced in the cell, or both.

Some hormones interact with specific receptor molecules on the cell surface to increase the production of intracellular **second messengers**, which are responsible for activation of the cell. The second messenger is often a cyclic nucleotide, either **cyclic adenosine monophosphate (cyclic AMP, cAMP)** or **cyclic guanosine monophosphate (cyclic GMP, cGMP)**. In other cases it is a phospholipid derivative, such as **diacylglycerol (DAG)** or **inositol triphosphate (IP$_3$)**. The cyclic nucleotide and lipid second messengers, in turn, commonly mediate their actions through stimulation of cellular enzymes, kinases, which phosphorylate cell-specific proteins; these phosphorylated proteins then function as the ultimate physiological effectors in the cell. Some hormones and growth factors bind cell surface receptors but do not exert their effects via cyclic nucleotide or lipid second messengers. Instead they activate intracellular **transcription factors**; these are then translocated to the nucleus, where they regulate the transcription of specific target genes.

Other hormones evoke transcriptional responses in cells through intracellular receptors. Specifically, the steroid and thyroid hormones activate **nuclear receptors**, which then function as hormone-induced transcription factors, typically producing slower, but more sustained actions.

Cellular Receptors and Hormone Action

Hormones regulate specific target tissues, not all cells in the body. One might ask what mechanism or characteristic of a cell determines whether it will be responsive to a particular hormone. In fact, it is those cell proteins that function as hormone receptors that provide the specificity for hormone–cell interaction. The receptor concept originated early in the previous century with the work of Langley, who proposed the existence of "receptive substances" that transduce the effects of a chemical messenger [20]. We now know, of course, that hormone receptors are protein molecules that are located on the cell surface, or in some cases the interior of the cell, and that their function is to recognize, bind, and convey the biological actions of a specific hormone in specific target cells and tissues.

Hormone Receptors Bind Specific Hormones

Each type of receptor is capable of binding only one specific hormone, or at most, a small number of closely related hormones. This ability of a receptor to distinguish between different ligands is referred to as its *ligand binding specificity*. While there may be several different molecular subtypes of receptors (*isoforms*) for a particular hormone, each of these nevertheless is highly selective for that hormone. Thus, at normal physiological levels each hormone primarily interacts only with its own specific cellular receptors. Estradiol, for example, interacts with estrogen receptors, not with other steroid receptors, such as those for cortisol or progesterone. Therefore hormone receptors possess a recognition function that must then be converted into an action function. Receptors recognize differences in hormone structure and thus provide receptor specificity. Norepinephrine and epinephrine are structurally similar (see Fig. 14.3), but norepinephrine preferentially interacts with certain types of adrenergic receptors, whereas epinephrine interacts more specifically with other adrenoceptor types (Chap. 14). The pharmaceutical industry capitalizes on receptor specificity to provide hormone analogs that can be used medicinally to activate or inhibit certain tissue-specific receptors. Hormone analogs that bind hormone receptors and mimic the actions of the hormone, sometimes with greatly enhanced potency, are referred to as receptor *agonists*. Those that occupy the receptor and prevent its activation by the hormone are referred to as receptor *antagonists*. The general term *ligand* is more broadly used to refer to a molecule that binds to a particular receptor, irrespective of its agonistic or antagonistic actions.

Binding of a hormone by a receptor occurs as a consequence of noncovalent interactions, for example ionic, hydrophobic, and van der Waals attractions between complementary components of the two molecules. The *affinity* of a receptor for a ligand is thus derived from the extent of these noncovalent interactions between them, and this in turn usually depends upon the biophysical properties conferred to both by their primary, secondary, and tertiary structures. Structural biologists study these biophysical properties, often by mutating key amino acid sequences in the receptors or ligands and analyzing the impact of these alterations on their three-dimensional structures, and on the ligand binding process. The binding of a hormone H to its receptor R can be considered as a reversible reaction that obeys the following chemical kinetics:

$$R + H \underset{k_{off}}{\overset{k_{on}}{\longleftrightarrow}} RH$$

where k_{on} is the rate constant for the association of the hormone with receptor and k_{off} is the rate constant for the dissociation of the hormone from its receptor. This reaction can be described by the simple equilibrium binding equation:

$$K_a = \frac{1}{K_d} = \frac{[RH]}{[R][H]} \tag{3.1}$$

in which [R] = concentration of free (unbound) receptor, [H] = concentration of free (unbound) hormone, and [RH] is the concentration of the bound receptor–hormone complex. The K_a is the *association constant*, and its reciprocal, the K_d, is the *dissociation constant* of the receptor–hormone complex. The K_d is commonly used to describe the *affinity* of the receptor for the hormone. For a receptor with high affinity for a hormone, the k_{off} would tend to be lower than the k_{on}, making the receptor–hormone complex more stable. Since the K_d is equal to the ratio k_{off}/k_{on}, a receptor with high affinity for hormone would thus be expected to have a relatively low K_d value. This is, in fact, the case—*the higher the affinity of a receptor for hormone, the lower is the K_d value.* Hormone receptors typically bind hormone ligands with affinities (K_d values) in the range of $10^{-11}-10^{-8}$ M.

The dissociation constant is specifically defined as the concentration of the hormone at which one half of the receptors are bound. The K_d value for a particular population of receptors is generally greater than the "basal" or unstimulated concentration of hormone in blood, and one can easily appreciate why this is the case; if the blood levels of a hormone [H] are lower than the K_d of the hormone receptor, then fewer than 50% of the receptors are occupied and activated. Physiological increases in hormone levels would thus be likely to produce proportional increases in receptor binding and activation without reaching 100% occupancy. However, if the blood levels of the hormone are considerably higher that the K_d value, then changes in hormone levels might not be faithfully reflected in corresponding changes in receptor binding and activation, because the receptor population may be completely occupied, or *saturated*, within the normal range of hormone values. On the other hand, K_d values cannot be too much greater than the basal concentration of hormone, as this would result in too little hormone bound to receptor to exert an appreciable effect on the target cell. Most endocrine systems have thus evolved an appropriate match between the affinity of receptors and the physiological range of concentrations of the corresponding hormone.

Tissue Responses to a Hormone are Determined by the Presence of Specific Receptors

Receptors provide the means by which hormones initially interact with cells. If each type of cell possessed all of the specific hormone receptors, then all cells might be expected to respond to all chemical messengers. If this were the case, each time a single hormone was released, all cells in the body would respond, and this would result in uncoordinated muscle contraction and relaxation and the uncontrolled secretion of numerous cellular products, such as hormones and enzymes. Therefore, cells do not possess receptors for all hormones, but rather only a limited number of receptor types. The magnitude of an individual tissue's response to a particular hormone is determined in large part by the number of receptors for the hormone that are present in those target cells.

Some hormones can simultaneously stimulate a number of different tissues, which implies that each of these diverse tissues possesses receptors for the hormone. Insulin stimulates glucose uptake by hepatocytes, fat cells, and certain muscle cells, and interacts with many other cell types. Thus, insulin is able to rapidly lower extracellular glucose levels, which is one of its major functions. If more than one tissue responds to a particular hormone at one time, it is often the case that all these different physiological responses would complement the physiological process being regulated. For example, parathyroid thormone (PTH) elevates serum Ca^{2+} levels by releasing Ca^{2+} from bone, stimulating Ca^{2+} uptake from the gut and preventing Ca^{2+} loss from the kidney. Each of these individual responses to PTH is important in elevating serum Ca^{2+} levels.

Some Hormones can Activate Multiple Receptor Isoforms

Although most hormone receptors exhibit a high degree of specificity for a given hormone, the reverse is not necessarily true; some hormones are capable of activating a number of different receptor *isoforms* (subtypes), and each of these may be coupled to the activation of different intracellular signal transduction pathways. In some cases different receptor isoforms for a particular hormone are produced by the transcription of different receptor genes. For example, two different genes encode two different receptors for the amino acid neurotransmitter glutamate; one of these receptor types (metabotropic glutamate receptors) is coupled to the activation of a second messenger pathway, while another type (ionotropic glutamate receptors) functions as a ligand-gated ion channel. In other cases, the RNA produced by transcription of a single receptor gene may be processed in alternate ways to produce multiple mRNA species, and some of these may encode alternate receptor protein isoforms.

Hormones that can exert several different physiological actions in different tissues, or multiple actions in the same tissue, are considered *pleuripotent*. The diverse physiological actions of a single hormone often depend upon its ability to simultaneously activate different receptor isoforms. Estrogen is one such hormone, as it serves as a natural ligand for at least two different estrogen receptors, known as estrogen receptor alpha (ERα) and estrogen receptor beta (ERβ). The same hormone ligand, estrogen, may thus evoke different responses in different tissues, or even different responses in the same tissues, depending upon the relative abudance of each of these two receptor isoforms in the target cells. In some mammary gland cells, for example, estrogen stimulates cell proliferation by activating ERα, while activation of ERβ in other cells can inhibit cell growth.

Characteristics of Physiological Receptors

Many proteins are capable of exhibiting weak molecular interactions with a variety of other biological molecules, yet very few of these represent *bona fide* receptor–ligand binding processes. What distinguishes a physiologically relevant receptor–ligand interaction from other intermolecular interactions? To conclude that the binding of a ligand to a putative receptor is a meaningful physiological event, several important critera must be met.

1. The binding of a hormone to its receptor is a process that almost always occurs with *high affinity*, with a K_d in a range appropriate for normal physiological concentrations of the hormone ligand.

2. Binding of a hormone by a receptor occurs with a high degree of *specficity*. This ensures the fidelity of the message conveyed by the hormone, and avoids inappropriate activation of the receptor by molecules other than the physiological ligand. Some receptors may be subject to binding by hormones that are closely related to the normal hormone ligand. Under normal conditions, however, this rarely occurs because the affinities of the receptor for these related molecules is low relative to the high affinity of the receptor for the normal receptor ligand. For example, oxytocin and vasopressin (AVP) are related in structure (see Fig. 7.2), and both hormones are capable of stimulating uterine smooth muscle contraction and activating renal tubular cAMP production. Uterine oxytocin receptors, however, have a greater affinity for oxytocin than for AVP, whereas renal AVP receptors have a greater affinity for AVP than for oxytocin. Thus, at normal circulating concentrations, each neurohypophysial hormone will only activate its appropriate target cell receptor.

3. Each hormone-responsive cell produces a finite number of receptors. It follows, then, that increasing concentrations of hormone ligand should reveal a *saturability* of the receptor binding process. Under normal conditions, a cell generally produces between 2,000 and 100,000 receptor molecules; this number of specific, high-affinity receptor sites is vastly outnumbered by the number of low-affinity, nonspecific binding sites that are normally present in cellular material. Thus, a physiological high-affinity receptor population would also be expected to show a relatively *low capacity* (fewer binding sites) compared to the virtually unlimited capacity of low-affinity, nonspecific binding sites.

4. The removal of hormone from target cells results in a rapid decay in the effects of the hormone. The reversibility of hormone action can thus be assumed to reflect the *reversible* nature of the receptor binding process that mediates the hormone effects.

5. The binding of a hormone by a receptor, if it is to be considered biologically meaningful, should be associated with some significant *physiological response* in the target cell.

Binding Assays are Used to Determine the Number, Affinity, and Ligand Specificity of Hormone Receptors

Many of these defining characteristics of physiological hormone receptors can be analyzed by means of radioligand binding assays. A saturation binding assay, for example, can be used to measure the number and affinity of hormone receptors in target cells. In these procedures, a fixed number of cells (or partially purified membranes, or cell extract) containing a constant number of receptors is incubated with increasing concentrations of radioisotopically labeled hormone which will bind in a concentration-dependent manner to the receptors present in the cells. The cells are then separated from the unbound radiolabeled hormone in the incubation solution, often by centrifugation or filtration. By counting the radioactivity bound to the cells, the total amount of hormone bound at each concentration of radiolabeled hormone can be deduced, and plotted as a curve representing *total binding* (Fig. 3.1c, top curve). The amount of radiolabeled hormone that remains free (unbound) in solution is also determined. This procedure is then repeated with the addition of 100–1000-fold excess of unlabeled hormone; the unlabeled hormone saturates the specific receptor sites and thus reveals the *nonspecific binding* (Fig. 3.1c, bottom line) sites, which are so numerous that they are not subject to displacement by the excess unlabeled hormone. The *specific binding* (Fig. 3.1, curve B) of hormone to receptor can thus

Figure 3.1 Figure 3.1 a-c Schematic representation of (a) hormone molecules binding to plasma membrane receptors, (b) hormone molecules present in increasing concentrations and corresponding increases in receptor binding, as in a typical saturation receptor binding assay, and (c) saturation receptor binding curves in a typical saturation binding assay. Shown are the hypothetical total binding and non-specific binding for increasing levels of radiolabeled hormone added to assay tubes. Specific binding at each level is derived by subtracting non-specific binding from total binding.

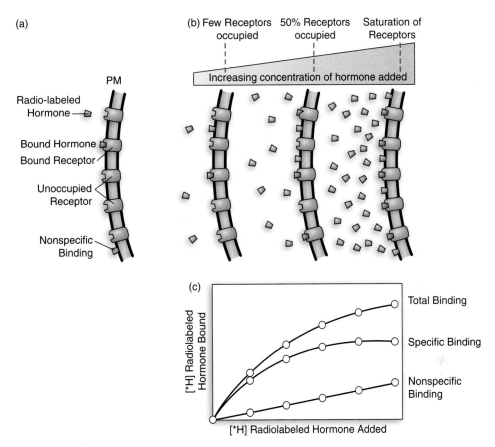

be calculated by simple subtraction of the nonspecific binding curve from the total binding curve. Fig. 3.1 demonstrates that, for most receptors, the amount of specific hormone binding increases with increasing concentrations of hormone, until it asymptotically reaches a saturation level of 100% receptor occupancy.

How can the specific binding curve be used to ascertain the total number and affinity of hormone receptors? One can use the data obtained in the saturation binding assay, specifically the *bound hormone* [HR] and *free hormone* [H] at each of the concentrations tested, to determine these important values. A convenient way of using these data points to obtain the number and affinity of receptors is to derive a *Scatchard plot* of the data. Recall that the binding of hormone to receptors obeys the kinetics described by equation 3.1, above, which can be rearranged to:

$$\frac{[RH]}{[H]} = K_a \times [R] \tag{3.2}$$

The total number of receptors, R_0 (also referred to as the initial receptor capacity), is equal to the number of receptors that are unoccupied by hormone, [R], plus the number that are occupied by hormone, [HR], that is:

$$R_0 = [R] + [HR]$$

(Note also that the number of bound receptor molecules is equal to the number of bound hormone molecules.) Solving for [R] this relationship is expressed as:

$$[R] = R_0 - [HR]$$

which can be substituted into equation 3.2 to yield:

$$\frac{[RH]}{[H]} = K_a \times (R_0 - [HR]) \tag{3.3}$$

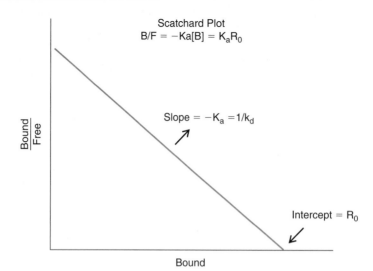

Figure 3.2 Schematic representation of a Scatchard plot of hypothetical data obtained from a saturation binding assay.

which is equivalent to:

$$\frac{[RH]}{[H]} = -K_a[HR] + Ka\,R_0 \qquad (3.4)$$

or, as commonly expressed:

$$\frac{\text{Bound hormone}}{\text{Free hormone}} = -K_a \times \text{Bound hormone} + K_a \times \text{Receptor number}$$

Using the data points obtained from the saturation binding assay, one can plot the ratio of bound hormone to free hormone as a function of bound hormone. This is a Scatchard plot (Fig. 3.2) that yields a straight line for a single population of receptors. Conveniently, the slope of this line is equal to the negative of the association constant, K_a (which is the reciprocal of the dissociation constant, K_d), and the receptor number is equal to the *x*-intercept. The Scatchard plot represented in Fig. 3.2 is typical for data obtained in most receptor binding

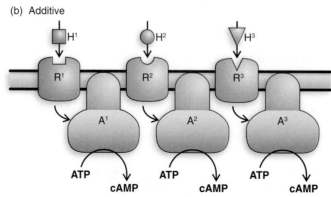

Figure 3.3 Although many hormones (H^1, H^2, H^3) mediate their effects through separate membrane receptors (R^1, R^2, R^3), transduction of their signals is funneled through only one adenylate cyclase (a), *not* through different cyclases (A^1, A^2, A^3) linked separately to each receptor (b).

assays. In practice, more complex regression analysis is sometimes required to analyze data obtained in receptor binding assays where multiple binding sites are present. For example, exponential Scatchard plots can result when the hormone reacts with multiple receptor types with differing affinities and/or numbers in the same target cells.

The number and affinity of receptors may thus be derived by means of saturation binding assays and Scatchard (or other) analysis. The ligand binding specificity of a receptor population, however, is commonly assessed by *competitive binding assays*. In these assays, a number of ligands of varying resemblance to the hormone are assessed for their ability to compete with the hormone for the receptor. Increasing amounts of the non-hormone ligand are incubated with cells expressing the receptor, as well as with a constant amount of radiolabeled hormone. A physiological receptor would be expected to show little, if any, inhibition of specific hormone binding by other endogenous biochemicals (especially other hormones) through their physiological concentration ranges.

Plasma Membrane Hormone Receptors

With the possible exception of steroid and thyroid hormones, other hormones stimulate cells by an initial interaction with specific plasma membrane receptors. This initial receptor interaction results in *transduction* of signals to the cytoplasmic side of the membrane where enzymes are activated, resulting in production of one or more intracellular second messengers. These membrane receptors are macromolecules, often glycoprotein in nature, which display a high affinity for a specific hormonal ligand. Peptide hormone receptors are localized, at least partially, to the outer surface of the cells, as shown by a number of experimental techniques. For example, ACTH covalently linked to a large polymer that cannot cross the membrane is still able to stimulate cAMP-mediated adrenal steroidogenesis. Other hormones have also been linked to sepharose beads, which are also too large to enter cells, and in all cases, the hormones still activate cAMP production in a variety of cells. In addition, specific antibodies that bind peptide hormones rapidly terminate their actions; since antibody molecules do not permeate the plasma membrane, this again indicates that the site of action of the hormones is extracellular.

Membrane Receptor Families have Characteristic Structures and Functional Properties

There are four main classes of membrane-bound receptors: (1) a "superfamily" of receptors coupled to G (GTP-binding) proteins (G-protein-coupled receptors, GPCRs), (2) receptors that are also enzymes (tyrosine protein kinases, serine/threonine kinases, or guanylate cyclase); (3) receptors that are associated with enzymes (cytokine receptors associated with tyrosine kinases), and (4) receptors coupled to ion channels. There are two structural classes of membrane hormone receptors [15, 17, 20]. The first group consists of receptors with multitransmembrane domains. The second group consists of hormone receptors with a single transmembrane domain (Fig. 3.4). Some hormone receptors with a single transmembrane domain and a cytoplasmic tail are often dimerized (bind together as pairs) on hormone binding, resulting in transmembrane signal transfer, as discussed in Chap. 12.

The majority of receptors for peptide hormones and neurotransmitters are linked to G proteins. The G-protein-coupled receptors contain a recognition site for the agonist (ligand) and a recognition site for a particular G protein (see discussion later in this chapter). These receptors are made up of a single chain consisting of 400 to 600 amino acid residues. The amino terminus contains sites for N-linked glycosylation, whereas the carboxy terminus has sites for phosphorylation by one or more protein kinases (e.g., protein kinase A, PKA). Seven stretches of 22–28 hydrophobic conserved residues, separated by hydrophilic segments, are characteristic structural features of these receptors [31]. Each transmembrane segment presumably forms closely packed helical bundles crossing the membrane one or more times (Fig. 3.5).

The N-terminal region, by virtue of its glycosylation, is extracellular and the carboxy-terminal domain is intracellular. The various portions between the seven hydrophobic stretches are either extra- or intracellular. The third intracellular segment and the carboxy-terminal segment display an extensive variability in length and sequence, which has led to the hypothesis that these parts

(a)

(b)

Figure 3.4   Schematic representation of (a) multi- and (b) single-transmembrane receptors.

Figure 3.5 Schematic model for insertion of G-protein-coupled receptors in the plasma membrane. From Strosberg [31], with permission.

of the receptors are responsible for the selective interaction with various regulatory G proteins required for information transfer [30, 32]. In general, the larger the ligand, the longer the N-terminal extension of the receptor (see Fig. 19.2). This superfamily of receptors containing seven transmembrane domains comprises several hundred distinct receptors for a variety of ligands: proteins, peptides, neurotransmitters (peptides and biogenic amines), odorants and even photons. In fact, the superfamily of GPCRs, with more than 1,000 different members, comprises the largest superfamily of proteins in the body [13].

Second Messengers of Hormone Action

How can so many chemically diverse hormones, neurotransmitters, and other signaling molecules activate receptors believed to share a similar overall tertiary structure? What is the nature of the physical changes linking agonist binding to receptor activation and subsequent transduction of the signal to the associated G protein on the cytoplasmic side of the membrane and to other signaling pathways? Many hormones acting as first messengers manifest their actions by stimulating the production of intracellular second messengers that then effect a physiological response [4, 6, 34].

Cyclic Nucleotides Function as Second Messengers in the Actions of Many Hormones

Receptors provide the recognition site for hormone–cell interaction [3]. This binding event must be translated into a cellular response. Binding of hormone to its membrane receptor often results in the activation of one or more nucleotide-cyclizing enzymes located on the inner surface of the membrane. Best studied is the enzyme adenylate cyclase, which, upon stimulation by a chemical messenger, converts ATP (adenosine triphosphate) to 3′,5′-cyclic adenosine monophosphate, cyclic AMP (cAMP). A signal transduction process was envisioned by Rodbell and coworkers as a key to the conversion of the hormone binding signal into increased adenylyl cyclase activity. Borrowing from information transfer theory, they coined the terms "discriminator" for the role played by receptor, "amplifier" for the role of the cAMP-forming enzyme, and "transducer" for the role of the intervening process [3]. Some hormones, on the other hand, activate guanylate cyclase that converts guanosine triphosphate (GTP) to cGMP [9, 10]. Enzyme cleavage of the cyclic ring of the nucleotides by a *phosphodiesterase* results in the production of inactive 5′AMP or 5′GMP (Fig. 3.6).

Each of the cyclic nucleotides produced intracellularly combines with a specific *cyclic nucleotide-dependent protein kinase* [16, 29, 32]. Cyclic AMP-dependent protein kinase (PKA), for example, is composed of two components, a *regulatory subunit* and a *catalytic subunit* [18, 20]. Interaction of cAMP with the regulatory subunit results in the release of the catalytic unit (Fig. 3.7) . The catalytic unit is thus free to function as a *kinase*, that is, a phosphorylating enzyme. Cyclic nucleotides therefore function by causing phosphorylation of

Adenylate
Cyclase

ATP

Cyclic AMP
Phosphodiesterase

Cyclic AMP

5′ AMP

Guanylate
Cyclase

GTP

Cyclic GMP
Phosphodiesterase

Cyclic GMP

5′ GMP

Figure 3.6 Cyclic nucleotide synthesis and inactivation.

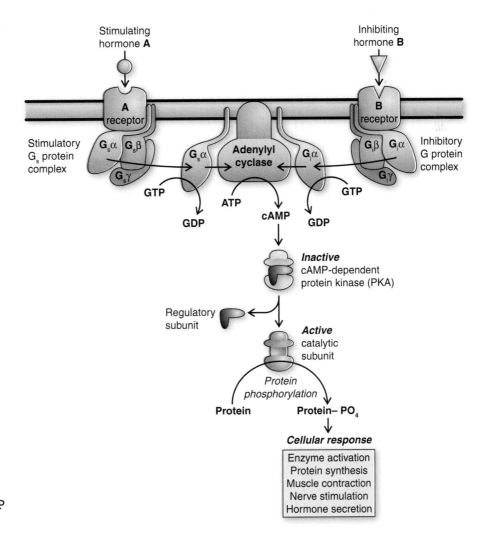

Figure 3.7 Cyclic AMP
production and action.

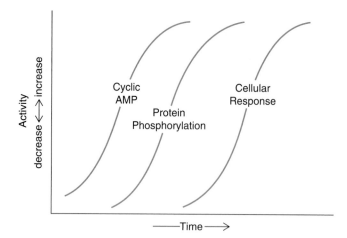

Figure 3.8 Temporal cellular events in homone-mediated cyclic AMP production and action.

Theophylline

Caffeine

l-Methyl-3-Isobutylxanthine

Figure 3.9

Methylxanthine structures: Theophylline, caffeine, and 1-methyl-3-isobutylxanthine (a synthetic xanthine analog).

some cellular component (substrate protein) of the cell (Fig. 3.8) , structural or enzymatic. Enzyme phosphorylation leads to a cascade phenomenon, whereby activation by phosphorylation of the first enzyme allows this enzyme to act as a kinase to phosphorylate a second enzyme, which may then phosphorylate another enzyme. At each step amplification occurs; thus, relatively few first messenger molecules acting on a limited number of receptors may produce a response several orders of magnitude greater. This cascade phenomenon has been studied in detail in the liver cell (see Fig. 11.11), but may be common to a number of cellular systems.

Cyclic nucleotides produced by hormone action are rapidly metabolized. Cyclic AMP- and cGMP-specific phosphodiesterases cleave the cyclic bonds within cAMP and cGMP to produce inactive 5′AMP and 5′GMP, respectively [5, 9]. *Phosphoprotein phosphatases* within the cell then dephosphorylate the proteins that were phosphorylated by the cyclic nucleotide-dependent protein kinases. Thus, cellular activity is rapidly returned to basal level.

Methylxanthines inhibit cAMP- and cGMP-dependent phosphodiesterase activity. Caffeine, theophylline, and theobromine are methylxanthines derived from coffee, tea, and cocoa, respectively (Fig. 3.9). Theophylline is the most potent of the three (but is less concentrated in tea than caffeine is in coffee). In the presence of relatively low concentrations of methylxanthines, the actions of hormones that stimulate adenylate cyclase are potentiated, as the cAMP generated by the hormones is degraded less rapidly by a phosphodiesterase. At high concentrations (e.g., 10^{-3} M), theophylline or caffeine alone may evoke a maximal response in a particular tissue. This suggests that adenylate cyclase is always active, but that the cAMP generated is continually being destroyed.

Sutherland was the first to demonstrate that extracellular chemical messengers, first messengers, activate production of intracellular cAMP, the so-called second messenger of hormone action [35]. Because many hormones interact with receptors to activate adenylate cyclase, which then causes a physiological response, Sutherland and his colleagues suggested criteria that should be satisfied before concluding that a particular effect of a hormone is mediated through cAMP.

1. The hormone should stimulate adenylate cyclase in broken cell preparations.
2. Physiological levels of the hormone should elevate cAMP before or concurrently with the physiological response (Fig. 3.7).
3. There should be a correlation between the activity of hormone analogs that elevate cAMP and their ability to activate the particular cellular response.
4. Methylxanthines or other drugs that inhibit phosphodiesterase activity should potentiate and, at high concentrations, mimic the hormone response.
5. Exogenous cAMP or its analogs should mimic the effect of the hormone.

The criteria have been satisfied for many cells studied. There is no convincing reason, however, that the first criterion should be met as, in the intact cell, information is generated from the receptor on the outer side of the plasmalemma to adenylate cyclase on the inner surface. The ionic environments of these two compartments are not similar and cannot be duplicated

Figure 3.10 Cyclic AMP and related analogs.

in vitro for both compartments at any one time. Calcium, for example, is inhibitory to adenylate cyclase, but may be necessary for transduction of signal from receptor to cyclase [1, 3]. It is difficult in vitro to provide Ca^{2+} for receptor binding or receptor signal transduction and, at the same time, not inhibit adenylate cyclase. The second criterion has been claimed not to have been satisfied in some systems. It is possible, however, that small changes in cAMP are undetectable, or that in some tissues the increase in cAMP is compartmentalized to a few cells. Thus, changes in cyclic nucleotide levels are not perceived among the larger cyclic nucleotide pool. The third and fourth criteria generally have been demonstrated in all cellular systems where cAMP plays a role as second messenger.

Cyclic AMP added to an in vitro preparation may induce the physiological response characteristic of the tissue, but only at very high concentrations. Apparently, this is because the nucleotide does not easily enter cells through the plasmalemma. To satisfy the fifth criterion, certain lipophilic analogs of cAMP (e.g., $(Bu)_2cAMP$) have been synthesized; they may produce a maximal response at relatively low concentrations in some tissues, but only at high levels in others (Fig. 3.10), depending upon the permeability of these different tissues to the analog.

Cyclic AMP also Initiates Signaling to the Genome

Many actions of second messengers initiate immediate cellular responses, such as opening or closing ion gates, stimulating cellular secretion, and stimulating muscle contraction or relaxation. Some of the actions are slower in commencement, but are more enduring. In some cells, the actions of cAMP are mediated at the level of the genome since the actions of some hormones that elevate intracellular cAMP levels are blocked by the actions of actinomycin D and cycloheximide, inhibitors of transcription and translation, respectively [19, 21]. Cyclic AMP mediates its action by way of PKA, which can phosphorylate a number of proteins depending on the particular cell type. One such protein common to the genomic actions of cAMP is the cAMP-responsive element-binding protein (CREB). This *transcription factor* is phosphorylated by cAMP-activated PKA. Phosphorylation of CREB by PKA allows the transcription factor to interact with the CRE (a DNA sequence) to activate transcription of a cell-specific mRNA for protein synthesis. Some genes do not have the CRE consensus sequence, yet their expression is regulated by the level of cAMP. For example, PKA also phosphorylates some structural proteins associated with chromatin to modify their interactions with DNA.

Membrane Receptor Signal Transduction

Hormone binding to receptors located on the outer side of the plasmalemma often results in an immediate activation of adenylate cyclase on the inner membrane of the cells. How does receptor occupation by hormonal ligands result in enzyme activation on the opposite side of the cell membrane? Receptor and enzyme were once thought to be structurally coupled, and binding of the hormone to the receptor then induced a conformational change in the enzyme, thus activating it. Actually, this model may be true in one instance; a membrane guanylate cyclase is apparently the receptor for certain hormones (e.g., atrial natriuretic factor, Chap. 15). However, most hormone receptors are discrete units, not components of the inner membrane nucleotide-cyclizing enzymes. Hormone binding induces a conformational change in the receptor, resulting in transduction of signal across the membrane to activate second messenger production. Demonstrating this fact were studies showing that fusion of cells that lack receptors but possess adenylate cyclase activity to a different species of cell, which possesses receptors but no adenylate cyclase activity, results in a hybrid cell that synthesizes cAMP in response to hormone stimulation.

G Proteins Mediate Dual Control of Adenylate Cyclase

The transduction of a hormone signal from receptor to adenylate cyclase typically requires the intermediate actions of one or more regulatory proteins [13, 38]. This regulatory protein is usually a guanylyl nucleotide regulatory protein that exhibits GTPase activity (converts guanosine triphosphate to guanosine diphosphate) in the activated state. Receptor signal transduction involves the mobilization and interaction of this protein with the hormone receptor, an event that then leads to adenylate cyclase activation [14, 15].

G proteins act as transducers by coupling membrane-bound receptors to intracellular effectors [3]. G proteins are heterotrimers and dissociate to liberate a nucleotide-bound α subunit and a complex of β and γ subunits when the α subunits are activated by the binding of GTP. Functional characterization provided the first basis for classification of G proteins: G_s is the G protein that activates adenylyl cyclase, and G_i is the G protein that inhibits adenylyl cyclase. Additionally, G_t (transducin) is the retinal G protein that activates a guanosine $3',5'$-monophosphate-specific phosphodiesterase. In each of these cases, the dissociated GTP-α subunit complex activates the effector enzyme (cyclase or phosphodiesterase). Thus, the concept arose that each G-protein oligomer contains a functionally specific α subunit in association with mixtures of a small number of different β and γ subunits. Nearly 20 distinct α subunits have now been described, as well as four or more β and γ subunits [3, 16, 19]. A model of the G-protein cycle is shown (Fig. 3.11).

The functional role of specific α subunits is not obvious from their structural classification. One of the most effective tools for implicating G proteins in specific functions in intact cells has been the use of pertussis toxin (PTX). The toxin uncouples the receptor from its G protein and thus blocks signal transduction by receptors that cause decreases in cAMP, regulate ion channels, and activate phospholipases. Members of the G_i class of α subunits contain sites susceptible to modification by PTX and are therefore expected to mediate activation of the PTX-sensitive processes. Activated $G\alpha_i$ subunits lower intracellular cAMP levels, and $G\alpha_o$ has been implicated in increasing phosphoinositide release.

Not all hormone receptor/G-protein interactions involve effects on intracellular second messenger production (e.g., increased cAMP or decreased cAMP) as a component of signal

Figure 3.11 Receptor–G-protein-mediated signal transduction. (a) Receptor (R) associates with a specific ligand (L), stabilizing an activated form of the receptor (R*), which can catalyze the exchange of GTP for GDP bound to the α subunit of a specific G protein. The $\beta\gamma$ heterodimer may remain associated with the membrane through a 20-carbon isoprenyl modification of the γ subunit. The receptor is desensitized by specific phosphorylation. (b) The G-protein cycle. Pertussis toxin (PTX) blocks the catalysis of GTP exchange by the receptor. Activated α subunits (αGTP) and $\beta\gamma$ heterodimers can interact with different effectors. Cholera toxin (CTX) blocks the GTPase activity of some α subunits fixing them in an activated form. (Modified from Simon et al., "Diversity of G proteins in signal transduction," *Science* 260:1072–1073, 1993.©1993 by the American Association for the Advancement of Science.)

transduction. Receptor/G-protein interaction may result in the direct activation of membrane ion channels (e.g., K^+, Ca^{2+}) [5, 11, 41]. Indeed, the $G\alpha_i$ and $G\alpha_o$ subtypes have been shown to function in regulating ion channels. The transmembrane movement of ions may then lead to depolarization or hyperpolarization of the cell membrane, resulting in a cellular response. It was initially thought that the α subunit of G proteins alone acts on enzymes and on ion channels. Evidence now indicates that the β and/or γ subunits also play a part in signal transmission. These individual subunits may activate specific isozymes of both phospholipase C (see what follows) and adenylate cyclase.

"Crosstalk" may Occur among Different Signal Transduction Pathways

Agonist-activated transduction pathways and second messenger formation are not entirely separate. Changes in concentration of one second messenger often lead to change in concentration of another—"crosstalk" [21, 40]. Activation of a single-receptor type may be able to activate G proteins of more than one family. The effect of a particular G protein might be attenuated by the activation of another G protein, which would provide free $\beta\gamma$ subunits [18]. Because $\beta\gamma$ subunits can combine with different α subunits, they would displace the equilibrium toward the trimeric inactive form of the G proteins [6, 14, 19].

Birnbaumer has succinctly summarized the landmarks in our understanding of the nature and roles of G proteins in signal transduction [3].

Phosphorylated Proteins as Physiological Effectors

The membrane actions of most hormones involve generation of an intracellular cyclic nucleotide, such as cAMP, as second messenger. The major site for the action of cAMP is the regulatory subunit of cAMP-dependent protein kinase (PKA). Two forms of the enzyme with slightly different regulatory properties have been isolated and are referred to as type I and type II. Both consist of two regulatory (R) and two catalytic (C) subunits. The regulatory units may differ in structure, but the catalytic units are believed to be identical. Cyclic AMP acts as the positive effector and causes the dissociation of the protein subunits and an activation of the enzyme according to the following scheme:

$$R_2C_2 \text{ (inactive)} + 4\,cAMP \longleftrightarrow (R - cAMP_2)_2 + 2\,C \text{ (active)}$$

The complete amino acid sequences of the catalytic and regulatory subunits of bovine cardiac muscle cAMP-dependent protein kinase have been elucidated [20, 33].

Within each cell type one or more specific proteins act as substrate for phosphorylation by PKA, with the amino acid serine being a common substrate for protein kinase action (see Fig. 3.17). Specific nuclear histone proteins may be the targets of the enzyme within hepatocytes. Within smooth muscle and nerve, specific membrane proteins become phosphorylated through the actions of cAMP or cGMP. In neurons, these substrate proteins may control the permeability of the postsynaptic membrane to ion flux [26]. In smooth muscle, phosphorylation of specific membrane substrate proteins, in response to cAMP or cGMP generated by receptor-specific agonists, may be related to the phenomena of membrane hyperpolarization and depolarization that accompany smooth muscle relaxation and contraction, respectively.

Cyclic nucleotide-independent substrate phosphorylation is important in the actions of certain hormones (insulin and other growth factors). Several of the intracellular effector molecules that activate the kinases involved in these substrate phosphorylations have been elucidated, and are discussed in succeeding chapters. Ca^{2+} may be a major stimulus to cyclic nucleotide-independent substrate phosphorylation. Once complexed with Ca^{2+}, the calcium-binding enzyme calmodulin (CaM) binds to and activates a wide variety of proteins, including a number of protein kinases and calcineurin, a phosphoprotein phosphatase. Initial characterizations of Ca^{2+}/CaM-dependent protein kinases in tissue extracts used a variety of exogenous protein substrates. A number of enzymes, including phosphorylase kinase, myosin light-chain kinase (MLCK) (see Fig. 7.13), and Ca^{2+}/CaM-dependent protein kinases I, II, and III (CaMK-I, II, and III, respectively) were resolved. Among these enzymes CaMK-II is unique in that it can phosphorylate a wide range of proteins in vitro and is widely distributed. These properties suggest that CaMK-II regulates many physiological responses to agonists that elevate intracellular Ca^{2+}. For this reason, it is also called the multifunctional Ca^{2+}/CaM-dependent protein kinase, or CaM-dependent multiprotein kinase. Thus,

CaMK-II plays a role in Ca^{2+}-mediated regulation analogous to the roles of PKA and protein kinase C (PKC) in the cAMP- and diacylglycerol-mediated systems, respectively [5, 7].

Protein Phosphatases also Play Important Roles in Cellular Regulation

It had been thought that only kinases required regulation and that they activated one another in sequence to overwhelm phosphatase activity in order to produce a temporary increase in phosphate content of key target proteins. Some kinases critical to cell growth also have sites for phosphorylation that cause inactivation, as well as activation. It is becoming clear that in addition to protein kinases, *protein phosphatases* are also important targets for cellular regulation [5, 31, 37]. The steady-state level of cellular protein phosphorylation is dependent on the balance of the activities of several protein phosphatases that act on protein substrates (see Fig. 3.18). Protein phosphatases reverse the action of protein kinases by hydrolyzing phosphoryl groups from proteins. In summary, not only kinases, but also some protein phosphatases, are probably involved in activating cellular responses to extracellular signals [5].

Multiple Membrane Messengers

Other messengers are involved in cellular regulation besides cyclic nucleotides. *Phosphoinositides* are phospholipids present within the plasma membrane of all eukaryotic cells. Some function as storage forms for potential messenger molecules and, in response to agonists, the phosphoinositides break down to liberate intracellular second messengers. At least three different messenger molecules are known to be produced from phospholipids: (1) *arachidonic acid* (a precursor to certain eicosanoids), (2) inositol triphosphate ($Ins(1,4,5)P_3$, or IP_3), and (3) 1,2-*diacylglycerol* (DG or DAG). Arachidonate is oxygenated to form several messengers, which include prostaglandins, prostacyclins, thromboxanes, and leukotrienes, as will be discussed later.

G Proteins also Couple Receptor Stimulation to Phosphoinositol Hydrolysis

Many hormones stimulate cellular processes through activation of G proteins whose α subunit ($G\alpha_o$) activates a specific phospholipase (PLC) that hydrolyzes the phosphodiester bond of phosphatidylinositol 4,5-biphosphate, providing the two messenger molecules $Ins(1,4,5)P_3$ and 1,2-diacylglycerol (Fig. 3.12) [10]. The water-soluble $Ins(1,4,5)P_3$ diffuses to intracellular Ca^{2+} stores where it induces the release of Ca^{2+} by binding to Ca^{2+}-channel-linked IP_3

Figure 3.12 Inositol phosphate and receptor signal transduction.

receptors [24, 30]. Diacylglycerol, being highly lipophilic, remains in the plasma membrane matrix where it activates protein kinase C (PKC). Two downstream signal cascades are thus initiated, involving both elevation of the cytosolic Ca^{2+} activity, resulting in modulation of Ca^{2+}-sensitive response elements, and Ca^{2+}/PKC-promoted protein phosphorylation. Removal of the agonist from the agonist–receptor complex results in the cessation of PLC-mediated phosphotidal inositol-(4,5) P_2 hydrolysis. Both IP_3 and DG are rapidly metabolized in cells; so in the absence of de novo synthesis the cellular levels of these two messengers rapidly decline; PKC is inactivated and cytosolic Ca^{2+} levels are brought back to resting levels by the membrane-associated Ca^{2+} transport systems.

Protein Kinase C is a Multifunctional Enzyme that Plays Important Roles in Signal Transduction

Protein kinase C (PKC) is a multifunctional enzyme present within the plasma membrane. This Ca^{2+}-activated, phospholipid-dependent enzyme has been shown in many tissues to be linked to signal transduction. Multiple subspecies of PKC have been described. These subspecies show subtle differences in enzymological properties, differential tissue expression, and specific intracellular localization. Many growth factors (Chap. 12) are stimulatory to cell proliferation, and PKC plays a role as a component of the factors acting on cellular differentiation and proliferation. In one model, hormone receptor activation results in the production of IP_3 (see earlier), as well as in an increase in intracellular Ca^{2+}. The intracellular Ca^{2+} may be derived from one or several sources, either from sequestration within the endoplasmic reticulum or from the extracellular compartment. In this model, PKC is activated by DG in the presence of Ca^{2+}. A model of hormone action involving IP_3 and DG is shown in Fig. 3.12 and summarized here:

1. Activation of the membrane receptor is coupled to phospholipase C (PLC) through guanylyl nucleotide-binding (G) proteins.
2. This leads to hydrolysis of phosphoinositol (PIP_2) and formation of two key metabolites, diacylglycerol (DG) and inositol triphosphate (IP_3).
3. IP_3, which is released into the cytoplasm, mobilizes intracellular Ca^{2+} from stores within the endoplasmic reticulum (ER) and, possibly, from transmembrane transport of Ca^{2+} into the cell [24, 25].
4. During the initial phase of cell activation, two signals, the rise in DG content of the plasma membrane and the rise in the Ca^{2+} concentration in the cell cytosol, act synergistically to cause binding of PKC to the plasma membrane.
5. The resulting association of the kinase with the membrane leads to its conversion to a Ca^{2+}-sensitive form.

Eicosanoids and Hormone Action

In the early 1930s, it was noted that human semen and extracts of seminal vesicles from animals caused uterine tissue to contract or relax. The purified substance was given the name *prostaglandin (PG)*, although it is now realized that the prostate glands are not a major source of PGs. The PGs belong to a family of chemically related substances, *eicosanoids*, which are produced by cells in response to a variety of extrinsic stimuli [33, 36]. They are generally known as paracrine regulators, and as such are referred to by some as locally acting hormones in their own right. However, they are also produced by cells in response to some hormones and therefore, they will be considered here as intracellular second messengers in the actions of hormones. The Nobel Prize in Physiology/Medicine for 1982 was awarded to Bergstrom, Samuelsson, and Vane for their "discoveries concerning prostaglandins and biologically related substances" [25, 26].

Eicosanoids are produced exclusively within the plasma membrane of cells and are derived mainly from arachidonic acid released from phospholipids by the action of phospholipase A_2(PLA_2). Arachidonic acid is formed from the essential fatty acid linolenic acid, by elongation and desaturation. Hormones and other stimuli (e.g., local hypoxia) may activate phospholipase activity and liberate arachidonic acid to serve as substrate for eicosanoid biosynthesis. The arachidonic acid may be used in one or more different pathways, depending on the tissue

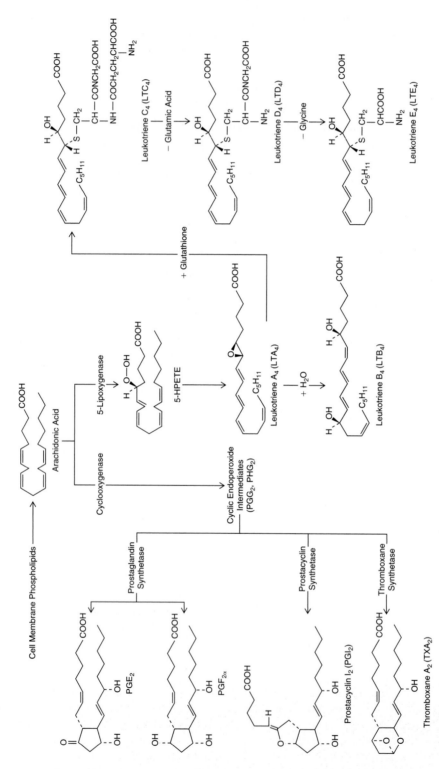

Figure 3.13 General scheme for prostaglandin, prostacyclin, thromboxane, and leukotriene biosynthesis.

concerned and particular nature of the extrinsic stimulus. In one pathway arachidonic acid is converted to unstable endoperoxide intermediates by a group of enzymes termed the cyclooxygenase system (Fig. 3.13). Then, depending on the action of other tissue-specific enzymes, these intermediates may be converted to one of a number of related products (prostanoids): prostaglandin E_2 (PGE_2), prostaglandin $F_{2\alpha}$($PGF_{2\alpha}$),prostacyclin I_2 (PGI_2), or thromboxane A_2 (TXA_2) (Fig. 3.13).

In some cells, arachidonic acid metabolism follows a second pathway to produce a group of biologically active *leukotrienes* (LTs). These are formed by the enzyme 5-lipoxygenase, which converts arachidonic acid to 5-hydroperoxy-6,8,11,14-eicosatetra-enoic acid (5-HPETE). 5-HPETE is then converted to the epoxy acid, LTA_4, which is subsequently changed to LTB_4 by the addition of water, or to LTC_4, by the addition of glutathione. LTD_4, is then formed by the loss of glutamic acid and LTD_4, is converted to LTE_4, by the loss of the glycine residue (Fig. 3.13).

Each of these definitive products of arachidonic acid metabolism may then act on nucleotide cyclases within the plasma membrane to stimulate cyclic nucleotide formation. PGE_2 and PGI_2 invariably stimulate adenylate cyclase [23, 24]. In cultured rabbit endometrial cells, $PGF_{2\alpha}$ exerts no effect on the levels of cAMP or cGMP; however, phosphatidic acid and phosphoinositide turnover can be stimulated by $PGF_{2\alpha}$. Some $PGF_{2\alpha}$ receptors may be associated with a specific guanine nucleotide regulatory protein linked to activation of PLC [37]. Leukotrienes and PGI_2 and TXA_2 are released from their cells of origin to act as humoral hormonal messengers (Fig. 3.14).

Steroidal anti-inflammatory agents, such as cortisone, block the release of precursor fatty acids (arachidonate) and thus the formation of all eicosanoids. Nonsteroidal anti-inflammatory agents, such as aspirin, inhibit cyclooxygenase and prevent the production of prostanoids. Therefore, these drugs may be used selectively to inhibit PG, prostacyclin, and thromboxane formation without a concomitant effect on leukotriene formation. It is also possible to modulate the precursor fatty acid component in cell membrane phospholipids by dietary means, which in turn can alter the types of eicosanoids formed endogenously. Some food constituents, such as vitamin C, vitamin E, garlic, onion, ginger, and alcohol, can affect the production of eicosanoids. Dietary manipulation may serve as a long-term strategy to favorably modify endogenous eicosanoid production.

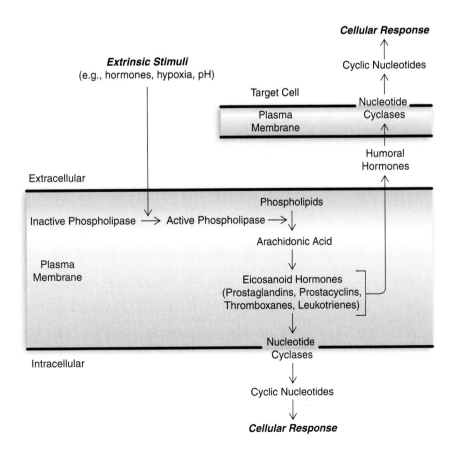

Figure 3.14 General scheme of eicosanoid biosynthesis and mechanisms of action.

Prostaglandins were the first of the arachidonic acid products to be discovered. All the PGs are variants of a basic 20-carbon carboxylic fatty acid (prostanoic acid) that is bent back on itself in the shape of a hairpin and is conformationally restricted by a five-membered cyclopentane ring. The number of double bonds present within the side chains determines whether the PG belongs to the 1, 2, or 3 series. Two particularly important PGs of the E and F series are $PGF_{2\alpha}$ and PGE_2 which differ by the presence of a hydroxyl or a keto group, respectively, at carbon 9 within the cyclopentane ring (see Figs 2.4 and 3.13).

A major physiological role of PGE_2 and $PGF_{2\alpha}$ is the control of vascular smooth muscle activity. Hormones that regulate smooth muscle relaxation or contraction stimulate the production of PGE_2 or PGI_2 and $PGF_{2\alpha}$ respectively. In response to tissue hypoxia, PGE_2 production may lead to a localized hyperemia in skeletal muscle. Thus PGs, by their localized actions on the microcirculation, adjust local blood flow in response to changing metabolic requirements of the tissue.

Prostacyclins (PGI_2) are produced by the blood vessel wall (endothelial cells), and PGI_2 is the most potent natural inhibitor of blood platelet aggregation known. PGI_2 binds to a specific platelet receptor and activates adenylate cyclase. Increased intracellular levels of cAMP are then inhibitory to platelet aggregation. The vascular endothelium therefore can be considered as an endocrine tissue that produces a humoral hormone, PGI_2, whose role may be to prevent blood platelet aggregation and to maintain vascular flow through its action as a local vasodilator. Whether PGI_2 is released into the general circulation to function as a hormone on more distant blood platelets and vascular endothelia is presently unresolved.

Thromboxane A_2 is a specific product of the blood platelet. In response to stimuli known to induce clotting (collagen substrate, thrombin, epinephrine), platelet TXA_2 levels are elevated, as are cGMP concentrations. It is believed that TXA_2 may act in some way as a Ca^{2+} ionophore (transport) to translocate this divalent Ca^{2+} from the extracellular environment or from sequestered intracellular organelles of the platelet. The free cytosolic Ca^{2+} may then be responsible for inducing the cellular shape changes associated with the platelet aggregation phenomenon. As noted before, PGI_2 is inhibitory to platelet aggregation through its action on increasing platelet cAMP levels. Inhibition of platelet aggregation may result from protein substrate phosphorylation and the subsequent uptake of Ca^{2+} into vesicular components of the cell.

Besides causing platelet aggrtegation, TXA_2 also induces constriction of vascular and bronchiolar smooth muscle and mitogenesis and hypertrophy of vascular smooth muscle. PGI_2, in contrast, inhibits platelet aggregation and relaxes vascular smooth muscle. TXA_2 and PGI_2 working in concert play a homeostatic role to regulate vascular blood flow and blood clotting. It is hoped that selective inhibitors of thromboxane synthesis will be developed so that the tendency toward platelet aggregation is reduced, while permitting normal rates of formation of the other PGs.

Leukotrienes are so named because they are made by leukocytes and contain three conjugated double bonds [23]. The subscript indicates the total number of double bonds in the molecule (Fig. 3.13). Leukotrienes are extremely potent in causing vascular contraction and inducing vascular permeability. Migratory leukocytes function in local inflammatory responses by releasing leukotrienes at the site of injury in response to noxious stimuli. The anti-inflammatory actions of glucocorticoids (Chap. 15) may be because these steroids inhibit phospholipase activity and, therefore, restrict the availability of arachidonic acid for leukotriene formation. Certain leukocytes may be considered as wandering endocrine cells that release chemical messengers, leukotrienes, at sites of injury or invasion by foreign proteins to induce inflammatory or allergic responses. Increased leukotriene production appears to be implicated in the pathophysiology of tissue trauma. There are increased concentrations of leukotrienes in blood plasma and bile subsequent to tissue injury.

Leukotrienes are a family of bioactive lipids that have a constellation of pharmacologic effects on respiratory, cardiovascular, and gastrointestinal systems. They produce smooth muscle spasm, cause myocardial depression, increase vascular permeability, enhance mucus production, decrease epithelial mucus transport, and have the chemotactic property to attract leukocytes to a site of cellular injury. The overwhelming evidence suggests that leukotriene synthesis and subsequent release in experimental animals and in humans are associated with certain pathophysiological events. Disorders such as asthma, adult respiratory distress syndrome, chronic bronchitis, cystic fibrosis, septic shock, psoriasis, inflammatory bowel disease, and myocardial ischemia have all been reported to be associated with increased levels of leukotrienes.

LTD_4/LTE_4 receptors appear to be linked to the turnover of inositol phosphates via activation of phospholipase C [23, 24]. Regulation of the activity of PLC appears to be coupled to the receptor via a G protein. Since the response to LTD_4 is inhibited by pertussis toxin, the G protein may be of the G_i (inhibitory) class. In a variety of tissues and cell culture systems, LTD_4/LTE_4 and agonist analogs produced a rapid increase in inositol phosphates after stimulation, an effect that was blocked stereoselectively by receptor antagonists. The agonist-induced increases in inositol phosphates correlated directly with the generation of lipoxygenase products (e.g., leukotrienes) and smooth muscle contraction. Current data support the hypothesis that, at least for LTD_4/LTE_4 receptors, phosphoinositide hydrolysis with subsequent Ca^{2+} mobilization constitute important transduction mechanisms.

Nuclear Hormone Receptors

In contrast to many polypeptide hormones, steroid and thyroid hormones initiate their actions by combining with intracellular receptors [36] that are present in the nucleus and, in some cases, perhaps also in the cytoplasm. Steroid hormones are generally bound by *steroid hormone binding globulins* as they circulate in blood. The small fraction of free steroid can diffuse through the plasmalemma and the nuclear membrane to bind its receptor. It is likely that these hormones enter all cells, but only manifest their action in those cells that possess receptors.

Steroid/Thyroid Hormone Receptors

Most steroid and thyroid hormones interact with their unoccupied receptors within the nucleus, although some may additionally bind receptors in the cytoplasm and be transported to the nucleus. Nevertheless, a two-step mechanism is involved, wherein the activated nucleoplasmic receptor must be translocated to the chromatin. The binding of the steroid–receptor complex to chromatin (DNA and associated proteins) results in de-repression of a specific DNA sequence and increased mRNA synthesis. The mRNA then codes for proteins specific to that cell type; in uterine muscle (myometrium), for example, estradiol induces the synthesis of actin and myosin, proteins necessary for the contractile machinery of uterine myometrial cells.

Each steroid hormone has its own specific intracellular receptor. Estrogens, but not androgens, bind at physiological concentrations to estrogen receptors in the uterus. Thus, as for membrane receptors, receptor specificity determines whether a particular cell type will respond to the steroid. The synthesis of mRNA and the subsequent production of proteins require a matter of hours or days to be fully manifested (Chap. 18). The actions of most hormones are on membrane receptors and, in contrast, result in an immediate production of one or more second messengers followed by rapid protein phosphorylation and a subsequent cellular response.

The effects of steroid and steroid-like hormones are mediated by specific receptors that belong to a superfamily of transacting "zinc finger" proteins. After binding of the specific ligand, these receptor proteins (so-called "ligand-induced transcription factors") influence gene expression via association with specific DNA elements, known as hormone-responsive elements (HREs). Specific HREs are known for estrogen-, thyroid hormone-, progesterone-, and glucocorticoid-responsive genes. The estrogen-response element (ERE) is similar to, but distinct from, the glucocorticoid-responsive element (GRE) and the thyroid hormone-responsive element (T_3RE). The progesterone- and glucocorticoid-responsive elements are so similar as to be functionally identical. 1,25-Dihydroxycholecalciferol ($1,25(OH)_2D_3$), or vitamin D_3, affects cellular replication and function in many cells and tissues through a typical steroidal hormone receptor and exerts its effects through a vitamin D-responsive element (VDRE). It is not clear whether opposing effects on gene expression by different steroidal hormones are elicited through the same or different HREs.

In summary, the sequential steps in the action of many steroid hormones, particularly gluco-corticoids, mineralocorticoids, androgens, progestins, and estrogens, involve the following:

1. The hormone enters into target cell by simple diffusion.

2. The steroid hormone binds to its cytoplasmic/nuclear protein receptor. Before binding of hormone, these intracellular receptors exist as monomers complexed with non-steroid-binding heat shock proteins, and they are incapable of binding DNA and regulating transcription. The receptor binds the ligand with high affinity and with a high degree of specificity, releasing the heat shock proteins.

3. Homodimers of hormone-bound receptor molecules are formed, and this greatly increases the affinity of the receptors for DNA HREs in the regulatory regions of hormone-responsive genes.

4. The receptor/steroid hormone complex translocates into the nucleus of the cell if it is not already in the nucleoplasm.

5. The receptor/steroid complex binds to DNA HREs and recruits other proteins called *coactivators*. This protein complex collectively regulates transcription initiation of the target gene, thus regulating the rate of RNA synthesis (transcription).

6. mRNA is translated into cell-specific proteins.

More specific details of this model (Fig. 3.15) are discussed in Chapters 9, 17, and 18. It is recognized that this model is an oversimplification of a much more complex mechanism of steroid/thyroid hormone action. Indeed, the sequence of events that mediate thyroid hormone, retinoic acid and vitamin D receptor signaling are known to differ substantially from the foregoing scheme. These receptors are bound to HREs in their free state and recruit co-repressor molecules that collectively inhibit gene transcription. Upon binding hormone,

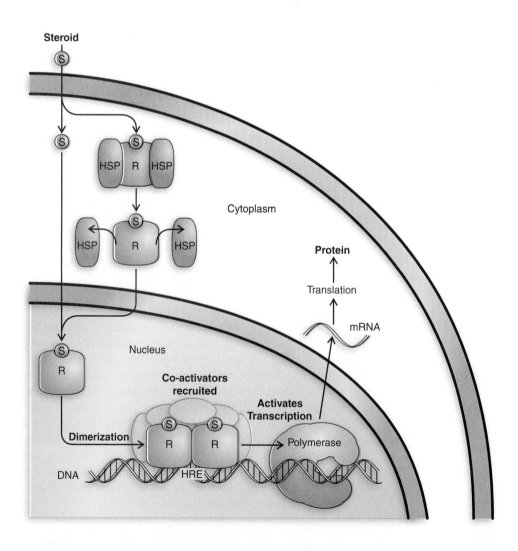

Figure 3.15
Mechanisms of steroid hormone action.

the co-repressors are released and replaced by coactivators, which facilitate stimulation of gene transcription.

Direct Membrane Actions of Steroid Hormone

The classical model of steroid action involves binding of the hormone to intracellular receptors that are members of a superfamily of ligand-induced transcription factors. The hormone receptor complexes then modulate the expression of target genes by binding to specific DNA sequences, the so-called hormone-response elements (HREs). There is increasing evidence for rapid, actinomycin-D- and cycloheximide-insensitive (therefore, presumably nongenomic) effects of some steroid hormones. For example, in rats, short-term exposure to the gonadal steroid progesterone is associated with rapid changes in behavior, and this effect occurs in the absence of new protein synthesis. Gonadal and steroid hormones can alter neuronal firing activity in certain neurons within milliseconds to minutes after administration [26].

Permissive, Additive, and Synergistic Actions of Hormones

Some hormones exert a *permissive* action, that is, they must be present for other hormones to exert their effects. Because many peptide hormones stimulate cells through activation of cAMP, one would not expect that the action of one peptide hormone could enhance the action of another peptide hormone, other than in an additive manner. Rather, it might be expected that for one hormone to potentiate the activity of another, the mechanisms of action of the two hormones would be different. The permissive effects of hormones are generally restricted mainly to the actions of steroid or thyroid hormones, where the ligands enhance each other's action or the action of other hormones working through membrane receptors. The following mechanisms, among others, could account for the permissive actions of steroid or thyroid hormones:

1. These hormones, through their actions on specific mRNA synthesis, could cause an increase in the number of membrane receptors, which might increase the production of cyclic nucleotides, thus leading to an increased cellular response to hormones acting on the plasmalemma.
2. Thyroid or steroid hormones could increase or decrease the amount of cyclic nucleotide-dependent protein kinases or the amount of substrate available for phosphorylation by cAMP- or cGMP-dependent protein kinases.
3. Thyroid and steroid hormones could enhance the synthesis of a protein that could act as an inhibitor of another protein (e.g., phosphoprotein phosphatase) whose action is antagonistic to cyclic nucleotide action (Fig. 3.16).

Two or more hormones may also exert simple *additive* effects on a cell, by virtue of the fact that the actions of both are mediated by the same signal transduction pathways. The hormones epinephrine and glucagon stimulate glycogenolysis and the release of glucose by liver cells. Because glucagon and epinephrine are not similar in structure, they would not be expected to mediate their effects through the same receptor, although they both activate hepatic adenylate cyclase activity. This can be demonstrated by the use of antagonists that are specific for a receptor. Propranolol, a β-adrenergic receptor blocking agent, antagonizes epinephrine-induced liver glycogenolysis, but not the glycogenolytic action of glucagon (Chap. 14). The action of glucagon, but not epinephrine, on the other hand, is blocked by specific antagonists of glucagon. Present evidence indicates that hormones with similar actions do not stimulate separate cyclases. Thus, at lower concentrations of the two hormones, their combined effects on adenylate cyclase activity and glycogenolysis would be additive through this common pathway. However, at high concentrations, the maximal production of cAMP produced by one hormone would not be augmented by the addition of another hormone given the limiting pool of cyclase (Fig. 3.3).

One might wonder why one cell, such as the hepatocyte (liver cell), possesses two separate receptors that activate the same ultimate physiological response. The reason is that different hormones, such as glucagon and epinephrine, are released under different

Figure 3.16 General scheme for the permissive actions of steroid hormones.

physiological states of an animal. Glucagon released from the pancreatic islets regulates the moment-by-moment breakdown of liver glycogen whenever blood glucose levels become slightly depressed (hypoglycemic). Under conditions of stress, however, epinephrine is released from the adrenal chromaffin tissue. This hormone not only stimulates hepatic glycogen breakdown into glucose, but it also increases vascular blood flow, respiratory rate, and many physiological processes associated with the stress response. Continuous stress, over time, would be detrimental to the welfare of the individual; thus, each hormone plays a specific temporal role in maintaining blood glucose levels (Chap. 14).

Synergism is a term often used to describe the physiological response of a tissue to a combination of two hormones that greatly exceeds the individual actions of either hormone. For example, the pituitary gonadotropic hormone, FSH, has no detectable effect on enzyme activity of testicular interstitial tissue, and the other major pituitary gonadotropin, LH, only minimally stimulates such activity. However, in the presence of FSH, the actions of LH are greatly enhanced. This might be caused by an FSH-induced increase in LH receptors known to occur in other steroid-synthesizing tissue in response to these two gonadotropins. Methylxanthines, when used at low concentrations, may only slightly increase the basal activity of cells. Used at a low concentration, a hormone might also have a minimal effect. When used in combination, however, a hormone and a methylxanthine may produce a dramatic response. The action of the hormone is to increase cyclic nucleotide levels, whereas the action of the methylxanthine is to inhibit degradation of cAMP by phosphodiesterase.

In summary, the action of one hormone may require the action of one or more other hormones that individually are relatively inactive, a phenomenon referred to as the permissive action of hormones. Additive effects of two hormones occur when their corresponding receptors are coupled to the activation of the same amplifying enzyme and second messenger.

Figure 3.17 Protein kinase phosphorylation of a protein substrate.

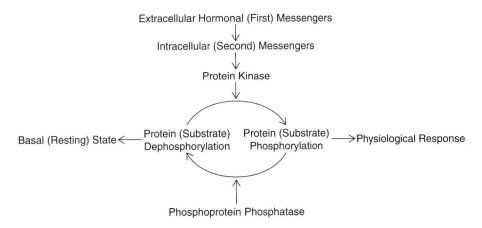

Extracellular Hormonal (First) Messengers

Intracellular (Second) Messengers

Protein Kinase

Basal (Resting) State ← Protein (Substrate) Dephosphorylation   Protein (Substrate) Phosphorylation → Physiological Response

Phosphoprotein Phosphatase

Figure 3.18 Role of protein kinases and phosphoprotein phosphatases in hormone action.

Synergistic effects, on the other hand, occur when a tissue's response to two or more hormones in combination is greater in magnitude than the sum of the individual actions of the hormones. The permissive, additive, and synergistic actions of a hormone may not easily be separated into distinct physiological entities.

Receptor Regulation

Receptors are not static components of the plasmalemma; rather, receptor number is in a constant state of flux and may change with the cell cycle or with the state of cellular differentiation. A cell therefore may become more or less responsive to a hormone, depending on the specific developmental or differentiated state of the tissue. Cells may even lose their capacity to respond to a certain hormone, but gain the ability to react to another, presumably because of the differentiated loss and gain of membrane receptors.

Hormones can Regulate Receptor Number

Hormones may regulate the number of their own (*homologous*) or other (*heterologous*) receptors. Receptor regulation may be negative or positive, resulting in so-called "down-" or "up"-regulation, respectively. Prolactin, for example, induces the appearance of PRL receptors (up-regulation) in the liver and certain other tissues. Continuous exposure of lymphocytes to insulin results in decreased binding (down-regulation) of the hormone to the cells. Some obese individuals have high concentrations of insulin in their blood, even though their blood sugar level is normal. Theoretically, glucose levels should be diminished in the presence of insulin. The cells of some of these obese individuals apparently possess fewer insulin receptors. When obese individuals diet, which lowers blood glucose and insulin levels, their cells are able to bind increased amounts of insulin due to restoration of receptor number.

Most hormones, like insulin, produce the same effect (e.g., down- or up-regulation) on receptors in the various tissues that they regulate. Angiotensin II (AII), however, appears to increase or decrease receptors depending on the particular cell type involved. For example, AII increases the number of its receptors on adrenal cells, but decreases its receptor population on certain smooth muscle cells. Thyrotropin-releasing hormone (TRH) acts on pituitary thyrotrophs to release thyroid-stimulating hormone (TSH), which then stimulates thyroid hormone (T_4 and T_3) production by the thyroid gland. Thyroid hormones then decrease the sensitivity of thyrotrophs by stimulating a loss of TRH receptors, a good example of negative feedback. Glucocorticoids, on the other hand, increase the number of pituitary TRH receptors. The latter two examples of heterologous receptor regulation demonstrate both down- and up-regulation. Changes in receptor number may provide an important mechanism for preventing hyperstimulation of cells to hormones under pathological states of hormone oversecretion. Receptor modulation may also provide a mechanism by which hormones act in sequence to amplify or diminish responses to other hormones. The gonadotropins, FSH and LH, are secreted and act on the ovaries in a sequential manner; it appears that LH action is dependent on induction of LH receptors by FSH.

Receptor Cooperativity Can Modulate Responses to Hormones

Hormone receptor studies suggest that mechanisms of hormone–receptor interaction are compatible with negative or positive models of *cooperativity*. There are two major events that govern the response elicited by a hormone: hormone binding, and the coupling between the binding event and the first biochemical signal elicited. The binding event can be described as being *noncooperative*, *positively cooperative*, or *negatively cooperative*. These terms describe how binding of a hormone to its receptors affects its subsequent binding to other receptors possessed by the cells. Although it was originally believed that binding to one site did not affect binding to others, it is now realized that subsequent binding events can also be affected in a positive or negative manner. Positive cooperativity is the phenomenon observed where the initial binding of the hormone to its receptor enhances the affinity of additional receptors of the same type to the hormone. This may be an important mechanism for sensitizing a cellular system when hormone levels are low and occupy only a few of the available receptors. Negative cooperativity, where binding of the hormone reduces the affinity of receptors for subsequent binding events, may provide a mechanism for desensitizing cells to abnormal concentrations of a hormone. The kinetics of negative and positive cooperativity in hormone binding depart from the typical law of mass action behavior. The affinity of insulin receptors, for example, is not fixed, but decreases as occupancy increases.

"Spare Receptors" are Commonly Present in Hormone-Responsive Cells

In most cells, a maximum biological response is achieved when only a small percentage of receptors is occupied. For example, maximal stimulation of steroidogenesis by Leydig cells of the testis occurs when only about 1% of LH receptors are occupied. The additional receptors are referred to as *spare receptors* and are considered to be fully functional. The role of this receptor reserve may be to increase the sensitivity of target cells to activation by low levels of hormone. It is recognized, however, that the term spare is used in a relative sense, as the degree of receptor excess differs according to the particular biological response measured. Generally, the magnitude of adenylate cyclase activation is closely correlated with the degree of receptor occupancy, but the more distal physiological response, such as muscle contraction or hormone secretion, is evoked when only a small percentage of the receptor population is occupied.

Termination of Hormone Action

Hormones that act at the plasmalemma are degraded within the blood by serum enzymes, and within certain organs such as liver. The declining circulating level of a hormone would result in a decrease in further stimulation of membrane adenylate or guanylate cyclase activities. In the absence of cyclic nucleotide production, the residual intracellular cyclic nucleotides would be destroyed rapidly by cytosolic phosphodiesterase action, and cellular activity would return to basal levels [4]. Effects of steroid and thyroid hormones and some peptide hormones may be of longer duration. The actions of these hormones involve transcription of DNA, translation of RNA, and protein synthesis. In the absence of further hormone stimulation, the newly synthesized RNA species and proteins are degraded by cytoplasmic enzyme actions.

After the initial stage in hormone–plasma membrane interaction, the hormone–receptor complexes cluster at specific sites on the cell membrane [12]. Clustering of hormone–receptor complexes apparently triggers vesiculation of the plasma membrane–hormone–receptor complex, followed by cellular internalization by endocytosis. The contents of the vesicle are either degraded by lysosomal or other enzymes, or they may undergo plasmalemmal vesiculization and endocytosis to provide a mechanism for hormone transport to intracellular target sites. Both events may be operative, depending on the particular hormone and cell type. Figure 3.19 summarizes some mechanisms that attenuate signaling by G-protein-coupled receptors.

Pathophysiological Correlates of Hormone Action

Syndromes of hormone deficiency are often associated with increased sensitivity to the missing hormone, and this is correlated with increased concentrations of receptors for the hormone. Conversely, exposure of cells to elevated levels of a hormone may result in a decrease in target

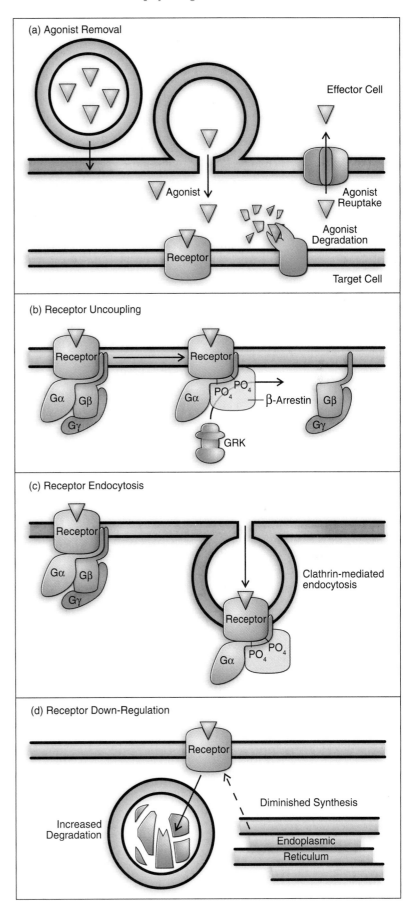

Figure 3.19 Mechanisms that attenuate signaling by G-protein-coupled receptors (GPCRs). (a): Agonist removal. Reuptake or enzymatic degradation in extracellular fluid is the first step in terminating the signal. (b): Receptor uncoupling. Phosphorylation of activated receptors by G-protein-receptor kinases (GRKs) and subsequent interaction of the receptor with arrestins interdicts interactions with G proteins and effectively terminates the signal, causing rapid desensitization. (c): Receptor endocytosis. Agonist-induced endocytosis depletes the plasma membrane of high-affinity receptors and may represent a second phase of desensitization. (d): Receptor down-regulation. Down-regulation occurs during prolonged exposure of cells to agonists and may be mediated by increased degradation and diminished synthesis of receptors. (From S. K. Böhm et al., "Mechanisms attenuating signaling by G-protein coupled receptors." *Am. J. Physiol.* 273:G586–G601, 1997.) Certain cellular elements may also exhibit specific affinities for non-hormonal agents, such as narcotics or other drugs; these affinities provide the basis for medicinal drug therapy. Some drugs interact with hormone receptors, which may result in activation of the cell, or, if the ligand (receptor-binding substance) lacks intrinsic biological activity, it may act as an antagonist to block the binding of the natural hormone.

tissue receptors for the hormone. Clinical evidence suggests that receptor modulation by circulating hormone concentrations is an important physiological adaptation. There are examples of heterospecific receptor modulation that can lead to adverse physiological responses. Thyroxine, for example, increases the number of β-adrenergic receptors in cardiac muscle and vascular tissues, as well as having a direct effect on the heart. This accounts for the enhanced sympathetic nervous activity that is usually a symptom of hyperthyroidism (Chap. 14).

Myasthenia gravis is an example of an *autoimmune disease* where antibodies to cholinergic receptors have been developed within the body. The antibodies block acetylcholine receptors at the neuromuscular junction. This, of course, leads to muscle dysfunction. In patients with Graves' disease, there are circulating immunoglobulins that bind to thyrotropin receptors in the thyroid gland. This immunoglobulin, the so-called thyroid-stimulating antibody (TSAb), enhances T_4–T_3 production, which results in hyperthyroidism (Chap. 13). A large number of human endocrinopathies are related to defects in hormone–receptor interaction. The hormone may be defective in structure, receptor number may be decreased, increased, or blocked as described, or there may be a defect in receptor-signal transduction. *Cholera* is a disease characterized by an enormous secretion of water and electrolytes by intestinal mucosal cells and often leads to death from dehydration. The affliction is caused by the cholera vibrio (*Vibrio cholerae*). The pathogen secretes a toxin that irreversibly binds to the guanylyl nucleotide regulatory protein. This leads to the continuous activation of adenylyl cyclase and production of cAMP, and the abnormal secretion of water and electrolytes.

That mutations of G proteins are involved in some pathological states is becoming increasingly clear [30]. It has been discovered that a subset of GH-secreting human pituitary tumors carry somatic mutations that inhibit the GTPase activity of the α_s subunit. This results in an increase in cAMP production by these cells and cell proliferation. Thus, mutated G proteins may behave as oncogenes in some specific cell types. The importance of understanding the role of G proteins in normal and abnormal cellular function is evident from the fact that two researchers won the Nobel Prize in Medicine/Physiology in 1994 for their discoveries of G proteins and their role in ligand-activated cellular signal transduction [3].

REVIEW EXERCISES

Compare and contrast each of the following terms. In what way are they related? How do they differ?

phosphorylaton/dephosphorylation (and hormone action)
regulatory/catalytic (subunits)
lipase/phospholipase
adenylate/guanylate (cyclases)
kinase/kininase
additive/synergistic (actions of hormones)
stimulus-contraction/stimulus-secretion/stimulus-response (coupling)
G_s/G_i
DAG/IP_3
G-protein-coupled receptor/nuclear receptor

Define or characterize each of the following terms:

receptor "crosstalk"	protein kinase A (PKA)
stimulus-response coupling	tyrosine kinase
methylxanthine	synergism
guanylcyclase	hormone analog
transacting zinc finger proteins	protein kinase C (PKC)

Think, analyze and discuss:

1. The binding of a hormone to its receptor is a process that occurs with high affinity and specificity.
   a. What type of molecular interactions mediate binding between a receptor and ligand?
   b. An individual inherits a genetic mutation in the gene that encodes a hormone receptor protein. The mutated gene encodes a receptor protein that contains a substitute amino acid in the "binding pocket" of the receptor—the portion of the molecule that is critical for normal binding of ligand. Would the amino acid substitution be likely to have an effect on the affinity, specificity, or both the affinity and specificity of the receptor for the ligand? Why?
   c. Tissue biopsies are obtained from the affected individual, and purified cell membranes are obtained from cells which express the mutated receptor. A membrane preparation is similarly derived from an unaffected individual. How might you experimentally determine and compare the affinities of the receptor for its ligand in both individuals? In which individual would you expect to see a higher K_d value? Why? How might you determine the specificity of the receptor in both individuals?

2. Vasopressin receptors bind the vasopressin molecule with high affinity, yet they are also capable of binding oxytocin with a relatively lower affinity. Would the K_d value for the binding of vasopressin to its receptor be higher, lower, or no different from the K_d value for oxytocin binding to the same receptors? Does oxytocin normally activate vasopressin receptors in vivo? Why or why not?

3. A hormone is found to bind with high affinity to membranes from a fixed number of cells. It is also determined, however, that the hormone binds to a second class of binding site with a considerably lower affinity. Which of the two types of binding sites is likely to be present in greater numbers? Why? Which of these two types of sites is more likely to represent binding to a physiological receptor?

4. When the sympathetic nerves to the heart are sectioned in an experimental animal, the response of cardiac tissue to drugs that stimulate adrenergic receptors becomes exaggerated. Formulate a hypothesis as to the reason for this *denervation supersensitivity*. How could you use a receptor binding assay to test your hypothesis? Draw a graph of the results that you would expect to obtain. What type of receptor regulation may mediate this effect?

5. Epinephrine and glucagon both stimulate glycogenolysis and glucose release from liver cells. The actions of both hormones are mediated by stimulation of cAMP production. Draw the signal transduction pathways that mediate their respective actions. Include in your diagrams the specific receptors, transducer proteins, amplifying enzymes, second messengers, and cyclic nucleotide-dependent kinases that likely mediate their effects. Which component(s) of their signal transduction pathways are different? Which are the same? Consider a situation in which the second messenger production is maximally stimulated by epinephrine. Would glucagon be likely to further stimulate cAMP production? Why or why not?

6. In adipocytes, epinephrine stimulates cAMP formation as described in (5), above, while certain prostaglandins, such as PGE_1, exert the opposite (inhibitory) effect in the same cells. Draw the signal transduction pathway that mediates the PGE_1 effect. Include in your diagram arrows indicating whether each component of the signaling cascade would be stimulated or inhibited as a consequence of PGE_1 action. Which components of the signal transduction pathway are different from the pathway mediating epinephrine's effects? Which are different? Which are regulated in a similar or opposite direction?

7. Epinephrine and norepinephrine can stimulate more than one type of adrenergic receptor. Each of the different types of adrenergic receptors can be coupled to the activation of different guanine nucleotide-binding proteins, or G proteins. Commonly, the β-adrenergic receptor couples to G_s, while the α_1-adrenergic receptor couples to G_i and the α_1-adrenergic receptor couples to G_q. For each of these receptors, list the amplifying enzyme, the second messenger(s), and a major effector enzyme that mediates signaling in their respective pathways.

8. Receptors for steroid hormones are proteins that are primarily located in the nucleus of the cell. Based on the chemical characteristics of steroid hormones, can you think of a reason why the steroid hormone receptors are located in the nucleus, as opposed to being positioned on the external surface of the plasmalemma?

9. Actinomycin D is a drug that blocks DNA-dependent RNA polymerase, and thereby blocks gene transcription. Would this drug be expected to block the major actions of estrogen on uterine cells? The actions of progesterone? The actions of oxytocin? Why or why not?

References

[1] Antoni, F. A. 1997. Calcium regulation of adenylyl cyclase. *Trends Endocrinol. Metab.* 8:7–14.

[2] Beck-Sickinger, A. G. 1996. Structural characterization and binding sites of G-protein-coupled receptors. *DDT* 1:502–13.

[3] Birnbaumer, L., and M. Birnbaumer. 1995. Signal transduction by G-proteins. *J. Recept. Signal Transduct. Res.* 14:213–52.

[4] Böhm., S. K., E. F. Grady, and N. G. Bunnett. 1997. Regulatory mechanisms that modulate signalling by G-protein-coupled receptor. *Biochem. J.* 322:1–18.

[5] Bradley, J., J. Reisert, and S. Frings. 2005. Regulation of cyclic nucleotide-gated channels. *Curr. Opin. Neurobiol.* 15:343–9.

[6] Cabrera-Vera, T. M., et al. 2003. Insights into G protein structure, function, and regulation. *Endocr. Rev.* 24:765–81.

[7] Chapman, D. E., and E. J. Neer. 1997. G protein βγ subunits. *Annu. Rev. Pharmacol. Toxicol.* 37:167–203.

[8] Colbran, R. J. 2004. Targeting of calcium/calmodulin-dependent protein kinase II. *Biochem. J.* 378:1–16.

[9] Conti, M., et al. 1995. Recent progress in understanding the hormonal regulation of phosphodiesterases. *Endocr. Rev.* 16:370–89.

[10] Drewett, J. G., and D. L. Garbers. 1994. The family of guanylyl cyclase receptors and their ligands. *Endocrinol. Rev.* 15:135–60.

[11] Drøbak, B. K. 1992. The plant phosphoinositide system. *Biochem. J.* 288:697–712.

[12] Grady, E. F., S. K. Böhm, and N. W. Bunnett. 1997. Turning off the signal: Mechanisms that attenuate signaling by G protein-coupled receptors. *Amer. J. Physiol.* 273:G586–G601.

[13] Hildebrandt, J. D. 1997. Role of subunit diversity in signaling by heterotrimeric G proteins. *Biochem. Pharmacol.* 54:32–9.

[14] Hille, B. 1992. G protein-coupled mechanisms and nervous signalling. *Neuron* 9:187–95.

[15] Ji, T. H., W. J. Murdock, and I. Ji. 1995. Activation of membrane receptors. *Endocrine* 3:187–94.

[16] Kisselev, O., et al. 1995. Receptor–G protein coupling is established by a potential conformational switch in the bg complex. *Proc. Natl. Acad. Sci. USA* 92:9102–6.

[17] Kleuss, C., et al. 1993. Selectivity in signal transduction determined by gamma subunits of heterotrimeric G proteins. *Science* 255:832–4.

[18] Knighton, D. R., et al. 1991. Crystal structure of the catalytic subunit of cyclic adenosine monophosphate-dependent protein kinase. *Science* 253:407–14.

[19] Kolb, A., et al. 1993. Transcriptional regulation by cyclic AMP and its receptor protein. *Annu. Rev. Biochem.* 62:749–95.

[20] Langley, J. N. 1906. On nerve endings and on special excitable substances. *Proc. Roy. Soc. B* 78:170–94.

[21] Lefkowitz, R. J. 1994. Rodbell and Gilman win 1994 Nobel Prize for Physiology and Medicine. *Trends Pharmacol. Sci.* 15:442–4.

[22] MacFarland, R. T. 1995. Molecular aspects of cyclic GMP signaling. *Zoological Sci.* 12:151–63.

[23] Metters, K. M. 1995. Leukotreine receptors. *J. Lipid Med. Cell Signal.* 12:413–27.

[24] Mikoshiba, K. 1997. The InsP$_3$ receptor and intracellular Ca^{2+} signaling. *Curr. Opin. Neurobiol.* 7:339–45.

[25] Oates, J. A. 1982. The 1982 Nobel prize in physiology or medicine. *Science* 218:765–8.

[26] Oichinik, M., T. F. Murray, and F. L. Moore. 1991. A corticosteroid receptor in neuronal membranes. *Science* 252:1848–51.

[27] Pierce, K. L., et al. 2002. Seven transmembrane receptors. *Nat. Rev. Mol. Cell Biol.* 3:639–50.

[28] Schuchard, M., et al. 1993. Steroid hormone regulation of nuclear proto-oncogenes. *Endocrinol. Rev.* 14:659–69.

[29] Spaulding, S. W. 1993. The ways in which hormones change adenosine 3′,5′-monophosphate-dependent protein kinase subunits, and how such changes affect behavior. *Endocrinol. Rev.* 14:632–50.

[30] Spiegel, A. M., A. Shenker, and L. S. Weinstein. 1992. Receptor-effector coupling by G-proteins—implications for normal and abnormal signal transduction. *Endocrinol. Rev.* 13:536–65.

[31] Stoker, A. W. 2005 Protein tyrosine phosphatases and signaling. *J. Endocrinol.* 185:19–33.

[32] Strosberg, A. D. 1996. G protein coupled R7G receptors. *Cancer. Surv.* 27:65–83.

[33] Su, Y., et al. 1995. Regulatory subunit of protein kinase A: Structure of deletion mutant with cAMP binding domain. *Science* 269:807–13.

[34] Sumida, C., R. Graber, and E. Nunez. 1993. Role of fatty acids in signal transduction: Modulators and messengers. *Prosaglandins. Leukot. Essent. Fatty Acids* 48:117–22.

[35] Sutherland, E. W. 1972. Studies on the mechanism of hormone action. *Science* 177:401–8.

[36] Tsai, M. J., and B. W. O'Malley. 1994. Molecular mechanisms of action of steroid/thyroid receptor superfamily members. *Annu. Rev. Biochem.* 63:451–85.

[37] Ushikubi, F., M. Hirata, and S. Narumiya. 1995. Molecular biology of prostanoid receptors: An overview. *J. Lipid Med. Cell Signal.* 12:343–59.

[38] Wettschureck, N., and S. Offermanns. 2005. Mammalian G proteins and their cell type specific functions. *Physiol. Rev.* 85:1159–204.

CHAPTER

4

Endocrine Methodologies

*S*ome of the methods presently used in endocrinological studies were developed for more practical purposes. In many cultures castration was practiced as a form of punishment. In the Middle and Far East castration was performed to provide servants (eunuchs) for harems; in Italy castrated young boys were trained to be adult sopranos. Castration is presently used to improve the flavor of meat from some domestic animals (e.g., castrated chickens produce capons). These "practical" operations were the forerunners of the gonadectomies of present-day endocrinological studies.

The idea that glands contained humors or substances that could act as replacement therapy for a lost function of a gland was first entertained seriously by a French physician, Charles Brown-Séquard. He injected himself with extracts from dog, guinea pig, and rabbit testicles and proclaimed that the extracts had remarkable rejuvenating effects. Brown-Séquard even recommended that extracts be obtained from the mature calf to give to men the vigor of horses and other larger animals. It is now believed that these extracts had only a placebo effect. Nevertheless, glandular extraction, purification, and injection into animals have become important methods in elucidating the hormonal role of particular tissues and organs.

Although hormones control a large variety of physiological events, their basic function is to act at the level of the cell to stimulate cellular physiological processes inherent in the cell. Melanocytes, for example, synthesize the pigment melanin. Melanocyte-stimulating hormone (MSH) enhances melanin formation by increasing the activity of the rate-limiting enzyme tyrosinase. Cortisol is a hormone produced by adrenal steroidogenic tissue. Corticotropin (ACTH) activation of adrenocortical enzyme activity leads to elevated cortisol biosynthesis. Thus effects of hormones are reflected in physiological processes in the many cell types present within an organism. This chapter summarizes some of the methods employed by endocrinologists to study endocrine glands and the target cells and tissues that they regulate.

General Considerations

The methods now employed to study endocrine systems are highly diverse [8, 9, 29]. Classical in vivo and in vitro methods include surgical manipulations, tissue extract preparation for hormone isolation and identification, histological methods for the localization of hormones, and numerous hormone and receptor assay methods. Modern endocrine research utilizes virtually any of the latest molecular, cellular, physiological, behavioral, and genetic approaches—often in combination with the classical techniques—to further our understanding of hormone synthesis, secretion, physiological roles, and mechanisms of action. The techniques described in what follows will be mentioned in more detail in later chapters.

What Do Endocrinologists Want to Know about a Hormone?

Following discovery of a hormone, endocrine studies usually focus on the following investigations (not necessarily in the order delineated):

1. *Source.* The distribution of the hormone will be determined. The hormone may be found in more than a single organ, tissue, or cellular source. For example, several gastrointestinal hormones are also found within the central nervous system.

2. *Structure determination and synthesis.* Depending on the type of hormone, the structure will be determined by any of a variety of methods. In the case of a peptide hormone, the primary (amino acid) sequence will be determined. From this information the peptide will then be synthesized and its biological activity, compared to the purified extract, will be determined. This will establish the substance and structure as the authentic hormone.

3. *Biosynthesis.* The biosynthetic pathway of hormone production should be delineated. Knowledge of the primary structure of a peptide hormone can be used to predict the corresponding sequence of the gene that encodes it; the gene can be cloned and the cDNA structure corresponding to the hormone mRNA can be used to predict the prohormone structure and possible enzymological events related to production of the mature hormone.

4. *Control of secretion.* The extrinsic or intrinsic factor(s) regulating the control of hormone secretion must then be determined. Endogenous stimuli may involve negative or positive feedback by other hormones, or the circulating products (other hormones, metabolic substrates), or consequences (blood volume, water and/or electrolyte composition of the blood) of its actions. The nervous system may directly or indirectly regulate hormone secretion from endocrine organs or tissues.

5. *Cellular mechanisms of secretion.* Once the first messengers regulating hormone secretion have been determined, it is then necessary to determine the nature of the second messengers and structural elements (ion channels, cytoplasmic organelles) that participate in the process of hormone release (secretion).

6. *Circulation and metabolism.* It is important to determine the half-life of the hormone in the systemic circulation. Steroid or peptide hormones may be noncovalently bound to circulating proteins. Fluctuations in the levels of the "binding" proteins may affect the total amount of hormone present in the blood and therefore available for hormone action. The half-life of the hormone in the circulation may be affected by degradation or other alterations of the hormone by serum enzymes. The retention time of the hormone in the circulation may also be affected by processes of filtration by the kidney.

7. *Biological actions and roles.* Removal of the hormone from the body by one or more methods usually will result in physiological effects in the animal that will predict one or more functions for the hormone. Administration of the hormone (replacement therapy) or related analog to the animal should confirm one or more roles for the hormone. Studies on other species of animals may suggest additional or alternate roles for the hormone.

8. *Mechanisms of action.* Following administration of the hormone, in vivo and in vitro cellular changes in biochemical processes and products should indicate one or more second messengers involved in hormone action. The receptor and signal transduction mechanisms involved in hormone action should define the temporal aspects between receptor activation and cellular response. Structure–activity studies will determine the essential features of the hormone required for hormone action, in the case of a peptide, the "message sequence."

9. *Pathophysiological aspects.* The existence of a hormone is sometimes gleaned from the symptoms of a human pathophysiological condition. In other cases the discovery of a hormone in experimental animals provides a new explanation for a previously misunderstood clinical condition. In either case, it is important to study the relationship between the normal biology of a hormone and the clinical consequences of alterations in synthesis, secretion, and actions of that hormone. These studies take place in animal models of human diseases, and to the extent that is ethically possible, in human clinical populations.

10. *Comparative endocrinology.* Some hormones are evolutionarily conserved in structure and/or function in organisms ranging from the most primitive to the most recently evolved. The structures and biological roles of other hormones, however, have clearly evolved and become specialized for particular adaptations in various species. In some cases, the responses to the same hormone molecule are specialized by the types of receptors and signaling mechanisms that are present in the responsive cells. In other cases, variations in the molecular structure of the hormone itself have arisen through gene mutations, and these can alter and/or expand the biological activities of a particular molecular variant, and even increase the number of different molecular variants produced within the same organism. Comparative endocrinologists attempt to track the evolution of hormone structure and function, and determine the adaptational significance of these evolutionary relationships for the physiological ecology of different animal species.

Surgical Methods

Surgical removal of a putative endocrine gland or tissue from an animal is followed by subsequent assessment of physiological alterations. A change in functional activity of suspected target organs (i.e., atrophy) suggests an endocrine function for the extirpated tissue. One might also monitor changes in blood or urinary levels of certain metabolites or electrolytes. Removal of the adrenals, for example, would result in lowered circulating levels of adrenal steroids and catecholamines and a reduction in the plasma Na^+ concentration. Transplanting an organ back into the same or a different animal also provides information on the functional role of the organ. In mammals, transplantation of an organ from a donor to a host is usually done in genetically related (inbred) strains of animals so that the transplant is not rejected by immunological processes. Endocrine organs can be transplanted to an *ectopic* (abnormal) site in the animal, usually beneath the kidney capsule or within the eye, where rapid vascularization often occurs. Removal of the pituitary is referred to as a *hypophysectomy.* The pituitary target organs of "hypox" animals become atrophic due to the absence of hormonal stimulation. In a few examples endocrine tissue is normally under a tonic inhibitory control; the tissue then becomes hypertrophic when transplanted to an ectopic site within the animal or when incubated in vitro.

Removal of both members of paired (bilateral) target organs (e.g., adrenal glands or gonads) usually leads to complete loss of dependent tissue/organ functions. If only one of the pair (unilateral) is removed, the remaining organ usually undergoes *compensatory hypertrophy.* In other words, there is an increase in cell size and number in the remaining organ to compensate functionally for the loss of hormone secretion from the ablated organ (Fig. 4.1). In endocrine systems in which one endocrine organ may control secretions by another, the feedback mechanisms that may operate are often studied by assessing the effects of organ removal and hormone replacement on the putative feedback target.

Other examples of endocrine ablations include pinealectomy (epiphysectomy), adrenalectomy, thyroidectomy, and thymectomy. The diverse nature of such endocrine tissues as the gastrointestinal hormone-secreting cells prevents such a surgical procedure. The pancreatic islets are similarly impossible to remove without removing concomitantly the exocrine tissue that comprises most of the mass of the pancreas. Islet ablation, however, can be accomplished by the use of alloxan or streptozotocin, drugs that specifically destroy the insulin-secreting cells of the islets. Cobalt chloride is similarly effective in the elimination of the glucagon-secreting cells of the pancreatic islets. In brain tissues, localized electrolytic lesions can be made to eliminate specific brain nuclei that contain cells of interest, and the consequences of these ablations can be functionally assessed.

Hormone Replacement Therapy

The undesirable effects of hormone loss following surgical ablation or loss due to certain disease states often can be adequately reversed by administration of the needed hormone or related analog. At menopause, for example, many women experience bone mineral loss (osteoporosis) due to declining levels of ovarian estrogens. Estrogen/progesterone

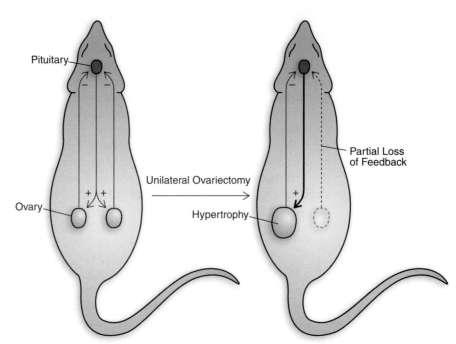

Figure 4.1
Compensatory ovarian hypertrophy in a unilaterally ovariectomized rat.

(contraceptive steroid) replacement therapy can be used to prevent increased risk of bone fractures in these women. Children lacking growth hormones can maintain normal stature (growth) when given this hormone, thus avoiding stunted growth, which will result due to the absence of the hormone. In animal experiments, many of these same pathological conditions can be mimicked by surgical, genetic or pharmacological means and then the effectiveness of hormone replacement regimens can be assessed in these pathophysiological animal models.

Immunological Neutralization of Hormone Activity

Antibodies can be prepared against most of the peptide hormones. Injected into the intact animal, these antibodies neutralize the biological activity of the endogenous hormones. This methodology may have clinical applications, since such an immunological approach may be useful for contraception in both the male and the female. For example, the mammalian zona pellucida, which surrounds growing oocytes and ovulated eggs, is a potential immunogen for a contraceptive vaccine. Immunization with sera against the zona produces reversible contraception in the mouse without obvious side effects [15, 16]. Many experimental uses of this methodology can be foreseen. For example, injections of antibodies to nerve growth factor (NGF, Chap. 12), a hormone required for growth and development of the sympathetic nervous system, result in failure of this system to develop. The injected animals are effectively immunosympathectomized (Chap. 14).

Tissue Extracts and Purification

Crude extracts of endocrine or other tissues were used by some early investigators to determine whether these materials could replace the excised endocrine tissue. With improved chemical techniques, the hormonal entities contained within the extracts were purified. This led eventually to the preparation of pure substances that were, and still are in many cases, marketed by pharmaceutical houses for medicinal or experimental use. Replacement therapy with these preparations can lead to full restoration of target organ function or even to hypertrophy (excessive enlargement), if too much of the preparation is provided. Many diabetics must receive daily injections of exogenous insulin to augment insufficient quantities produced endogenously by the pancreatic islets. For many years, the only source of peptide/ protein hormones, such as insulin, that is too large to synthesize was generally from endocrine glands obtained from the abattoir (slaughterhouse). Generally, the hormones extracted are of *bovine* (cattle), *ovine* (sheep), *porcine* (pig), or even *equine* (horse) origin. Often these foreign proteins are immunologically neutralized within the body following administration, therefore necessitating a change in the type (source) of the hormone used. Steroid hormones are commonly extracted from the urine of large domestic animals, for example horses, and used in the preparation of hormone replacement therapies, such as the estrogen-containing treatments taken by some postmenopausal women.

Chemical Identification and Synthesis

Before the advent of modern molecular biological techniques, the structures of most protein hormones were identified by painstaking purification of the source tissues, followed by meticulous biochemical analysis of the hormone's amino acid sequence. A purified hormone was chemically identified, and then subjected to a simple analysis of the percentage of carbon, hydrogen, oxygen, nitrogen, sulfur, or other atoms present, thus providing an empirical formula. Further analysis of the protein then indicated the number and nature of amino acids present (an amino acid analysis). This was followed by a determination of the *primary sequence* (exact amino acid sequence) of the peptide or protein under study. This is not easy if a large protein hormone is being studied. Nevertheless, one might obtain information on the N-terminal or C-terminal sequences of these large protein hormones.

In the more recent past, hormone structures have been determined by screening of cDNA libraries, cloning cDNAs representing candidate hormone genes, and determining the predicted amino acid sequence of the putative hormone. In some cases, the gene encoding the hormone was identified using *forward genetic* methods (from phenotype to genotype); these approaches generally involve the genetic analysis of mutant mouse strains that exhibit phenotypic evidence for disruption of a gene of interest. For example, the gene encoding the adipocyte-derived hormone, leptin, was "positionally cloned" by analyzing genomic markers and deducing the genomic location of the heritable DNA sequence linked to the obese phenotype in the mutant (ob/ob) mouse [41]. With the sequencing of the human, mouse, and other animal genomes, it has also become possible to screen sequence data banks and identify putative hormone and receptor nucleotide and amino acid sequences based on the presence of characteristic structural motifs. All of the foregoing methods have similarly been used to characterize hormone receptors and their corresponding genes.

From the primary hormone structure, the secondary (α-helical or β-pleated sheet) and tertiary (folding, intrachain bonding) structures may often be implied from the distribution of basic or acidic amino acids or the presence of sulfhydryl (–SH) groups within the protein. Some peptide hormones, such as insulin, possess a quaternary structure, that is, the hormone is made up of two peptide chains folded together into a three-dimensional structure (conformation). A number of the larger peptide hormones, for example, follicle-stimulating hormone (FSH), luteinizing hormone (LH), and thyroid-stimulating hormone (TSH), are composed of two chains, the so-called α and β subunits of their structures.

Chemical analysis may indicate that proteins are modified through sulfation or conjugation to carbohydrate moieties. The pituitary hormones, FSH, LH, and TSH, are examples of *glycoproteins* (Chap. 5). Determination of steroid or other hormone structures requires different chemical and physical methods of analysis. After determination of the putative hormone structure, it is necessary to synthesize the proposed structure and demonstrate that the natural and synthetic structures are identical with respect to chemical, physical, and biological characteristics. One can then synthesize related structural analogs of the hormone to determine the structural basis for the biological activity of the hormone. Table 4.1 provides the abbreviations used to symbolize the amino acids present within the primary structure of a peptide hormone. (See, e.g., Figs 5.8 and 11.5.)

Histological-Cytological Studies

The early endocrine studies were, as expected, anatomical and purely descriptive in nature. The light microscope was used to determine the histological nature of the endocrine glands. Many early observations were made on these tissues even before their endocrine role was suspected. Much of this work was accomplished by the great German, Italian, and other

TABLE 4.1   Abbreviations used for amino acids

Amino Acid	Three-Letter Code	One-Letter Code
Alanine	ala	A
Cysteine	cys	C
Aspartic acid	asp	D
Glutamic acid	glu	E
Phenylalanine	phe	F
Glycine	gly	G
Histadine	his	H
Isoleucine	ile	I
Lysine	lys	K
Leucine	leu	L
Methionine	met	M
Asparagine	asn	N
Proline	pro	P
Glutamine	gln	Q
Arginine	arg	R
Serine	ser	S
Threonine	thr	T
Valine	val	V
Tryptophan	trp	W
Tyrosine	tyr	Y

European cytologists of the nineteenth century. Although light microscopic methods are still important, the electron microscope is now the tool in the investigation of cellular function at the ultrastructural level. The scanning electron microscope bridges the gap between light and electron microscopy.

Gross observations of endocrine tissue provide only general details of anatomical localization, organ size, vascularization, and innervation. Severe alterations from the normal in organ size may provide clues to an underlying pathophysiology. The thyroid gland, for example, may become enlarged (goitrous) under certain conditions of hyperstimulation (see Fig. 13.11). At the histological level, one is able to discern the cytological characteristics of endocrine tissues. The cells may be *hypertrophic* (enlarged) or *atrophic* (diminished) depending on whether they are hyperactive or hypoactive, respectively. Hypertrophic cells contain an abundance of endoplasmic reticulum and Golgi bodies, as these organelles function in many cellular synthetic processes. Atrophic cells, on the other hand, lack this synthetic machinery and contain a much diminished cytoplasmic mass. Endocrine cell hypertrophy is usually accompanied by *hyperplasia*, an increase in cell number.

Histological stains are available to provide further information on chemical components of cells. Hematoxylin and eosin are two popular dyes for staining cells for routine histological observation. Hematoxylin, a basic dye, interacts with acidic components of the cell, such as the phosphoric acid of DNA and RNA. These components are said to be *basophilic* or to exhibit basophilia. On the other hand, eosin, an acidic dye, interacts with the basic components of the cell, which are then said to be *acidophilic* or to exhibit acidophilia. Used in combination, hematoxylin and eosin usually stain the nucleus and cytoplasm blue and pink, respectively.

By the use of a battery of histological stains, one can characterize each cell present in the pituitary. With hematoxylin and eosin, it is only possible to separate the basophils from the acidophils and chromophobic (nonstaining) cells (*chromophobes*). Other histological stains are needed to further differentiate the several types of basophils. Certain stains can be used to demonstrate the presence of specific organic constituents, such as glycoproteins, in gonadotrophs of the pituitary, or glycogen in hepatocytes [29].

Immunohistochemistry can be Used to Visualize the Expression Pattern of a Hormone or Receptor

Immunological methods have been used for many years to characterize and analyze the expression of hormones in endocrine cells. They are also used to characterize the specific distribution of receptors, cell signaling molecules, transcription factors, and other proteins that mediate

Figure 4.2 Principle of immunohistofluorescence methods for the microscopic detection of a protein of interest in individual cells.

hormone actions in target tissues. *Immunohistochemistry* refers to the use of specific antibodies to detect and label specific antigens (molecular targets of immune mediators), for example hormones, in a tissue of interest. This term is often used interchangeably with *immunocytochemistry*, which is a narrower and perhaps more accurate description of those techniques that allow identification of a particular antigen at the level of individual cells, or even within specific subcellular compartments (Fig. 4.2). These powerful procedures make use of antibodies that specifically recognize and bind to a specific epitope (portion of a particular molecule), thereby allowing one to visualize and identify which cells in a tissue contain that specific molecule. Either *polyclonal* or *monoclonal* antibodies can be used in immunohistochemical procedures. Polyclonal antisera are generated by immunizing animals with a suspension containing the target molecule, and subsequently obtaining the hyperimmune serum from those animals that mount a robust and specific immune reaction to the antigen. The polyclonal antiserum, as its name implies, contains several different clonal strains of immunoglobulins that may contribute to varying degrees to the total antibody titer. Monoclonal antibodies are produced by immunizing a mouse with a specific antigen, obtaining spleen cells from the animal, and fusing these cells with chemically selectable myeloma cells to produce *hybridomas*. Each hybridoma is capable of expanding to produce a homogeneous clonal line of cells that produce chemically and immunologically homogeneous antibodies. Most importantly, the selected clonal cell line produces large quantities of a single antibody species that recognizes and binds to a single antigenic determinant.

Irrespective of the type of antibody utilized, the success of any immunohistochemical approach depends upon the specificity and the affinity of the antibody for a particular antigen. In a version of immunohistochemistry referred to as *immunohistofluorescence*, antibodies to peptide or protein hormones are conjugated to a fluorescent dye and used to identify cells that produce the molecule of interest. The tissue to be examined is first treated with a fixative, such as glutaraldehyde, and sectioned into thin slices. After the tissue is placed on a microscope slide, a solution of the antibody conjugate is added to the tissue, and the excess solution is then rinsed from the slide several times. Microscopic observations usually reveal that the fluorescent antibody is bound only in those cells that produce the hormone, the antigen (see Fig. 10.8). Specificity is determined by prior incubation with a "blocking peptide", a synthetic peptide that is identical to the portion of the target hormone or receptor that is known to be bound by the antibodies. The blocking peptide interacts with the antibody and thus prevents it from binding the endogenous antigen. The absence of fluorescent labeling of tissue following preincubation with the blocking peptide confirms the specificity of the antibody for the intended antigen target.

In immunoenzyme histochemistry, an antibody to a hormone is conjugated to an enzyme, such as peroxidase. The antibody–enzyme conjugate is then allowed to interact with the tissue slice. When substrate for the enzyme is added, the conjugated enzyme catalyzes very localized reactions that yield a color or opaque product in the vicinity of the antigen (the hormone). By this immunoperoxidase method and use of the electron microscope, it is even possible to localize the site of the enzyme activity to the secretory vesicles/granules of a cell, which provides strong evidence that these organelles contain the hormone under investigation.

In *double-labeling* immunocytochemical procedures, two antibodies can be used to simultaneously examine the expression of two antigens in a single tissue section. The two antibodies possess specificity for the two different antigens, respectively, and they are linked to two different labels for differential visualization under the microscope. The utility of these procedures is far-ranging, and includes the ability to characterize the expression of specific hormone receptors to specific subsets of potential target cells in a complex tissue, such as the brain.

Immunohistochemical methods have also proven to be useful in functional studies of hormone secretion and action. The activation of a neurohormone-secreting cell, for example, is often accompanied by the expression of *immediate early genes*, such as those encoding the proto-oncogene c-Fos [11]. With immunocytochemical methods, cells that express this gene product can be identified as those that are activated under certain experimental conditions. For example, brain cells that are activated by physical or behavioral stress have been "mapped" by means of c-Fos immunocytochemical methods. Similarly, some hormone actions are mediated by intracellular messengers that become phosphorylated upon activation; antibodies can be developed that specifically recognize the phosphorylated form of signaling molecule, and thus they can be used to immunocytochemically map the cell groups in which hormone treatments activate that particular signaling pathway.

Assay Methodologies

Endocrine studies utilize all the modern tools of physiology, molecular biology, and genetics to understand hormone function. Below are considered those quantitative methods that have proven to be particularly important in analyzing the synthesis, secretion, and actions of specific hormones.

Bioassays Measure Levels of a Hormone on the Basis of its Biological Activity

The physiological activity of a hormone was originally determined by bioassay. Although some assays have been replaced by more modern methods, in some instances, the only method available is bioassay. In a bioassay, the activity of a hormone is studied on living cells, tissues, or organs. Physiological responses such as muscle contraction and relaxation or glandular secretion are monitored. The assay may be performed in vitro or in vivo (in situ) depending on the assay used. Usually, the tissue or organ selected is naturally responsive to the hormone. These biological preparations are usually responsive to hormones in the nanomolar (10^{-9} M) to picomolar (10^{-12} M) range [25]. Other hormones may also affect these tissues, but usually in pharmacological (micromolar, 10^{-6} M) doses.

The frog skin bioassay for melanocyte-stimulating hormone (MSH) is simple, specific, and exquisitely sensitive. Melanin granules within melanophores of frog skin disperse in response to the hormone, causing the skin to turn from light green to dark brown (Chap. 8). This change can be measured in a number of ways, but one objective method is to monitor changes in light reflectance off the surface of the skin [25]. The toad bladder, and such epithelial structures as frog skin and the mammalian renal nephron, have been used in vitro to study the actions of vasopressin on transport of water and other components, such as Na^+ and urea, across these organs. Studies of ion transport in the toad bladder have contributed detailed information on the mechanisms involved in vasopressin action (Chap. 7).

The steroid-primed uterus of the rat has been used in vitro to study the mechanisms of oxytocin-induced contraction of this organ. Mammary tissue from the lactating mouse is used in vitro to determine milk-ejecting potency of oxytocin and related analogs. Other bioassays include in vitro adrenal steroidogenesis and secretion in response to ACTH: prostate and seminal vesicle growth in vivo in response to testosterone in the castrated male rodent; measurement of iodide uptake by the thyroid after exogenous TSH injections; measurement of epiphyseal plate (cartilage) growth in the young rat in response to growth hormone. Many investigators now use primary cell culture systems or immortalized cell lines rather than intact animals or removal of organs from such animals.

Bioassays can be Used in Conjunction with Structure–Activity Analyses

Bioassays determine whether a putative hormone or hormone analog possesses biological activity. Structure–activity studies determine the amount of activity, usually compared with some standard hormone. The minimal effective dose (MED) and maximal activities within the particular assay are usually determined first. Then, intermediate concentrations of the hormone between the two extremes (maximum and minimum) can be utilized to provide a dose–response curve. Usually, the half-maximal activity of the hormone is compared with a similar half-maximal control response (e.g., to the parent hormone or to an analog) and expressed as a potency ratio. The hormone or hormone analog may possess one or more times greater or lesser activity (potency) than the native hormone (see Fig. 8.18).

Bioassays are Used with Site-Directed Mutagenesis to Analyze Functional Domains of Hormone Receptors

Although the primary sequence of many hormone receptors is known, how the receptors function cannot be readily discerned from the amino acid sequence. One would like to know the sequence(s) responsible for ligand (hormone) binding and the sequence(s) responsible for signal transduction leading to a cellular response. A mutant receptor can be synthesized from the original normal receptor cDNA and the mutated DNA introduced into "immortalized" (usually cancer) cells. For example, single base changes, multiple base changes, additions, or deletions (subtracting amino acids) can be made. Then, a functional response to a hormone by these cells containing mutated DNA can be measured [26]. For example, one can measure changes in levels of a second messenger, such as cAMP, following addition of the hormone to the cells.

Radioimmunoassays Measure Levels of a Hormone on the Basis of its Antigenic Properties

The development of the radioimmunoassay (RIA) has allowed the detection of hormones in minute concentrations and with a high degree of specificity [40]. RIA has provided greatly increased diagnostic accuracy of pathological states characterized by hormonal excess or deficiency. These assays are routinely employed to determine the concentration of hormones and other molecules in blood or other body fluids. As with the immunohistochemical methods, the success of RIA procedures is dependent upon the use of antibodies that specifically recognize and bind the hormone with high affinity. Both polyclonal and monoclonal antisera can be used in an RIA. The second important reagent for an RIA is radiolabeled hormone. In most RIAs, the hormone is iodinated or tritiated; in peptide hormones or in other proteins, the tyrosine moiety incorporates iodide. The typical RIA procedure depends upon the binding of the specific antibody to the radiolabeled antigen (e.g., hormone) with the same kinetics as described for receptor binding to ligand in the previous chapter:

$$*[H] + [Ab] \underset{k_{off}}{\overset{k_{on}}{\longleftrightarrow}} [H][Ab]$$

where $*[H]$ = radiolabeled hormone, [Ab] = antibody, [H][Ab] = hormone bound by antibody, and k_{on} and k_{off} are association and dissociation rate constants, respectively. Like the binding of ligand with receptor, this is a reversible reaction in which k_{on} is greater than K_{off}. At a fixed concentration of $*[H]$ and [Ab], the reaction equilibrates at a maximum level of $*[H][Ab]$. This is referred to as the maximum binding, or B_0. The principle of the RIA is that the unlabeled hormone, [H], when it is added to such a reaction mixture, will *compete* with the radiolabeled hormone, $*[H]$, for binding to the antibody, [Ab].

$$[H] + *[H] + [Ab] \underset{k_{off}}{\overset{k_{on}}{\longleftrightarrow}} [H][Ab] + *[H][Ab]$$

	Maximum Binding	Standard 1	Standard 2	Standard 3	Standard 4	Unknown X	Unknown Y	etc.
Antibody	+	+	+	+	+	+	+	
*Hormone	+	+	+	+	+	+	+	
Hormone	–	+	++	+++	++++	–	–	
Unknown	–	–	–	–	–	?	?	

Figure 4.3 Schematic representation of a typical RIA procedure with hypothetical standard curve.

Since the amount of radiolabeled hormone and antibody is fixed, then increasing levels of unlabeled hormone will increasingly bind to the antibody, and displace labeled hormone from doing so. Thus, the higher the concentration of [H] in the reaction solution, the more the [H] [Ab] and the less the *[H] [Ab] will be formed. The RIA is therefore considered a *competitive inhibition assay*. In practice, the RIA is executed by adding reagents to a series of test tubes, as depicted in Fig. 4.3. An initial set of tubes constitutes the standard curve, in which increasing standard (known) amounts of unlabeled hormone are added to the fixed amount of radiolabeled hormone and antibody. Remaining tubes contain the same amounts of *[H] and [Ab] as do tubes in the standard curve, but in place of a standard amount of hormone, a given amount of the fluid containing unknown amounts of the hormone (e.g., serum) is added. The reaction is allowed to proceed to equilibrium. In some RIA procedures, a second antibody is then added that recognizes and binds to the first antibody, creating a larger protein complex that is more easily separated by the final step, which is centrifugation to separate *[H] [Ab] from unbound *[H]. The amount of *[H] [Ab] in the pellet following centrifugation is determined by monitoring the radioactivity emitted by the tubes in a gamma radiation counter, and plotted versus the standard amounts of [H] added to yield a standard curvilinear plot (Fig. 4.2). The amount of radioactivity from *[H] [Ab] in the sample (unknown) tubes is then used to extrapolate the value for the unknown from the standard curve. In addition to protein hormones, cyclic nucleotides and many other nonprotein substances are also measured by these RIA procedures with remarkable sensitivity, precision, and specificity. The non-proteinaceous substances are, however, usually conjugated to an antigenic carrier protein to produce antibodies for their assay.

Non-Radioisotopic Immunoassays are Now Widely Used by Endocrine Researchers and Clinicians

The availability of monoclonal antibodies was a major enabling step in the development of newer immunoassays, many of which can be performed without the use of radiolabeled reagents. *Immunometric assays* are those which utilize chemically labeled, monoclonal antibodies to directly measure hormone levels in a non-isotopic procedure. These assays usually utilize two different monoclonal antibodies that recognize two separated epitopes on the same target hormone molecule. The first antibody is attached to a solid phase (e.g., the surface of a well in a test plate) and it is used to "capture" the hormone by binding to its corresponding epitope. A second "signal" antibody is chemically attached to a fluorescent, chemiluminescent, or enzymatic label. When this signal antibody is subsequently added to the incubation, it attaches to a second epitope on the captured hormone. The chemical signal

Substrate

Enzyme

Primary Antibody 2

Antigen

Primary Antibody 1

Capture Assay
"Sandwich"

Figure 4.4 Principle of a typical immunometric "sandwich assay."

provided by the signal antibody can then be read as a direct reflection of the amount of bound hormone. Figure 4.4 depicts the principle of this type of immunometric assay, which is sometimes referred to as a "sandwich immunoassay." Many other variations of immunometric assays have been developed, and their ease of use and sensitivity has prompted their widespread use in research and in medical diagnostics. Many of the home pregnancy tests, for example, make use of an immunometric assay principle to detect the early pregnancy associated hormone, human chorionic gonadotropin (hCG), in urine.

Analysis of Hormone Actions

Radioisotopes can be Used to Assay Cellular Responses to a Hormone

A number of endocrine methods use the radioactive isotopes of various elements (e.g., ^{125}I, ^{45}Ca, ^{35}S, ^{32}P, ^{23}Na, ^{14}C, ^{3}H) to determine physiological and biochemical responses within a cell. The half-life of a hormone, for example, can be ascertained by radiolabeling the hormone and then determining its distribution, excretion rate, and metabolism within the body of an animal. Iodide [^{125}I] is taken up by thyroid cells and incorporated into thyroid hormones (T_4 and T_3). Radiometric methods can be used to measure uptake of radioactive iodide atoms by the thyroid. Information obtained often reflects the biosynthetic activity of the thyroid gland, and this method is also used to localize hyperplastic thyroid tissues.

The radioisotope of carbon [^{14}C] can be incorporated synthetically into the structure of a molecule such as glucose. Subsequent metabolism of glucose with the concomitant evolution of radioactive carbon dioxide [^{14}C]O_2 is a measure of the metabolic activity of the cell. Insulin, for example, increases release of radioactive CO_2 by stimulating the uptake of radiolabeled glucose into diaphragm muscle where it is metabolized. This is also a good example of a bioassay. Tritium, a radioisotope of hydrogen [^{3}H], is widely used in autoradiography and in enzyme assays. The tritium isotope is generally used as a component of some organic structures, such as an amino acid or nucleotide (e.g., thymidine). The sodium radioisotope [^{23}Na] most often used to measure Na^+ uptake into nerve or muscle cells during studies on transmembrane potential changes in response to chemical messengers or other stimuli. Radioactive calcium [^{45}Ca] is often used to measure uptake of this divalent cation during muscle contraction and relaxation, nerve stimulation, or cellular secretion. Moreover, this isotope can localize Ca^{2+} sequestration within mitochondria or in the sarcoplasmic reticulum. Incorporation of sulfur [^{35}S] into the amino acid cysteine has been particularly productive in the study of neurohypophysial hormone synthesis because neurohypophysial peptides contain a high percentage of this amino acid. Such labeling of newly synthesized neurohypophysial hormones has greatly advanced studies on the movement of these proteins by axoplasmic transport down the neuronal secretory axons (Chap. 7).

Radioactive phosphorus [^{32}P] in the form of phosphate can be used to monitor protein phosphorylation as induced, for example, by hormonal stimulation of cells (see Fig. 3.17). A variety of assays use radioisotopes to determine the concentration of a hormone in an endocrine tissue, in the blood, or in the urine. Radioisotope assays can also be used to determine enzyme activation or inhibition by a hormone. In each of these assays specialized equipment capable of measuring the decay of the isotope is used (e.g., liquid scintillation counters or gamma counters).

Radioligand Binding Assays Assess Physiological Regulation of Hormone Receptor Number or Affinity

The actions of hormones in target cells may be subject to physiological regulation, such as up- or down-regulation, and endocrine researchers use a variety of methodologies to investigate how these adjustments occur. In many cases, it has been shown that alteration in the responsiveness of a tissue to a hormone may occur as a result of alterations in the number or affinity of active receptors that are present in the tissue. Chronic hyperinsulinemia, for example, can induce a pronounced reduction in plasma membrane insulin receptor number, a phenomenon that results from a high rate of ligand binding and subsequent internalization and degradation of receptors in target cells. The reduced number of insulin receptors, in turn, is associated with a reduction in the responsiveness of the target tissues to insulin. Radioligand binding assays can be used to document changes such as these in receptor number or affinity for ligand.

Different Receptor Number

(a)

Different Receptor Affinity

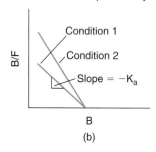

(b)

Different Receptor Number
and Affinity

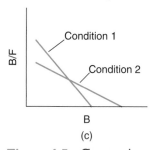

(c)

Figure 4.5 Comparison of hypothetical Scatchard plots derived from pairs of receptor binding data sets in which two receptor populations differ in (a) number, (b) affinity, or (c) both number and affinity.

The saturation binding assay, as discussed in the context of receptor binding concepts in Chapter 3, is the most common radioligand binding assay method for assessing the number and affinity of a specific hormone receptor in a given target tissue. A typical saturation receptor binding assay method (see Fig. 3.1) can be used to derive a Scatchard plot that permits the calculation of the binding affinity, K_d, and the initial receptor capacity (number of receptors), R_0, for a population of receptors in a given number of cells or mass of tissue. How can this method be used to assess physiological or pathophysiological changes in receptor affinity or number? This can be accomplished by comparing the results of separate binding assays performed on cells or tissues obtained under different experimental or clinical conditions. The K_d and R_0 values for each condition can be derived from the corresponding Scatchard analysis, and these can then be compared to determine if either are regulated as a function of the experimental or clinical variable. Figure 4.5a-c depicts two Scatchard plots of assay data obtained under different conditions, where the receptors for the hormone are altered in either number, affinity, or both number and affinity.

In some experimental circumstances, an endocrine researcher may wish to determine the anatomical distribution or amount of a receptor protein in a target tissue, without the need for assessing its binding activity. Immunohistochemistry is commonly used to characterize the expression patterns of hormone receptors. Often the availability of monoclonal antibodies that recognize extracellular domains of plasma membrane receptor molecules makes these procedures possible. The total content of receptor protein in target tissues or cells per se can likewise be directly measured using immunoblot procedures, as described below.

Immunoblots Permit Analysis of Specific Proteins in Hormone-Responsive Cells

Hormones exert their effects by inducing changes in the activity or amount of specific signaling molecules in target cells. Both types of actions can be studied by means of *immunoblotting* techniques, which are also referred to as *Western blotting*. A protein mixture derived from a tissue or cell culture is first size-fractionated via sodium dodecyl sulfate (SDS)–polyacrylamide gel electrophoresis, and then the resolved protein bands are transferred to a porous nitrocellulose membrane. The membrane is then incubated in a solution containing an antibody that binds to the specific protein of interest. The membrane is then washed to remove unbound antibody, and then incubated with a second antibody that recognizes and binds to the first antibody. The second antibody is covalently linked to an indicator molecule, such as alkaline phosphatase, which catalyzes the formation of a colored precipitate upon addition of substrate. The bands containing the target protein are thus indicated by this chromogenic reaction. The intensity of the band is generally proportional to the amount of antibody bound, and hence the amount of the specific protein contained within the band. Using these procedures, alterations in the amount of a receptor or post-receptor signaling molecule can be detected. Immunoblots can also be used to detect changes in the phosphorylation state of a signaling molecule, which can often provide presumptive evidence for the activation of that protein. Thus, increased phosphorylation can sufficiently alter the electrophoretic mobility of the protein, so that the antibody can detect the appearance of a separate band of immunoreactivity on the immunoblot.

Some Cellular Responses to Hormones can be Assessed by Enzyme Assays

Enzyme activity can also be measured by radioisotope methods. Adenylate cyclase or guanylate cyclase is measured by quantitation of the conversion of an appropriately radiolabeled precursor, ATP or GTP, respectively, to a radiolabeled cyclic nucleotide. This is a true measure of cyclizing activity of the membrane fractions, as measurements of cyclic nucleotide levels in the cell fail to indicate how the nucleotide levels are altered. Cyclic AMP levels, for example, may be altered by a number of processes, such as increased or decreased phosphodiesterase activity, which are unrelated to cyclase activity and cAMP formation. Measurement of tyrosinase activity of melanocytes is monitored by production of radiolabeled water from the appropriately labeled precursor, tyrosine (Fig. 4.6).

Autoradiographic Techniques Determine the Cellular Site of Radiolabeled Substrate Incorporation

This technique determines the cellular site of radiolabeled substrate incorporation [7, 14]. A radioisotope is injected into an animal or added to the medium within which cells are

Figure 4.6
Radioisotope enzyme
assay; tyrosinase assay.

[³H]-Tyrosine   — Tyrosinase →   Dihydroxyphenylalanine C [³H]-Water

Tyrosinase Assay

grown. A sample of tissue/organ from the animal or the cell culture is then placed on a microscope slide, as is done for routine microscopy. In the darkroom the slide is now immersed in a photographic emulsion and kept in the dark for a period of time. Decay of the isotope (usually tritium) leads to reduction of the silver bromide in the overlying emulsion to silver crystals. Because the *beta* particles released by the tritium travel only a short distance, the silver grains directly over the emulsion are preferentially exposed, since they are closest to the source of isotope decay. The tissue with emulsion is then placed in developer and stained, if desired. By this method, for example, one can determine the incorporation of tritium-labeled thymidine into DNA [14]. This nucleotide is generally used to determine the mitotic activity of cells. After orchidectomy, for example, there is enhanced hypothalamic activation of pituitary gonadotrophs (due to the lack of negative feedback inhibition by testosterone). This leads to increased incorporation of radiolabeled thymidine into the DNA of these cells, which can be visualized by autoradiographic methods.

The action of steroid hormones involves interaction with nuclear DNA. Autoradiography using tritium-labeled steroids provides a method for demonstrating the cellular site of steroid action (Fig. 4.7). Radiolabeled peptide hormones can be used to determine the topographical localization of hormone receptors in an organ or tissue (see Fig. 7.7). Some hormones mediate their effects through stimulation of RNA synthesis. This is demonstrated by the use of tritium-labeled uracil, which is incorporated specifically into RNA rather than DNA. Using giant chromosomes of the dipteran fly (midge), *Chironomus*, for example, it is possible to localize tritium uptake to specific Balbiani rings (large "puffs") of the chromosomes [2], sites known to be responsible for very active RNA synthesis (Fig. 4.8).

Analysis of Gene Expression in Endocrine Systems

The processes by which the DNA sequence encoding a protein is decoded, leading to the production of that protein, are collectively referred to as gene expression. Hormones often exert their effects by inducing alterations in the gene expression of specific proteins in a target tissue. Moreover, hormone genes themselves are typically subject to physiological

Figure 4.7   (a) Heavily labeled cells in the medial preoptic nucleus of the mouse after injection with [³H]estradiol; × 850. (b) Labeled neurons, at a higher magnification, showing the concentration of silver grains over the cell nuclei; × 1,360. (c) Guinea pig anterior pituitary cells; radioactivity is retained in nuclei of certain cells after injection of [³H]estradiol; × 1,360. (From Warembourg [36], with permission.)

Figure 4.8 Pattern of [³H]uridine incorporation into RNA produced by larval salivary chromosomes of a dipteran fly. Note intense labeling of Balbiani rings 1 and 6. (From Beermann [2], with permission.)

regulation. In many endocrine studies, therefore, the analysis of changes in the expression of specific genes provides critically important information about hormone synthesis and action. There are several potential ways in which gene expression may be regulated, including the stimulation or inhibition of (1) transcription of DNA to RNA, (2) processing of RNA to mRNA, (3) rate of mRNA turnover (conversely, its stability), (4) translation of mRNA to protein, and/or (5) post-translational processing of the translated protein. Some methods permit assessment of the rate of transcription, while others rely on steady-state mRNA levels as a summary indicator of processes 1–3. Measurements of mature protein accumulation can give an estimate of the overall rate of synthesis, although these values may be difficult to interpret if the rate of degradation or release of the protein is also regulated independently of synthesis.

Steady-State mRNA levels are Analyzed as a Measure of Gene Expression

Hybridization, or annealing, involves pairing of complementary strands of nucleic acids. Hybrids can form between DNA-DNA, DNA-RNA, or RNA-RNA strands. DNA is analyzed on a solid support such as a membrane (Southern hybridization, or *Southern blot*). The oldest and most common method for the analysis of RNA is the *Northern blot.* In this procedure, RNA is isolated from a group of cells or a tissue, electrophoretically fractionated by size in an agarose gel, and then transferred to a nylon or nitrocellulose membrane. A radiolabeled cDNA probe corresponding to the mRNA of interest is then hybridized to the RNA on the blot. The bands of hybridization are then detected via exposure of apposed X-ray film, and the magnitude of the specific autoradiographic band thus serves as a valid index of the amount of the specific RNA sequence present in the sample [33]. Another common method for mRNA analysis is the *ribonuclease protection assay,* in which a radiolabeled RNA probe and the corresponding target mRNA are hybridized in a solution, and then treated with a ribonuclease that digests single-stranded but not double-stranded RNA. The remaining probe–mRNA hybrids are then electrophoresed and autoradiographically quantified [21] (Fig. 12.15).

The most sensitive methods for measurement of mRNAs include *reverse transcriptase-polymerase chain reaction* (RT-PCR) and *real-time polymerase chain reaction* (real-time PCR) techniques. Both approaches provide powerful alternatives for the measurement of mRNAs that are expressed in low abundance, such as those that encode many hormone receptors or intracellular signaling molecules. A reverse transcriptase enzyme is first used to reverse transcribe the mRNA contained within a sample cDNA, and then the sequence of interest is amplified (copied thousands of times) by the polymerase chain reaction. The PCR makes use of a pair of ~20-mer oligonucleotide primers that are designed to hybridize

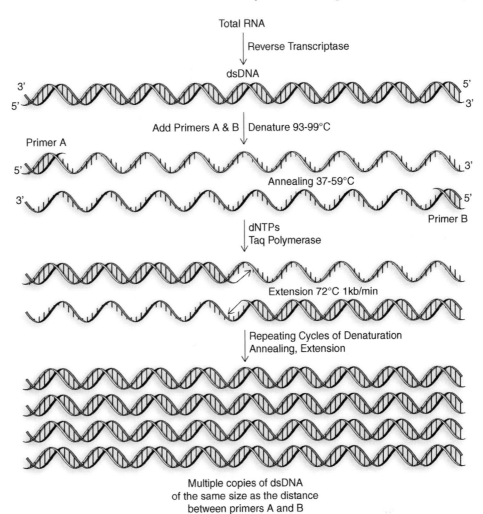

Total RNA

Reverse Transcriptase

dsDNA

Add Primers A & B | Denature 93-99°C

Primer A

Annealing 37-59°C

Primer B

dNTPs
Taq Polymerase

Extension 72°C 1kb/min

Repeating Cycles of Denaturation
Annealing, Extension

Multiple copies of dsDNA
of the same size as the distance
between primers A and B

Figure 4.9 Schematic representation of the principle of the polymerase chain reaction (PCR).

with nucleotide sequences that flank the DNA sequence to be amplified (Fig. 4.9). The reaction mixture contains the sample cDNA, specific oligonucleotide primer pair, a DNA polymerase enzyme, and deoxynucleotide triphosphate (dNTP) precursors, and is subjected to repeated cycles of heating and cooling in a *thermocycler* apparatus. During each cycle, the following occurs: (1) heating causes the double-stranded DNA to be denatured, i.e., rendered single-stranded, (2) the primers anneal with the corresponding flanking sequences on each DNA strand, (3) the primer sequences are elongated by the actions of DNA polymerase, which incorporates the dNTPs into the extensions, thus producing (4) two double-stranded DNA molecules that correspond to the original double-stranded DNA. These cycles of denaturing, primer annealing, and extension are repeated to yield two-fold amplification of the PCR product, or "amplimer," per PCR cycle. Thus, thirty cycles of PCR would be expected to increase the amount of DNA corresponding to the sequence between the two primers by 2^{30} or ~1 billion times! For semi-quantitative RT-PCR, the amplified product is electrophoresed and either stained or autoradiographically analyzed for the extent of radiolabeled dNTP incorporation. The amount of the amplified product is then considered to be proportional to the amount of the specific cDNA sequence originally present in the sample. Often the results are normalized to those obtained from the amplification of an mRNA sequence of unvarying abundance, for example a "housekeeping" gene, as an internal procedural control.

More accurate quantitation of mRNA can now be achieved using real-time PCR procedures. Several versions of this basic method have been developed, but all use a fluorescence-sensitive apparatus that monitors in real-time the progress of a PCR that emits fluorescence signal in proportion to the amplification of product. Often the relative amounts of the target sequence present in a sample are indexed as a function of the number of PCR cycles or cycle times (C_t) required to reach a minimum threshold of fluorescence.

Figure 4.10 In situ hybridization. The probe (RNA or DNA) is labeled with a radioactive or nonradioactive detection system. The DNA probe in this example (5'-CATG-3') is hybridizing with the messenger RNA associated with the rough endoplasmic reticulum. After hybridization to cells or tissue sections, the RNA or DNA of interest can be detected by autoradiography or non-isotopic methods. Advantages of in situ hybridization include more precise intracellular localization of the RNA or DNA of interest and direct visualization of positive cells in relationship to surrounding cells and tissues (From Lloyd, with permission. *Endocrine Pathophysiology* 4:64–72, 1993.)

Tissue- and Cell-Specific mRNA Expression Patterns are Analyzed by In Situ Hybridization

The nucleotides can also be localized within cells and tissues by *in situ hybridization* (ISH) [20, 32, 38, 39] (Fig. 4.10). This powerful technique used to localize mRNA involved in hormone synthesis is beautifully demonstrated in Fig. 8.5. Most ISH methods utilize radiolabeled cDNA or cRNA probes to hybridize to an mRNA sequence present in the cells of a slide-mounted tissue slice. The location of the hybridized probe is indicated by development of apposed photographic film, or more precisely, by exposure of radiographic emulsion coating the mounted tissue. Thus, the identity and location of cells expressing the mRNA of interest are indicated by the appearance of silver grains in the overlying emulsion. The number of silver grains that develop over an individual cell is proportional to the number of mRNAs encoding the protein of interest that hybridized with the radiolabeled probe. The ISH method can therefore permit semi-quantitation of mRNA expression; the principal advantage of the ISH technique is that it permits both quantitation and cellular resolution of mRNA expression patterns—an advantage not shared by total RNA hybridization methods. With in situ hybridization, it is also possible to address questions regarding differential gene regulation within different nuclei in a given brain region or within different cell populations in a specific nucleus. This level of resolution can reveal subtleties of gene regulation that cannot be detected with Northern blots or RNase protection assay methods. Moreover, it is also possible to determine if specific colocalized genes are coordinately regulated in brain nuclei in which some or all of the neurons display such colocalization. The principal disadvantages of in situ hybridization methods are that they are time- and labor-intensive and that absolute quantification cannot be ensured [6].

Hormone Effects on Gene Expression can be Profiled using DNA Microarrays

Many hormones exert their actions on a particular target tissue by simultaneously altering the expression of many different genes. The development of DNA microarray technologies has enabled endocrine researchers to identify hormone-responsive genes among thousands of candidates in single experiments. Several versions of these technologies have been developed. In general, however, either oligonucleotides or cDNA probes corresponding to large numbers of genes—in some cases encompassing the great majority of genes in a particular genome—are covalently attached to specified sites in a micronized grid on glass chips. The RNA sample is converted to cRNA or cDNA, labeled with a fluorescent marker, and hybridized to the immobilized probes on the chip. A specialized chip reader measures the intensity of the fluorescence at each probe position on the chip, reflecting the level of the corresponding mRNA. Computer analysis and comparison of the data among chips then permits identification of those genes that are expressed to a different extent in hormone-stimulated versus untreated conditions [27].

Transcriptional Regulation can be Studied using Reporter Gene Constructs

The techniques of molecular biology also enable endocrine researchers to analyze the mechanisms controlling transcription of genes that encode hormones, receptors, and proteins that are regulated by hormone action in target tissues. Often the objective of these studies is to identify promoter regions of a particular gene that regulate its transcription, and analyze regions within the promoter that are targets of specific transcriptional regulators. Reporter gene constructs are often used in these studies to obtain a "read-out" of promoter activity. Such a construct might be made by cloning the putative promoter region of a gene, and fusing it to a common reporter gene, such as the firefly luciferase gene. The promoter–reporter construct can be transfected (chemically introduced) into cells in culture, and the transcriptional activity of the promoter is monitored by measurement of reporter gene expression. In the case of the luciferase reporter construct, transcriptional activity is reported by luciferase enzyme activity; this is easily quantitated by lysing the cells, adding luciferin and the luciferase substrate, ATP, and monitoring the luciferase-catalyzed luminescence with a luminometer. Endocrine researchers often study the features of a promoter by "bashing" it: making truncations or specific sequence mutations or deletions in the promoter sequence, and then assessing changes to its basal activity and/or responses to putative transcriptional regulators. A sequence that normally mediates a positive or negative regulation of transcription can thus be identified by the loss or gain of transcriptional activity in its absence.

Electrophysiological Methods

Most cells are excitable, that is, they will respond to stimuli by becoming depolarized or hyperpolarized, which results, for example, in relaxation or contraction, respectively, of smooth muscle. These potential transmembrane changes can be monitored by intracellular or extracellular microelectrodes. The response of the cells to hormonal or other stimuli therefore can be detected. Most stimuli depolarize cells, but some chemical messengers,— for example gamma-aminobutyric acid (GABA), a central nervous system neurotransmitter, hyperpolarize cells. Chemical messengers can be applied to the surface of a cell by *microiontophoresis* and resulting transmembrane potential changes recorded downstream by microelectrode recordings. Electrophysiological methods have been important in studying electrical properties of the neurosecretory neurons of the neurohypophysis (see Fig. 7.3) and the response of pituitary cells to hormones (see Fig. 6.19).

Pharmacological Methods

Many exogenous substances (e.g., drugs) interact with molecular components of cells, and they therefore can be used to study the physiological activity of cells or the mechanism by which chemical messengers stimulate or inhibit such activity [10]. For example, at the level of the plasmalemma, cardiac glycosides, such as ouabain, are used to inhibit the Na^+/K^+ pump. Certain hormone secretions are enhanced or inhibited by ouabain, and this suggests that active transport (Na^+/K^+ ATPase) systems may be involved in the secretion mechanism of these hormones.

Many agents are inhibitors of intracellular enzyme activity. Of particular interest are the methylxanthines, such as theophylline (from tea) and caffeine (from coffee), which are phosphodiesterase inhibitors. These drugs mimic the actions of many hormones because they elevate intracellular cAMP levels (see Fig. 3.7).

There are a number of metabolic inhibitors that affect utilization of substrates for ATP formation. Iodoacetic acid blocks glycolysis, dinitrophenol (DNP) uncouples oxidative phosphorylation, and oligomycin prevents mitochondrial phosphorylation of ADP to ATP. The false substrate, 2-deoxyglucose, can be used to slow down glucose utilization within cells. These inhibitors provide information on the degree to which the glycolytic (Embden–Meyerhof) pathway or the citric acid cycle (Krebs cycle) contributes to cellular function.

Colchicine, a plant alkaloid, inhibits microtubule assembly by binding with tubulin, the protein subunit of these intracellular filaments. Inhibition of hormone action by colchicine or related microtubule inhibitors (vincristine and vinblastine) might suggest, therefore, that the hormone works through a cellular mechanism in which microtubules are involved. Insulin secretion is inhibited by colchicine, suggesting that microtubules may function in the secretion of this hormone. Cytochalasin B is a fungal metabolite that specifically interferes with microfilament function and is without effect on microtubule integrity. Cytochalasin B is inhibitory to the secretion of a number of hormones, suggesting that these filamentous organelles may be involved in the secretory process of these hormones.

At the level of the nucleus, actinomycin D inhibits RNA production. Puromycin and cycloheximide, on the other hand, inhibit protein synthesis. Thus inhibition of hormone action by actinomycin D implies that the hormone works through a transcriptional process of RNA synthesis. Inhibition of hormone action by puromycin or cycloheximide, in contrast, is interpreted to implicate a translational process of protein synthesis in the action mechanism of the chemical messenger.

Rather specific cation *ionophores* have been discovered and synthesized. These organic cation transport molecules specifically incorporate certain cations into their structure. They cross biological membranes and carry ions into cells. Ionophore A23187, for example, is specific for Ca^{2+} and, because many hormones activate cells by a calcium ion mechanism, this ionophore is in some systems hormone-mimetic. Valinomycin is an ionophore with relatively high specificity for K^+ transport. Some agents, on the other hand, are specific inhibitors of ion transport into cells. Verapamil, a Ca^{2+} channel antagonist, blocks Ca^{2+} entry into cells. Used concomitantly with a hormone, verapamil's inhibitory action may suggest that a particular hormone action is Ca^{2+}-dependent. Local anesthetics, such as procaine and tetracaine, may also block the action of some hormones by their antagonism of Ca^{2+} flux into cells.

Phospholipid vesicles (liposomes) have proved to be suitable carriers for many biologically active molecules. These transport vehicles fuse with and become incorporated into the plasma membrane, thereby transferring their contents into the cytoplasm. Liposomes loaded with Ca^{2+}, for example, are incorporated into the mast cell plasma membrane, which results in localized cell surface secretion of histamine [30]. Liposomes therefore provide a novel method of studying mechanisms of stimulus-secretion coupling, particularly as it relates to the release of a chemical messenger such as histamine.

Some agents are hormone receptor agonists, although in some cases they may not appear to bear any structural similarity to the true receptor agonist, the hormone. Certain ergot alkaloids, for example, stimulate dopamine receptors and inhibit MSH and prolactin secretion, thus providing some evidence that dopamine may be the natural hypothalamic inhibitor of these hormones. Certain structures related to acetylcholine (e.g., carbachol) exhibit intrinsic cholinergic activity, and they are of particular usefulness because they have a longer duration of activity as they are more resistant to enzymatic degradation.

Hormone action can be blocked by receptor antagonists, which are compounds that specifically act with hormone receptors but lack intrinsic agonistic activity [3]. For example, chlorpromazine and related antidepressant drugs block dopamine receptors. Acetylcholine action can be blocked by atropine (on smooth muscle) and curare (on skeletal muscle) and other cholinergic receptor antagonists. Cimetidine is a specific inhibitor of histamine (H_2) receptors and markedly inhibits histamine-stimulated gastric acid secretion. Cyproterone acetate and spironolactone are specific antagonists (antihormones) of testosterone and aldosterone receptors, respectively. Cyproterone acetate is a valuable tool in the treatment of cancer or hyperplasia of the prostate, hirsutism in the female, and precocious puberty in both sexes, as these maladies are often due to excess androgen secretion and action.

Synthetic analogs of peptide hormones may be used to block receptor occupancy by the native hormone. Hormone antagonists might prove useful in blocking the actions of excessive amounts of the native hormone in certain disease states (e.g., Cushing's disease). So-called "beta blockers," for example, have proved clinically useful in reducing the activity of the heart [3]. In women, the steroid hormone progesterone plays a central role in the establishment and maintenance of pregnancy (Chap. 19). A synthetic progesterone analog has been developed that possesses antiprogesterone activity (see Fig. 19.11). It has been used successfully as a medical alternative for early pregnancy interruption and other clinical applications.

As mentioned earlier, cobalt chloride and alloxan can be used specifically to destroy the alpha (glucagon-secreting) or beta (insulin-secreting) cells, respectively, of the pancreas. Monosodium glutamate (MSG) administered neonatally causes degeneration of neurons of the arcuate nucleus of the hypothalamus [12]. The neurotoxicity of MSG appears to be useful for investigative purposes because it is difficult to produce such lesions by electrolytic and radiofrequency methods without damage to other neurons or fiber tracts. The use of MSG, therefore, offers the opportunity to study the endocrine and morphological manifestations of destruction of specific neurons within the brain. Some pharmaceutical agents used in endocrine studies are described in Table 4.2.

Behavioral Methods

Many endocrine researchers study the effects of hormones on behavior. In some comparative studies, the roles of various hormones and their receptors are examined in wild animal populations, so as to determine how hormones may mediate behavioral adaptations to certain environmental niches. Mechanistic studies of hormone function, particularly those focusing on biomedical issues, most commonly employ quantitative behavioral tests in laboratory mice, rats, and monkeys. Standardized measures have been developed for the analysis of hormone effects on virtually any type of behavior displayed by these animals. Some behavior tests are relatively straightforward, such as those that monitor food consumption or drinking behavior. Other tests, such as those that examine interactions between two or more conspecific animals (reproductive behavior, parental behavior, pair-bonding) require use of more specific testing arenas and simultaneous monitoring of several variables. Analysis of sexual behavior in rodents, for example, may require measurements of both

TABLE 4.2 Some pharmaceutical and other agents used in cell physiology studies

Agent	Application
Actinomycin D	Inhibits RNA synthesis (transcription)
Alloxan	Destroys beta (insulin-secreting) cells of pancreatic islets
Chlorpromazine	Dopamine receptor antagonist
Cobalt chloride	Destroys alpha (glucagon-secreting) cells of pancreatic islets
Colchicine	Disrupts microtubules
Cycloheximide	Inhibits protein synthesis
Cyproterone acetate	Testosterone receptor antagonist
Cytochalasin B	Disrupts microfilaments
2-Deoxy-D-glucose	Metabolic inhibitor: inhibits glucose uptake and utilization
Dexamethasone	Synthetic glococorticoid agonist
Dinitrophenol	Metabolic inhibitor: uncouples oxidative phosphorylation
Ergot alkaloids (e.g., ergocryptine)	Dopamine receptor agonist (inhibits prolactin secretion)
Iodoacteic acid (or iodoacteamide)	Metabolic inhibitor: inhibits glycolysis
Ionophore A23187	Calcium (Ca^{2+}) transport carrier (ionophore)
Liposomes	Drug carriers
Local anesthetics (procaine, tetracaine)	Inhibit cellular uptake of Ca^{2+}
Methylxanthines (theophyline, caffeine)	Phosphodiesterase inhibitors (elevate cAMP)
Oligomycin	Metabolic inhibitor: inhibits phosphorylation of ADP to ATP
Puromycin	Inhibits protein synthesis (translation)
Saralasin	Angiotensin II receptor antagonist
Spironolactone	Aldosterone receptor antagonist
Thiouracil	Inhibits thyroid iodide uptake and T_4–T_3 synthesis
[³H]Thymidine	Studies on DNA synthesis
[³H]Uracil	Studies on RNA synthesis
Valinomycin	Potassium transport carrier (ionophore)
Verapamil	Inhibits cellular uptake of Ca^{2+}

proceptive (e.g., hopping and darting in females) as well as consummatory behaviors (e.g., mounting, intromission and ejaculation by the male, or lordotic behavior of the female). Specific behavioral assay methods are considered in subsequent chapters as they are used to study hormone effects on specific behaviors. Sensitive and sophisticated behavioral assays have been developed to assess the effects of hormones on feeding, drinking, sexual behaviors.

Recombinant DNA Techniques

Recombinant DNA technologies are now used to express recombinant proteins in a variety of in vitro expression systems. In some cases the purpose of the recombinant protein expression is to analyze its biological activity or its structure–function relationships in a biological context. In other circumstances, larger amounts of purified protein are required for biophysical studies of its molecular structure. Expression and purification at the largest scale, and perhaps posing some of the biggest technical challenges, is required for the production of hormones for medical and/or commercial purposes.

Hormones play important roles in regulating the activity of most cells of the body; indeed, some hormones are necessary for life. Parathormone and aldosterone, two hormones that regulate the electrolyte composition of the body fluids, are examples. Growth hormone (GH) is necessary for growth, and its absence in the young animal results in short stature. Failure of the pancreas to produce insulin results in diabetes mellitus. Insulin replacement therapy requires obtaining these hormones from other animal sources, but some individuals develop antibodies to these nonhuman sources of the hormone. In the case of GH, only pituitaries obtained from human cadavers or primates can be used, since GH from other animals is ineffective.

Recombinant DNA techniques offer the hope that a number of human hormones can be synthesized by bacteria in large amounts and at reasonable prices. Recombinant DNA

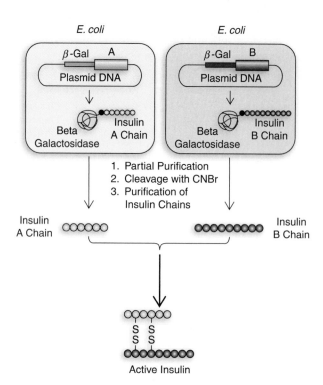

Figure 4.11
Recombinant DNA technique for the microbial production of insulin. (From Riggs et al. [23], with permission.)

Figure 4.12 Photograph of gigantism produced in the mouse by injection of metallothionein–growth hormone fusion genes into the pronucleus of the fertilized egg followed by implantation within the uterus of a recipient mother. Giant mice (left) became almost twice as heavy as littermates (not bearing the GH gene). (Reprinted by permission from Palmiter et al. [18]. *Nature,* 300 [5893]: 611–15.©1982 by Macmillan Journals, Limited.)

techniques are essentially in vitro extensions of natural phenomena. These methods involve purification or synthesis of genetic material and its insertion into a bacterial host. Several bacterial strains have been constructed that can produce human hormones, and genetically engineered bacteria now provide important sources of peptide hormones [23]. Two methods have been used to provide the genetic material to be cloned. For shorter peptides (e.g., insulin, somatostatin), DNA synthesis is used to make a gene of the desired hormone. In the case of the two chains of insulin, the 21-amino-acid A chain and the 30-amino-acid B chain are made in separate bacterial strains as tails on a larger precursor protein, the enzyme β-galactosidase. The individual insulin chains are then clipped from the precursor proteins and, after purification of the separate insulin chains, they are joined by air oxidation (Fig. 4.11). The method used for larger proteins utilizes mRNA and reverse transcriptase to make a DNA copy that is then inserted into the bacterial genome and cloned. For example, cDNA for proinsulin is inserted into *Escherichia coli* cells, which are then grown by fermentation to produce proinsulin. The connecting peptide is then cleaved enzymatically from proinsulin to produce human insulin.

Genetic Engineering

The functions of hormones and their receptors are now routinely studied using the powerful and remarkably informative approaches afforded by genetic engineering. These methods are commonly used to produce a desired genetic modification in a mouse and observe the phenotypic consequences of the genetic alteration. Most often, genetic engineering is used to generate animals in which either a foreign gene is expressed (a *transgenic* animal), or a specific gene is inactivated (a gene "*knockout*" animal).

In the early 1980s, endocrine researchers first injected foreign genes into mammalian embryos and found that this transgenesis approach could provide a powerful tool for use in endocrine research. Foreign DNA can be introduced into the mammalian genome by microinjection of DNA molecules of interest into pronuclei of fertilized cells, followed by the implantation of the eggs into the reproductive tracts of recipient mothers. The integration of the foreign DNA into one of the host chromosomes at an early stage of embryonic development results in the development of a transgenic animal [1, 13, 22, 34, 35]. In the earlier experiments, microinjection of the structural gene for rat growth hormone into the pronuclei of fertilized mouse eggs resulted in the development of some offspring that grew significantly larger than their littermates (Fig. 4.12). This methodology has important implications for studying the biological effects of growth hormone: as a way to accelerate animal growth, as a model for gigantism, and possibly as a means of correcting genetic disease. In the years following these original studies, transgenesis has been used in myriad ways to study hormone and receptor function. Transgene expression can be *targeted*, such that the transgene is only active in a desired cell or tissue. This can be accomplished by placing the coding region of the transgene under the control of a promoter sequence that is active only in the desired target cells. In some cases this is done to assess the consequences of overexpression of a hormone or receptor by the specific targeted cell group; in other circumstances, the transgenic protein is designed to be functionally inactive and serve as a *dominant negative* (inhibitory) modulator of its endogenous counterpart in a targeted cell group. Transgenesis is also used to label cells of a certain phenotype, such that they may be visualized in the living state. For example, the promoter sequence for the hypothalamic neurohormone, gonadotropin-releasing hormone (GnRH), can be fused to a gene encoding the jellyfish green fluorescent protein (GFP) to create transgenic mice in which the transgene, and hence the fluorescent GFP molecule, are only expressed in GnRH neurons. This particular animal model has been used to permit visualization of these few neurons in living brain tissues for electrophysiological experiments [28].

Transgenic technologies have been studied in several commercially important animal species with emphasis on growth enhancement as a strategy to shorten long production cycles. For the production of transgenic Pacific salmon, an "all-salmon" genetic construct consisting of a metal-lothionein-β promoter fused with the full-length type 1 GH gene was developed. The pOn-MTGH1 DNA was injected into coho salmon eggs with extraordinary results (Fig. 4.13). On average, the transgenic salmon were more than 11-fold heavier than the nontransgenic controls. Most interesting was the observation that the transgenic fish precociously developed a silver body coloration typical of salmon undergoing the physiological preadaptation (smoltification) necessary for the spring migration from freshwater to the marine environment.

Gene knockout animals have provided a wealth of vital information about the physiological roles of hormones and their receptors. Indeed, the loss of function in a gene deletion mutant animal can confirm the essential role of a protein in a specific endocrine process, or even recapitulate a disease state that is believed to arise from an analogous gene mutation in humans. The first step in the gene targeting procedure is the introduction of a disrupted allele of the target gene into cultured embryonic stem cells. The targeting construct is fashioned to contain a selectable marker, such as the gene encoding a protein that confers resistance to a cytotoxic drug. Only those cells in which the homologous recombination event occurs will therefore survive growth in media containing the toxic drug. Using this process, the cells heterozygous for the targeting construct are selected, grown in culture, and then injected into mouse blastocysts. These embryos are then

Figure 4.13
Nontransgenic (left) and transgenic (right) coho salmon siblings at 14 months old showing size difference and silver appearance of transgenic individuals, indicative of transformation to seawater adaptability. Length of top large fish (fork length), 41.8 cm. (Used by permission from Devlin et al., "Extraordinary salmon growth." *Nature* 371:209–10, 1994.)

surgically transferred into the uteri of pseudopregnant female mice. The resultant progeny are chimeric for the targeted cells. Breeding of these founder animals produces some mice carrying a single copy of the disrupted gene in all cells, and thus, subsequent breeding of two heterozygous mice will produce some mice that are homozygous for the inactivated gene sequence. These homozygous "knockouts," if they are physiologically viable, can then be studied to assess the potential loss of function that accompanies the loss of the specific hormone, receptor or other protein of interest.

In some cases, mice carrying a germline mutation in a vital gene have lethal defects that preclude their use. To circumvent this problem, geneticists have developed methods that permit cell-specific gene targeting, in which the gene mutation can be induced in a specifically targeted subset of cells in the body. The loxP-Cre recombination system is one such method. This strategy involves the generation of mice bearing site-specific recombination sites, called loxP sites, in the intronic sequences that flank an essential exon of the target gene. A second line of mice is produced that harbor a transgene construct containing a gene promoter fused to the Cre recombinase gene; importantly, the promoter is known to be active only in the cells of interest. Mating of the two mouse lines results in the expression of Cre protein only in the targeted cells, where it acts at the loxP sites to delete the exon of the targeted gene. Thus, the specific gene deletion only occurs in the target cells, avoiding the potentially lethal complications of total germline gene deletion. Many striking examples of the successful use of this system are found among studies of the tissue-specific actions of insulin. Conditional disruption of the insulin receptor gene in brain, for example, recently provided unambiguous confirmation that insulin acts centrally to regulate feeding behavior and energy homeostasis [4].

Animal Models for Research

Both vertebrate and invertebrate animals are used as model systems for endocrine research. A few examples of vertebrate models are discussed.

Cyclostomes

These most primitive vertebrates, which include the hagfish and lampreys, have not been extensively studied. These eel-shaped animals spend their lives in both marine and freshwater environments and therefore most likely possess a complex endocrine system as in other more evolved ("higher") vertebrates.

Cartilaginous Fishes

These ancestors of the bony fishes include sharks, skates, and rays and, although prevalent in numbers and readily available, they have not been the subject of much endocrine research.

Bony Fishes

These fish represent the largest and most diverse group of vertebrates. They have evolved adaptive features that enable them to survive in a multitude of ecological niches. Many of their specialized physiological functions are under endocrine regulation [20]. Migration to and from the sea by some species requires unique roles for some hormones. Prolactin, for example, is essential for survival in some fish transferred from saltwater to freshwater (as happens in salmon migrations). The control of color change in fish is much more complex than in other vertebrates and may, in some species, use a recently discovered melanin-concentrating hormone, whose function may be limited to more recent (teleost) fishes (Chap. 8). The corpuscles of Stannius are also unique to certain bony fishes and produce a hormone, teleocalcin, not found in other vertebrate species. The urotensins derived from the urophysis of certain species provide another example of hormones whose roles may be restricted to certain bony fishes (Chap. 7).

Amphibians

Amphibians include urodeles (salamanders, e.g., "mudpuppies," newts) and anurans (frogs and toads), as well as less well-known representatives. Their ready availability, their relatively small size, and the fact that they go through a dramatic metamorphic change from larval to adult life has made them important models for endocrine research. Our understanding of the roles of the thyroid gland and its hormones in endocrine physiology has been greatly influenced by studies on amphibians (Chap. 13). The amphibian egg has always been an important model for an understanding of early vertebrate development. These eggs have provided evidence for roles of hormones (growth factors and steroid hormones) during the earliest developmental stages.

Reptiles

Snakes, lizards, turtles, and tortoises, as well as the crocodilians and related species, compose this vertebrate group. There has been relatively little research done on these animals, but important information on some unique reproductive and behavioral strategies under endocrine control have been discovered (see Fig. 7.12).

Birds

These descendants of the reptiles include a large variety of birds that occupy a great diversity of ecological niches. It is not surprising, therefore, that these animals have evolved some unique endocrine strategies. Both wild and domesticated birds (chicken, quail) are available in substantial numbers for experimental studies. Birds have provided unique models for understanding the neuroanatomical substrates controlling behavior (e.g., bird song, courtship; Chap. 16). The role of the kidney in vitamin D hormone production has been best studied in birds because of the important relationship between the hormone and the control of Ca^{2+} metabolism necessary for eggshell formation (Chap. 9).

Nonprimate Mammals

The mouse, rat, hamster, and guinea pig have been particularly important animals for the advancement of our knowledge of endocrinology. Use of the mouse has predominated in molecular genetics, and the rat has perhaps proven most effective in the study of endocrine physiology. The hamster has proved to be a particularly useful model for understanding the role of the pineal gland and its hormone, melatonin, in the control of reproductive cycles (Chap. 20). The nude mouse has been a useful model for supporting the growth of human tumors, since it lacks an active immune system necessary to reject the transplants. The Brattleboro rat lacks the hormone vasopressin and therefore is a unique model of "diabetes insipidus" (Chap. 7).

Primates

Monkeys, because of their close evolutionary relatedness to humans, have played important roles in understanding the human endocrine system. For example, our knowledge of the structure and function of the corpus luteum of the ovary has been aided by use of primate models.

Animal Welfare

Most endocrinologists would probably strongly agree that studies in animals have been essential for the progress of endocrinology. Surgical removal of various organs has provided key insights into the existence and origin of hormones. Most endocrinologists would also probably agree that animals are still absolutely essential for basic studies in endocrinological research. Only recently, for example, an atrial natriuretic factor (ANF) was isolated from the heart of rats. This atrial peptide probably plays a pivotal role in the pathophysiology of several disease states. Nevertheless, most endocrinologists probably would agree that not all animals have always been treated humanely and, in many cases, the numbers of animals used may have been in excess of the actual numbers needed. The past indiscretions are being remedied at most or all research centers.

Molecular biology has now provided a variety of nonanimal model systems wherein the actions of hormones can be studied in vitro using cell cultures [37]. Although these methods will not entirely supplement studies on living animals, they will provide some alternate, less intrusive, methods of study.

Perspectives

As in other subdisciplines of biology, endocrinological research faces some interesting ethical issues. Controversies regarding the use of embryonic stem cells or fetal tissues are similar to those of other bioethical debates, but with a novel twist because of the contested status of the fetus and abortion. Fetal tissue transplants hold great hope for many patients. Extensive work with animal models has shown that human fetal brain cells transplanted into the substantia nigra of monkeys with exogenously produced Parkinson's disease have had beneficial effects. Researchers think that the time has come for expanded clinical trials. Clinical trials, conducted either abroad or with private funding, have shown that fetal tissue implants can significantly improve the symptoms of Parkinson's disease in some individuals. Transplantation of fetal brain cells from 6- to 8-week-old fetuses into multiple sites on each side of the patient's brain resulted in an increase in brain dopamine production and, more importantly, symptoms were greatly reduced for a considerable period of time [31]. Experimental evidence is also strong that fetal islet cell transplants can restore normal insulin function in diabetics. And fetal thymus and liver transplants may have utility for blood and immune system disorders. Many other examples could be cited to document the urgent need of fetal tissues for use in clinical medicine. Unfortunately, "respect for the needs of such patients appears to conflict with respect for prenatal human life and larger societal concerns" [24]. More recently, many of the same hopes and concerns have arisen regarding the use of embryonic stem cells. These cells possess the capacity to be differentiated into any type of cell (totipotent), or at least a number of different types of cells (pluripotent). Embryonic stem cells are potentially derivable from thousands of unused, fertilized human eggs stored in the freezers of in vitro fertilization clinics. Advances in developmental cell biology have opened up a new frontier of biomedical science, in which these cells may be induced to differentiate into cells that may be capable of restoring specific tissue function in several devastating disease states. As of the writing of this edition of this textbook, the United States Congress is considering legislation to permit the use of federal funding for research with embryonic stem cell lines beyond the limited number that are currently approved. Regardless of the legislative outcome, concerns on the part of some citizens about the use of these cells makes it likely that the public debate on this issue will continue into the foreseeable future.

REVIEW EXERCISES

Compare and contrast each of the following terms. How are they related? How do they differ?

orchidectomy/ovariectomy
basophilic/acidophilic
atrophy/hyperplasia
immunoassay/
  radioimmunoassay
Northern blot/real-time PCR

teleost/cartilaginous
  (fishes)
hypertrophy/
  hyperplasic
unilateral/bilateral
immunocytochemistry/
  in situ hybridization
transgenesis/gene
  targeting

Define or characterize each of the following terms:

ectopic transplantation
axoplasmic transport (flow)
atrophy
sandwich assay
immunosympathectomy
reverse transcriptase PCR
Western blot
reporter construct
conditional gene targeting

binding protein
immunocytochemistry
glycoprotein
hormone analog
ion channel
immunohistofluorescence
transfection
gene knockout animal
stem cells

Think, analyze and discuss:

1. Short stature in children may occur as a normal inherited trait, or it may result from a clinically identifiable pathology or endocrine pathophysiology. Growth hormone deficiency (GHD) is an example of an endocrine pathophysiology in which the abnormally low secretion of GH can be the apparent cause of short stature in children. How would a clinical endocrinologist determine if serum levels of GH are abnormally low in a child with short stature? What method would he or she use to analyze GH levels in blood? What reagents would be required? How does the method work?

2. Estrogen (ER) and progesterone (PgR) receptors are prognostic factors in breast cancer. The expression of ERs and PgRs in breast cancer cells is also commonly analyzed to guide decisions regarding therapeutic options to pursue. What method would be used to characterize the cell-specific expression of the ER or PgR proteins in breast tumor tissue sections? Describe the procedure, and list the specific reagents and major equipment that would be required.

3. Gene targeting methods have been used to assess functional consequences of hormone receptor gene ablation, and to thereby clarify the functional roles of the targeted hormone receptor. The targeting of the receptor gene

is presumably accompanied by a loss of the receptor protein. In studies such as these, it is incumbent upon the investigator to demonstrate that the binding of hormone to the targeted receptor is indeed eliminated, or at least significantly diminished, in target tissues of the "gene knockout" animals.

  a. Describe a receptor binding assay method that could be used to measure the number and affinity of receptors in the wild-type (normal) animals and those in the receptor gene knockout animals. What reagents would be required? How would the receptor binding assay procedure be performed?

  b. Assume that you have performed the assay methods described in (a), on tissues from the wild-type and (homozygous) receptor gene knockout animals, as well as from a heterozygous group of animals in which the receptor numbers may only be partially reduced, but not eliminated by the disruption of only one allele of the receptor gene. For each of the three analyses, draw approximations of the saturation binding curves that you would expect to derive from the binding assays. Include total, specific, and non-specific binding curves for each. How would they differ among the three groups? Additionally, draw schematic representations of the Scatchard plots of each set of data on the same graph. How would they differ? How would they be similar?

4. The decline in estrogen levels in menopausal women is associated with increased risk of excessive bone demineralization, a condition commonly known as osteoporosis. Many investigators are attempting to understand where and how estrogen normally acts to protect the skeleton from bone demineralization, with the hope of developing new drug therapies for patients with osteoporosis.

  a. There are known to be two isoforms of the estrogen receptor, ERα and ERβ, that are encoded by separate genes. Which molecular methods could you use to determine the relative amounts of the respective receptor isoform mRNAs that are expressed in bone cells? Which method would you use to ascertain which specific types of bone cells, e.g. osteoblasts or osteoclasts, express the mRNAs encoding ERα or ERβ?

  b. Consider how you might investigate the effects of estrogen decline on bone mineralization in an experimental animal. What surgical method might be used to induce a loss of circulating estrogen in a female rat?

  c. Suppose you have available to you both a specific ERα agonist and a specific ERβ agonist. You wish to determine if one or the other, or both, of the ER isoforms is more important in mediating the effects of estrogen on bone density. Using the experimental animal model in (b), above, design an experiment in which you could use these new drugs to assess the relative involvement of the two receptors in mediating estrogen's protective effects on the skeleton.

5. Insulin activates the insulin receptor (IR) in hepatic cells, prompting it to become phosphorylated on key tyrosine residues. The receptor, in turn, is a tyrosine kinase that phosphorylates downstream signaling molecules, such as the insulin receptor substrate 1 (IRS1) protein, thereby activating this intracellular messenger. What method might you use to assess the degree of IR and IRS1 activation in cultures of hepatic cells? For your experiments, you have available to you a panel of monoclonal antibodies that recognize total IR, phosphotyrosine-IR, total IRS1, and phosphotyrosine-IRS1, respectively. Describe the method that you would use.

6. Anabolic steroid abuse has been anecdotally linked to a variety of pathophysiologies and behavioral disorders, but their molecular actions in the brain remain poorly understood. It is likely that these androgens, like other steroid hormones, exert their actions in the brain by simultaneously altering the expression of many different genes, and in several different parts of the brain.

  a. What method could be used to simultaneously identify genes whose expression levels are altered by testosterone in the brains of experimental animals? Describe the experimental method and technologies that might be used.

  b. If specific testosterone-responsive genes were identified by this method, then what methods could be used to specifically identify which brain cell populations exhibit testosterone-induced alterations in the expression of these genes?

References

[1] Aguzzi, A., et al. 1994. Transgenic and knockout mice: Models of neurological disease. *Brain Pathol.* 4:3–20.

[2] Beermann, W. 1973. Direct changes in the pattern of Balbiani ring puffing in *Chironomus:* Effects of sugar treatment. *Chromosoma* 4:297–326.

[3] Black, J. 1989. Drugs from emasculated hormones: The principle of syntropic antagonism. *In Vitro Cell. Develop. Biol.* 25:311–20.

[4] Bruning J. C., et al. 2000. Role of brain insulin receptor in control of body weight and reproduction. *Science* 289:2122–5.

[5] Burgoyne, R. D., and A. Morgan. 1993. Regulated exocytosis. *Biochem. J.* 293:305–16.

[6] Camp, P., et al. 1992. Gene expression of peptidergic signals: Effects of steroids. *Neuroprotocols* 1:67–76.

[7] Chirguin, J. M. 1990. Molecular biology for nonmolecular biologists. *Diabetes Care* 13:188–97.

[8] Davis, J. R. E. 1996. Molecular biology techniques in endocrinology. *Clin. Endocrinol.* 45:125–33.

[9] Fukamizu, A. 1993. Transgenic animals in endocrinological investigation. *J. Endocrinol. Invest.* 16:461–73.

[10] Gilman, A. G., L. S. Goodman, and A. Gilman. 1990. *Goodman and Gilman's the pharmacological basis of therapeutics.* New York: Macmillan.

[11] Hoffman, G. E., M. S. Smith, and J. G. Verbalis. 1993. c-Fos and related immediate early gene products as markers of activity in neuroendocrine systems. *Front. Neuroendocrinol.* 14:173–213.

[12] Holzwarth, M. A., J. R. Sladek, Jr., and K. M. Knigge. 1976. Monosodium glutamate induced lesions of the arcuate nucleus. *Anat. Rec.* 186:197–205.

[13] Kudlow, J. E. 2002. Transgenic animal models of pituitary function. In: J. D. Baxter, S. Melmed, and M. I. New, eds. *Genetics in endocrinology.* Modern Endocrinology Series (L. Martini, series ed.).– Philadelphia: Lippincott Williams & Wilkins, pp. 27–36.

[14] Leblond, C. P. 1991. Time dimension in cell biology. A radioautographic survey of the dynamic features of cells, cell components, and extracellular matrix. *Protoplasma* 160:5–38.

[15] McCabe, J. T., et al. 1986. *Front. Neuroendocrinol.* 9:149–67.

[16] Millar, S. E., et al. 1989. Vaccination with a synthetic zona pellucida peptide produces long-term contraception in female mice. *Science* 246:935–8.

[17] Mumby, M. E., et al. 1985. Monoclonal antibodies as probes of structure, function and isoenzyme forms of the type II regulatory subunit of cyclic AMP-dependent protein kinase. *Pharmacol. Ther.* 28:367–87.

[18] Palmiter, R. D., et al. 1982. Dramatic growth of mice that develop from eggs microinjected with metallotionein–growth hormone fusion genes. *Nature* 300:611–15.

[19] Parmentier, M., et al. 1989. Molecular cloning of the thyrotropin receptor. *Science* 246:1620–2.

[20] Powers, D. A. 1989. Fish as model systems. *Science* 246:352–8.

[21] Prediger, E. A. 2001. Detection and quantitation of mRNAs using ribonuclease protection assays. *Methods Mol Biol.* 160:495–505.

[22] Reventós, J., and F. Munell. 1997. Transgenic animal models in reproductive endocrine research. *Eur. J. Endocrinol.* 136:566–80.

[23] Riggs, A. D., et al. 1980. Synthesis, cloning, and expression of hormone genes in *Escherichia coli. Rec. Prog. Horm. Res.* 36:261–76.

[24] Robertson, J. A. 1988. Rights, symbolism, and public policy in fetal tissue transplants. *Hastings Ctr. Rpt.* 5–12.

[25] Shizume, K., A. B. Lerner, and T. B. Fitzpatrick. 1954. In vitro bioassay for melanocyte stimulating hormone. *Endocrinology* 54:553–60.

[26] Simonsen, H., and H. F. Lodish. 1994. Cloning by function: expression cloning in mammalian cells. *Trends Pharmacol. Sci.* 15:437–41.

[27] Soulet, D., and S. Rivest. 2002. Perspective: how to make microarray, serial analysis of gene expression, and proteomic relevant to day-to-day endocrine problems and physiological systems. *Endocrinology* 143:1995–2001.

[28] Spergel, D. J., et al. 2001. Using reporter genes to label. selected neuronal populations in transgenic mice for gene promoter, anatomical, and physiological studies. *Prog. Neurobiol.* 63(6):673–86.

[29] Spicer, S. S. 1993. Advantages of histochemistry for the study of cell biology. *Histochem. J.* 26:531–47.

[30] Theoharides, T. C., and W. W. Douglas. 1978. Secretion in mast cells induced by calcium entrapped within phospholipid vesicles. *Science* 201:1143–5.

[31] Thompson, L. 1992. Fetal transplants show promise. *Science* 257:868–70.

[32] Tong, Y., et al. 1990. Glucocorticoid regulation of proopiomelanocortin mRNA levels in rat arcuate nucleus. *Mol. Cell. Neurosci.* 1:78–83.

[33] Trayhurn, P. 1996. Northern blotting. *Proc. Nutr. Soc.* 55:583–9.

[34] Wall, R. J., D. E. Kerr, and K. R. Bondioli. 1997. Transgenic dairy cattle: Genetic engineering on a large scale. *J. Dairy Sci.* 80:2213–24.

[35] Wall, R. J., et al. 1997. Transgenic animal technology. *J. Androl.* 18:236–9.

[36] Warembourg, M. 1976. Detection of diffusible substances. *J. de Microscopie et de Biologie Cellulaire* 27:277–80.

[37] Weiss, J., and J. L. Jameson. 1993. Perifused pituitary cells as a model for studies of gonadotropin biosynthesis and secretion. *TEM* 4:265–70.

[38] Wilcox, J. N. 1993. Fundamentals of in situ hybridization. *J. Histochem. Cytochem.* 41:1725–33.

[39] Woodruff, T. K. 1998. Cellular localization of mRNA and protein: in situ hybridization histochemistry and in situ ligand binding. *Methods Cell Biol.* 57:333–51.

[40] Yalow, R. S. 1978. Radioimmunoassay: A probe for the fine structure of biologic systems. *Science* 200:1236–45.

[41] Zhang, Y., et al. 1994. Positional cloning of the mouse obese gene and its human homologue. *Nature* 372:425–32.

CHAPTER 5

Pituitary Hormones

The pituitary has often been referred to as the master endocrine gland of vertebrates. This perceived importance may have arisen because the pituitary is located near the brain and controls such important endocrine glands as the adrenals, thyroid, and the gonads. The pituitary gland is now known to be subservient to hormonal stimuli derived from the brain and other endocrine glands [3]. Indeed, in many ways it can be regarded as relaying and amplifying signals originating from the overlying brain tissue, i.e., the hypothalamus.

The pituitary gland of the human male is somewhat smaller than the tip of the little finger and weighs between 0.5 and 1.0 g; its size in the human female becomes larger during pregnancy. The pituitary is recessed within the sella turcica of the sphenoid bone, beneath the hypothalamus near the optic chiasm. In this position, the pituitary is one of the most inaccessible of the mammalian endocrine glands. Early anatomists considered the pituitary to be a part of the brain and, in fact, the gland does possess a neural component.

In 1886, Marie, a French physician, made an important observation that acromegaly often occurred along with a tumorous condition of the pituitary [13]. Other physicians noted that the pituitary gland of the male and the female often became enlarged following gonadectomy. Cushing, an English physician, was the first to note the association between tumors of the pituitary and the resultant disease that bears his name. Cushing showed in 1909 that partial removal of the anterior pituitary of an acromegalic patient resulted in rapid recovery. Much later, it was established that pituitarigenic Cushing's disease was associated with elevated secretion of corticotropin.

Smith noted that hypophysectomy (removal of the pituitary gland) in the rat resulted in complete stasis of growth and a rapid regression of the size of the adrenals (mainly the steroidogenic cortex), the thyroid, and the gonads [13]. Ablation of the posterior lobe of the pituitary alone failed to produce these effects. Smith also observed that daily intramuscular injections of fresh rat or bovine anterior pituitary homogenates into hypophysectomized rats brought about a nearly normal growth rate. In addition, this replacement therapy caused a partial restoration of the size of the adrenals, thyroid, and gonads. Evans and Long noted that extracts of bovine pituitaries enhanced the growth rate of intact rats over that of their littermates [13]. Treatment of rats with such extracts for 9 months or more resulted in the production of experimental gigantism. This exaggerated increase in growth was due to generalized overgrowth of the skeleton and to an enlargement of most tissues and organs. These results provided experimental evidence for the existence of a growth hormone (somatotropin) of hypophysial origin.

Smith and Allen, working independently, demonstrated that growth and metamorphosis of larval amphibians (frog tadpoles) were prevented by removal of the structure that gives rise to the anterior pituitary [13]. The larval animals were also light in color compared to normal intact tadpoles. These early experiments provided evidence for the existence of a pituitary thyroid-stimulating hormone and a melanocyte-stimulating *hormone (MSH). Subsequently, other researchers provided evidence for the existence of other pituitary hormones regulating adrenal and gonadal function and numerous other physiological processes. This chapter will discuss the nature and endocrine role of the pituitary hormones.*

Anatomy of the Pituitary Gland

The pituitary gland (also known as the hypophysis) is composed of tissues that are derived from two diverse origins [12]. An understanding of the origin and development of the pituitary is critical to an understanding of the structure–function relationships of this endocrine gland. Early anatomists believed that the structural components of the pituitary (from the Latin *pituita*, or phlegm) gland were concerned with the removal of phlegm or mucus from the cavities of the brain. The comparative anatomy of the pituitary of many vertebrates has been reviewed in an important monograph by Holmes and Ball [16]. The ultrastructural characteristics of the anterior pituitary cells have been described in detail elsewhere [10].

The Adenohypophysis and Neurohypophysis have Separate Embryonic Origins

The human pituitary is composed of the *adenohypophysis*, alternatively referred to as the *anterior lobe*, and the *neurohypophysis*, also called the *posterior lobe* (Fig. 5.1). The adenohypophysis is primarily glandular tissue, while the neurohypophysis consists of neuronal processes that originate from neurons in the hypothalamus. The embryological origins of the adenohypophysis and neurohypophysis are distinct. The former derives from an inward invagination of the oral ectoderm of the stomodeum (primitive mouth cavity) known as Rathke's pouch (Fig. 5.2). The neuronal component arises from the neural ectoderm of the floor of the forebrain. Rathke's pouch elongates and becomes constricted at its attachment to the oral epithelium. A remnant of the connection between Rathke's pouch and the stomodeal ectoderm may persist as a "pharyngeal" pituitary. An infundibular (funnel-shaped) process develops as a diverticulum (pouch) of the floor of the diencephalon. The infundibulum increases in size because of neuroepithelial cell proliferation. Nerve fibers grow into the infundibulum from hypothalamic nuclei. The neuroepithelial cells then differentiate into *pituicytes* (neuroglial-like elements), which are dispersed between the neuronal endings within the infundibulum.

Cells of the anterior wall of Rathke's pouch proliferate to give rise to the pars distalis [10]. Continued proliferation of these cells leads to reduction of the lumen of Rathke's pouch to a *residual cleft* and a separation of the cells of the posterior wall from the anterior pituitary. Those cells adjacent to the infundibulum may proliferate to give rise to a pars intermedia of considerable size in some species. Failure of the adenohypophysis to contact the developing neurohypophysis results in the inability of the pituitary cells to form a pars intermedia. In birds, the adenohypophysis is separated from the neurohypophysis by a layer of connective tissue and a pars intermedia does not develop. In humans, the fetal pars intermedia regresses and is absent in the adult (Chap. 8). Dorsal extensions of the anterior pituitary surround the infundibular stalk to give rise to the *pars tuberalis*, which provides the anatomical link between the pars distalis and the hypothalamus. The definitive pituitary in many species consists of the pars distalis, the pars intermedia, the pars tuberalis, and the pars nervosa (Fig. 5.3). The intimate anatomical relationship between the pituitary gland and the overlying brain provides an important clue to understanding the essential functional relationship of the components of the brain–pituitary axis [9, 10, 14, 17].

The major endocrine cell types of the adenohypophysis emerge in a temporally and spatially specific manner during development. In recent years, the molecular mechanisms that determine pituitary cell fate have been studied intensely [23], and many of the key signals that guide cell proliferation, placement, and differentiation have been elucidated. It is clear

Pituitary Gland (Hypophysis)

Adenohypophysis
 Pars Distalis ----------- Anterior Lobe
 Pars Tuberalis
 Pars Intermedia --------- Intermediate Lobe
                                              Neurointermediate Lobe
Neurohypophysis
 Pars Nervosa ------------ Posterior Lobe
 Infundibulum

Figure 5.1 Anatomical components of the pituitary gland.

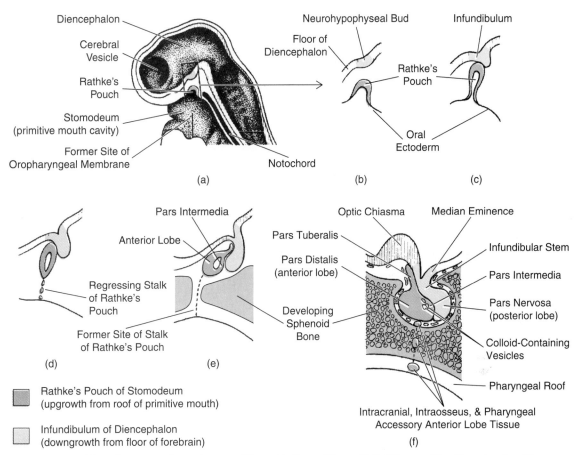

Figure 5.2 Developmental anatomy of the pituitary. (From K. L. Moore, *The Developing Human, Clinically Oriented Embryology*, 2nd edn, 1977. Courtesy of W. B. Saunders Company.)

that molecular cues elaborated by the developing ventral diencephalon and oral ectoderm are required for proper pituitary organogenesis. All of these factors appear to be produced in specific gradients in the extracellular environment of the developing Rathke's pouch, and the presence of a given cell at a given point among these gradients dictates its fate in the nascent pituitary. These extracellular growth signal gradients induce the expression of specific sets of intracellular transcription factors in the developing pituitary cells, and these, in turn, activate specific genetic programs for differentiation into one of the six endocrine cell phenotypes. Many of the transcription factors known to be important in cell type

Figure 5.3 The pituitary gland of humans. In the adult human, unlike most mammals, the pars intermedia is absent. (From R. Guillemin and R. Burgus, "The hormones of the hypothalamus," with permission [14]. ©1972 by Scientific American, Inc. All rights reserved.)

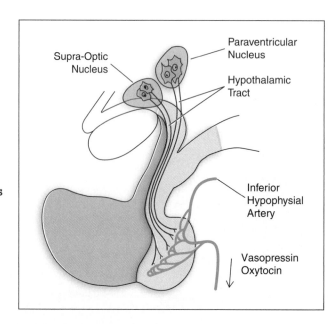

Figure 5.4 Vascular connections between the pituitary gland and the hypothalamus [14]. (From R. Guillemin and R. Burgus, "The hormones of the hypothalamus," with permission [14]. ©1972 by Scientific American, Inc. All rights reserved.)

determination are among the families of structurally related *homeodomain* protein regulators that operate as developmental signals in a variety of tissues.

Lobation, Vascularization, and Innervation of the Pituitary can Differ among Species

The size of each lobe of the pituitary gland varies between different species, and may be related to the particular environmental niche occupied by the species [12]. Animals that rapidly change color may possess a relatively large pars intermedia; the pars nervosa of aquatic species may be small, but relatively large in land-dwelling species, particularly those inhabiting arid climates. These size differences in pituitary gland components reflect the hormonal output of the glands required for successful adaptation to a particular habitat.

The pituitary gland receives its blood supply from the superior and inferior hypophysial arteries. The anterior and posterior branches of the superior hypophysial artery penetrate the hypophysial stalk, as well as the hypothalamus (Fig. 5.4). The pars distalis is vascularized by *hypophysial portal vessels* that arise from the capillary beds within the median eminence of the hypothalamus. This hypophysial portal vessel system provides the link for carrying hormonal information from the central nervous system (CNS) to the pituitary (Chap. 6). Whether the anterior lobe receives blood exclusively from the portal circulation, or whether some additional direct arterial blood supply is available, is unresolved. The pars nervosa receives a separate blood supply from the inferior hypophysial artery (Fig. 5.5). The pars

Figure 5.5 Neural components of the pituitary gland of humans [14]. (From R. Guillemin and R. Burgus, "The hormones of the hypothalamus," with permission [14]. © 1972 by Scientific American, Inc. All rights reserved.)

intermedia, if present, is relatively avascular. Physiologists have generally assumed that all hormones produced by the adenohypophysis are released directly into the efferent portal veins to be carried through the systemic circulation to distant target tissues. There is evidence that some adenohypophysial venous blood may be shunted to the neurohypophysis [3]. This circular path of blood flow may permit adenohypophysial venous blood to be carried up the infundibular process to the brain. This observation carries the important implication that pituitary hormones might be able to modify CNS function.

Except for neurovascular elements, there is no evidence that neurons innervate or otherwise directly influence the cell activity of the pars distalis of humans or most other mammals. Neuronal elements may affect cellular hormone secretion within the pars distalis of some teleost fishes. The cells of the pars intermedia of amphibians and some mammals are surrounded by a plexus of catecholaminergic neurons that regulate MSH secretion from the melanotrophs (MSH-secreting cells). Such a direct neuronal innervation is absent from the pars intermedia of some reptiles. The pars nervosa is composed of axonal endings of neurons whose cell bodies are located in hypothalamic nuclei. In mammals, these are the *paraventricular* and *supraoptic* nuclei (Fig. 5.5).

The gross morphology of the pituitary differs considerably between the vertebrate classes and often between species of the same class. At the cytological level the individual cell types may be intermingled to varying degrees (as in tetrapods) or separated into zones (as in most teleost fishes). There is no distinct neural lobe in fishes. The neural lobe is, however, characteristic of tetrapods, and this may be related to the terrestrial manner of life of these vertebrates, where one or both neurohypophysial hormones may be of adaptive importance (see Fig. 8.2). The size of the pars intermedia varies considerably between species, and all birds lack a pars intermedia. This is not a unique feature, as the pars intermedia is not present in some mammals (elephants, whales, adult humans).

Cytological Methods Distinguish Different Pituitary Cell Types

Histochemical and immunocytochemical methods have provided definitive information on the specific cellular sources of each pituitary peptide hormone [28]. The cells of the pars distalis have been differentiated into somatotrophs, lactotrophs (mammotrophs), corticotrophs, thyrotrophs, and gonadotrophs [22]. These terms relate to the particular hormonal product synthesized by each of these cells. The individual cell types are also referred to as *acidophils*, *basophils*, or *chromophobes*, depending on their affinity for certain dyes used in histological stains (Table 5.1). Somatotrophs and lactotrophs are acidophils, whereas the thyrotrophs and gonadotrophs are basophils. The corticotrophs are basophils but are often referred to as chromophobes. The cells of the mammalian pars intermedia are also considered to be chromophobes. The extent to which a cell exhibits acidophilia, basophilia, or chromophobia may depend on the granular content (hormone-containing vesicles) of the cell, which often varies with the temporal secretory activity of the cell. These secretory vesicles may become depleted after continued secretory activity of the cells; in contrast, these granules may accumulate, at least transiently, if the cells stop releasing hormone. Granule synthesis may eventually decline if the cell is no longer stimulated to secrete its hormonal product. Except for the sparse pituicytes (glial-like cells), the pars nervosa contains only neuronal axonal endings.

Nongranulated, presumably nonsecretory cells are also present in the pars distalis, pars intermedia, and neurohypophysis. These elements have been referred to as glial cells,

TABLE 5.1   Histochemical classification of pituitary pars distalis cells

Cell Type	Hormone		Staining Characteristic
Corticotroph[a]	Corticotropin	(ACTH)	Basophil
Thyrotroph	Thyrotropin	(TSH)	Basophil
Gonadotroph			
FSH-gonadotroph	Follitropin	(FSH)	Basophil
LH-gonadotroph	Lutropin	(LH)	Basophil
Lactotroph (mammotroph)	Prolactin	(PRL)	Acidophil
Somatotroph	Growth hormone	(GH)	Acidophil

[a]Cytological classification uses either the suffix -troph or -trope (e.g., corticotrope).

glial-like cells, stellate cells, and follicular cells. The processes of these cells often separate one pituitary cell from contact with another. In some species, they may form the lining of minute ductules or follicles within the adenohypophysis. A variety of putative functions have been suggested for these cells, and it is possible that they modulate pituitary hormone secretion in response to regulatory cues [24].

Although each of the pituitary hormones is localized to a particular cell type, as determined by ultrastructural and immunocytochemical analysis, most gonadotrophs (human, rat, quail, frog) contain both of the gonadotropic hormones, lutropin and follitropin (see below). Nevertheless, subpopulations of gonadotrophs contain only one of the gonadotropins. This may contribute to the nonparallel release of gonadotropins in response to certain stimuli (see Fig. 18.11). Individual gonadotrophs vary in their staining intensity for labeled antibodies to each of the gonadotropins, suggesting that gonadotrophs may represent a fluid, heterogeneous population of cells capable of synthesizing and storing both or one of the hormones. Immunocytochemical observations have revealed that all cell types of the pars distalis are present within the pars tuberalis of the human and monkey. The hormonal function of the pars distalis therefore may be augmented by secretory contributions from the pars tuberalis.

Hormones of the Pituitary

A number of peptide hormones are produced by the pituitary. These hormones regulate such target organs as the gonads, the adrenals, and the thyroid gland. The mammary glands, uterus, kidneys, and other tissues are also controlled by hypophysial hormones. Two gonadotropins are present: *follicle-stimulating hormone* (FSH), or *follitropin*, and *luteinizing hormone* (LH), or *lutropin*. A *thyroid-stimulating hormone* (TSH), or *thyrotropin*, regulates thyroid activity, and an *adrenal cortical-stimulating hormone* (ACTH), or *adrenocorticotropin (corticotropin)*, regulates adrenal activity. A *growth hormone* (GH), which has generalized growth-promoting effects, and a *prolactin* (PRL), which has more specific growth-promoting action on the mammary glands, are also present in some species. A melanocyte-stimulating hormone (α-MSH, α-melanotropin) is produced by cells of the pars intermedia, or possibly by cells within the pars distalis (of birds). The neurohypophysial hormones, *oxytocin* and the *vasopressin,* are elaborated within neurons of the neurohypophysis, whose cell bodies originate within the hypothalamus. A melanin-concentrating hormone (MCH) is also present within the neurohypophysis of teleost fishes [5] (see Chap. 8). The pituitary hormones are released into the bloodstream where they circulate to interact with their cells of target organs.

Pituitary Hormones can be Grouped into Families of Structurally Related Proteins

The hormones of the pituitary can be classified into four groups based on their structural similarity and presumed evolutionary origin: (1) Growth hormone and prolactin possess numerous similar sequences of amino acids within their individual structures, and they are also structurally related to placental lactogen. (2) Thyrotropin, follitropin, and lutropin are glycoproteins and are related in structure to each other and to chorionic gonadotropin (choriogonadotropin, CG), a hormone of placental origin. (3) α-Melanotropin and corticotropin contain a sequence of amino acids in common, which accounts for their overlapping actions and suggests a related evolutionary origin. (4) The two neurohypophysial hormones, oxytocin and vasopressin, are present in the neurohypophysis, and they are structurally related to each other.

Growth Hormone and Prolactin are Structurally Related Hormones that Stimulate Growth and Development

These hormones of the pituitary exert profound effects on body growth. In the young animal, GH plays an essential role in general body growth, whereas PRL stimulates the growth of specialized tissues such as the mammary gland during pregnancy and lactation.

Growth Hormone.   The existence of a hormone that is responsible for general somatic growth was suggested by the early experiments of Evans and Long (1922) and Smith (1926) [13]. Hypophysectomized young rats failed to grow to adult size, but extracts of the pituitary stimulated growth in these rats and in rats of normal growth. Human GH is also effective in promoting linear growth in children with congenital GH deficiency. In young animals, the epiphyses of the long bones are separated from the shaft of the bones by an epiphyseal cartilaginous plate. Chondrogenesis is accelerated by GH, which results in a widening of the epiphyseal plates as more extracellular matrix (chondroitin sulfate) is synthesized and released by chondrocytes. This widening has been used as a bioassay for GH (tibia test).

Growth hormone accounts for 4% to 10% of the wet weight of the anterior pituitary in the human adult (5 to 10 mg per gland). GH circulates in the plasma complexed to one or more binding proteins, and basal (resting or nonstressed) levels of immunoassayable GH in the plasma range from 1 to 5 ng per milliliter. The circulating levels of the hormone decline during the first 2 or 3 weeks after birth to then reach the basal levels characteristic of the adult human. Age-related changes in total 24-hour secretion of GH have been described. Although GH levels remain rather constant during the period of accelerated growth in early childhood, there is an appreciable increase during the period of maximal growth in adolescence. Interestingly, a substantial part of the 24-hour secretion of GH occurs during the first 90 minutes of nocturnal sleep. In every mammalian species studied so far, spontaneous episodes of GH secretion occur several times over a 24-hour period. Particularly in the rat, GH release follows a rhythm with high-amplitude GH secretory bursts occurring at regular 3.3-hour intervals. In the intervening trough periods, basal plasma GH levels are undetectable. Both a hypothalamic growth hormone-releasing hormone (GHRH/somatocrinin), as well as a GH release-inhibiting factor (somatostatin, SST) control GH secretion (Chap. 6).

Growth hormone is a polypeptide synthesized by somatotrophs of the pars distalis. GH is derived from a prohormone in the pituitary cells but is rapidly converted to GH by proteolysis. The human hormone consists of 191 amino acids with two intramolecular disulfide bonds. The hormone is strikingly similar in structure to PRL and placental lactogen (PL). The latter molecule also contains 191 amino acids and possesses S–S bonds in exactly the same locations as in GH; in 161 positions, the amino acids are identical. The structural homologies between GH, PRL, and PL suggest a single progenitor molecule that arose early in vertebrate evolution (see Fig 12.12).

Growth hormone is an anabolic hormone that enhances amino acid incorporation into muscle protein and stimulates extracellular collagen deposition (Chap. 12). Thus, it produces a positive nitrogen and phosphorus balance and a concomitant fall in blood urea nitrogen and amino acid levels. Urinary excretion of Na^+ and K^+ is also decreased, probably due to the increased uptake of these ions by growing tissue. These effects of GH on protein metabolism and electrolyte balance are mediated indirectly through the actions of *somatomedins* released from the liver in response to GH stimulation of hepatocytes. These somatomedins (insulin-like growth factors, IGFs) stimulate cellular growth in a variety of tissues and organs (see Fig. 12.2). In addition to the growth-promoting effects of somatomedins, GH itself has direct anti-insulin effects on metabolism.

The absence of GH secretion leads to short stature in the young child, whereas overproduction of GH during early postnatal development leads to gigantism. In the adult, excess GH secretion leads to acromegaly. Short stature may result from a pituitary failure of GH production (hypopituitary short stature) or from a failure of the liver to respond to GH and synthesize somatomedins (Laron syndrome). The pathogenesis of acromegaly has been explained by either a "pituitary" or a hypothalamic mechanism. In the former view, overproduction of GH may result from GH-secreting tumors of the adenohypophysis (intrasellar tumors). The hypothalamic hypothesis implicates the defect as residing within the central nervous system, possibly from an overproduction of GHRH or an underproduction of somatostatin. The secretion of either of these hypophysiotropic factors is controlled by other neural inputs (e.g., dopaminergic neurons) that may contribute indirectly to the etiology of acromegaly. Nevertheless, the vast majority of patients with acromegaly have identifiable pituitary tumors, but whether these tumors arise from long-term overstimulation by the hypothalamus or are independent of hypothalamic influence, possibly due to cellular mutagenesis of somatotrophs or a related stem cell, is still unclear [18, 19].

The acromegalic characteristics of GH overproduction probably result from the direct effects of GH on target tissues, as well as growth effects mediated through the somatomedins. The growth changes in bones and soft tissues are most noticeable in the hands, feet, and face. Proliferation of connective tissue and interstitial fluid results in thickening of the skin and in an increase in subcutaneous tissues. The viscera and related organs, the lungs, liver, heart, and kidneys, are usually enlarged. Individuals with acromegaly may display increased metabolic rates, and the lipolytic actions of GH on adipose tissue combined with anti-insulin actions on other tissues result in hyperglycemia as a symptom of a developing diabetes mellitus.

The etiology of GH deficiency may also relate to a pituitary or hypothalamic dysfunction. Intrasellar tumors or other destructive processes, as well as familial (genetic) or congenital (birth) defects, may result in a lack of GH production that could lead to short stature if initiated at a young age. Lack of GH secretion may be accompanied by a total lack of pituitary hormone production (panhypopituitarism) or may be an example of an isolated GH deficiency of unknown etiology. Short stature may also result from pituitary deficiency secondary to hypothalamic dysfunction, possibly related to an absence of GHRH. Suprasellar (CNS) lesions may also result in GH deficiency, and there are even examples of psychosocial short stature. GH of mammalian origin is active in many species, but human subjects are responsive only to human or primate GH. However, GH has become available commercially for the treatment of short stature by gene-splicing techniques within bacteria (Chap 12).

Prolactin.   Mammary growth and development and lactogenesis in the human female are regulated, in part, by a lactotropic hormone from the pituitary [2]. Prolactin plays diverse roles in other vertebrates. In fact, no other known peptide hormone has such a repertoire of biological actions. Because the varied effects of this hormone usually bear some relationship to physiological responses essential for reproductive success, PRL has been referred to as the "hormone of maternity." Roles for PRL in the male and nonpregnant female been recognized (Chaps 17 and 18).

In 1928, Stricker and Grueter discovered that an extract of the anterior pituitary gland could stimulate milk secretion in rabbits. The control of mammary gland development and the stimulation of milk synthesis are complex processes that involve the participation of many hormones. The mammotropic action of PRL requires the participation of several hormones, which, in some species, include estrogens, insulin, glucocorticoids, progesterone, and GH. The direct action of PRL on the mammary gland was shown in ovariectomized rabbits first given estrogen and progesterone to produce lobuloalveolar growth (Chap. 19). When PRL was injected into the individual ducts of the mammary gland, only the alveoli connected to the injected duct produced milk. Riddle, Bates, and Dykshorn discovered that a specific fraction of bovine pituitary extracts, which they named prolactin, stimulated crop sac growth in pigeons [21].

During pregnancy or in the postpartum lactational period prolactin cells comprise as much as 50% of the acidophil population of the pituitary. Production of PRL by lactotrophs in the pituitary is affected by estrogens, and during pregnancy and lactation serum PRL levels rise substantially. Estrogens stimulate PRL secretion by the anterior pituitary gland and stimulate PRL synthesis by a direct effect on PRL gene transcription. Estrogens increase mitotic activity and cell number of pituitary lactotrophs. Hyperprolactinemia and PRL-secreting pituitary tumors are relatively common in women of reproductive age, and this has raised the question of the role of endogenous estrogens in their pathogenesis.

Serum PRL levels increase at puberty, but only modestly compared to the rise in FSH and LH concentrations that also occur. Estrogen infusions are stimulatory to PRL secretion, which may explain the increase in PRL secretion at puberty, a time when ovarian steroid biosynthesis is enhanced. During pregnancy, there is a progressive increase in serum PRL concentrations reaching maximal values at term. In mothers who do not nurse their young, the postpartum concentrations of PRL rapidly fall back to normal by 3 weeks, unless breast-feeding is commenced. Concentrations of PRL in the amniotic fluid exceed those in the maternal or fetal circulation early in pregnancy and at term. By biological, chemical, and immunological criteria, human amniotic fluid PRL is similar or identical to that of the pituitary hormone. The chorion-decidua may be the source of amniotic prolactin, but the possible physiological function, if any, of the placental PRL is unknown.

PRL is luteotropic in some mammalian species, and it may act in concert with LH or FSH on the corpus luteum to stimulate progesterone biosynthesis and secretion. Progesterone production by the ovarian corpus luteum is required for growth and development of the uterus and for suppression of further ovum maturation and ovulation (Chap. 19). PRL has a profound effect on the growth, differentiation, and function of a number of integumental structures: hair and sebaceous glands in mammals; brood patch and feather development in certain birds; epidermal sloughing in lizards; and integumental mucous gland secretion in certain teleosts. Because the mammary gland is an integumental derivative and is considered to be phylogenetically related to sweat glands, one may conclude that the highly specialized mammotropic action of PRL in humans and most mammals may have evolved from the more generalized action of PRL on a variety of integumentary functions.

In certain birds (pigeons and doves), PRL controls the production of a so-called crop sac "milk." In response to PRL, the epithelium of the two lateral lobes of the crop wall thickens in both the male and the female at the time the eggs are hatched. The epithelium proliferates, and the cells accumulate lipid and begin to degenerate. The layers of cells are sloughed off to form a mass of material that is regurgitated to feed the young birds. Besides its effect on the integument, PRL controls many other physiological processes. Considering its versatility, the name given to the hormone, prolactin, is obviously restrictive and only refers to one of its many roles.

Although the major role of PRL in humans is the control of lactation, evidence suggests that PRL may control testicular function, at least in some rodents. Hypophysectomy of adult rats causes a loss of testicular LH receptors and this, as expected, is associated with a loss in testicular responsiveness to LH. Inhibition of LH or FSH secretion from the pituitary is not, however, associated with a loss of LH receptors. Inhibition of pituitary PRL release, on the other hand, is associated with a loss of testicular LH receptors. Thus, PRL may be essential for the maintenance of LH receptors. This view is substantiated by the observation that PRL treatment increases LH receptor number in the gonads of dwarf male mice and in atrophic testes of light-deprived hamsters (Chap. 20). Prolactin also stimulates growth of the testosterone-stimulated prostate gland of the castrated rat.

Plasma levels of PRL in humans are slightly higher in females than males, although there is considerable overlap of the ranges of PRL concentration in the two sexes. PRL is secreted episodically and has a half-life in the blood of about 15 to 20 minutes. There is a nighttime surge of PRL secretion, which, like GH, is associated with sleep (Fig. 5.6). The times of onset and duration of the PRL peak are not identical to those of GH. The most potent stimulus to PRL secretion is nursing. Release of the hormone is mediated by cutaneous sensations arising from the breast and nipple, not by psychic factors associated with the presence of the infant. Breast stimulation of the human male has no effect on PRL release. Secretion of PRL from the pituitary is controlled by PRL-inhibiting factors (PIFs), and the major PIF is known to be dopamine, which is primarily elaborated by a set of tuberoinfundibular dopaminergic neurons. This inhibitory control is somehow diminished during late pregnancy and lactation. The existence of PRL-releasing factor has been suggested in mammals, and PRL secretion in birds is mainly under a stimulatory control (Chap. 6).

PRL is a single-chain polypeptide of 23 kDa composed of three intramolecular disulfide bridges and N-linked glycosylation sites. The 60% to 100% sequence homology of PRL between animal species reflects their phylogenetic relationship. Many structural variants (isoforms) of PRL are known and may arise by differential splicing. Glycosylated PRL is found in the pituitary and plasma. The carbohydrate moieties vary among species, and this heterogeneity accounts for differences in bio-activity [25].

Although PRL and GH share structural similarity, their physiological actions in humans are discrete. Acromegalic patients with elevated GH levels only occasionally develop galactorrhea; individuals with galactorrhea or women who are breast-feeding have normal serum

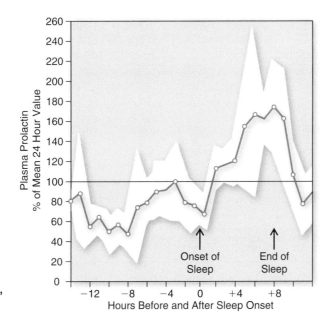

Figure 5.6 Human plasma levels of PRL during a 24-hour period [11]. (Reprinted by permission of *The New England Journal of Medicine*, Frantz, A. G. "Prolactin," vol. 298, pp. 201–207, 1978.)

GH concentrations. Some patients with a hereditary form of isolated GH deficiency lactate normally, although GH is absent.

Luteinizing Hormone, Follicle-Stimulating Hormone, and Thyrotropin are Glycoprotein Hormones

Three hormones of the anterior pituitary are glycoproteins [27], containing up to 33% carbohydrate by weight. Thyrotropin (TSH), follicle-stimulating hormone (FSH), and luteinizing hormone (LH) contain covalently bound carbohydrate moieties at one or more positions within their structures [15]. Each of these pituitary glycoproteins is composed of two chains, so-called α and β subunits. The α subunits of the three pituitary glycoproteins within a species are identical to each other, whereas the β subunit of each hormone is structurally distinct [4]. The α subunit consists of a polypeptide of 92 residues in humans and 96 residues in the other mammalian species studied. Although α subunits exhibit identical amino acid sequences in a given species, their N-linked oligosaccharide chains are generally different. Seventy-one of the 96 positions are occupied by the same amino acid residue in most mammals. Ten of the half-cystine residues of these molecules are conserved, which suggests that the five disulfide bridges are likely to be identical, thus leading to a common conformation in all α subunits. This hypothesis is strengthened by the observation that hybrid heterodimers can be obtained with α and β subunits from different species.

Although related in structure, the β subunits exhibit different amino acid sequences within and between species. The β subunits are composed of 110–111 residues (LHs), 112–118 residues (TSHs), 117–121 residues (LHs), or 145 residues (human chorionic gonadotropin; hCG). Each subunit possesses 12 Cys residues at highly conserved positions among species. The six disulfide bridges within the β subunits probably result in similar overall three-dimensional structures. Amino acid sequences that are identical in the glycoprotein β subunits represent intersubunit contact sites, whereas the nonidentical residues contribute to interaction with target tissue receptors and therefore provide hormonal specificity. The α and β subunits of the glycoprotein hormones are independently synthesized; some pituitary tumors, for example, exhibit isolated or unbalanced α-subunit secretion. Also, isolated or unbalanced ectopic secretion of α or β subunits of choriogonadotropin by malignant uterine neoplasms has been noted. Two separate mRNA species have been identified from mouse thyrotropic tumors, each coding for a different subunit of the hormone. A single gene per haploid DNA complement codes for the α subunits of the glycoprotein family of hormones in any one species. The peptide component of the glycoproteins is first synthesized under direct genetic control. Glycosylation, the attachment of carbohydrate moieties, is a postribosomal event controlled by glycosyltransferase enzymes localized in the Golgi cisternae of the cells.

The constituent sugars of glycoprotein hormones are D-mannose, D-galactose, L-fructose, N-acetylneuraminic acid, D-glucosamine, and N-acetylated D-galactosamine. All α subunits contain two oligosaccharides that are N-linked to asparagines. All pituitary glycoprotein hormones may contain O-sulfated (attached through serine to the peptide chain) hexosamines. The carbohydrate moieties of the α subunit in the gonadotropic hormones are important for biological function. Their specific removal, without affecting the polypeptide primary structure, causes an uncoupling of the receptor–adenylate cyclase system in target cells of the testis. The integrity of the carbohydrate in the α subunit is directly or indirectly involved in receptor–signal transduction. Removal of 70–75% of the total carbohydrate in gonadotropins leads to derivatives that are still able to bind to their specific receptors, but are unable to stimulate adenylate cyclase. In addition, it has been shown for oLH, bLH, hCG, and oFSH that deglycosylated gonadotropins specifically antagonize the action of the corresponding native hormones. The protein and carbohydrate components of gonadotropins clearly have different roles in the expression of biological activity. The role of the glycosylated α subunit in signal transduction could be of evolutionary significance, as there is a high degree of structural conservation of the α subunit among different species, and an identical α subunit is used in the assembly of the three glycoprotein hormones in all species [1, 27].

One may question the individual role of each subunit in cellular interaction. It has been suggested that the α subunit endows the β subunit with a conformation necessary for binding to the receptor and that the α subunit itself is necessary for stimulation of adenylate cyclase. It has also been proposed that domains in the α subunit, in combination with domains in the β subunit, are responsible for interaction with receptors. In the latter case conformational changes contributing to the specificity of binding could also be induced in an α subunit by the β subunit. Molecular

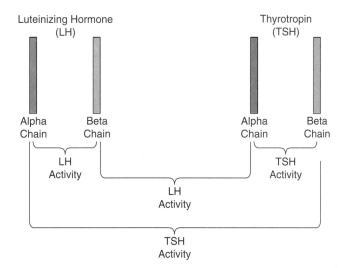

Figure 5.7
Glycoprotein subunit hybridization studies.

hybridization studies involving recombinations of α subunits with β subunits demonstrate that hormonal specificity is conferred upon the hybrid by the β subunit (Fig. 5.7).

Thyrotropin.   The early work of Allen and of Smith (described in Greep [13]) demonstrated that thyroidectomy resulted in failure of tadpoles to metamorphose into frogs. This effect could also be duplicated by hypophysectomy of tadpoles. Metamorphosis of thyroidectomized tadpoles could be accomplished, however, by addition of thyroid gland extracts to the water in which the larvae swam. Pituitary extracts stimulated metamorphosis of hypophysectomized, but not thyroidectomized, tadpoles. These observations suggested that the pituitary gland might be the source of a substance that was stimulatory to thyroid production of a metamorphic hormone. Thyroxine and triiodothyronine are the hormones produced by the thyroid (Chap. 13). A thyroid-stimulating hormone (TSH, thyrotropin) has been isolated from the pituitary and its structure determined in a number of mammalian species. Thyroid-stimulating activity has been found in pituitaries of all vertebrates examined. Thyrotropin is synthesized within basophilic thyrotrophs of the pars distalis. The number of secretory granules present within the thyrotrophs is increased if animals are treated with thyroxine, confirming that thyroid hormones exert a negative feedback preventing TSH secretion.

As the name implies, the most important role of TSH is the control of thyroid gland function. By its action on the thyroid to liberate thyroid hormones, TSH is responsible for the control and coordination of many biological processes. In the amphibian, for example, TSH is responsible for inducing metamorphosis; in the mammal, TSH plays an important role in thermogenesis. Thyrotropins of mammalian origin stimulate thyroid activity in all vertebrates except cyclostomes, and pituitary extracts of nonmammalian vertebrates stimulate mammalian thyroid glands. The amino acid composition of turtle TSH is strikingly similar to that of bovine TSH. Purified lutropin of mammals possesses intrinsic TSH activity when tested on teleost thyroid glands. This observation supports the suggestion that the primitive glycoprotein may have been an LH-like molecule that became modified during evolution into a TSH-like molecule.

Luteinizing hormone.   The gonads—the ovaries and the testes—secrete steroid hormones that regulate the growth and development of a variety of target tissues. In many animals, hypophysectomy leads to atrophy of the gonads, and extracts of the pituitary cause recrudescence of the gonads of hypophysectomized animals. These experiments implicate the pituitary gland in the control of gonadal function. Originally two pituitary fractions possessing gonadotropic activity were obtained. One of these stimulated follicular growth in the ovaries and increased spermatogenic activity in the testes. This hormone is now referred to as follicle-stimulating hormone (FSH) or follitropin. The other factor, referred to as luteinizing hormone (LH) or lutropin, stimulated corpora lutea formation and ovulation in the female and stimulated testosterone secretion and development of secondary sexual characteristics in the male.

Luteinizing hormone stimulates testosterone synthesis by the interstitial cells of Leydig of the testes. The action of LH is dependent on FSH induction of Leydig cell LH receptors. Indirectly LH stimulates spermatogenesis by way of its effect on testosterone biosynthesis, which is required for maturation of the germ cells. In the human female LH induces ovulation and is necessary for the initial development of the corpus luteum (Chaps 18 and 19).

Follicle-stimulating hormone. After many initial difficulties, a gonadotropic hormone separate from LH was obtained. FSH is responsible for the early development of the ovarian follicle in the female and for the initial steps of spermatid maturation in the male [29]. The role of FSH in the male is twofold: to increase the LH receptor population of testicular Leydig cells so that they are sensitive to the actions of LH and to act in concert with LH to stimulate spermatogenesis. Specifically FSH stimulates synthesis of a testicular (Sertoli cell) androgen-binding protein as well as the aromatase enzyme that converts testosterone to estradiol. FSH interacts with granulosa cells of the developing follicle, and its actions are mediated through cAMP. The biological roles and mechanisms of action of FSH are discussed later (Chaps 17 and 18).

Corticotropin and Melanotropins are Hormones Derived from a Common Precursor, Proopiomelanocortin

A lipotropic hormone, β-lipotropin (β-LPH), of pars distalis origin was first described by Li in 1964, but the physiological significance of this polypeptide was not discerned until many years later. β-LPH is now realized to be one of several peptide components of the large prohormone molecule proopiomelanocortin (POMC) (see Fig. 8.4). Corticotropin and α-melanocyte-stimulating hormone (α-MSH) are structurally related peptide hormones that are both derived from POMC. Corticotropin, also called adrenocorticotropic hormone (ACTH), is produced by corticotroph cells of the pars distalis [6] and functions as the major pituitary hormone controlling the synthesis and secretion of corticosteroid hormones by the adrenal cortex. The α-MSH, as well as other related melanotropic peptides, are primarily produced by cells of the pars intermedia, and control integumental melanocyte (melanophore) melanin production in many vertebrates. Both corticotrophin and α-MSH, as well as several other biologically active hormones, are first expressed as separate peptide sequences within POMC. In the pars distalis, enzymes within corticotrophs split the ACTH sequence from the precursor protein. In the pars intermedia, on the other hand, enzymes release the tridecapeptide sequence of α-MSH (see Fig. 8.3) from POMC. The remaining components of POMC protein are released along with ACTH or α-MSH during vesicular exocytosis. Thus, the differential activities of the proteolytic processing enzymes in cells of the pars distalis and pars intermedia dictate the predominance of ACTH production in the former and α-MSH in the latter. The POMC protein is also expressed in hypothalamic neurons, where melanocortins play important roles in the regulation of food intake and energy homeostasis, as discussed in Chap. 11.

In addition, within the molecule of β-LPH (and thus, within POMC) is found the amino acid sequence of a so-called β-melanotropin (β-melanocyte-stimulating hormone, β-MSH). There is no evidence, however, that this melanotropic peptide is cleaved from the POMC within the pituitary and plays any normal hormonal role (Chap. 8). The C-terminal 61–93 sequence of bovine β-LPH is referred to as β-endorphin, and the smaller 61–65 sequence is referred to as methionine enkephalin. Both β-endorphin and Met-enkephalin function within the nervous system as neurohormones, in part as endogenous analgesic hormones of humans.

Both α-MSH and ACTH possess similar sequences within their structures (see Fig. 8.1), which is why each hormone can stimulate the target tissues of the other hormone, melanocytes and adrenal glands, respectively. β-Lipotropin was originally isolated from the fin whale pituitary and chemically characterized. The proposed primary structure of whale β-LPH differs from the ovine LPH only at four amino acid residues. The β-endorphin segment (residues 61–91) is identical to that of ovine β-LPH. The total number of residues in β-LPH differs among species: human (89), ovine (91), bovine (93), porcine (91), ostrich (90), and fin whale (91).

Corticotropin. The steroidogenic tissues of the adrenal glands secrete a number of steroid hormones that profoundly affect carbohydrate and mineral metabolism. In most mammals steroidal tissue surrounds the adrenal medulla to form the so-called adrenal cortex. Hypophysectomy results in atrophy of the adrenal cortex. The steroidogenic tissue of the hypophysectomized animal is restored in animals receiving replacement therapy with pituitary extracts. Purification of pituitary preparations led to the isolation and structural characterization of an adrenal cortical-stimulating hormone (ACTH), adrenocorticotropin or corticotropin, as it is also designated.

```
              5                    10                   15                   20
Ser–Tyr–Ser–Met–Glu–His–Phe–Arg–Trp–Gly–Lys–Pro–Val–Gly–Lys–Lys–Arg–Arg–Pro–Val–Lys–Val–Tyr–Pro ┐
                                           35                   30                   25
          Human    Phe–Glu–Leu–Pro–Phe–Ala–Glu–Ala–Ser–Glu–Asp–Glu–Ala–Gly–Asn ┘
          Bovine                           –Glu–       –Ser–
          Ovine                            –Gln–       –Ser–
          Porcine                          –Glu–       –Leu–
```

Figure 5.8 Comparative primary structures of some corticotropins.

Corticotropin is synthesized within basophils of the pars distalis [6]. Unlike the glycoprotein-containing basophils that synthesize TSH, FSH, and LH, the corticotroph cells are often chromophobic and are sometimes considered to be chromophobes. Certain chromophobic basophils may represent very active corticotrophs that are essentially degranulated, and therefore do not stain. Certain adenoma cells associated with Cushing's disease are, on the other hand, intensely PAS-positive. The glycoprotein present within these cells is not directly related to ACTH but is apparently a component of the precursor molecule, POMC.

Corticotropin is the smallest peptide hormone of the anterior pituitary and is composed of a single linear chain consisting of 39 amino acids. Thus far, this chain length is a consistent feature of all species of ACTH. Structural differences between species are found only between residues 24 and 33, and these differences in mammals amount to only one or two residue differences (at positions 31 and 33) between any two species (Fig. 5.8). A shark (*Squalus acanthias*) corticotropin is also 39 amino acids long but differs at 11 positions from the human hormone. Ostrich (*Struthio camelus*) ACTH is similar in length to other corticotropins and differs from human ACTH at only five residues. The synthesis of a biologically active nonadecapeptide, corresponding to the first 19 amino-terminal residues of ACTH, and the subsequent total synthesis of the porcine ACTH were landmarks in the field of peptide hormone synthesis. $ACTH_{1-24}$ is commercially available and is the form generally used for studies on ACTH action, as the biological activity resides within this invariant 1–24 sequence of the hormone.

As its name implies, the major role of ACTH is to stimulate steroid biosynthesis within adrenal steroidogenic tissue. Cortisol and corticosterone are the major glucocorticoids produced by the adrenal gland in response to ACTH stimulation. These steroid hormones are important in carbohydrate metabolism. Excessive secretion of ACTH in humans leads to Cushing's disease (syndrome), which is characterized by excessive plasma levels of cortisol and, therefore, pathological alterations in glucose metabolism. The absence or diminished secretion of ACTH results in Addison's disease, a disorder characterized by deficits in cortisol production with severe consequences on cellular metabolism. Because the first 13 amino acids are similar to those comprising α-MSH, it is not surprising that ACTH possesses considerable melanotropic activity. Nevertheless, there is no evidence that ACTH plays any normal role in the control of integumental melanocyte function. On the other hand, in primary Addison's disease and in Cushing's syndrome of secondary origin, where ACTH is secreted in excessive amounts, hyperpigmentation is also a visually obvious symptom, a so-called "cardinal symptom" of the disease. The hyperpigmentation is probably due to the excessive levels of circulating ACTH. The heptapeptide sequence, -Met-Glu-His-Phe-Arg-Trp-Gly-, an active sequence of α-MSH, is mainly responsible for the melanotropic activity of ACTH as well as that of β-lipotropin. In some species, ACTH also possesses lipolytic activity, an action shared by other melanocortins. It is unknown, however, whether this action represents a physiological role of the hormone.

Melanocyte-Stimulating Hormone. The pars intermedia is the source of a melanocyte-stimulating hormone (α-MSH, α-melanotropin). The pituitary gland of the adult human lacks a pars intermedia, and this is correlated with the absence of α-MSH in the pituitary and plasma in humans. α-melanotropin is present in the pituitary of other vertebrates and plays an important role in the skin coloration of many animals. α-MSH is composed of 13 amino acids (see Fig. 8.1). The physiological roles of α-melanotropin are discussed in detail in Chap. 8.

Vasopressin and Oxytocin are the Major Neurohypophysial Hormones

Two nonapeptides, oxytocin and arginine vasopressin (AVP), are present in the neurohypophysis of humans. Each of these hormones is separately synthesized in different neurohypophysial neurons. Each neurohypophysial hormone is derived from a prohormone, oxyphysin or pressophysin, synthesized in cell bodies located within the paired paraventricular and supraoptic nuclei, respectively, of the hypothalamus (Fig. 5.5). Oxytocin- and AVP-containing vesicles travel from the sites of synthesis within the hypothalamic nuclei by axoplasmic transport to axon terminals within the pars nervosa, where they are stored until released.

The neurohypophysial hormones are released into the circulation to travel to their distant target tissues. Oxytocin plays an instrumental role in stimulating milk release from the mammary gland through an action on contractile elements (myoepithelial cells) of the breasts. Oxytocin also stimulates uterine contraction at term and therefore provides a major endocrine stimulus to the process of parturition. Vasopressin plays an essential role in water retention (and therefore blood pressure) by its action on the collecting tubules of the kidney. Two or more neurohypophysial hormones are present in the neurohypophysis of each vertebrate species except cyclostomes (lampreys and hagfishes), which possess but a single such peptide, arginine vasotocin (AVT). The structures of the individual neurohypophysial hormones (oxytocin, lysine and arginine vasopressin, vasotocin, mesotocin, isotocin, and others) have been determined from a number of species (see Table 7.1) and the possible pathways of their structural evolution described. The roles and actions of the neurohypophysial hormones are discussed in Chap. 7.

Pituitary Pathophysiology

Pituitary dysfunction may involve undersecretion or oversecretion of one or more hypophysial hormones [26]. Table 5.2 summarizes the major physiological defects related to the pathophysiology of the pituitary gland. Hyposecretion of pituitary hormones may result from destruction of normal glandular cells within the pituitary by an expanding tumor, disruption of hypothalamo-pituitary vascular connections, or damage to or disease of the hypothalamus. Hypersecretion, on the other hand, may result from neoplasia (pituitary tumors) or from hypertrophy and hyperplasia, resulting from enhanced hypothalamic stimulation of the pituitary. Hypersecretion of α-MSH or PRL could result, plausibly, from loss of a tonic hypothalamic inhibitory input to the pituitary (see Chap. 6).

TABLE 5.2   Some examples of pituitary pathophysiology

Hormone	Etiology	Symptom
All hormones	No pituitary hormones (empty sella syndrome)	Panhypopituitarism
Growth hormone (GH)	Deficiency (childhood)	Short stature
	Excess	
	child	Gigantism
	adult	Acromegaly
Prolactin (PRL)	Deficiency	No disease states reported
	Excess	Hyperprolactinemia: galactorrhea–amenorrhea syndrome
Thyrotropin (TSH)	Deficiency	
	child	Hypothyroidism (cretinism)
	adult	Hypothyroidism (myxedema)
	Excess	Hypothyroidism (thyrotoxicosis, Graves' disease)
Follitropin (FSH)	Deficiency	Hypogonadism: failure of germ cell maturation
	Excess	No information available
Lutropin (LH)	Deficiency	Hypogonadism: failure of sexual maturation
	Excess	No information available
Corticotropin (ACTH)	Deficiency	Addison's disease
	Excess	Cushing's disease/syndrome (hypercortisolism)
Oxytocin	Deficiency	No information available (necessary for milk secretion)
	Excess	No disease states reported
Vasopressin (AVP, ADH)	Deficiency	Diabetes insipidus (excessive water loss, dehydration)
	Excess	Syndrome of inappropriate ADH secretion (hypertension)

Panhypopituitarism, which involves total loss of hypophysial hormone secretion, could be due to a congenital dysfunction—failure of the pituitary to develop—or to destruction of the pituitary at a later stage in life. It is also possible that the pars distalis might fail to secrete only one of its many hormones. Hypopituitary (pituitarigenic) short stature may result, for example, from the specific failure of the pituitary to secrete GH. Growth hormone is being used in medicine to stimulate growth in GH-deficient patients. Recombinant human GH is quite effective in permitting children to attain normal growth. Its development and application, therefore, have been significant advances in medicine. In the future, GH may be used clinically for a wide variety of other applications, such as aiding wound healing, repartitioning fat into muscle, reversing certain aspects of aging, and immunopotentiation in conjunction with vaccines. There is evidence, however, that GH promotes the proliferation of certain types of transformed cells. Furthermore, immunoreactive GH can be found in prostatic tumors, and GH can be elevated in human cancer patients. Other health concerns about the use of growth hormone have been raised, ranging from diabetes to hypertension. Although the use of GH appears to be safe and is actually improving the quality of life for some patients, its use must be monitored to learn whether it causes any significant long-term side effects.

Microadenomas (tumors) may be responsible for the excess secretion of a particular pituitary hormone [7, 8]. Microadenomas composed of PRL-secreting cells are the most common pituitary neoplasms of rats and humans. Although some patients may have very high levels of serum PRL, not all develop galactorrhea (excess discharge of milk from the breast). Other hormones, such as estrogens and corticosteroids, along with PRL, are necessary for stimulation of lactogenesis. Amenorrhea, anovulation, and galactorrhea are all common sequelae of excess PRL secretion, and hypogonadism occurs in many hyperprolactinemic adult females. Hypersecretion of PRL is inhibitory to pituitary gonadotropin secretion, which accounts for the loss of gonadal function associated with the galactorrhea–amenorrhea syndrome. If PRL-secreting adenomas are selectively removed by surgical techniques, normal menses return. The pivotal role of PRL in mammary gland growth and differentiation is well established. In addition, there is substantial evidence that PRL is a causative factor in mammary gland neoplasia of rodents and possibly of humans. There is evidence that PRL, in conjunction with sex steroids, contributes to accelerated malignant mammary growth as indicated by the more fulminant course of breast cancer during pregnancy.

There are no reported examples of overproduction or underproduction of oxytocin. Vasopressin may, however, be excessively secreted or not secreted at all. In the Brattleboro strain of rats, for example, the animals do not secrete any vasopressin, and this defect is correlated with an absence of AVP within neurons of the neurohypophysis. In the syndrome of inappropriate AVP secretion, excess amounts of the hormone are secreted without relationship to plasma osmolality (Chap. 7). A common cause of excessive AVP secretion is malignancy, where AVP is secreted ectopically from a carcinoma of the lung.

Although excess secretion of pituitary hormones may result from a defect at the pituitary or hypothalamic level, pituitary hormones may be secreted by tumors of nonpituitary origin. Thus ectopic production of excessive amounts of ACTH by small cell or oat cell lung tumors may be responsible for the etiology of Cushing's syndrome, where the adrenal cortex releases excessive amounts of cortisol in response to the ACTH of ectopic tumor origin. Elevated plasma levels of β-LPH and ACTH are frequently observed in blood and tumor tissue of patients with various types of carcinoma. Because β-LPH and ACTH are components of a larger POMC precursor, it is not surprising that both these peptides are elaborated simultaneously by neoplastic tissues.

Tumors of patients with acromegaly may secrete GH and PRL, which suggests that these tumors may represent mixed adenomas. When more than one hormone is found within a certain tumor, they are usually those most related structurally, that is, PRL and GH, or TSH, FSH, and LH. During the induction and progression of pituitary neoplasms, secretion of more than one hypophysial hormone is common. Ectopic secretion of PRL occurs from cancers of nonhypophysial origin (e.g., bronchogenic or nephrogenic sources). The molecular basis of pituitary hormone under- or oversecretion is being increasingly better understood [7, 18, 19].

MOLECULAR MEDICINE CASE STUDIES

Development of the pituitary gland and expression of the PRL, GH, and TSH genes is dependent on the Pit-1 gene, which encodes the POU homeodomain transcription factor, PIT-1 [20]. The POU homeodomain group of transcription factors was so-named as an acronym of the original four members of this subfamily of homeodomain factors, *Pit-1*, *Oct-1* and *Oct-2*, and *Unc-86*, which all contain similar molecular motifs that confer characteristic DNA binding properties to this group. Pit-1 is the first member of the POU homeodomain transcription factor family discovered, and has been shown to be required for the normal development of anterior pituitary cell types and proper expression of PRL, GH, and TSHβ genes. PIT-1 contains a DNA-binding site consisting of a POU homeodomain essential for DNA-binding and a POU-specific domain that are required for both high-affinity and high-specificity binding on the GH, PRL, and TSH genes. In the Snell and Jackson dwarf mouse strains, which are inherited in an autosomal recessive mode, it has been shown that these dwarf phenotypes result from mutations in the Pit-1 gene. Mutation of the Pit-1 gene results in hypoplasia of the pituitary gland and deficiencies of GH, PRL, and TSH secretion.

In a DNA sample from a 3-month-old girl with severe growth deficiency from birth, a single-base mutation in codon 271 (CGG to TGG) that changes arginine to tryptophan (R271W) in the POU homeodomain was discovered. The patient presented with distinct facial features with prominent forehead, marked midfacial hypoplasia with depressed nasal bridge, deep-set eyes and a short nose with ante-verted nostrils (Fig. 5.9). During GH treatment, the dysmorpic facial features in the patient became less pronounced (Fig. 5.9). These facial features are also encountered in some forms of inherited isolated GH deficiency (e.g., IGHD type 1A) and also in infants with Laron dwarfism, which is caused by receptor resistance to GH (Chap. 12).

Anterior pituitary gland hypoplasia has been documented in a number of other patients with the R271W mutation. These observations suggest that the Pit-1 transcription factor is important for the normal development and function of the pituitary gland, as has been demonstrated in several animal models [1].

(a)   (b)   (c)   (d)

Figure 5.9 Pituitary dwarfism. Figures (**a**) and (**b**) show the patient at 3 months of age before treatment with thyroxine and GH; (**c**) at 2.5 years of age after 1.5 years of GH treatment; (**d**) at 3 years of age after 2 years of GH treatment. Note that the dysmorphic facial features become less pronounced. (From A. Aarskog, H. G. Eiken, R. Bjerknes, and O. L. MyKing. "Pituitary dwarfism in the R271W Pit-1 mutation," *European Journal of Pediatrics* 156:829–834, 1997, with permission.)

REVIEW EXERCISES

Compare and contrast each of the following terms. In what way are they related? How do they differ?

corticotroph/lactotroph
follitropin/lutropin
somatocrinin/somatostatin

adenohypophysis/
 neurohypophysis
heterodimer/homodimer
pars distalis/pars nervosa

lactotroph/prolactin
ACTH/α-melanotropin

gonadotropin/basophil
growth hormone/prolactin

Define or characterize each of the following terms:

anterior lobe
chromophobe cells

ectopic secretion
myoepithelial cells

corticotroph glycoprotein
vasopressin Rathke's pouch

Describe the etiological bases (causes) for each of the following endocrinopathies:

acromegaly galactorrhea
Addison's disease hypopituitarigenic dwarfism
goiter Laron dwarfism
cretinism panhypopituitarism
Cushing's disease pituitarigenic gigantism

Think, analyze and discuss:

1. What were the early observations that the pituitary gland might be considered the "master" endocrine gland?
2. In classical studies, lesion methods (these produce damage in a localized tissue area) were used to determine that the anterior pituitary does not function as a "master" gland, but is instead largely controlled by neurosecretory neurons in the hypothalamus. Design such a study in which you could test the hypothesis that this is the case. What structure(s) would you lesion? What measurements would you make? Describe the results you would expect to obtain, and how you would interpret them.
3. When pituitary tumors develop in an individual, they often arise from the proliferation of one particular endocrine cell phenotype. Among the most common of these microadenomas (benign tumors) are prolactinomas, which produce excess prolactin.
   a. What would be a likely physiological symptom of a prolactinoma?
   b. What method could be used to confirm the presence of high levels of prolactin in the bloodstream of an individual with a prolactinoma?
   c. If a suspected prolactinoma were surgically removed, how could the excised tumor tissue be definitively confirmed as a prolactinoma? What method(s) could be used, and what specific reagents would be required?
   d. Consider the case of a patient who exhibits the symptoms of a hyperprolactinemia, yet does not present any radiological evidence of pituitary tumor. To reduce prolactin levels in lieu of surgical intervention, what type of drug treatment might be considered for this patient?
4. The POMC molecule serves as a precursor molecule for the production of several different biologically active peptides. Consider the recent development of a mutant mouse strain bearing a null mutation, or "knockout," of the POMC gene. Can you predict some of the pathophysiological phenotypes that would likely arise in these animals? Which features of the predicted phenotype would be attributable to the loss of which POMC-derived peptides?

References

[1] Aarskog, A., et al. 1997. Pituitary dwarfism in the R271W Pit-1 mutation. *Eur. J. Pediatr.* 156:829–34.

[2] Ben-Jonathan, N., et al. 1996. Extrapituitary prolactin: distribution, regulation, functions, and clinical aspects. *Endocr. Rev.* 17:639–69.

[3] Bergland, R. M., and R. B. Page. 1979. Pituitary–brain vascular relations: A new paradigm. *Science* 204:18–24.

[4] Bousfield, G. R., W. M. Perry, and D. N. Ward. 1994. Gonadotropins: chemistry and biosynthesis. In: E. Knobil

and J. D. Neil, eds. *The physiology of reproduction*, New York: Raven Press, pp. 1749–920.

[5] Castrucci, A. M. L., et al. 1989. Melanocyte stimulating hormone (MSH) and melanin concentrating hormone (MCH) may be structurally and evolutionarily related. *Regul. Pept.* 24:27–35.

[6] Childs, G. Y. 1992. Structure–function correlates in the corticotropes of the anterior pituitary. *Front. Neuroendocrinol.* 3:271–317.

[7] Davis, J. R. E., and N. Hoggard. 1993. Towards the pathogenesis of human pituitary tumours. *J. Endocrinol.* 136:3–6.

[8] Dötsch, J., et al. 1996. G_s-mutation at codon 201 in pituitary adenoma causing gigantism in a 6-year-old boy with McCune–Albright syndrome. *J. Clin. Endocrinol. Metab.* 81:3839–42.

[9] Dubois, P. M., and A. El-Amraoui. 1995. Embryology of the pituitary gland. *TEM* 6:1–7.

[10] Dubois, P. M., and F. J. Hemming. 1991. Fetal development and regulation of pituitary cell types. *J. Electron Microsc. Technique* 19:2–20.

[11] Frantz, A. G. 1978. Prolactin. *N. Engl. J. Med.* 298:201–7.

[12] Green, J. D. 1951. The comparative anatomy of the hypophysis with special reference to its blood supply and innervation. *Am. J. Anat.* 88:225–311.

[13] Greep, R. O. 1974. History of research on anterior hypophysial hormones. In: R. O. Greep and E. B. Astwood, eds. *Handbook of physiology* (sec. 7, vol. 4, part 2–). Washington, DC: American Physiological Society, pp. 1–27.

[14] Guillemin, R., and R. Burgus. 1972. The hormones of the hypothalamus. *Sci. Am.* 227:24–33.

[15] Hartree, A. S., and A. G. C. Renwick. 1992. Molecular structures of glycoprotein hormones and functions of their carbohydrate components. *Biochem. J.* 287:665–79.

[16] Holmes, R. L., and J. N. Ball. 1974. *The pituitary gland*. Cambridge: Cambridge University Press.

[17] Omeljaniuk, R. J., H. R. Habbi, and R. E. Peter. 1989. Alterations in pituitary GnRH and dopamine receptors associated with the seasonal variation and regulation of gonadotropin release in the goldfish (*Carassius auratus*). *Gen. Comp. Endocrinol.* 74:39–99.

[18] Parks, J. S., E.-I. Kinoshita, and R. W. Pfaffle. 1993. Pit-1 and hypopituitarism. *TEM* 4:81–5.

[19] Pfaffle, R. W., et al. 1992. Mutation in the POU-specific domain of Pit-1 and hypopituitarism without pituitary hypoplasia. *Science* 257:1118–21.

[20] Radovick, S., et al. 1992. A mutation in the POU-homeodomain of Pit-1 responsible for combined pituitary hormone deficiency. *Science* 257:115–18.

[21] Riddle, O., R. W. Bates, and S. W. Dykshorn. 1933. The preparation, identification and assay of prolactin—a hormone of anterior pituitary. *Am. J. Physiol.* 105:191–216.

[22] Schwartz, J., and F. Gracia-Navairo. 1996. Ain't misbehavin': Reflections on the functional differences among anterior pituitary cells. *Mol. Cell. Endocrinol.* 123:1–6.

[23] Scully, K. M., and M. G. Rosenfeld. 2002. Pituitary development: regulatory codes in mammalian organogenesis. *Science* 295:2231–5.

[24] Semoff, S., and M. E. Hadley. 1978. Localization of ATPase activity to the glial-like cells of the pars intermedia. *Gen. Comp. Endocrinol.* 35:329–41.

[25] Sinha, Y. N. 1995. Structural variants of prolactin: Occurrence and physiological significance. *Endocr. Rev.* 16:354–69.

[26] Spada, A., and G. Faglia. 1996. G-protein dysfunction in pituitary tumors. *Front. Horm. Res.* 20:108–21.

[27] Thotakura, N. R., and D. L. Blithe. 1995. Glycoprotein hormones: Glycobiology of gonadotropins, thyrotropin and free α subunit. *Glycobiology* 5:3–10.

[28] Tixier-Vidal, A., and M. G. Farquhar (eds.). 1975. *The anterior pituitary.* New York: Academic Press.

[29] Ulloa-Aguirre, A., et al. 1995. Follicle-stimulating isohormones: Characterization and physiological relevance. *Endocrinol. Rev.* 16:765–87.

CHAPTER

6

The Endocrine Hypothalamus

I n the embryonic development of the pituitary gland, ectoderm from the oral cavity and neuroectoderm from the brain evaginate and move toward each other to form the pituitary gland. There must be some physiological significance that these two different tissues have become integrated into one functional glandular component. As we have noted (see Chap. 5), the pituitary gland is a rich source of hormones that controls a variety of physiological functions. Adrenocorticotropin secretion exhibits a diurnal (daily) rhythm; it is also released in response to a variety of stresses. Follicle-stimulating hormone (FSH) and luteinizing hormone (LH) secretion fluctuates in a predictable pattern throughout the female ovarian cycle and, midway through the cycle, there is a surge of LH release that is responsible for initiating ovulation. Oxytocin is released from the pituitary in response to suckling or sometimes during coitus. Pituitary growth hormone is secreted due to the ingestion of certain metabolic substrates.

Pituitary hormone secretions are clearly adaptive in nature, as hormones play essential roles under conditions of special need. For example, the reproductive cycles of many animals are linked to seasonal changes in day length. The pelage color of the weasel is white in winter and brown the rest of the year. The weasel's coat color is regulated by pituitary melanocyte-stimulating hormone (MSH). What are the cues that dictate whether a particular pituitary hormone will be secreted? Metabolic substrates, such as glucose, fatty acids, and amino acids, might serve as intrinsic cues to inform the pituitary of circulating levels of these substrates. But in vitro studies reveal that the pituitary is not directly sensitive to these substrates. Cold temperature is a stimulus to thyroid-stimulating hormone (TSH) secretion, and day length affects pituitary gonadotropin secretion. Obviously, these extrinsic stimuli must be initially intercepted by the nervous system. A vast body of experimental data supports the view that the control of secretion of each of the pituitary hormones is regulated by the brain. This would explain the embryological processes related to the early development of the pituitary. In this chapter, the evidence for a central nervous system control of pituitary function is reviewed, and the specific roles of the **hypophysiotropic** hormones that control pituitary hormone secretion are explained.

The Neurovascular Hypothesis

Removal of the pituitary gland leads to atrophy of the adrenal cortex, thyroid, and gonads. Transplantation of the pituitary to an ectopic site in an animal, such as in the eye or under the kidney capsule, leads to a similar end-organ atrophy. Transplantation of the pituitary back under the hypothalamus, however, is followed by revascularization and functional reactivation of the pituitary. Transection of the pituitary stalk or placement of a barrier between the hypothalamus and the pituitary leads to atrophy of the pituitary and its target organs. Subsequent revascularization of the pituitary leads to functional reactivation of the gland and its target organs. From these observations, Geoffrey Harris, an English endocrinologist, concluded that it is "difficult to escape from the conclusion that the hypophysial portal supply has some specific effect in activating anterior pituitary tissue" [18]. Transplantation of pituitary tissue from young rats under the pituitary stalk of adult female rats resulted in the recurrence of normal, regular estrus cycles at a time when the donor young were still immature. The onset of pituitary-gonadotropic activity, it was concluded, probably depends on a hypothalamic influence rather than a maturation of pituitary or ovarian tissues. Even a pituitary from a young male animal could reactivate the pituitary-gonadal axis when transplanted into an adult female. According to Harris, the anterior pituitary tissue is plastic in nature and "its pattern of secretory activity is not due to any intrinsic property of the tissue itself, but to some outside 'drive' or stimulus, derived probably from the central nervous system."

These observations led Harris to elaborate the *neurovascular hypothesis*. He suggested that humoral factors released by the hypothalamus were carried by the portal blood vessels to the pituitary to regulate hormone secretion. Extracts of the brain, specifically of the hypothalamus, will stimulate or inhibit secretion from the pituitary whether studied in vivo or in vitro. Lesions of specific areas of the hypothalamus, as induced by electrocautery, lead to specific defects in pituitary hormone secretion. Electrode stimulation of these same anatomical sites within the hypothalamus, on the other hand, leads to the release of a particular pituitary hormone.

Crude extracts of the hypothalamus provided early evidence that the hypothalamus contained factors inhibitory or stimulatory to pituitary hormone secretions. These extracts were further purified to yield subfractions that by bioassay inhibited growth hormone (GH) release or stimulated thyrotropin or gonadotropin secretion. Further purification and physical methods of analysis provided the definitive structures of the so-called *hypophysiotropic factors* present in these extracts. These studies revolutionized the field of endocrinology [15].

Structure-Function of the Endocrine Hypothalamus

The hypothalamus is the basal part of the diencephalon lying below the thalamus, as its name implies [46]. The hypothalamus forms the walls and lower part of the third ventricle of the brain (Fig. 6.1). It includes the optic chiasm, the tuber cinereum, the infundibulum, and the mammillary bodies. The tuber cinereum is the part of the third ventricle floor that extends downward toward the infundibulum. The lower part of the tuber cinereum, which is richly supplied with blood vessels that drain into the pituitary stalk and then in turn empty into a secondary plexus in the anterior pituitary, is referred to as the *median eminence*. The vascular link between the median eminence and the pituitary gland is known as the *hypophysial portal system* (Fig. 6.2). Within the hypothalamus are clusters of neurons, *hypothalamic nuclei*, which are symmetrically located around the third ventricle. The *supraoptic* nuclei (SON) and *paraventricular* nuclei (PVN), for example, are composed of

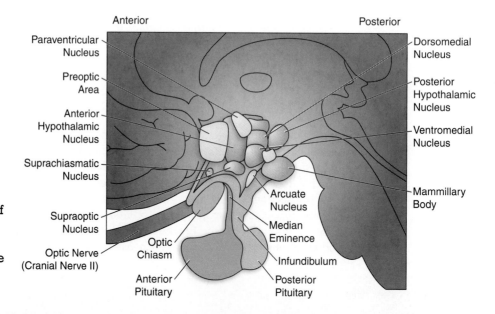

Figure 6.1   Frontal section through the cerebral hemispheres of the human brain; the principal hypothalamic nuclei present within the plane of transect are indicated.

Anterior   Posterior

Paraventricular Nucleus
Preoptic Area
Anterior Hypothalamic Nucleus
Suprachiasmatic Nucleus
Supraoptic Nucleus
Optic Nerve (Cranial Nerve II)
Optic Chiasm
Anterior Pituitary

Dorsomedial Nucleus
Posterior Hypothalamic Nucleus
Ventromedial Nucleus
Mammillary Body
Arcuate Nucleus
Median Eminence
Infundibulum
Posterior Pituitary

Figure 6.2
Hypophysial portal system. (From Porter et al. [36], with permission.)

cell bodies whose axons extend into the median eminence and then into the neurohypophysis (see Fig. 5.5). This particular nerve tract, consisting of neuronal axons from the SON and PVN, is the *supraopticoparaventriculohypophysial tract*. Other major nuclear groups within the hypothalamus include the ventromedial nuclei, arcuate nucleus, lateral tuberal nuclei, and dorsomedial nuclei (Fig. 6.1).

The endocrine hypothalamus consists of *neurosecretory neurons* whose secretory activity provides the neurohormones (hypophysiotropic factors) that regulate adenohypophysial function [6]. These neurons are the elements of the *parvocellular* (from the Latin *parvus*, or small) *neurosecretory system* and are distinguished from the *magnocellular system* of neurosecretory neurons that compose the supraoptic and paraventricular neurons that synthesize oxytocin and vasopressin. The neurons of the parvocellular neurosecretory system converge toward the pituitary stalk to form the *tuberoinfundibular tract*. These neurons abut on the endothelium of the primary plexus of the portal system of the median eminence. Immunocytochemical methods have demonstrated hypophysiotropic factors (*hypophysiotropins*) within these neurons [24]. Electron microscopic studies provide evidence that these cells release their chemical messengers into the hypophysial portal system.

When pieces of pituitary tissue were grafted into various regions of the basal forebrain of rats, the *medial basal hypothalamus* (MBH) was capable of maintaining the normal structure and function of the pituitary grafts. Therefore, the MBH was named the *hypophysiotropic area* [17]. Apparently the integrity and secretory activity of pituitary cells implanted within this area is due to the local release of hypophysiotropins from the parvocellular neurons. The hypophysiotropic area extends from the median eminence upward and forward, through the anterior hypothalamus, to the suprachiasmatic region.

The endocrine hypothalamus is connected to the rest of the central nervous system by synaptic contacts from other neuronal elements. Information flow from other brain centers is relayed to hypothalamic parvocellular neurons, which then secrete their hypophysiotropins into the pituitary portal vasculature of the median eminence. The median eminence therefore can be considered the final point of convergence of the central nervous system (CNS) on the peripheral endocrine system. The hypophysial portal system provides a restricted vascular link between the neurosecretory cells of the hypothalamus and the anterior pituitary gland.

Figure 6.3 Technique for cannulation of the hypophysial portal system. (From Porter et al. [36], with permission.)

The most rigid proof that the hypothalamus does indeed release hormones into the hypophysial portal system to regulate pituitary function would be the demonstration that such hormones are found in the portal vessels in higher concentrations than in the systemic circulation. Elegant methods involving cannulation of the hypophysial portal system and selective collection of portal blood have verified this thesis (Fig. 6.3) [34, 36, 37]. Each of the hypophysiotropins has been demonstrated within portal blood; the concentration of these hormones is increased after stimulation of certain hypothalamic sites. In addition, infusion of hypophysiotropins by portal cannulation induces secretion of pituitary hormones.

To determine the functional relationship of the medial basal hypothalamus (MBH) and adjacent preoptic area (POA) tissues to the rest of the brain, a knife was designed by Halász and colleagues to cut all the neural connections between the MBH-POA tissues and the remainder of the forebrain. This knife left the MBH-POA in continuity with the pituitary gland and supposedly left most of the blood supply to the MBH and the pituitary intact. Nevertheless, the hypophysiotropic area remained almost fully functional after this hypothalamic deafferentation. This suggests that the cells of origin of the hypophysiotropins reside mostly, if not entirely, within the MBH and POA tissues [17].

The importance of hypothalamic humoral factors in the control of pituitary function was uniquely demonstrated by ectopic transplantation of the adenohypophysis under the kidney capsule [11]. Although the adenohypophysis becomes well vascularized in this site, most of the gland atrophies due to generalized hypoactivity of most cellular elements of the gland. The lactotrophs, however, become hypertropic and hyperplastic (increase in size and cell number). As discussed later, this reflects the fact that hypothalamic control of the lactotroph is predominantly inhibitory. The systemic effects of adenohypophysial inactivity include end-organ atrophy of the gonads, adrenals, and thyroid gland. On the other hand, there is "functional reactivation and cytological restoration of pituitary grafts by continuous local intravascular infusion of median eminence extracts" [18]. It was concluded that hypothalamic humoral factors of median eminence origin control the structure and function of the pituitary gland.

The Hypophysiotropic Hormones

Stimulatory and inhibitory factors of hypothalamic origin control pituitary hormone secretion as previously discussed. The structures of most vertebrate gonadotropin-releasing hormone, thyrotropin-releasing hormone, GH release-inhibiting hormone, corticotropin-releasing hormone and prolactin (PRL) and MSH release-inhibiting hormones have been characterized. There is less information available relative to the existence of putative PRL- and MSH-releasing factors. In many cases, the distribution of hypophysiotropins within the CNS has been determined by radioimmunoassay (RIA) of brain tissue. Brain tissue can be cut in a rostral–caudal direction, as well as laterally from side to side, to provide a series of tissue slices. A small, round (Palkovits) punch is used to obtain small samples of tissue from the brain slices. By RIA, one can determine the concentration of hypophysiotropins within these punch biopsies and then map

NH₂–His–Pro–Glu–OH
NH₂–Pro–Glu–His–OH
NH₂–Pro–His–Glu–OH
NH₂–His–Glu–Pro–OH
NH₂–Glu–Pro–His–OH
NH₂–Glu–His–Pro–OH

(pyro)–Glu–His–Pro–NH₂

Figure 6.4 Six synthetic peptides related to thyrotropin-releasing hormone (TRH).

the distribution of the neuropeptides within the brain. Using immunohistochemical methods involving antibodies against neuropeptides, one can also localize hypophysiotropins to specific neurons within the brain. In situ hybridization methods are likewise used to localize mRNAs encoding hypophysiotropic neurohormones to specific neuronal populations.

Thyrotropin-Releasing Hormone (TRH) Stimulates Synthesis and Secretion of TSH

The structure of the hypothalamic hormone controlling TSH secretion was determined in 1969 independently by Guillemin and Schally and their colleagues. For this monumental work and the elucidation of the structures of the GH release-inhibiting hormone (somatostatin) and the gonadotropin-releasing hormone (GnRH), they received a Nobel Prize in Physiology/Medicine. The task of elucidating the structure of TRH was not easy, but its eventual determination provided important insights into present-day methods of endocrine research. The episodes relating to the so-called race to Stockholm have been dramatically described [48].

From about 25,000 ovine and porcine hypothalamic fragments, about 1 mg of TRH was obtained. These purified preparations, extremely potent in stimulating TSH release from the pituitary, both in vivo and in vitro, consisted of a simple peptide composed of three amino acids: glutamic acid, histidine, and proline in equimolar ratios. What was the exact sequence of the amino acids in the peptide? There was not enough material left to answer this essential question. It was decided, therefore, to synthesize the six possible putative isomers of the peptide (Fig. 6.4). Most surprisingly, none of the tripeptides possessed the chromatographic or biologic characteristics of TRH. It was discovered that there was no free N-terminal amino group in the natural tripeptide; in other words, the amino-terminal group was protected in some way. The peptides were then treated with acetic anhydride in an effort to protect the NH₂ terminus, as in the natural TRH that lacked a free NH₂ group (Fig. 6.5). Only one of the peptides, Glu-His-Pro-OH, possessed biological activity, which was, however, lower than that of the natural TRH. This product proved to be pyro-Glu-His-Pro-OH. The α-amino group of glutamic acid had condensed with the carboxyl group of the glutamic acid to give the pyroglutamic acid form of the peptide. This structure, however, was not identical to natural TRH, which was more basic in nature. A more basic, less acidic compound could be obtained by protecting the free carboxyl group of the proline. Amidation of the C-terminal proline then yielded pyro-Glu-His-Pro-NH₂, whose activity was indistinguishable from that of natural TRH (Fig. 6.5). The structures of porcine, ovine, bovine, and human TRH proved to be identical. The arduous task just outlined for determining the structure of TRH illustrates the important contributions of chemistry to the emerging field of neuroendocrinology.

Figure 6.5 Synthesis of thyrotropin-releasing hormone.

Figure 6.6   The cDNA sequence of the TRH precursor encodes a protein of 255 amino acids. The sequence **Gln-His-Pro-Gly** occurs five times and each tetrapeptide is flanked by paired basic residues (Lys Arg or Arg Arg). Thus, the prohormone generates five TRH molecules from each precursor protein.

The mode of TRH biosynthesis in the mammalian brain is by post-translational cleavage of a larger precursor protein. Processing proTRH yields several copies of the biologically active peptide (Fig. 6.6). Only the repeated TRH coding units dispersed throughout the precursor are maintained between amphibian and mammalian prohormones [23]. Conservation of this pattern throughout evolution suggests that the ability of a precursor to generate multiple bioactive peptides may be an important mechanism in the amplification of hormone production.

TRH immunoactive cell bodies have been localized within the brain. The highest concentration of TRH cells is found in the paraventricular nucleus of the hypothalamus and the preoptic area. Many of these TRH neurons project their axonal processes into the median eminence, where they make neurovascular junctions with capillaries of the primary portal plexus. The densest network of TRH-containing fibers is thus found in the medial part of the external layer of the median eminence, with some processes also found in the pituitary stalk. Electrical stimulation of the paraventricular nucleus or median eminence can elevate portal vessel concentrations of TRH and peripheral plasma levels of TSH.

Somatostatin (SST) Inhibits GH Secretion from Somatotrophs

Pituitary GH is secreted episodically in all species, including humans. The pulsatile pattern of GH release from the pituitary gland is the net result of a delicate interplay between two hypothalamic hormones, a stimulatory, GH-releasing factor and a GH release-inhibiting hormone [12]. A hypothalamic peptide that inhibits the release of GH from the anterior pituitary was isolated and its primary sequence determined. This tetradecapeptide, referred to as somatostatin (SST), has been synthesized and has been determined to be chemically and biologically identical to the hypophysiotropic peptide (Fig. 6.7). The oxidized (ring) and the reduced (linear) forms of the peptide both have full biological activity in vitro and in vivo.

Somatostatin has been localized to secretory granules of neurons located within the hypothalamus by electron microscopic immunohistochemistry. Although originally isolated from the hypothalamus, this peptide has been shown to have widespread effects on brain, endocrine and exocrine pancreas, and gut function [13]. Furthermore, SST has a widespread distribution in the CNS and is also found localized to the D cells of the gut and the endocrine pancreas. Somatostatin has an inhibitory effect on GH release in response to every known stimulus. Action of SST is directly on the pituitary somatotrophs. A high density of SST-producing neurons is located in the anterior periventricular area of the hypothalamus, and many of these neurons project to the median eminence, where they form neurosecretory contacts.

A 28-residue prosomatostatin, a putative SST precursor from the porcine hypothalamus, has been isolated, chemically characterized, and its primary structure determined (Fig. 6.8). The last 14 amino acids of the precursor are identical in structure to SST. After synthesis, it

Ala–Gly–Cys–Lys–Asn–Phe–Phe–Trp–Lys–Thr–Phe–Thr–Ser–Cys

Figure 6.7   Primary structure of mammalian somatostatin.

1   14
Ser–Ala–Asn–Ser–Asn–Pro–Ala–Met–Ala–Pro–Arg–Glu–Arg–Lys–

28
–Ala–Gly–Cys–Lys–Asn–Phe–Phe–Trp–Lys–Thr–Phe–Thr–Ser–Cys

Figure 6.8 Primary structure of porcine prosomatostatin.

was found to be chemically and biologically identical to the prosomatostatin isolated from the brain and gut. This peptide possesses high GH and PRL release-inhibiting activity and has been shown to be a hormone in its own right.

Somatostatin has been found in the brain and pancreas of the frog, catfish, torpedo (an elasmobranch), and hagfish (a cyclostome). It is also present in the skin and bladder of the frog. Incubation of pituitary glands of the teleost tilapia (*Sarotherodon mossambicus*), in the presence of synthetic SST, resulted in a dose-dependent decrease in GH secretion. These results suggest that GH secretion in teleosts may be controlled by SST or an SST-like peptide, indicating that this action of the molecule has been fully conserved throughout vertebrate evolution.

GH-Releasing Hormone and Ghrelin Stimulate GH Secretion

A 44-amino-acid peptide was isolated from a human pancreatic tumor that specifically stimulated GH secretion, both in vitro and in vivo, from the rat pituitary gland (Fig. 6.9)[38]. The synthetic replicate had full biological activity and was similar in physicochemical properties to GH-releasing hormone (GHRH) present in hypothalamic tissues [14, 38]. GHRH possesses sequence homologies to several gut peptides of the secretin-glucagon family of peptides. Some GHRH-like immunoreactivity has been found in hypothalamo-hypophysial regions of many mammals, amphibians, and a variety of teleost fishes. There is a high degree of sequence similarity in the first 29 residues of GHRH from various species. The 1–29 residues possess similar activity to the entire 1–44 sequence. The highly conserved bioactive core of the peptide therefore accounts for the lack of species specificity of the molecule [5]. Almost all GHRH-producing neurons are found in the arcuate and ventromedial hypothalamic nuclei.

The existence of a second GH secretogogue was inferred many years ago from the observation that a synthetic hexapeptide could stimulate GH secretion independently of the GHRH receptor. The receptor mediating the actions of this exogenous peptide was identified as a G-protein-coupled receptor separate from the GHRH receptor, and recently a endogenous peptide ligand for the receptor was isolated and characterized from stomach tissue. The 28-amino-acid peptide, termed ghrelin, is produced by the stomach, small intestine, and to a lesser extent, by a small set of hypothalamic neurons. In addition to its significant GH-releasing activity, ghrelin appears to regulate brain circuitries controlling feeding behavior and energy homeostasis.

Gonadotropin-Releasing Hormone (GnRH) Stimulates LH and FSH Secretion from Gonadotrophs

A vast amount of experimental evidence has established that the hypothalamus regulates pituitary gonadotropin (LH and FSH) secretion via neurosecretion of the decapeptide GnRH [8]. The structure of GnRH was determined from extracts of 250,000 porcine hypothalami. The peptide was subsequently synthesized and found to act in an identical physiological manner to the putative hypothalamic peptide in all animals studied. The peptide was originally named luteinizing hormone-releasing hormone (LHRH) for its greater potency in stimulating release of LH versus FSH; this name also presupposed the discovery of a separate FSH-releasing

5   10   15   20
Tyr–Ala–Asp–Ala–Ile–Phe–Thr–Asn–Ser–Tyr–Arg–Lys–Val–Leu–Gly–Gln–Leu–Ser–Ala–Arg–Lys–Leu

25   30   35   40
Leu–Gln–Asp–Ile–Met–Ser–Arg–Gln–Gln–Gly–Glu–Ser–Asn–Gln–Glu–Arg–Gly–Ala–Arg–Ala–Arg–Leu–NH₂

Figure 6.9 Primary structure of a growth hormone-releasing hormone.

| (pyro)Glu | — | His | — | Trp | — | Ser | — | Tyr | — | Gly | — | Leu | — | Arg | — | Pro | — | Gly | — | NH₂ |
| 1 | | 2 | | 3 | | 4 | | 5 | | 6 | | 7 | | 8 | | 9 | | 10 | | |

Figure 6.10 Primary structure of mammalian gonadotropin-releasing hormone (GnRH).

factor (FSH-RF). However, most endocrinologists now refer to the neurohormone as GnRH, as it appears to be the primary neural regulator for both gonadotropins, and the existence of a separate FSH-RF has remained controversial. GnRH has been detected in the nerve fibers and terminals in proximity to the portal vessels in the median eminence of the hypothalamus. Mammalian GnRH is a decapeptide whose primary structure appears to be similar between mammalian species (Fig. 6.10).

Early studies showed that deafferentation of the rat hypothalamus causes a marked reduction in the GnRH content of the MBH, suggesting that GnRH arises from, or is controlled by, cells in more rostral areas of the brain [16, 17]. Subsequent immunohistochemical studies confirmed that most GnRH neurons in the rat are indeed located in the preoptic and septal regions, and that most of these neurons extend axons into the external layer of the lateral median eminence, where neurosecretion of the peptide into the hypophysial portal vessels occurs. In some species, notably the guinea pig, monkey, and human, most GnRH neurons are located more caudally in the arcuate nucleus of the MBH. As would be expected for a hypophysiotropic hormone, GnRH is present in high concentrations in hypophysial portal blood, whereas it is virtually undetectable in the systemic circulation. The role of GnRH in the control of pituitary gonadotropin secretion was confirmed by the use of immunization and later, by pharmacological techniques; Injections of antibodies to GnRH or GnRH receptor antagonists are followed by prompt drops in LH secretion and gonadal atrophy. Similarly, when GnRH antiserum or receptor antagonist is injected into female rats on the morning of proestrus, the preovulatory surge of LH release that normally follows in the afternoon does not occur, and ovulation is prevented (Chap. 18). Furthermore, administration of anti-GnRH serum to normal or castrated rats lowers not only LH but also FSH levels, thus revealing the key role of the hypophysiotropin in maintaining the secretion of both gonadotropins. The essential role of GnRH in regulating reproduction has also been confirmed in studies of the hypogonadal mouse. This mutant mouse bears a mutation in the GnRH gene, and consequently it does not produce biologically active GnRH decapeptide and it is sterile. Remarkably, reproductive capacity can be fully restored in these mice with GnRH gene therapy [27] or GnRH neuron transplantation in the hypothalamus [25].

In all animals studied to date, GnRH has been found to be released in an intermittent, "pulsatile" manner. This mode of release appears to be of critical importance in maintaining continued responsiveness of the gonadotroph to the GnRH stimulus. Thus, intermittent administration of GnRH can reestablish gonadotropin secretion in monkeys with hypothalamic

Figure 6.11 The primary structures of some known forms of GnRH [22]. The amino acid residues that differ from the mammal appear enclosed here.

	1	2	3	4	5	6	7	8	9	10
Mammal	pGlu	His	Trp	Ser	Tyr	Gly	Leu	Arg	Pro	Gly–NH₂
Chicken I	pGlu	His	Trp	Ser	Tyr	Gly	Leu	Gln	Pro	Gly–NH₂
Catfish	pGlu	His	Trp	Ser	His	Gly	Leu	Asn	Pro	Gly–NH₂
Chicken II	pGlu	His	Trp	Ser	His	Gly	Trp	Tyr	Pro	Gly–NH₂
Dogfish	pGlu	His	Trp	Ser	His	Gly	Trp	Leu	Pro	Gly–NH₂
Salmon	pGlu	His	Trp	Ser	Tyr	Gly	Trp	Leu	Pro	Gly–NH₂
Lamprey	pGlu	His	Tyr	Ser	Leu	Glu	Trp	Lys	Pro	Gly–NH₂

lesions, while constant infusions of GnRH fail to do so. Constant GnRH administration may lead to a desensitization or down-regulation of the processes responsible for gonadotropin release (Chap. 18).

Both LH and FSH are synthesized within the same gonadotroph following stimulation with GnRH and modulation by gonadal hormones (steroids and polypeptides). The frequency of the GnRH stimulus may be the major regulator of the relative proportions of FSH and LH synthesized and secreted, with less frequent GnRH pulses leading to preferential FSH secretion and more frequent GnRH pulses to LH secretion. Within the gonadotroph, the rate at which the α and β subunits are synthesized is regulated by the amount of translatable mRNA, and the actual amount of β subunit mRNA may be the rate-limiting step in gonadotropin synthesis. Different frequencies of GnRH pulsatility may therefore be transduced in the gonadotroph to differentially stimulate LH versus FSH β subunit gene transcription by cellular mechanisms that remain unknown.

Synthetic GnRH has significant gonadotropic activity in mammals, birds, and amphibians. In the amphibian, hypothalamic concentrations of GnRH vary with the seasonal reproductive cycle. A physiological role for GnRH has been demonstrated in teleosts. Although GnRH functions in the reproductive processes in mammals, the demonstration of the presence of the peptide in the brain of nonmammalian species need not restrict its function to a reproductive role.

Multiple molecular forms of the peptide have evolved, but all bear striking structural similarity [22]. The major mammalian GnRH is referred to as GnRH-1, and at least 15 variants of this decapeptide have been documented among many nonmammalian species. All of these are decapeptides with at least 50% sequence identity [43]. Between 800 and 2,000 neurosecretory GnRH-1 neurons are contained with the mammalian brain, scattered along a bilateral continuum from the olfactory bulbs to the MBH [51]. It has been convincingly demonstrated that GnRH-1 neurons originate in the nasal placode during development, and undergo a stereotyped migration into the forebrain during fetal development, ultimately assuming their postnatal septal-preoptic-hypothalamic positions. A second decapeptide, referred to as GnRH-2, differs from GnRH-1 by three amino acid residues and is expressed in virtually all vertebrates. Recent studies have shown that GnRH-1 and GnRH-2 are encoded by separate genes in mammals, and that their distributions in the brain are distinct. GnRH-2 is primarily expressed in midbrain and hindbrain neurons, as well as in certain parts of the hypothalamus, and its functions are not well characterized [22].

Corticotropin-Releasing Hormone (CRH) Stimulates ACTH Secretion from Corticotrophs

The first of the hypophysiotropic hormones to be investigated with great vigor was the putative corticotropin-releasing hormone (CRH) [10]. A peptide with high potency for stimulating the secretion of ACTH from cultured rat pituitaries was isolated from ovine hypothalami and synthesized [39]. The structure of this 41-residue peptide is shown (Fig. 6.12) and is partially similar in structure to urotensin I, a peptide found within the spinal cord (urophysis) of certain teleost fishes (Chap. 7). Antisera to CRH and CRH receptor antagonists significantly lower ACTH levels in adrenalectomized rats, and ACTH levels are diminished in mice bearing targeted deletions of the CRH gene. These findings confirm that endogenous CRH plays a major physiological role in regulating pituitary ACTH secretion [7, 49].

Characterization of CRH from a number of species indicates that its structure is highly conserved; the molecules in humans and rats are identical and differ by seven amino acids from the bovine sequence and by only two amino acids from the porcine structure. CRH shares homologies with a number of peptides found in primitive vertebrates, suggesting a common ancestral precursor. The CRH peptide is considered to be a member of a family of structurally related peptides that includes urocortin-I, -II, and -III. Neurons producing CRH

1   20
Ser–Gln–Glu–Pro–Pro–Ile–Ser–Leu–Asp–Leu–Thr–Phe–His–Leu–Leu–Arg–Glu–Val–Leu–Glu–Met⌐

30   41
└ Thr–Lys–Ala–Asp–Gln–Leu–Ala–Gln–Gln–Ala–His–Ser–Asn–Arg–Lys–Leu–Leu–Asp–Ile–Ala–NH$_2$

Figure 6.12 Primary structure of a corticotropin-releasing hormone (CRH).

are primarily located in the parvocellular region of the paraventricular nucleus (PVN) of the hypothalamus, while the urocortins are expressed more widely in extrahypothalamic areas. Many of the parvocellular CRH neurons of the PVN co-express the neurohypophysial neurohormone arginine vasopressin (AVP), which has been shown to act synergistically with CRH in releasing ACTH. Extrahypothalamic neuronal circuitries expressing CRH and the urocortins have also been characterized, where these peptides may mediate behavioral stress responses and modulate mood and affect. As such, there is considerable interest in developing pharmaceutical products that might exploit the emerging CRH receptor pharmacology to develop new anti-anxiety and/or antidepressant therapies.

Dopamine is a Major Prolactin-Release-Inhibiting Factor (PIF)

There is abundant evidence that PRL secretion from the pars distalis is under an inhibitory control by the hypothalamus. When female rat anterior pituitaries are autotransplanted to extracranial sites, they selectively maintain functional corpora lutea while the remainder of the ovary atrophies, as do the adrenals and thyroid gland [31, 32]. In the rat, PRL is required for functional activation of the corpora lutea and progesterone biosynthesis. These results demonstrate that PRL secretion continues uninterrupted, whereas FSH, LH, and other anterior pituitary hormones are discontinued following ectopic transplantation. If after being autotransplanted under the kidney capsule for a month, pituitaries are retransplanted back into close anatomical relationship with the median eminence, female rats return to normal cycling, which includes ovulation. If these recycling rats are mated, they will successfully carry litters to term.

Patients with pituitary stalk section or hypothalamic lesions have elevated plasma levels of PRL. In the rat, electrolytic lesions in the median eminence result in a large increase in PRL secretion. If anterior pituitary glands are incubated in vitro, PRL secretion commences immediately and continues uninterrupted almost indefinitely. Cytologically, the lactotrophs hypertrophy under such conditions. None of the other hormones of the pars distalis is secreted and, with the exception of the lactotrophs, the other secretory elements of the glands atrophy and disappear from the incubated glands. Taken together, all these observations, both in vivo and in vitro, support the hypothesis that the hypothalamus is the source of a PIF.

The evidence is overwhelming that this PIF is dopamine (DA). The presence of DA in hypophysial portal blood, as well as in the anterior pituitary gland, has been demonstrated. DA inhibits PRL secretion from pituitary glands incubated in vitro. In addition, apomorphine or ergot alkaloids (e.g., ergocryptine), known DA receptor agonists, are inhibitory to PRL secretion in vitro or in vivo. This inhibition by DA and related agonists can be antagonized by chlorpromazine, haloperidol, and other DA receptor antagonists. Injections of DA receptor antagonists result in increased PRL secretion. On the other hand, injections of levodopa, a substrate for DA biosynthesis, are inhibitory to PRL secretion. Bromocriptine, a long-acting dopamine receptor agonist, is highly effective in reducing serum PRL levels in over 90% of patients with hyperprolactinemia, regardless of etiology. This drug has also been found to reduce the size of some prolactinomas in humans.

A Physiological Prolactin-Releasing Factor (PRF) has yet to be Demonstrated

There is some experimental evidence for TRH, vasoactive intestinal polypeptide (VIP), and oxytocin as potential prolactin-releasing factors. For example, is a potent stimulus to PRL secretion in virtually every vertebrate species studied. It is unclear, however, whether any of these regulators is a true physiological prolactin-releasing hormone (PRH). Recently a preproprotein molecule was identified in brain that is proteolytically processed to produce a 30-amino-acid peptide and a 21-amino-acid peptide, with both molecules exhibiting specific prolactin-releasing activity [19]. It has been suggested that these prolactin-releasing peptides (PRPs) are bona fide PRHs of physiological importance. However, it was recently determined that the expression of these putative PRHs is absent in fibers innervating the median eminence, suggesting that the major physiological PRH has yet to be identified.

Dopamine May Function as an MSH Release-Inhibiting Factor (MIF)

The role of the pars intermedia as the source of a melanotropin (α-MSH) that regulates color change in many non-human vertebrates is well established (Chap. 8). Like PRL, MSH is under an inhibitory control by the hypothalamus. Stalk transection or damage to the hypothalamus results in enhanced MSH secretion. Transplantation of the pars intermedia to an ectopic site in the animal also leads to enhanced MSH secretion. In addition incubation of neurointermediate lobes in vivo results in a sustained secretion of MSH. These results suggest that the hypothalamus exerts a tonic inhibitory control of MSH secretion.

What is the mechanism by which the hypothalamus tonically represses MSH secretion? In many vertebrates (e.g., frog and mouse), the pars intermedia is penetrated by aminergic neurons whose cell bodies are located within the hypothalamus. The axons of these neurons form a plexus around and between the pars intermedia cells. The release of a neurotransmitter, most likely DA, from these neurons is apparently responsible for inhibition of MSH secretion. In vitro, DA inhibits MSH secretion from isolated pituitary glands (Chap. 8). Present evidence suggests that DA is the physiological MSH release-inhibiting factor (MIF, melanostatin). There is minimal evidence for the existence of any putative hypothalamic MSH-releasing factor (MRF) of a peptidergic nature. In some species, serotonin may be a factor regulating pars intermedia MSH secretion (Chap. 8).

Control of Hypothalamic/Hypophysial Hormone Secretion

In response to cold, many mammals release TSH, and in response to stress, ACTH is secreted from the pituitary gland. Suckling of the mammary glands stimulates PRL and oxytocin secretion, and GH is released in response to intake of certain dietary metabolic substrates. These pituitary responses are regulated by hypophysiotropic factors. What factors and mechanisms regulate the secretion of the hypophysiotropins? Because the brain is composed mainly of neurons and supporting elements, other neurons within the brain would be expected to regulate the hypophysiotropin-secreting neurons. These other neurons, in turn, are linked to yet other neuronal inputs such as sensory neurons that are receptive to endogenous (intrinsic) and exogenous (extrinsic) cues.

Neurohormone Secretions are Governed by Central Neurons and their Neurotransmitters

Extrinsic and intrinsic stimuli received through sensory neurons are conducted through neuronal routes to the brain where this information may be inhibitory or stimulatory to hypophysiotropic hormone secretion. Conduction of sensory information is via neuronal elements, and each nerve must release a neurotransmitter to effect synaptic transmission. These neurohormones include the monoamine neurotransmitters (Fig. 6.13) and the amino acid neurotransmitters (Fig. 6.14). There are well-defined aminergic (monoamine) pathways within the brain that are composed of serotonergic, dopaminergic, noradrenergic, and even epinephrine-containing neurons. Axons from these neurons project from extrahypothalamic sites into the hypothalamus where they innervate hypophysiotropic hormone-producing cells. Depending on the nature of the receptors possessed by these neurons, the neurotransmitters may inhibit or stimulate hypophysiotropin secretion from these peptidergic neurons. This will then be reflected in enhanced or inhibited pituitary

Figure 6.13 The monoamine neurotransmitters.

H H H
HO — C — C — C — C — NH$_2$
‖ ‖ ‖ ‖
O H H H

Gamma-Aminobutyric Acid

H
HO — C — C — NH$_2$
‖ ‖
O H

Glycine

H H H O
HO — C — C — C — C — C — OH
‖ ‖ ‖ ‖
O H H NH$_2$

Glutamic Acid

Figure 6.14 **The amino acid neurotransmitters.**

hormone secretion. For example, inhibitory inputs to hypophysiotropic neurons containing inhibitory factors (MIF, PIF, SST) would be expected to enhance pituitary secretion of MSH, PRL, and GH, respectively.

Specific Neurotransmitters Regulate Hypophysiotropin Secretions

A brief discussion of the neuroendocrine control of each hypothalamic hypophysiotropin is provided.

Control of CRH Secretion. A number of different neurotransmitters are involved [49] in regulating ACTH secretion. Stress is a potent stimulus to ACTH secretion. This response is diminished by atropine implantations at sites within the hypothalamus, thus implicating one or more cholinergic pathways (involving acetylcholine as neurotransmitter) in the control of ACTH secretion. Stimulation of CNS cholinergic structures provokes pituitary ACTH release [33]. Central catecholamines induce release of both CRH and AVP into the portal capillary plexus. These findings support the hypothesis that stress induces release of catecholamines from axons projecting to the paraventricular nucleus, thus activating adrenergic receptors that may selectively stimulate an AVP-containing subpopulation of CRH neurosecretory cells [48].

Control of PIF Secretion. Suckling is the normal stimulus to PRL secretion. This neuroendocrine reflex involves the inhibition of dopaminergic neurons whose release of PIF maintains a tonic inhibition of PRL secretion. A number of neurotransmitters participate in the control of PRL secretion. PRL secretion increases during sleep and is entrained to sleep, as a shift in the sleep cycle will shift the rhythm of PRL secretion (see Fig. 5.6). The nocturnal rise in PRL secretion apparently involves activation of hypothalamic serotonergic (5-HT) neurons because administration of the 5-HT blocking agent, methysergide, blunts the increase in PRL secretion. In addition, inhibitors of serotonin synthesis (e.g., p-chlorophenylalanine) abolish suckling-induced PRL release. There is an increased metabolism of brain 5-HT in suckled female rats, and PRL secretion is enhanced following administration of 5-HT receptor agonists.

Gamma-aminobutyric acid (GABA) may also control PRL secretion. Injections of GABA stimulate or inhibit PRL secretion depending on the concentrations employed. The stimulating effect of large doses of GABA is blocked by the GABA receptor antagonist, bicuculline. Vasoactive intestinal peptide (VIP) is localized to nerve endings in the hypothalamus and is present in the hypothalamo-hypophysial portal blood. VIP receptors have been identified in a PRL-secreting tumor; the peptide stimulates cAMP production in the pituitary gland while stimulating PRL secretion. VIP, therefore, may play a physiological role in the control of PRL secretion. There is evidence for the role of the histaminergic system in the regulation of PRL secretion because intraventricular injections of histamine stimulate PRL secretion in rats, whereas blockage of histamine H$_1$ receptors prevents stimulation of PRL secretion in response to stress or suckling.

Control of Growth Hormone Secretion. A variety of stimuli elevate GH secretion, presumably through inhibition of somatostatin secretion or by an enhancement of GHRH secretion [44]. Some of the GHRH-immunoreactive nerve cell bodies within the arcuate nucleus of the rat hypothalamus possess SST binding sites. The finding of SST receptors on GHRH-containing arcuate neurons provides a morphological substrate for the concept of direct "cross-talk" between SST and GHRH neuronal systems within the CNS. Such intrahypothalamic interactions between these two neuropeptides may be a vital component in the generation and maintenance of the ultradian (cycle more frequent than 24 hours) rhythm of GH secretion [2, 28]. The dynamic role of SST and GHRH in the control of GH secretion is depicted (Fig. 6.15).

Control of GnRH Secretion. Several transmitters and neuropeptides participate in the regulation of gonadotropin secretion [3]. At the hypothalamic level, control of gonadotropin-releasing hormone (GnRH) involves norepinephrine, GABA, glutamate, angiotensin II, neuropeptide Y, neurotensin, and 5-hydroxytryptamine, as well as interleukins 1 and 2 [26]. Hypothalamic dopaminergic neurons are clearly stimulatory to GnRH secretion from parvocellular neurons. Dopamine secretion itself is inhibited by enkephalinergic neurons.

Figure 6.15 Rebound GH secretion following somatostatin withdrawal involves GHRH release. Regular rebound GH secretion can be elicited by intermittent infusions of somatostatin in conscious rats. The figure shows two groups of four animals given intravenous somatostatin infusions interrupted for 30 minutes every 3 hours. The lower panel shows that injection (arrowed) of 0.5 ml normal rabbit serum has no effect on GH rebound release, whereas injection of 0.5 ml antirat GHRH serum in another group of rats (upper panel) greatly attenuates the subsequent GH rebounds. (From Robinson, with permission, *Acta Paediatrica Scandinavica* 372:70–8, 1991.)

Therefore, an enkephalin such as Met-enkephalin is indirectly in control of GnRH secretion and ultimately FSH and LH secretion. Ovarian steroids can interfere with gonadotropin regulation by either direct effects on GnRH release or by increasing the sensitivity of anterior pituitary cells to GnRH, thus potentiating the release of pituitary hormones.

Control of TRH Secretion. Apparently noradrenergic neurons stimulate TSH secretion by a stimulatory action on TRH-secreting neurons. Evidence in both humans and rats suggests that glucocorticoid excess inhibits thyroid function at a suprapituitary level. A glucocorticoid response element may be present on the TRH gene, and a glucocorticoid receptor has been identified on TRH neurons in the paraventricular nuclei. These observations provide a molecular basis for the effects of glucocorticoids on TRH gene expression (and TRH synthesis). A complex array of other factors influence TRH production [23].

Peripheral Hormones Exert Feedback Actions in the Hypothalamus

In response to a hypophysiotropin, adenohypophysial hormones, such as TSH, ACTH, and the gonadotropins, are released into the general circulation where they circulate to their target tissues. Target tissue stimulation results in increased secretion of target tissue hormones, such as thyroid hormones (T_4 and T_3), adrenal glucocorticoids (e.g., cortisol), and gonadal steroids (e.g., estradiol, testosterone, progesterone). These hormones then circulate to their respective target tissues to mediate their actions. The pituitary gland and the hypothalamus are themselves target organs of these steroid or thyroid hormones (Fig. 6.16). Three mechanisms of feedback control of hypophysiotropin and hypophysial

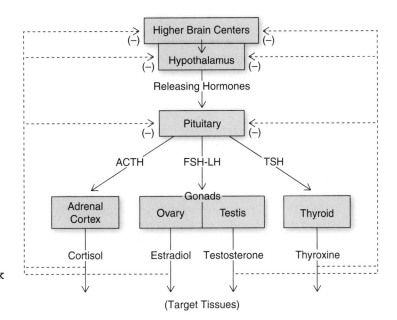

Figure 6.16 Feedback control of pituitary hormone secretion.

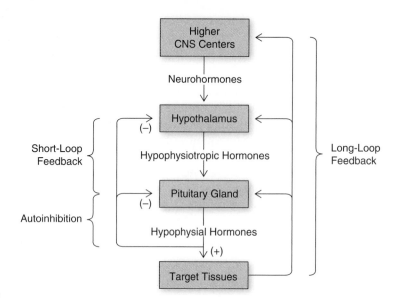

Figure 6.17 Model of long-loop and short-loop mechanisms and autoregulation of pituitary hormone secretion.

hormone secretion are recognized. Peripheral target tissue hormones may feed back through a so-called *long-loop* system to act at the level of the pituitary, at the level of the hypothalamus, or even at higher brain centers (Fig. 6.17). Hypophysial hormones may also circulate by retrograde portal system blood flow to affect hypothalamic hypophysiotropic hormone secretion by a so-called *short-loop* mechanism. There is even evidence that secreted hypophysial hormones may feed back on their cells of origin to inhibit their own secretion, referred to as *autoinhibition* or *autofeedback inhibition* (Fig. 6.17).

Although some of the pituitary hormones, such as PRL, the neurohypophysial hormones, and α-melanotropin, stimulate peripheral target tissues, these target tissues do not themselves secrete hormones. The secretion of these hypophysial hormones therefore is not controlled by long-loop hormonal feedback mechanisms. The secretion of these hormones, however, may be controlled by reflex mechanisms and other sensory stimuli reaching the hypothalamus from sensory receptors. For example, suckling of the breast by the infant leads to secretion of oxytocin from the neurohypophysis. A decreased blood volume or increase in plasma electrolyte concentration is stimulatory to vasopressin secretion. It is becoming more evident that certain metabolic substrates (e.g., glucose, amino acids, free fatty acids) may also act at the level of the hypothalamus to affect hypophysiotropin secretion.

Steroid hormones implanted in the hypothalamus also modulate pituitary hormone secretion. It can be demonstrated, using autoradiographic methods, that steroid hormones localize to specific sites within the CNS. Immunocytochemical methods have been used to confirm that these same cell groups express the cognate steroid receptor proteins. These feedback sites for steroid hormones may also represent production sites of the hypophysiotropins. Indeed, immunocytochemical methods have localized hypophysiotropins, such as GnRH and SST, to these same hypothalamic steroid-binding sites.

Corticotropin Secretion. ACTH stimulates adrenal glucocorticoid production and secretion. Glucocorticoids, such as cortisol and corticosterone, and dexamethasone (a synthetic glucocorticoid) exert a negative feedback on ACTH secretion. Their locus of action is apparently at the level of both the pituitary and the hypothalamus, as determined by the following experiments. Dexamethasone injected into the adenohypophysis inhibits ACTH secretion. Given prior to microinjection of exogenous CRH or hypothalamic extract directly into the pituitary, dexamethasone abolishes ACTH release in response to the hypophysiotropin. Finally, CRH stimulation of ACTH secretion from pituitary glands incubated in vitro is inhibited by addition of corticosterone to the medium. CRH levels in the brain are increased after bilateral adrenalectomy; this change can be prevented by administration of exogenous glucocorticoids. Thus, glucocorticoids act on the hypothalamus to modulate the turnover of hypothalamic CRH, as well as acting directly on the pituitary.

Gonadotropin Secretion.   Gonadectomy of an animal, such as the rat, results in an increased secretion of gonadotropins. Injections of gonadal steroids—estrogens or androgens—result in decreased circulating levels of gonadotropins in gonadectomized animals. These results suggest that gonadal steroids exert a negative feedback inhibition of gonadotropin secretion. Where are the sites of action of gonadal steroids in this feedback mechanism? Gonadectomy results in an acceleration of pulsatile GnRH neurosecretion, and steroid hormone replacement can reverse this process. Thus, the brain is clearly a target of steroid hormone negative feedback. The specific population of steroid-responsive cells mediating these effects is still unknown. This issue was only partially answered by the use of radiolabeled gonadal steroids as well as steroid receptor immunocytochemistry. Injections of [^{3}H]estradiol, for example, result in an accumulation of the ligand within the hypothalamus; autoradiographic studies demonstrate that the hormone localizes over the nuclei of neurons in specific hypothalamic sites (see Fig. 3.3). The radiolabeled hormone localizes to the same preoptic and hypothalamic neurons that have been implicated in the control of pituitary gonadotropin secretion. Immunocytochemical analyses of steroid receptor expressing neurons are in agreement with these receptor binding studies. These results indicate that gonadal steroids regulate pituitary gonadotropin secretion through long-loop feedback to the hypothalamus. The intracellular pathways mediating steroid feedback actions in the brain are not well understood, and are the subject of much current study. Gonadal steroids may also exert negative feedback effects directly at the level of pituitary gonadotrophs (Chap. 18). The positive feedback actions of ovarian steroids are also likely exerted at both hypothalamic and pituitary levels, as discussed in Chapter 18.

Prolactin Secretion.   Injection of PRL or implantation of PRL into the median eminence of rats reduces the secretion of PRL from the pituitary. In some of these studies, the hypothalamic content of PIF (dopamine) was found to be increased; these results suggested that a short-loop feedback system might regulate pituitary PRL secretion. There is other evidence that PRL can inhibit its own secretion by a direct action on the lactotrophs of the anterior pituitary gland.

Growth Hormone Secretion.   The CNS control of pituitary growth hormone secretion is believed to be mediated by a balance between somatostatin and GHRH. There is evidence that GH acts at the level of the hypothalamus to stimulate the synthesis and release of SST. GH mediates most of its effects indirectly through the stimulation of somatomedin production and release by the liver. The somatomedins then act on many tissues and organs to enhance growth. There is also evidence that insulin-like growth factor I (IGF-I) acutely stimulates SST release by the hypothalamus. IGF-I also exerts a much slower direct inhibitory effect on pituitary GH secretion. These observations suggest that IGF-I participates in a long-loop negative feedback action on SST secretion by the hypothalamus, as well as a slower long-loop action at the level of the pituitary.

Immunoneutralization of endogenous GHRH causes a significant increase in arcuate GHRH mRNA levels with a concomitant decrease in pituitary GH levels. Both GH and IGF-I replacement are effective in antagonizing the effect of GHRH-ab treatment on hypothalamic GHRH mRNA levels. These findings indicate that GH and/or IGF-I represent major factors in the negative regulation of GHRH synthesis.

Thyrotropin Secretion.   TSH secretion is enhanced following thyroidectomy or inhibition of thyroid hormone (T_4/T_3) production by drugs. This enhanced TSH secretion is abolished by the concomitant administration of T_4 or T_3 to an animal. Thyroid hormones also control TRH synthesis by regulating gene expression of the TRH prohormone in the "thyrotropic area" of the hypothalamus. Regulation of TRH production by thyroid hormones occurs primarily at the transcriptional and translational levels rather than by post-translational processing. Experimental data support the view that hypothalamic TRH production is regulated by thyroid hormones and that the rise in plasma TSH in hypothyroidism is likely due to increased release of TRH from the median eminence [4]. TSH secretion from isolated pituitaries in culture induced by TRH is also inhibited by thyroid hormones. These results demonstrate control of pituitary TSH secretion by actions at the level of the hypothalamus, as well as the pituitary.

Hypophysiotropic Hormones are Usually Secreted in a Rhythmic Pattern

During the process of evolution, certain physiological processes of animals have become regulated by endogenous rhythms that are closely attuned to the daily periodicities of the light–dark cycle. The term *circadian* (from the Latin for *circa*, about, and *dies*, day) was coined to describe these diurnal rhythms of activity. These endogenous rhythms undoubtedly evolved in response to the daily environmental light cycle. Daily exogenous light cues, however, no longer act as the immediate cause of the *biologic rhythm*, but only as a synchronizing mechanism or *Zeitgeber* (time-givers). In the absence of environmental information, the biological rhythm free-runs with its own frequency and can be entrained to a range of frequencies, however limited, that differ slightly from the 24-hour cycle.

Systemic biological rhythms are regulated by a so-called *biological clock* whose anatomical site may be the *suprachiasmatic nucleus* of the hypothalamus. Within recent years the cellular and molecular mechanisms that mediate the generation of circadian rhythmicity have been discovered, as described subsequently in this text (Chap. 20). Because seasonal changes in animals may be triggered by changes in the length of the day, some mechanism must also exist whereby the duration of the daylight period can be measured and translated into changes in pituitary hormone secretion. The mechanisms involved in measurement and translation are unknown, but they appear to involve both secretion of melatonin by the pineal gland as well as neural inputs to hypophysiotropin-secreting cells (Chap. 20).

In humans, the plasma concentration of cortisol rises in the morning and declines in the afternoon and evening. A similar adrenocortical rhythm, present in many mammalian species, may be associated with a 24-hour variation in secretion rates of CRH and ACTH as the plasma concentration of ACTH and the hypothalamic content of CRH exhibit a similar circadian rhythm. The secretion of GH has been shown to be pulsatile in nature in every species of animal studied, from rats to humans. For example, in human male and female subjects at various stages of pubertal development, nonsleep-related bursts of GH secretion occur. Generally, two episodes of GH secretion are observed during a 6-hour sampling period.

Neurohormones are also commonly secreted in a pulsatile manner, as rhythmic bursts of release with frequencies ranging from 1 pulse/20 minutes to 1 pulse/3 hours, depending upon the species and physiological circumstances. Pulsatile release of GnRH, as described above, is perhaps the best characterized of neurohormone release patterns. Functionally, this relates to the fact that some hormone receptors and post-receptor, intracellular signals, are down-regulated in the presence of continuous hormone secretion. An understanding of neurohormone pulsatility is essential if certain hypophysiotropins are to be used in clinical medicine.

Neuropharmacogogical Agents are Used to Probe the Neural Regulation of Hypophysiotropin Release

Pharmacological methods have been used successfully to determine the particular neural components involved in hypophysiotropin regulation of pituitary hormone secretion. For example, it was demonstrated that reflex ovulation in the rabbit could be blocked by rapid postcoital intravenous injections of dibenamine, an α-adrenoceptor (Chap. 14) blocking agent. Infusions of norepinephrine into the third ventricle of the brain resulted in an ovulatory surge of pituitary gonadotropins that was blocked by an α-adrenoceptor blocker and also by pentobarbital (a CNS-acting anesthetic), indicating that norepinephrine was acting within the brain [1].

Many drugs are available that can specifically modify neuronal activity and, in turn, hormonal secretion. The neuronal events are classified as presynaptic, synaptic, and postsynaptic. There are drugs that can modify the presynaptic events by affecting availability of neurotransmitter precursors, synthesis of neurotransmitters, transport of neurotransmitters along the axon, storage of neurotransmitters within secretory vesicles, exocytotic release of neurotransmitters from these vesicles, and inhibition of reuptake of neurotransmitters by presynaptic neurons. There are drugs that specifically interfere with the synaptic event by inhibiting the action of enzymes normally responsible for neurotransmitter inactivation within the synapse, thereby prolonging the action of neurotransmitters. Drugs can also affect postsynaptic events by blocking neurotransmitter receptors, by mimicking

Culture Medium   Peristaltic Pump   Cell Chamber   Fraction Collector

the receptor-mediated actions of the neurotransmitter, and by interfering with second messenger production and degradation within presynaptic or postsynaptic neurons. Increased or decreased release of a pituitary hormone by one of these drugs is interpreted to imply that a particular neurotransmitter is involved somewhere in the hypothalamic pathway of control of the hormone.

Mechanisms of Hypophysiotropin Action

Attempts to determine the mechanisms of action of hypophysiotropic hormones on pituitary target cells are complicated due to the heterogeneity of the pituitary cell population [6]. Nevertheless, the action of hypophysiotropins directly on hypophysial cells has been demonstrated [20, 47]. Pituitaries or pituitary cell cultures can be studied using a perifusion system (Fig. 6.18) wherein the actions of a hormone or drug on hormone secretion can be monitored. Electrophysiological activities of individual pituitary cells have been monitored. Early experiments showed that application of TRH by micropipette to individual dissociated anterior pituitary cells elicited action potentials in a subset of previously silent cells and increased the frequency of such potentials in a subset spontaneously active cells (Fig. 6.19). The respondent cells probably represent thyrotrophs (or possibly lactotrophs). TRH-induced depolarization of thyrotrophs is Ca^{2+} dependent, which suggests that the hypophysiotropic factor stimulates thyrotropin secretion through a stimulus-secretion coupling mechanism [47]. In recent years, immortalized pituitary cell lines have been developed using targeted tumorigenesis techniques [50]. The availability of these homogeneous cell populations has greatly facilitated the study of hypophysiotropin actions, signal transduction, hormone secretion, and gene expression in pituitary hormone-producing cells. The immortalized LβT cells, for example, are a gonadotroph cell line developed by Mellon and colleagues [29, 35] that has been used to assess the mechanisms by which GnRH regulates gonadotropin secretion and gonadotropin subunit gene expression.

The hypophysiotropic hormones exert their effects via G-protein-coupled receptors that are present only in the plasma membranes of their target pituitary cells. For example, GnRH stimulates gonadotropin secretion and subunit gene expression by activating GnRH receptors in the plasma membranes of gonadotrophs; few, if any, of the other pituitary cell types express appreciable numbers of GnRH receptors, and thus the gonadotroph is uniquely equipped to respond to the decapeptide. The GnRH receptors are primarily coupled to the activation of phospholipase C (PLC) via a G protein, $G_{q/11}$, leading to stimulation of phosphoinositide turnover as well as mobilization and influx of Ca^{2+}, activation of protein kinase C (PKC) and mitogen-activated protein kinase (MAPK).

Hypophysiotropic regulation of the somatotroph is particularly complex, as at least three different peptides—GHRH, SST, and ghrelin—and their corresponding cognate receptors simultaneously control GH synthesis and secretion in these cells. In somatotrophs, the effects of GHRH, SST, and ghrelin are mediated by activation of G-protein-coupled GHRH receptors, SST receptors, and the GH-secretogogue (GHS) receptors, respectively. GHRH stimulates and SST inhibits adenylate cyclase activity, cAMP production, and GH secretion from anterior pituitary cells [20]. GHS receptor stimulation activates PLC, phosphoinositol hydrolysis, PKC, and intracellular Ca^{++} mobilization. The mechanisms by which these three signals are transduced and integrated within the somatotroph remain to be clarified.

In subsequent chapters, the GPCRs and signal transduction pathways mediating effects of GnRH in gonadotrophs, GH, SST and ghrelin in somatotrophs, DA in lactotrophs, TRH in thyrotrophs, and CRH in somatotrophs are discussed in more detail.

Steroid and Thyroid Hormones can Directly Modulate Pituitary Hormone Secretion

Thyroid hormones and adrenal and gonadal steroids secreted in response to hypophysial hormones exert feed back at the level of the pituitary to modulate the action of hypophysiotropins. These feedback effects are discussed in the context of respective hormone systems later in this text, but their general actions are mentioned here. Thyroid hormones, thyroxine and triiodothyronine, are inhibitory to TSH secretion through actions mainly at the level of the pituitary gland. For example, TRH is stimulatory to TSH release from pituitary glands incubated in vitro, but the release of TSH from pituitaries is prevented by prior incubation of the glands in the presence of T_4 or T_3. The inhibitory effects of these thyroid hormones are, in turn, abolished by concomitant incubation of the glands in the presence of actinomycin or cycloheximide (inhibitors of RNA and protein synthesis, respectively), suggesting that the thyroid hormones stimulate the synthesis of an inhibitor of TRH action.

CRH stimulation of pituitary ACTH secretion is abolished by the synthetic glucocorticoid dexamethasone, both in vivo and in vitro. The negative feedback of adrenal glucocorticoids therefore is mediated, in part, directly at the level of the pituitary. Androgens have an inhibitory action on LH release at the hypothalamic and pituitary levels; their inhibitory effect on FSH release is restricted to the hypothalamus. Progesterone can exert stimulatory and inhibitory effects on gonadotropin secretion at the pituitary and hypothalamic levels. Modulation of hypophysiotropin action can occur by an alteration of hypophysial cell receptor number (and possibly receptor sensitivity). Estradiol increases the sensitivity of FSH- and LH-secreting cells to GnRH by a direct action at the level of the pituitary. The effect of estradiol can be stimulatory or inhibitory, depending on the dose and time of administration of the estrogen. The number of pituitary GnRH receptors is positively correlated with concentrations of estradiol in the serum. Modulation of gonadotroph GnRH receptors may be a necessary component of increased pituitary sensitivity to the hypophysiotropin during the estrous cycle. Estradiol may also increase PRL secretion in humans and in rats, and the steroid is also stimulatory to TSH secretion in rats. Daily injections of estradiol increase the number of pituitary TRH binding sites (see Fig. 19.9). Thyroxine injections in the rat, on the other hand, lead to a progressive decrease in pituitary TRH binding sites. Binding of the TRH to thyrotroph plasma membranes is enhanced by prior treatment with propylthiouracil, a drug that reduces thyroid hormone production by the thyroid (Chap. 13).

Pathophysiology of Hypothalamic Dysfunction

Because each of the pituitary hormones is under stimulatory or inhibitory control by hormones of the hypothalamus, adrenal, thyroidal, and gonadal hypoactivity or hyperactivity may often relate to defects at the level of the hypothalamus, rather than at the pituitary gland [30]. Abnormal pituitary hormone secretion may be related to defects in hypophysiotropic hormone synthesis and secretion or to altered activity of the neuronal inputs to hypophysiotropin neurons. Overproduction or underproduction of dopamine within CNS neurons, for example, is believed responsible for the etiology of schizophrenia and Parkinson's disease, respectively.

In 1943, Kallmann first described patients with hypogonadism and anosmia. Patients with the Kallmann syndrome fail to secrete gonadotropic hormones; the disorder is an example of hypogonadotropic hypogonadism. In Kallmann's syndrome, there appears to be a failure of migration of GnRH neurons due to deletion of a gene that encodes a protein necessary for controlling normal migration of GnRH neurons (and olfactory neurons). The deleted gene region (referred to as KAL) encodes a protein that is homologous to members of the fibronectin gene family, known to control neural chemotaxis, cell adhesion, and apparently in this case GnRH/neuronal migration during embryogenesis [9].

GnRH has been used therapeutically to induce ovulation in amenorrheic females. The hormone has also been used to treat oligospermia and hypogonadotropic hypogonadism in males. Highly potent analogs of GnRH have been developed for use in the treatment of hypogonadal function in the male and the female [9]. Although administration of GnRH causes an initial large release of gonadotropins in females, prolonged treatment results in disturbances in gonadotropin secretion, irregular follicular maturation, and a low incidence of ovulation (Chap. 18). A single dose of certain long-acting GnRH analogs is effective in decreasing gonadotropin secretion [8]. These peptides may prove useful as antifertility (contraceptive) agents.

Some tumors may secrete hypothalamic hormones. For example, ectopic secretion of a CRH-like peptide may be responsible for certain cases of Cushing's disease. A number of mechanisms may be invoked to explain the hyperprolactinemia associated with pituitary prolactinomas. First a hypothalamic disorder, involving decreased secretion of PIF or increased secretion of a PRL-releasing factor, could lead to eventual tumor formation. Second, PRL could be produced autonomously by a tumor whose cells, by loss of dopamine receptors or other mechanisms, have become partially or wholly independent of hypothalamic control [21].

Hypophysiotropins as Diagnostic Agents. Because synthetic hypophysiotropic hormones are commercially available, one can differentiate hypothalamic dysfunction from defects related to pituitary pathophysiology [40]. Administration of thyrotropin-releasing hormone with subsequent measurement of the TSH response, probably the most widely used of these tests, is used to diagnose subclinical hypothyroidism or hyperthyroidism. Repeated administration of GnRH usually is necessary to determine whether functional gonadotrophs are present [2]. Similarly, GHRH has been administered to GH-deficient patients to determine whether functional somatotrophs are present [40]. Although a single intravenous dose of GHRH may stimulate GH release in some patients with idiopathic GH deficiency, repetitive intermittent administration may be necessary to "prime" the somatotroph before significant GH stimulation occurs.

The specificity of releasing factors to stimulate respective target cells in the anterior pituitary has been shown. There is also convincing evidence that the hypothalamic-releasing factors do not interact at the level of the pituitary gland to enhance, inhibit, or modify each other's biological actions. These observations are of significance to clinical medicine. It is expected that a single bolus administration of several releasing factors (e.g., GnRH, TRH, CRH, and GHRH) will be used to determine pituitary reserve (ability to release appropriate hormones; e.g., FSH, LH, TSH, ACTH, GH). It might be expected that any single or multiple pituitary non-response or unexpected response will be due to single or multiple pituitary abnormalities, rather than to an interaction of the secretogogues administered.

Therapy with GHRH. The traditional treatment of GH-deficient children is administration of GH. Because Creutzfeldt–Jakob disease developed in a few young adults who received GH extracted from prion-contaminated human pituitary glands, these biological preparations are no longer available in the United States. Fortunately, the development of techniques for biosynthesis of GH by recombinant DNA technology has provided an ample supply of human GH for treatment of these children. Clinical trials of a methionyl-GH and

MOLECULAR MEDICINE CASE STUDY

$G_s\alpha$ mutation at codon 201 in pituitary adenoma causing gigantism in a 6-year-old boy with McCune–Albright syndrome (J. Dötsch, W. Kiess, J. Hänze, R. Repp, D Lüdecke, W. F. Blum, and W. Roscher. *J. Clin. Endocrinol.* Metab. 81:3839–42, 1996). Mutations of the α subunit of stimulatory GTP-binding proteins, $G_s\alpha$, are related to the development of pituitary adenomas. These mutations lead to a constitutive activation of the G-protein-coupled receptors resulting in increased adenylate cyclase activity and cAMP production. This increased second messenger production is believed to be tumorigenic. Activating point mutations for the human $G_s\alpha$ gene have been shown in codon 201 (Arg) and 227 (Glu) of exons 8 and 9, respectively. The oncogene generated by these mutations is termed *gsp*. In children, pituitary tumors causing gigantism are very rare, and

$G_s\alpha$ mutations in tumor tissue have not previously been reported. In adult acromegalic patients, on the other hand, the frequency of $G_s\alpha$ mutations may be 30–45% in GH-secreting adenomas.

The patient also presented with other endocrine abnormalities associated with the McCune–Albright syndrome (MAS). MAS is a sporadic disease characterized by abnormalities of bone growth, café-au-lait spots, precocious puberty, and multiple endocrinopathies. Overactive growth and secretion by affected tissues/organs is correlated with the multiple expression of activating mutations of the stimulatory G protein, *gsp*. Mutation of the $G_s\alpha$ gene early in development (postzygotic somatic mutation) accounts for the expression of multiple endocrine neoplasia.

pure GH indicate that these preparations are effective in promoting linear growth and are not associated with toxicity. An alternative treatment for GH deficiency is administration of GHRH to stimulate GH release [30], GH-deficient children have been treated with GHRH-40, GHRH-44, and a 29-amino-acid GHRH analog, with inconsistent results. Despite variations in GHRH preparations, total daily dose, and frequency of administration, a substantial proportion of children showed increased growth velocity during therapy with these GHRHs.

Conclusions and Speculations

The hypothalamus, the coordinating center of the brain, controls endocrine, behavioral, and autonomic nervous system functions. Specifically, it plays an important role in thermoregulation, feeding and drinking behaviors, cardiovascular activity, pituitary gland regulation, and certain types of motivation and learning. The experimental affirmation of the neurovascular hypothesis of Harris [18] was particularly important in establishing the functional role of hypothalamic hypophysiotropic factors in the control of endocrine function. Indeed, the hypothalamus provides the final common neuroendocrine pathway in the control of the peripheral endocrine system. The endocrine hypothalamus is itself regulated by the peripheral endocrine system, as well as by autonomic nervous system afferent inputs. Thus, the concept of neuroendocrinology has emerged that emphasizes the reciprocal integrated roles of the nervous and endocrine systems in the control of physiological processes. Table 6.1 summarizes the evidence that hypophysiotropic factors control pituitary hormone production and secretion.

The progressive elucidation of the presence and precise distribution of neurohormones within the hypothalamus and other brain centers may provide the exact neuroanatomical-neurohormonal correlates related to normal and abnormal neuroendocrine-physiology. An understanding of the structure of the hypophysiotropins and their subsequent synthesis has provided the clinician with new tools for enhancing pituitary hormone secretion under conditions of hypothalamic dysfunction. Of great interest is the discovery that the hypophysiotropins are not restricted to the hypothalamus, but rather are found throughout the nervous system, the gut, and other peripheral organs. Each of these hypophysiotropins may function in the control of a diverse number of physiological processes. A study of the comparative endocrinology of these peptides reveals that their role in the hypothalamus may indeed be a rather late evolutionary acquisition.

TABLE 6.1 Experimental evidence supporting a hypothalamic control of pituitary hormone secretion

1. Pituitary stalk section or placement of a mechanical barrier between the hypothalamus and the pituitary gland leads to diminished or enhanced secretion of certain pituitary hormones.
2. Ectopic transplantation of the pituitary gland leads to decreased or increased secretion of pituitary hormones.
3. Retransplantation of ectopically transplanted pituitaries under the hypothalamus leads to reactivation of pituitary hormone secretion (e.g., reestablishment of ovulatory cycles).
4. Specifically placed discrete lesions in the hypothalamus lead to diminished or enhanced secretion of specific hypophysial hormones.
5. Electrode stimulation of discrete hypothalamic sites leads to inhibition or release of certain pituitary hormones.
6. Pituitary hormone secretion is inhibited by implantation of target organ tissues or their hormones into discrete sites within the hypothalamus.
7. Hypothalamic extracts injected into intact animals or added to pituitary glands incubated in vitro enhance or inhibit pituitary secretions.
8. Ectopic pituitary grafts are reactivated (after partial atrophy) by local infusions of extracts of the median eminence.
9. Fragments of the pituitary gland transplanted within a specific site (hypophysiotropic area) of the hypothalamus remain functionally active.
10. Administration of pharmaceutical agents that enhance or inhibit neurotransmitter production by hypothalamic neurons leads to enhanced or inhibited pituitary hormone secretion.
11. Synthetic peptides identical in structure to the putative hypophysiotropic hormones mimic the activity of the hypothalamic peptides on pituitary hormone secretion.
12. Pituitary hypophysiotropic hormones are found in the hypophysial portal blood in greater concentration than in the systemic circulation.
13. Radiolabeled gonadal steroids localize to hypothalamic sites known to control pituitary gonadotropin secretion.
14. Electrode stimulation of hypothalamic tissue in vitro leads to a Ca^{2+}-dependent release of putative hypophysiotropins.
15. Electrical stimulation of the hypothalamus elevates plasma levels of hypophysiotropins.
16. Adrenalectomy, gonadectomy, and thyroidectomy, procedures which alter levels of pituitary hormone secretion, also alter hypothalamic levels of hypophysiotropins.
17. Immunocytochemical techniques localize hypophysiotropins to specific hypothalamic neurons.
18. Administration of antisera to hypophysiotropic hormones leads to enhanced or inhibited pituitary hormone secretion.

REVIEW EXERCISES

Compare and contrast each of the following terms. How are they related? How do they differ?

hypertrophy/hyperplasia
parvocellular/magnocellular (neurons)
ectoderm/neuroectoderm
hypophysiotropin/ hypophysiotropic area
hypogonadism/ hypergonadism
primary/secondary (hypothyroidism)
circadian/ diurnal rhythms

Define or otherwise characterize each of the following terms (then use each of the terms in a sentence):

neurovascular hypothesis
hyperprolactinemia
portal blood vessels
portal system
ectopic site
median eminence

Match each hypophysiotropin to its corresponding pituitary hormone(s), indicating (+) or (−) control:

CRH   LH
TRH   GH
GnRH   ACTH
GHRH   FSH
SST   PRL
DA   TSH

Think, analyze and discuss:

1. Suckling is a powerful stimulus for the release of prolactin from lactotrophs in the anterior pituitary gland. Research has demonstrated that the act of suckling stimulates nerve endings in the breast, sending nerve impulses up the neuroaxis. The neural signals reach neurohormone-secreting cells in the hypothalamus, which can, in turn, direct changes in prolactin secretion.
   a. Which neurohormone-producing cells might be modulated as a result of suckling? Would suckling stimulate or inhibit secretion of this neurohormone into the hypophysial portal vessels?
   b. In lactotrophs, the receptor that mediates the actions of the neurohormone in (a) is a G-protein-coupled receptor that is, in turn, coupled to the modulation of adenylate cyclase activity. Would stimulation of this receptor produce an increase or decrease in intracellular cAMP formation?
   c. Nursing of young is associated with an inhibition of gonadotropin (LH, FSH) secretion. This is thought to be the basis of "nature's contraception," viz. the physiologically-induced infertile state that often occurs during lactation, ensuring maximum allocation of maternal energy to a new infant. Can you think of a mechanism by which elevated prolactin levels may inhibit gonadotropin secretion, and thereby suppress ovulatory cyclicity during lactation?

2. Infertility can occur in both men and women as a result of impaired or completely absent GnRH neurosecretion. Describe a GnRH replacement therapy that might be prescribed for a patient with this condition. What pattern of GnRH administration might be most effective in restoring LH and FSH secretion? Why?

3. Secretion of each of the hypophysiotropic hormones is known to be subject to negative feedback regulation.

   a. Which hormones in the systemic circulation mediate the major feedback regulation of CRH, dopamine, GHRH, GnRH, TRH, and somatostatin, respectively? For each, note whether the feedback action would be manifest as an inhibition or stimulation of release of that neurohormone.

   b. Feedback loops governing hypophysiotropin secretion have been demonstrated in experimental animals. This has most often been accomplished by assessing the consequences of surgical removal of the source of the feedback regulator, and "replacement" of the putative feedback regulator, on secretion of the neurohormone. Design a set of experiments that test the hypothesis that one of the hypophysiotropic hormones (e.g. GnRH, CRH, TRH, etc.) is homeostatically regulated by the corresponding feedback regulator named in (a), above. You may assume that you have the ability to monitor levels of the hypophysiotropin in the hypophysial portal vessels in experimental animals. Graphically depict the results that you would expect to obtain.

   c. Menopause is a stage of life in which the ovaries of a woman produce declining levels of estrogen and progesterone. Which anterior pituitary hormone(s) might be measured in the serum of a woman, specifically as a sensitive indicator that she is perimenopausal? Why? Which hypophysiotropin would you expect to be secreted at a higher rate in a postmenopausal vs. premenopausal woman?

4. Which of the hypophysiotropic hormones, and the pituitary hormone it regulates, is released in response to stress? In response to cold temperature? In a circadian rhythm? For each of these three stimuli, propose and draw the neural pathways that might deliver these stimulatory signals to the respective hypophysiotropic neurons.

5. Growth hormone deficiency and resultant short stature can be due to hyporesponsiveness of pituitary somatotrophs, or it may be secondary to insufficient neurohormone secretion. What diagnostic tool might be used to differentiate between these two possibilities? How would it be used? What would be measured and what would be the outcome of the tests in each of the two scenarios?

References

[1] Al-Damluji, S. 1993. Adrenergic control of the secretion of anterior pituitary hormones. *Baillière's Clin. Endocrinol. Metab.* 7:355–92.

[2] Blunt, S. M., and W. R. Butt. 1988. Pulsatile GnRH therapy for the induction of ovulation in hypogonadotropic hypogonadism. *Acta Endocrinol. (Copenh.)* 288:58–65.

[3] Brann, D. W., and V. B. Mahesh. 1997. Excitatory amino acids: Evidence for a role in the control of reproduction and anterior pituitary hormone secretion. *Endocr. Rev.* 18:678–700.

[4] Bruhn, T. O., J. H. Taplin, and I. M. D. Jackson. 1991. Hypothyroidism reduces content and increases in vitro release of pro-thyrotropin-releasing hormone peptides from the median eminence. *Neuroendocrinology* 53:511–15.

[5] Campbell, R. M., and C. G. Scanes. 1992. Evolution of the growth hormone-releasing factor (GRF) family of peptides. *Growth Reg.* 2:175–91.

[6] Childs, G. V., et al. 1991. Hypothalamic regulatory peptides and their receptors: Cytochemical studies of their role in regulation at the adenohypophyseal level. *J. Electron Microsc. Technique* 19:21–41.

[7] Chrousos, G. P. 1992. Regulation and dysregulation of the hypothalamic-pituitary-adrenal axis. The corticotropin-releasing hormone perspective. *Endocrinol. Metab. Clin. North Am.* 21:833–58.

[8] Conn, P. M., and W. F. Crowley. 1991. Gonadotropin-releasing hormone and its analogues. *N. Engl. J. Med.* 324:93–103.

[9] Crowley, W. F., Jr., and J. L. Jameson. 1992. Gonadotropin-releasing hormone deficiency: Perspectives from clinical investigation. *Endocr. Rev.* 13:635–40.

[10] Cutler, G. B., Jr. 1996. Corticotropin-releasing hormone (CRH): Clinical studies and use. *The Endocrinologist* 7:105–65.

[11] Evans, J. W., and M. B. Nikitovitch-Winer. 1969. Functional reactivation and cytological restoration of pituitary grafts by continuous local intravascular infusion of median eminence extracts. *Neuroendocrinology* 4:83–100.

[12] Gillies, G. 1997. Somatostatin: The neuroendocrine story. *TiPS* 18:87–95.

[13] Guillemin, R. 1992. Somatostatin: The early days. *Metabolism* 41:2–4.

[14] Guillemin, R., et al. 1982. Growth hormone-releasing factor from a human pancreatic tumor that caused acromegaly. *Science* 218:585–7.

[15] Guillemin, R., and R. Burgus. 1972. The hormones of the hypothalamus. *Sci. Am.* 227: 24–33.

[16] Halász, B., J. Kiss, and J. Molnar. 1989. Regulation of the gonadotropin-releasing hormone (GnRH) neuronal system: Morphological aspects. *J. Steroid Biochem.* 33:663–8.

[17] Halász, B., L. Pupp, and S. Uhlarik. 1962. Hypophysiotropic area in the hypothalamus. *J. Endocrinol.* 25:147–54.

[18] Harris, G. W. 1955. *Neural control of the pituitary gland.* London: Edward Arnold.

[19] Hinuma, S., et al. 1998. A prolactin-releasing peptide in the brain. *Nature* 393:272–6.

[20] Horváth, J. E., K. Groot, and A. V. Schally. 1995. Growth hormone-releasing hormone stimulates cAMP release in superfused rat pituitary cells. *Proc. Natl. Acad. Sci. USA* 92:1856–60.

[21] Jameson, J. L. 1996. Inherited disorders of gonadotropin hormones. *Mol. Cell. Endocrinol.* 125:143–9.

[22] King, J. A., and R. P. Millar. 1995. Evolutionary aspects of gonadotropin-releasing hormone and its receptor. *Cell. Mol. Neurobiol.* 15:5–23.

[23] Lechman, R. M., et al. 1986. Thyrotropin-releasing hormone precursor: Characterization in rat brain. *Science* 231:159–61.

[24] Liposits, Z. 1993. Ultrastructure of hypothalamic paraventricular neurons. *Crit. Rev. Neurobiol.* 7:89–162.

[25] Livne, I., M. J. Gibson, and A. J. Silverman. 1992. Brain grafts of migratory GnRH cells induce gonadal recovery in hypogonadal (hpg) mice. *Brain Res. Dev. Brain Res.* 69:117–23

[26] Martini, L., et al. 1997. LHRF, LHRH, GnRH: What controls the secretion of this hormone? *Mol. Psychiat.* 2:373–5.

[27] Mason, A. J., et al. 1986. The hypogonadal mouse: reproductive functions restored by gene therapy. *Science* 234:1372–8.

[28] McCarthy, G. F., A. Beaudet, and G. S. Tannenbaum. 1992. Colocalization of somatostatin receptors and growth hormone-releasing factor immunoreactivity in neurons of the rat arcuate nucleus. *Neuroendocrinology* 56:18–24.

[29] Mellon, P. L., J. J. Windle, R. I. Weiner. 1991. Immortalization of neuroendocrine cells by targeted oncogenesis. *Recent Prog. Horm. Res.* 47:69–93.

[30] Moghissi, K. S. 1992. Clinical applications of gonadotropin-releasing hormones in reproductive disorders. *Endocrinol. Metab. Clin. North Am.* 21:125–40.

[31] Nikitovitch-Winer, M., and J. W. Everett. 1958. Comparative study of luteotropin secretion by hypophysial autotransplants in the rat: Effects of site and stages of the estrous cycle. *Endocrinology* 62:522–32.

[32] Nikitovitch-Winer, M., and J. W. Everett. 1959. Histologic changes in grafts of rat pituitary on the kidney and upon retransplantation under the diencephalon. *Endocrinology* 65:357–68.

[33] Palkovits, M. 1977. Neural pathways involved in ACTH regulation. *Ann. N. Y. Acad. Sci.* 297:455–76.

[34] Paradisi, R., et al. 1993. Adenopituitary hormones in human hypothalamic hypophysial blood. *J. Clin. Endocrinol. Metab.* 77:523–7.

[35] Pernasetti, F., et al. 2001. Cell-specific transcriptional regulation of follicle-stimulating hormone-beta by activin and gonadotropin-releasing hormone in the LbetaT2 pituitary gonadotrope cell model. *Endocrinology* 142:2284–95.

[36] Porter, J. C., et al. 1970. A procedure for the cannulation of a pituitary stalk portal vessel and perfusion of the pars distalis in the rat. *Endocrinology* 87:197–201.

[37] Porter, J. C., et al. 1980. Neural control of gonadotropin secretion. *Fed. Proc.* 39:2896–901.

[38] Rivier, J., et al. 1982. Characterization of a growth hormone-releasing factor from a human pancreatic islet tumor. *Nature* 300:276–8.

[39] Sawchenko, P. E., et al. 1993. The functional neuroanatomy of corticotropin-releasing factor. *Ciba Found. Symp.* 172:5–21.

[40] Schally, A. V. 1994. Hypothalamic hormones: from neuroendocrinology to cancer therapy. *Anticancer Drugs* 5:115–30.

[41] Schwartz, J., and R. Cherny. 1992. Intercellular communication within the anterior pituitary influencing the secretion of hypophysial hormones. *Endocr. Rev.* 13:453–75.

[42] Sealfon, S. C., H. Weinstein, and R. P. Millar. 1997. Molecular mechanisms of ligand interaction with the gonadotropin-releasing hormone receptor. *Endocr. Rev.* 18:180–205.

[43] Sherwood, N. M., D. A. Lovejoy, and I. R. Coe. 1993. Origin of mammalian gonadotropin-releasing hormones. *Endocr. Rev.* 14:241–54.

[44] Smith, R. G., et al. 1997. Peptidomimetic regulation of growth hormone secretion. *Endocr. Rev.* 18:621–45.

[45] Stojilkovic, S. S., J. Reinhart, and K. J. Catt. 1994. Gonadotropin-releasing hormone receptors: Structure and signal transduction pathways. *Endocr. Rev.* 15:462–99.

[46] Swaab, D. F., et al. 1993. Functional neuroanatomy and neuropathology of the human hypothalamus. *Anat. Embryol.* 187:317–30.

[47] Taraskevich, P. A., and D. W. Douglas. 1977. Action potentials occur in cells of the normal pituitary gland and are stimulated by the hypophysiotropic peptide thyrotropin-releasing hormone. *Proc. Natl. Acad. Sci. USA* 74:4064–7.

[48] Wade, N. 1978. Guillemin and Schally. *Science* 200:279–82; 411–15; 510–13.

[49] Whitnall, M. H. 1993. Regulation of the hypothalamic corticotropin-releasing hormone neurosecretory system. *Prog. Neurobiol.* 40:573–629.

[50] Windle, J. J., R. I. Weiner, and P. L. Mellon. 1990. Cell lines of the pituitary gonadotrope lineage derived by targeted oncogenesis in transgenic mice. *Mol. Endocrinol.* 4:597–603.

[51] Wray, S. 2002. Development of gonadotropin-releasing hormone-1 neurons. *Front. Neuroendocrinol.* 23:292–316.

Neurohypophysial Hormones

As early as 1895, extracts of pituitaries were discovered to cause a rapid rise in blood pressure when injected into animals [46]. An important advance was made with the subsequent discovery by Howell (1898) that the pressor principle of pituitary extracts resided in the posterior lobe [26]. Dale, an eminent English pharmacologist, was the first to note that an extract of dried bovine pituitary glands caused a contraction of the uterus in addition to an elevation in blood pressure [13]. In 1909, posterior pituitary extracts were first used in clinical obstetrics to induce labor at term. In the years following, it was discovered that posterior lobe extracts caused a rapid flow (release) of milk. **Antidiuresis** *as a response to injections of posterior pituitary extracts was demonstrated in 1913. The injections reduced urine flow, increased the osmolality of the urine, and alleviated thirst. Extracts of the neurohypophysis then became established as the clinical method of controlling the polyuria of* **diabetes insipidus**, *although the etiology of the syndrome was not yet understood.*

In the early 1950s, the two physiologically active principles of the posterior pituitary, **oxytocin** *(OT) and* **vasopressin** *(AVP), were completely separated so that their individual activities could be studied. Du Vigneaud and his colleagues determined the structures of the oxytocic and antidiuretic principles of the neurohypophysis [29]. European chemists also determined the structures of OT [64] and AVP [2] at about the same time. Among the first peptide hormones to be completely chemically characterized, oxytocin and vasopressin were then synthesized; for this work, du Vigneaud was awarded a Nobel Prize. This merging of pure chemistry with physiology provided the foundation for modern endocrinology.*

The Neurohypophysis

Unlike the adenohypophysis, which derives from an upward evagination of the oral (buccal) epithelium, the posterior pituitary develops from a downward growth of the neural ectoderm. Therefore, the neurohypophysis mainly consists of neural endings and associated blood vessels (Chap. 5). There are only a few cellular elements present within the pars nervosa and they are referred to as pituicytes. Their function is unknown, but they are probably glial cells and may function like the neuroglia of the central nervous system (CNS). This paucity of cell bodies was a puzzling observation to the early investigators who ascribed an endocrine role to the pars nervosa. Where or what were the secretory elements of the posterior pituitary?

Lesions within specific areas of the hypothalamus led to degeneration of the pars nervosa and to a disturbance in water balance. These and other observations revealed that the nerve endings in the pars nervosa originate in two pairs of hypothalamic nuclei. These magnocellular (Chap. 6) neurons contain a stainable material that allows easy identification of the pathways from the hypothalamic nuclei, through the median eminence, and down the infundibular stalk of the neurohypophysis (Fig. 7.1). The stainable material is composed of granules that

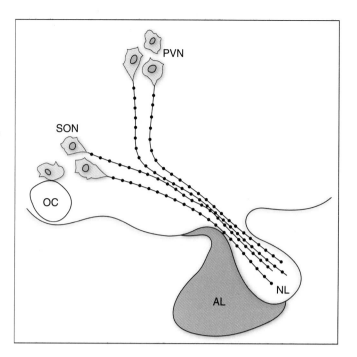

Figure 7.1 Diagram of a sagittal section through the pituitary gland. The relationship of the neurons that compose the supraoptic nuclei (SON) and the paraventricular nuclei (PVN) to the hypothalamo-hypophysial tract and the neural lobe (NL), and anterior lobe (AL), is revealed. OC, optic chiasm. (From Pickering [49], with permission.)

are now known to contain the hormones of the neurohypophysis. These large granules are referred to as *neurosecretory granules*; the process of granule formation and release is called *neurosecretion* [57].

The discovery that the neurohypophysis is the terminal organ of a CNS neurosecretory system, that it is mainly composed of hormone-containing nerve terminals, and that these axonal endings secrete their products into the bloodstream to act as hormones on distant target tissues, was an important landmark in understanding the role of neurons in endocrine function [4]. Thus, the discipline of vertebrate neuroendocrinology was established. The concept of neurosecretion in the vertebrate provided information that furthered understanding of the role of the brain in the control of pituitary and other endocrine functions. Neuroendocrinology in the vertebrate began with the study of the neurohypophysis and its hormones [16, 25].

Anatomically, the vertebrate neurohypophysis is considered to be a storage organ for the products of individual neuronal syntheses. The stored hormones are released into the adjacent vascular network. Such a functional unit is referred to as a *neurohemal organ* and is structurally analogous to the *corpus cardiacum* of some invertebrates. The study of these depot-release structures, the neurohypophysis and corpus cardiacum, and their release of neurohormones has been crucial in understanding brain–endocrine relationships in vertebrates and invertebrates.

Synthesis and Chemistry

Two nonapeptides, oxytocin (OT) and arginine vasopressin (AVP, also referred to as antidiuretic hormone, ADH), are found within the pars nervosa of most mammalian species. These neurohypophysial hormones are closely related structurally, but they serve quite different physiological roles. Oxytocin, for example, controls milk release from the mammary gland and contraction of the uterus, whereas AVP is concerned with water balance. The neurohypophysial hormones consist of nine amino acids folded into a ring through a disulfide bridge at positions 1 and 6 of the molecule, leaving a terminal tripeptide side chain (Fig. 7.2). AVP differs from OT in possessing a phenylalanine and an arginine at the 3 and 8 positions, respectively, of the molecule and is usually referred to as arginine vasopressin (AVP). Other structurally related neurohypophysial principles are found within the neurohypophysis of nonmammalian vertebrates (Table 7.1).

The neurohypophysial hormones are localized within the axonal endings that make up the pars nervosa. These hormones, however, are synthesized within the cell bodies of the pars nervosa neurons, which are located a long distance away in the hypothalamus. In mammals, birds, and reptiles, these cell bodies are found principally within the paired supraoptic nuclei (SON) and paraventricular nuclei (PVN) of the magnocellular neurosecretory system (Fig. 7.1).

Figure 7.2 Primary structures of oxytocin and arginine vasopressin (AVP). The individual amino acids are numbered by the conventional method.

In other vertebrates, this system consists of a single group of neurons in the anterior hypothalamus, the *preoptic nucleus*. In the amphibian, immunocytochemical studies have demonstrated separate hormone-producing neurons within the magnocellular preoptic nucleus, suggesting that the two types of neurosecretory neurons are intermingled. Although there is evidence that individual neurons synthesize only one species of hormone, both types of neurons are found intermingled within each of the hypothalamic nuclei. OT-synthesizing cells predominate in the PVN and AVP-synthesizing cells in the SON. In rats the number of neurosecretory neurons is, however, more than three times greater in the SON than in the PVN, and the contribution of OT from the former structure may be several times greater than that from the latter during reflex stimulation of OT release. In humans numerous large- and medium-sized neurons contain AVP mRNA in the PVN, SON, and accessory magnocellular nucleus. Small, lightly labeled AVP neurons are also found in the suprachiasmatic nucleus. Oxytocin mRNA is found in the SON, PVN, accessory magnocellular nucleus and, less frequently, in neurons of the lateral hypothalamus [62]. The relative contribution of oxytocinergic and vasopressinergic neurons within the PVN and SON varies considerably between species; the individual contributions of these two nuclear centers to neurohypophysial hormone secretion, therefore, remain unresolved. Whether OT or AVP is preferentially secreted from either the SON or PVN in response to a particular physiological need remains to be determined.

Radioisotope studies using [^{35}S]cysteine injected into the third ventricle reveal that incorporation of the radiolabel into protein occurs first within the cell bodies of the neurosecretory neurons. The label is then transported rapidly (2.5 mm/hour) down the axons to terminals within the pars nervosa. Studies revealed that radioactive amino acids injected into the SON appear in the posterior pituitary incorporated into AVP and its precursors within 2 hours of injection. In vitro studies showed that hypothalamo-median eminence tissue, but not neurohypophysial tissue, incorporated [^{35}S]cysteine into AVP. These experimental observations documented the origin of the neurosecretory material of the pars nervosa.

Each of the hormones is found in close association with a larger protein, referred to as a *neurophysin*. There is a specific neurophysin for each hormone, oxytocin-neurophysin (*oxyphysin*) and vasopressin-neurophysin (*pressophysin*). Neurophysins and their associated hormones are derived from the post-translational cleavage of precursor proteins, propressophysin and pro-oxyphysin. Inhibitors of neurophysin formation also repress formation of the associated hormones. In the homozygous state of the Brattleboro strain of rat (which has hereditary diabetes insipidus), there is an absolute lack of AVP secretion, but no comparable defect in OT synthesis and secretion. Pressophysin is also absent from the hypothalamus of

TABLE 7.1   Primary structures of the vertegrate neurohypophysial hormones

Hormone	Positions of Amino Acid Residues	Animal Group
Ancestral molecule	1 2 3 4 5 6 7 8 9 Cys–Tyr–X – X – Asn–Cys–Prp – X –Gly–NH_2	
Oxytocin	1 2 3 4 5 6 7 8 9 Cys–Tyr–Ile–Gln–Asn –Cys–Pro–Leu–Gly–NH_2	Mammals
Arginine vasopressin	1 2 3 4 5 6 7 8 9 Cys–Tyr–Phe–Gln–Asn–Cys–Pro–Arg–Gly–NH_2	Mammals except domestic pigs and macropodidae
Lysine vasopressin (Lysipressin)	1 2 3 4 5 6 7 8 9 Cys–Tyr–Phe–Gln–Asn–Cys–Pro–Lys–Gly–NH_2	Plaental mammals (Suidae) Marsupials (Macropodidae, Didelphidae)
Phenypressin	1 2 3 4 5 6 7 8 9 Cys-Phe-Phe-Gln–Asn–Cys–Pro–Arg–Gly–NH_2	Marsupials (Macropodidae)
Arginine vasotocin	1 2 3 4 5 6 7 8 9 Cys–Tyr–Ile–Gln–Asn–Cys–Pro–Arg–Gly–NH_2	Birds, reptiles, amphibians, bony fishes, and cartilaginous fishes
Isotocin	1 2 3 4 5 6 7 8 9 Cys–Tyr–Ile–Gln–Asn–Cys–Pro – Ile – Gly–NH_2	Bony fishes (teleosts)
Mesotocin	1 2 3 4 5 6 7 8 9 Cys–Tyr– Ile–Gln–Asn–Cys–Pro– Ile –Gly–NH_2	Marsupials, birds, reptiles, amphibians, lung-fishes
Glumitocin	1 2 3 4 5 6 7 8 9 Cys–Tyr– Ile–Ser–Asn –Cys–Pro–Gln–Gly–NH_2	Cartilaginous fishes (rays)
Asvatocin	1 2 3 4 5 6 7 8 9 Cys–Tyr– Ile–Asn–Asn–Cys–Pro–Val–Gly–NH_2	Cartilaginous fishes (spotted dogfish shark)
Phasvatocin	1 2 3 4 5 6 7 8 9 Cys–Tyr–Phe–Asn–Asn–Cys–Pro–Val–Gly–NH_2	

these rats, providing further evidence for the common origin of the neurophysin and its associated neurohypophysial hormone. The concept that peptide hormones may arise from the proteolytic cleavage of a precursor prohormone (in this case, a *proneurophysin*) is now recognized to be of more general significance for the production of most other peptide hormones.

The structural genes for the human preproarginine vasopressin neurophysin II (prepro-AVP-NPII) and prepro-oxytocin neurophysin I (prepro-OT-NPI) are closely linked. These two loci have been assigned to chromosome 20. Prepro-AVP-NPII consists of a single polypeptide chain containing a secretory signal sequence, the nonapeptide AVP, the hormone-carrier protein neurophysin II (NPII), and another peptide of unknown function. Prepro-OT-NPI consists of the same configuration, except that the AVP moiety is replaced by OT and the neurophysin moiety is NPI instead of NPII. Although the prepro-AVP and OT genes have been shown to be physically very close, their transcription occurs on opposite DNA strands and is not coupled to the same stimuli. AVP, OT, and their respective neurophysins are cleaved within neurosecretory granules and are reassembled into a hormone-binding protein complex before excretion from the posterior pituitary gland.

The amino acid sequences of the two neurophysins are similar within and between species [1, 12]. This suggests that they have arisen from a common ancestral neurophysin by gene duplication. These two neurophysins have been found in the pituitary of each of the mammals studied. The precursor molecule, with associated proteolytic enzymes, is present within the granules of the neurosecretory cells. These enzymes split the neurophysin from the precursor molecule inside the granule after it begins migration from the Golgi regions in the hypothalamic perikarya to the axon terminals in the neural lobe. AVP and OT bind noncovalently in a specific manner to neurophysins. Thus, the neurophysins are believed to function as transport proteins for the neurohypophysial hormones. Neurophysin is secreted with its hormone into the bloodstream in response to physiological stimulation. The secreted neurophysins are considered to function only as intraneuronal carrier proteins for the hormones and to lack any systemic hormonal/physiological function.

The early work of Bargmann and Scharrer [4], which used staining techniques for neurosecretory material, established the site of origin of the pars nervosa hormones. It was noted that some axons of the supraopticohypophysial tract project to the external zone of the median eminence and also to the third ventricle. Both AVP and neurophysin are present in granules of axons that are in contact with the hypophysial portal system, and these peptides are secreted into the portal blood. These observations suggest a possible role of AVP in the control of anterior pituitary function, such as in the facilitation of CRH actions on corticotrophs [15]. Neurohypophysial hormone secretion into the cerebrospinal fluid may also be important physiologically, for example in the regulation of cerebrospinal electrolyte composition.

Control of Neurohypophysial Hormone Secretion

Stimuli received by sensory receptors in the breast or vascular system result in release of OT or AVP, respectively, from the neurohypophysis. Neural afferents to the spinal cord connect with other neural pathways to the neurosecretory cell bodies localized within the PVN and SON. The neurosecretory neurons are in synaptic contact with neurons from these afferent pathways. There may be excitatory (cholinergic) and inhibitory (noradrenergic) connections from the rostral midbrain to the neurosecretory neurons. Destruction of noradrenergic neurons in the rabbit brainstem, for example, elevates plasma AVP, resulting in hypertension. There may also be interneurons that synchronize the activity of the neurosecretory neurons within the hypothalamic nuclei. Release of an excitatory neurotransmitter from afferent neurons onto the neurosecretory neurons results in depolarization of the cells. Action potentials can be recorded from mammalian neurosecretory cells of the SON and PVN. The pattern of firing of OT cells can be distinguished from that of AVP-secreting cells during appropriate stimulation, such as suckling or hemorrhage, respectively [50]. The putative AVP-secreting cells show a rhythmic bursting-type discharge that is increased by high osmotic pressure, whereas OT-producing cells appear to discharge continuously and in a random fashion. This pattern of firing, characteristic of the rat, may not be typical for all species.

Depolarization of neurosecretory cell bodies is propagated along the axons of the hypothalamo-hypophysial tract to the neuron terminals in the pars nervosa. Calcium ions enter the neurosecretory neurons during depolarization, and are required for the secretory process, as neurohypophysial hormone secretion is inhibited in the absence of Ca^{2+}. Neurosecretory granules fuse with the plasmalemma of the cells and are extruded via vesicular exocytosis. The secreted hormone and associated neurophysin enter the bloodstream in the vessels passing out of the neurohypophysis.

A specific facilitatory effect of OT on OT release has been demonstrated for SON and PVN neurons in various electrophysiological studies. In addition, the morphological finding of oxytocinergic synapses impinging on OT neurons in the SON provides evidence for a facilitatory action of OT on OT release. The stimulatory effect of OT on OT release could be functionally meaningful as a mechanism for enhancement of the burst discharges under conditions of OT demand [17]. Prolactin is also implicated in the control of OT release during suckling (Chap. 19).

Physiological Roles

Oxytocin is involved in the control of milk release and in uterine contraction during labor [16]. Vasopressin, or antidiuretic hormone as its name implies, is important in the homeostatic control of the extracellular fluid volume. The antidiuretic response is of

Figure 7.3 Scheme for measuring the electrical activity of hypothalamic neurosecretory neurons associated with reflex release of OT during suckling in the rat. The upper trace (supraoptic unit) shows the action potentials recorded from a cell in the supraoptic nucleus, and the lower trace is a recording of intramammary pressure. Note the burst of potentials that occurs 12 seconds before the increase in pressure. (From Lincoln and Wakerley [36], with permission.)

survival value to individuals of both sexes. OT, on the other hand, apparently functions only during specific times in the reproductive cycle of the adult female. No function for OT in the male has been clearly established.

Oxytocin Controls Milk Release and Uterine Contractions

Oxytocin is an example, along with several others (progesterone and chorionic gonadotropin, Chap. 19), of a hormone that plays only a transitory role, possibly specific to the female, and then, in some cases, only if she becomes pregnant and delivers a child at term.

Milk Release (Let-Down). OT functions in the control of milk release after parturition. Sensory nerve endings, which are localized to the areolae and nipples of the breasts, are stimulated by suckling (Fig. 7.3), and afferent neural pathways conduct these stimuli to the neurohypophysis [33]. From studies on different animals, the various components of these neural pathways have been traced. The pathways are ipsilateral (same side) to the teat being suckled. Neural impulses conducted along the sensory neurons enter the spinal column and ascend via dorsal, lateral, and ventral spinothalamic tracts to the mesencephalon of the brain. These stimuli are then transmitted via a diencephalic route to the hypothalamus. The neural pathways controlling OT secretion have been determined by electrode stimulation and lesioning experiments [63]. Stimulation of the ventral diencephalon in anesthetized animals results in ejection of milk. On the other hand, lesions in the PVN in lactating animals result in marked diminution in the quantity of milk released from the mammary gland. Electrophysiological recordings from putative oxytocinergic neurons in unanesthetized, freely moving rats established that the electrical activity displayed by these magnocellular neurons, some 10 to 12 seconds before milk ejection, is responsible for OT release under normal physiological conditions.

At parturition, dilation of the cervix (vaginal stretching) may also be a stimulus to OT secretion. Cross-circulation experiments have been carried out with pairs of unanesthetized ewes in which the jugular veins had previously been crossed so that each member of a pair received blood only from its partner. Mechanical distension of the vagina in one of the ewes resulted in a milk-ejection response only in the other ewe. Similar results were obtained when the roles were reversed. There is increased uterine activity during mating, and milk ejection during coitus in the human female and other animals has been reported. Auditory and optic sensory stimuli also affect milk let-down in some animals. (Ask any farmer who has milked a cow.)

The major target organ of OT is the mammary gland of the pregnant female. The alveolar and ductal system of the mammary gland is depicted in Fig. 7.4. OT released from the pars nervosa elicits contraction of cellular muscle-like elements [37, 51], myoepithelial cells (Fig. 7.5), which results in increased intramammary pressure and the expression of milk from the alveoli and ducts out through the teats (Fig. 7.6). The effect of OT on milk release from isolated mammary gland tissue in vitro is easily demonstrated [8]. High-affinity sites that bind [^{3}H]-labeled OT are present in membrane fractions of mammary gland from the

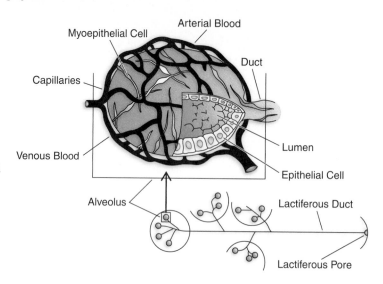

Figure 7.4 Alveolus and mammary gland ductal system. (From Rillema, "Development of the mammary gland and lactation." Reprinted by permission of the publisher from *Trends in Endocrinology and Metabolism* 5:149–54, © 1994 by Elsevier Science Inc.)

lactating rat [61]. OT-binding activity is specifically localized by autoradiography to the plasma membrane of myoepithelial cells of mammary tissue (Fig.7.7).

Male and female mice deficient in OT have been generated (knockout mice) to study the functional consequences of oxytocin absence on reproductive behavior, fertility, parturition, and nursing [45]. These mice are both viable and fertile and did not exhibit any behavioral or other physiological defects in the absence of the hormone. Although OT-deficient females exhibit normal maternal behavior, all offspring died shortly after birth due to the inability of the mothers to nurse. OT injected postpartum restores milk ejection and survival of the young. So, despite the numerous reproductive functions that have been ascribed to OT (see what follows), OT appears to play an essential role only in milk ejection in the mouse [45].

Uterine Contraction.   OT has been used for years to induce labor in human females at term. OT contracts the myometrium (uterotropic action), which can be demonstrated in vitro. Whether OT is responsible for initiating labor has been debated. Although OT is found in the maternal circulation throughout pregnancy, OT concentrations in the blood increase only during the final stages of labor, not before. It is suggested that parturition may be triggered not only by an increase in OT secretion per se, but also by an increase in the sensitivity of the myometrium of the uterus to the hormone [60]. The response of the myometrium to OT is, indeed, maximal at or near parturition.

It has been demonstrated that specific binding of [³H]oxytocin to uterine receptors of pregnant rats increases dramatically at term and is maximal during labor [60, 61]. In contrast, there is only a gradual increase in binding of [³H]oxytocin to mammary tissue, but this binding does become maximal during lactation. Changes in the ratio of plasma estradiol to

Figure 7.5 Silver-stained section of lactating mammary gland of the goat. A surface view of a contracted alveolus shows a myoepithelial cell with nucleus and branching processes. (From Richardson [51], with permission.)

progesterone concentration closely parallel the changes in OT binding: Estradiol is elevated and progesterone diminished at term. Estrogens increase myometrial sensitivity to OT and increase the number of OT receptors in the uterus. Progesterone, on the other hand, suppresses the appearance of OT receptors. Decreased synthesis of progesterone, therefore, may indirectly increase production of OT receptors. Thus, it appears that parturition is preceded by a dramatic increase in myometrial OT receptors, which may render the myometrium more sensitive to OT [21]. The meager number of OT receptors before term might make the myometrium insensitive to the circulating hormone. Therefore, parturition may be triggered by an increase in myometrial receptor number, as well as an increase in OT levels in the blood during labor (but see below). This hypothesis unites many observations and arguments on the role of OT in parturition.

Circulating OT, however, is not essential for the initiation or maintenance of spontaneous labor. Parturition can begin in the absence of circulating OT, and although OT antiserum suppresses lactation, it fails to affect parturition. There is no universal agreement as to whether there is an increase in circulating OT levels prior to the onset of labor. OT of pituitary origin therefore may not play a physiological role in parturition. Oxytocin mRNA and peptide in rat uteri are increased more than 150-fold during pregnancy, exceeding that of hypothalamic mRNA (Fig. 7.8). These observations suggest that the rat uterus itself is the major site of OT gene expression during the later stages of pregnancy [32, 33, 70]. OT therefore may act as a local paracrine or autocrine mediator of parturition, rather than as a circulating hormone. It appears that the uterus contains an intrinsic OT system in which both ligand and receptor are subject to strict regulation. The rise in uterine OT gene expression, in concert with the rise in uterine OT receptors, may represent the "trigger for parturition." OT gene expression has also been observed in the human uterus. Dysregulation of uterine OT gene expression may be an underlying cause of premature or delayed labor.

Vascular Smooth Muscle Actions. Neurohypophysial hormones contract or relax vascular smooth muscle [39]. The exact type of response depends on species, vascular bed, and region within a vascular bed. Thus, within a single species of animal, the neurohypophysial peptides can exert vasoconstrictor actions in one peripheral vascular bed and vasodilator actions in another. There may be two distinct kinds of neurohypophysial hormone receptors, one that subserves contraction and the other that subserves relaxation. There may even be different relative proportions of both receptors that vary in number depending on blood vessel segment and species. In addition, OT may act on a distinctly different vascular receptor from that of AVP. For example, OT is highly effective in contracting human umbilical arteries and veins, whereas AVP is relatively inactive. Rat aortic strips, in contrast, are extremely sensitive to the contractile effects of AVP, but are insensitive to OT. Synthesis of neurohypophysial analogs can provide peptides with unique and selective microcirculatory effects that may be clinically useful in the treatment of low vascular flow rates.

Figure 7.6 Disposition of myoepithelial cells (black) around alveoli and ducts. (Top) Myoepithelial cells relaxed, alveoli full. (Bottom) Myoepithelial cells contracted, alveoli emptied, ducts widened. (From Linzell [37], by permission of John Wright & Sons.)

Figure 7.7 Autoradiographic localization of tritium-labeled OT to myoepithelial cells of the rat mammary gland. Radioactivity was accumulated in the regions corresponding to the location of myoepithelial cells in the alveoli (left) and along the ducts (right). (From Soloff et al. [61], with permission.)

Figure 7.8   Immunocytochemical staining of sections of rat uterus with an antibody to OT. (a) Uterus of 21-day-pregnant rat. (b) Same as (a), but non-immune serum was used instead of primary antiserum. (c) Uterus, stained with immune serum, of nonpregnant, diestrous female rat. Sections were immunostained with an avidin-biotin complex. (From Lefebvre et al., with permission. *Science* 256:1553–5, 1992. ©1992 by the American Association for the Advancement of Science.)

Effects on Adenohypophysial Function.   OT exerts an inhibitory effect on CRH-mediated ACTH secretion when infused into the human male. No effects on other adenohypophysial hormone responses under conditions of submaximal stimulation by hypothalamic-releasing factors could be demonstrated. OT may play a part in the neuroendocrine response to stress in humans [47].

A possible regulatory role of OT in PRL secretion during suckling has been suggested. Although secretion of OT and PRL is not absolutely correlated, it was reported that OT-stimulated release of PRL from dispersed rat pituitary cells in vitro, and immunoneutralization of rats with antiserum specific to OT, significantly reduced PRL release during suckling or after estrogen treatment. Superfusion of rat pituitary cells with OT resulted in a significant PRL-releasing activity. It is likely that OT plays an important role in PRL release, especially during suckling, as reported by several investigators [40].

Maternal Behavior.   Intact (nonovariectomized) virgin female rats given OT through lateral ventricular cannulae displayed full maternal behavior toward foster pups [48]. Saline- or AVP-treated animals did not display full maternal behavior. Estrogens also induce maternal behavior, and it was suggested that elevated or recently elevated levels of estrogens may be necessary for the induction of full maternal behavior by OT. Intracerebroventricular- (ICV-) injected OT in ovariectomized female rats failed to induce maternal behavior, whereas most estrogen-primed animals became fully maternal in response to the hormone.

Ovarian estrogens may promote maternal behavior by increasing OT release or OT binding within the brain, or both. OT levels do rise markedly around the time of parturition. Maternal behavior is significantly reduced following ICV infusion of antibodies to OT. These observations suggest that OT endogenous to the brain may mediate the onset of maternal behavior. OT is widely distributed within neurons of the brain, and cerebrospinal fluid levels of OT rise markedly around the time of parturition. It is possible that OT may be released at many sites within the brain to activate maternal behavior [48].

Mating Behavior.   The ventromedial nuclei (VMN) of the hypothalamus are important for the control of female mating behavior, and hormone action within these nuclei has been causally related to behavior. Estradiol induces receptors for OT in the VMN and in the area lateral to these nuclei over the course of 1 to 2 days, and progesterone causes, within 30 minutes of its application, a further increase in OT receptor binding and an expansion of the area covered by these receptors lateral to the VMN. The rapid progesterone action appears to be a direct and specific effect of this steroid on membrane receptors, because it was produced in vitro as well as in vivo and was not mimicked by a variety of other steroids. The effect of progesterone occurred in the posterior part of the VMN, where OT infusion facilitated female mating behavior; it did not take place in the anterior part of the VMN, where OT infusion had no effect on mating behavior [58].

Human Sexual Response. Plasma OT levels increase during sexual arousal (self-stimulation) in both women and men and are significantly higher during orgasm/ejaculation than during prior baseline testing [11, 16]. OT is secreted specifically at the time of ejaculation in men. This is preceded by a rise in AVP secretion during arousal, which returns to baseline values by the time of ejaculation. AVP release during arousal may be associated with specific suppression of OT until ejaculation. OT may play a role in the physiology of sexual responses by facilitating contractions of the smooth muscles of the uterus and vagina in women. Likewise, release of OT during sexual responses in men may be related to increased contractility of reproductive smooth muscle tissue [42]. Thus, OT may enhance both sperm and egg transport, thereby promoting reproductive success [10].

Ovarian hormones affect the levels of neurohypophysial hormones in the pituitary of the rat. The firing rates of paraventricular neurons are increased during proestrus and estrus and after estrogen treatment in ovariectomized rats. Estrogen treatment also facilitates the activation of paraventricular secretory cell units and the reflex release of OT by genital tract stimulation. Therefore, ovarian hormones may not only promote the expression of sexual receptivity (Chap. 18), but may also increase levels of neurohypophysial hormones and facilitate release of these hormones during mating. Because these hormones have potent stimulating effects on uterine and oviduct smooth muscle, they might also enhance the likelihood of fertilization by promoting sperm transport.

Social Behaviors. In addition to their functions as neurohormones, oxytocin and AVP are also released as neurotransmitters at certain synaptic terminal fields in the brain, where they may affect a variety of neural processes and behavior. It has been demonstrated that both peptides are particularly important as neuromodulators that regulate various components of social behaviors, including social recognition, social memory, and affiliative behaviors, such as "pair-bonding" [3, 5, 69]. Oxytocin's involvement in social memory has been evidenced by the findings that mice with a null mutation of the oxytocin gene exhibit profound deficits in social processing and social recognition [19], if not complete social amnesia; when OT is given to these same mice before an encounter with a male, it restores the animal's ability to acquire the social memory. These effects of OT appear to be mediated by cells located in the medial amygdala [18]. In female prairie voles, oxytocin appears to be especially important in the process of pair-bonding with males. Prairie voles are a monogamous species that show high levels of social behaviors, including the formation of strong pair bonds with mates. Infusion of OT into the cerebral ventricles accelerates pair-bonding in the female prairie vole, while infusion of an OT receptor antagonist prevents pair-bond formation in these animals [66, 69]. Non-monogamous vole species that do not exhibit pair-bonding behaviors have been shown to have different oxytocin distribution patterns in the brain than do the monogamous prairie voles [27]. Taken together, these findings suggest that social behaviors in the female rodent depend upon a certain pattern of oxytocinergic neuronal development. That social behaviors are disturbed in animals with altered oxytocinergic function may have important implications for the understanding of human syndromes of disturbed social recognition, such as autism.

Vasopressin (AVP) Mediates Osmoregulation and Blood Pressure Responses

AVP has two major physiological actions: It induces the contraction or relaxation of certain types of smooth muscle, and it promotes the movement of water (and Na^+) across responsive epithelial tissues, notably the distal tubule of the mammalian kidney and the skin and urinary bladder of amphibians. Radioimmunoassay of circulating AVP under varying experimental conditions and pathophysiological states has provided detailed information on the role of AVP in the control of water balance [52].

Figure 7.9 Schematic representation of possible modes of organization of the neurohypophysis (NH) and its regulatory afferents from osmoreceptors (OR) and baroreceptors (BR). Supraoptic and paraventricular nuclei are designated as SON. (From Robertson, Athar, and Shelton [52], with permission.)

Osmoregulation. When body fluid osmolality decreases, AVP levels fall; this causes the excretion of free water via copious volumes of hypotonic urine. In contrast, when body fluid osmolality rises, AVP is released, stimulating free-water retention and excretion of small volumes of hypertonic urine. Blood osmolality is important in the control of AVP secretion [52, 53], and injections of small volumes of hypertonic solution into the carotid artery of the dog result in an immediate antidiuresis. Osmoreceptors are localized in the anterior hypothalamus. These osmoreceptors were thought to be near or identical to the magnocellular neurons of the neurohypophysis. It is now believed that the osmoreceptor function is not performed by the neurosecretory cells. An antidiuretic response is evoked only when hypertonic saline is infused in small volumes at sites some distance from the SON. Small lesions in the medial preoptic area of the hypothalamus, which do not involve the neurohypophysis, prevent AVP secretion in response to fluid deprivation. In addition, in the rare clinical syndrome of adipsic hypernatremia, patients have a complete lack of osmotically mediated AVP secretion, but they secrete AVP in response to hemodynamic (baroreceptor) stimuli. The osmoreceptors in humans would therefore appear to be totally separate from the neurosecretory cells and are apparently not an integral component of the neuronal pathways by which AVP secretion is affected by hemodynamic variables [52].

In summary, the physiologically important osmoreceptor control mechanism is near but neither identical to nor intermixed with the cell bodies of the neurohypophysial neurons (Fig. 7.9A$_1$). Because osmotically mediated AVP release can be totally ablated without altering in any way the hormonal response to hypotension, this excludes the possibility that hemodynamic stimuli are transmitted to the neurohypophysis by way of osmoreceptor neurons (Figs. 7.9A$_1$ and A$_2$). Possibly the AVP-secreting cells of the neurohypophysis are functionally heterogeneous; that is, they are divided into different units that receive afferents from the osmoregulatory or the baroregulatory systems (Fig. 7.9B). If so, one might expect that the function of one unit should have no effect on the other. This is not the case. In addition, electrophysiological recordings from neurosecretory cells in the anterior and lateral hypothalamus revealed firing rates that could be altered by both volume and osmotic stimuli. Thus, the control system may be organized as depicted (Fig. 7.9C).

In normal individuals, the *osmostat* appears to be set so that AVP secretion is suppressed to low or undetectable levels whenever plasma osmolality falls to 280 mOsm/kg or below [53]. Above this concentration, AVP secretion rises (Fig. 7.10, left) in direct proportion to the osmolality, affecting maximal antidiuresis at a plasma osmolality around 295 mOsm/kg. Changes in plasma osmolality as small as 1% will increase or decrease plasma AVP levels and affect urinary osmolality (Fig. 7.10, right), suggesting that the osmoreceptors are extraordinarily sensitive to changes in blood electrolyte concentration. Osmoreceptors exhibit a specificity for certain solutes. For example, hypertonic saline or sucrose, but not urea or glucose, induces an antidiuretic response. Because well over 90% of the osmotic activity of plasma is normally contributed by Na^+ and its anions, the osmoreceptors would be expected to function mainly in the detection of Na^+ osmolality changes. Oral saline intake reduces the AVP content of the SON and PVN but is without effect on the AVP content of the median eminence. Salt loading also increases the mRNA content of the neural lobe, suggesting increased synthesis of the hormone. This supports the concept of an independent control of AVP biosynthesis in the median eminence.

Blood Volume–Pressure Regulation. Changes in blood volume and pressure affect AVP secretion. Hemodynamic influences are exerted via neural afferents originating in pressure-sensitive receptors (baroreceptors) in the left atrium of the heart, aortic arch, and the carotid sinus ([68], Fig. 7.11). Afferent stimuli in response to changing blood volume or pressure reach the brainstem through the vagal and glossopharyngeal nerves. The central pathways integrating these signals are unidentified, but they may involve a primary synapse in the nucleus tractus solitarius with a secondary relay in the posteromedial nucleus of the hypothalamus.

Significant increases in plasma AVP (in rats) are not detected until blood volume is reduced by more than 8%. The relationship between AVP and blood volume in humans

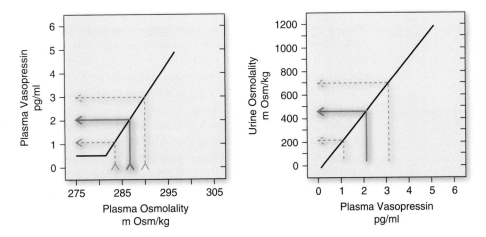

Figure 7.10 Effect of small alterations in basal plasma osmolality on plasma vasopressin and urine osmolality in normal humans. (From Robertson, Shelton, and Athar [53], with permission.)

follows an exponential pattern similar to that of rats. Under more unphysiological conditions, as in excessive hemorrhage, AVP causes maximal antidiuresis and may exert significant pressor effects on certain vascular beds. In humans and other animals, there is an exponential relationship between plasma AVP levels and the degree of hypotension produced. Enhanced AVP secretion ensues after a reduction in mean arterial pressure as small as 5%. Volume and Na^+ concentration may also affect AVP secretion through the renin–angiotensin system (Chap. 15). Angiotensin II, an octapeptide, may act on the brain to stimulate AVP secretion. Thus, a complex set of factors control AVP secretion and, subsequently, water and electrolyte balance.

Central AVP may play a role in the control of blood pressure and heart rate in both normotensive and hypertensive animals [54]. Administration of AVP into the CNS produces changes in arterial pressure and heart rate that can be reversed by competitive receptor antagonists. AVP is also a potent releasing factor for corticotropin and corticosterone, which in turn act on the cardiovascular system. Central administration of AVP produces cardiovascular responses attributable to stimulation of sympathetic outflow. AVP, in early stages of hypertension, may alter sympathetic outflow via an effect on central neural structures controlling the CNS. Central administration of AVP also causes an increase in heart rate; thus, the peptide appears to override the ability of the baroreceptor reflex to buffer changes in arterial pressure. AVP may therefore participate in baroreceptor reflex resetting in hypertension and alter sympathetic outflow via effects on the baroreceptor reflex system [5].

Adenohypophysial Function.   In the monkey, AVP is present in high concentrations in the portal blood of the anterior pituitary [38]. There is an increase in neurosecretory material in the median eminence of the rat after adrenalectomy. Specifically, there is an increase in both neurophysin and AVP, but not OT, in the external zone of the median eminence, and the increase appears to be due to a lack of glucocorticoids.

Figure 7.11 Effects of periodically increased pressure in the isolated carotid sinus on the activity of a SON neuron. Upper, middle, and bottom traces show the blood pressure, unit activity, integrated record of the number of spikes per second, and carotid sinus pressure. (From Yamashita [68], with permission.)

Vasopressin stimulates the release of ACTH and, subsequently, cortisol from the pituitary and adrenal glands, respectively. This has been described in rats, in humans, in isolated pituitary glands, and in dispersed anterior pituitary cells. The greatest response to AVP occurs when it is coadministered with corticotropin-releasing hormone. In this situation, there is *synergism* between the two releasing factors to cause an augmented release of ACTH. Thus, it is now thought that if AVP plays a role in the release of ACTH it is probably through the potentiation of the CRH action.

AVP at physiological concentrations acts specifically on anterior pituitary cells to enhance the release of TSH. The finding that AVP is equipotent with TRH in stimulating TSH release strongly suggests that AVP may indeed be a physiological regulator of TSH secretion. In the hypothalamus, however, AVP may function as a negative autofeedback agent to regulate signals for TSH release. The fact that centrally administered AVP lowers plasma TSH, but not other hormones, is consistent with observations that hypothalamic releasing or inhibiting factors, at the appropriate ventricular dose, produce effects that oppose their direct actions on their respective target cells of the adenohypophysis. Others have supported this concept of negative ultrashort-loop feedback for hypothalamic releasing and inhibiting factors in vitro.

Social Behaviors. Both OT and AVP have been found to be of importance in a variety of social behaviors in both sexes; however, AVP and the AVP receptor 1a (V1aR) appear to play a more critical role in males than in females [9]. Studies in male rats and mice have demonstrated that vasopressin release in the lateral septum is a necessary component of circuitries mediating social recognition. When given intracerebroventricularly to a male rat after an initial social encounter, AVP facilitates consolidation of the social memory [7]. Infusions of AVP have similarly been found to facilitate several male-typical social behaviors, such as aggression, scent marking, and courtship; by contrast, mice lacking the V1aR exhibit severe deficits in social processing and social recognition [20, 23]. Remarkably, transfer of the V1aR gene into the lateral septum of V1aR-deficient mice can completely rescue social recognition in these animals, demonstrating that the V1aR is both necessary and sufficient for normal social recognition [6]. Central infusion of AVP enhances pair-bond formation in male prairie voles, while treatment with V1aR antagonist prevents pair-bond formation in this species [35]. Thus, AVP and the V1aR appear to be of critical importance in the neural processes underlying the social recognition and affiliative behaviors in the males of several rodent species. The potential implications of these findings for social behaviors and social bond formation in other species, including humans, may prove to be profound [34].

Vasotocin (AVT) is a Major Nonapeptide Hormone in Nonmammalian Vertebrates

AVT rather than AVP is present in the pituitary gland of nonmammalian vertebrates. Only a few of the many putative roles of this hormone can be discussed here.

Sexual Behavior. Intracerebroventricular injections of AVT induce sexual activity (amplectic clasping) in male newts (salamanders), a response that was blunted by an AVT antagonist or by an anti-AVT immune serum. Intracranial implants of certain gonadal steroids in castrated male newts maintained the behavioral response to AVT. Systemic injections of the steroid hormones failed to increase the incidence of sexual behavior. These observations suggest that AVT induces sexual behavior in newts by acting on cells in the brain. In male newts, high concentrations of AVT in the cerebrospinal fluid, dorsal preoptic area, ventral infundibular nucleus, and optic tectum are associated with the propensity to exhibit sexual behavior. This is the first direct evidence that the motivational state of an animal to initiate reproduction is regulated, in part, by the concentrations of particular neuropeptides in specific brain areas [71].

Oviposition. There is evidence, in some reptiles and birds [59] at least, that AVT regulates oviductal muscle contraction. Marine turtles are oviparous reptiles that emerge from the water to construct a nest and deposit a clutch consisting of 100 to 200 eggs. The nesting process can be clearly divided into a series of nine discrete nesting behaviors. Nesting begins when the animal strands (emerges from the water) and proceeds through the production of a body pit (a shallow depression into which the animal positions itself for oviposition); nest construction; digging the egg chamber; depositing the first, middle, and last eggs; covering the nest; and ends when the animal returns to the water. The entire process consumes

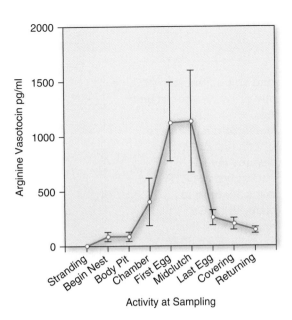

Figure 7.12 Mean serum AVT levels in olive Ridley sea turtles (*Lepidochelys olivacea*) throughout nesting. (Figure provided by Robert A. Figler, Texas A&M University.)

approximately 1 hour. Circulating levels of AVT were shown to increase dramatically prior to the onset of oviposition and decrease rapidly following its conclusion. The time span of this transient increase is approximately 45 minutes (Fig. 7.12). The elevation of systemic AVT coincident with a period of increased oviductal motility indicates a role for AVT in reptilian reproduction analogous to the known reproductive roles of the neurohypophysial peptides in birds and mammals.

Oviposition, the expulsion of the egg from the oviduct, is accompanied by a marked increase in contractions of the oviductal smooth muscle in the hen and generally takes place each day. AVT may play a physiological role in the regulation of oviposition since an increase in plasma levels of AVT and a decrease in AVT content in the neurohypophysis have been demonstrated during egg expulsion from the oviduct. An increase in oviductal contractility may be a stimulus for AVT release during normal oviposition. The mechanisms that initiate an increase in contractions of the oviduct are not known [59].

Circulation and Metabolism

A number of enzymes exist in a variety of tissues that can degrade the neurohypophysial hormones in a specific manner. For example, an enzyme capable of inactivating OT appears in human blood during pregnancy. It is produced in the placenta and is referred to as plasma *oxytocinase*. This amino peptidase produces a rupture of the ring of OT by hydrolysis of the hemicystinyl-tyrosyl bond. The colostrum also contains enzymes, apparently produced in the mammary gland, which inactivate neurohypophysial hormones. The kidney, which is also a target organ for neurohypophysial hormones, contains a variety of enzymes that degrade and inactivate these hormones.

Mechanisms of Hormone Action

As for other peptide hormones, OT and AVP interact with target tissue cellular membrane receptors. All of the known OT and AVP receptor types and isoforms are members of the G-protein-coupled receptor family. Some of the earliest evidence for a role of cyclic nucleotides in hormone action derived from studies on the mechanism of AVP action.

Oxytocin Actions. OT interacts not only with myometrial, but also with endometrial receptors. OT stimulates the synthesis of prostaglandin $F_{2\alpha}$ ($PGF_{2\alpha}$) in the ovine uterus by interacting with the endometrium, which is the principal source of uterine PGs. Estrogens also enhance uterine synthesis of PGs by increasing the activity of PG synthetase in rats.

Figure 7.13 Scheme of contraction in uterine smooth muscle [67]. A rise in Ca^{2+}, produced either spontaneously or by an agonist such as OT interacting with its receptor (R), causes Ca^{2+} to bind to calmodulin (Ca^{2+}/CaM). This activates myosin light-chain kinase (MLCK). This kinase then phosphorylates light chains on myosin (P-myosin). This allows actin binding and activates myosin Mg-ATPase, thus contraction can occur with hydrolysis of ATP. P-myosin is dephosphorylated by phosphatases, leading to relaxation. If MLCK is phosphorylated, for example by Ca^{2+} calmodulin-dependent protein kinase II, then it is much less efficient at phosphorylating myosin, and force falls. Reduction of Ca^{2+} will also promote relaxation. (Modified from [67].)

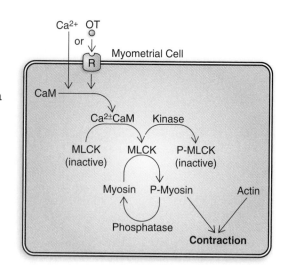

Estrogens also increase the number of endometrial and myometrial OT receptors. Progesterone antagonizes these estrogen effects in rats. Thus estrogen-induced development of endometrial OT receptors would enhance endometrial $PGF_{2\alpha}$ production in the presence of OT. Myometrial contractions, a mechanical event, also induce endometrial $PGF_{2\alpha}$ production; thus, OT may affect $PGF_{2\alpha}$ synthesis directly and indirectly.

Prostaglandins of uterine origin are believed to control luteolysis in some species of mammals. OT could induce luteal regression via regulation of uterine synthesis of PGs. The normal course of labor might depend on an early increase in uterine synthesis of PGs to inhibit luteal or placental production of progesterone. Decreased progesterone levels would remove the block to OT-induced uterine contractions, which are maintained up to that time by the steroid hormone (Chap. 19). The uterotropic actions of OT have now been clarified in some detail. OT exerts its myometrial contractile effect by increasing intracellular levels of Ca^{2+}. OT binding to myometrial receptors inhibits Ca^{2+} extrusion at the sarcolemma by inhibiting a Ca^{2+}-ATPase. OT receptor binding also produces a rapid Ca^{2+} influx (measured with ^{45}Ca) through receptor-mediated Ca^{2+} channel activation. The inhibition of Ca^{2+} extrusion and the concomitant uptake of the cation prolongs the elevation of intracellular Ca^{2+}, thus promoting myometrial contraction. Inositol triphosphate (IP_3) causes release of Ca^{2+} from internal stores of myometrial cells and from sarcoplasmic reticulum (SR) microsomal fractions. Oxytocin stimulates IP_3 production by human gestational myometrial cells. OT also elevates IP_3 in a dose-dependent manner in the pregnant uterus but is ineffective in the nonpregnant uterus. A model for OT-induced uterine contraction is shown (Fig. 7.13).

Vasopressin Actions. Vasopressin receptors display a diversity in pharmacological, functional, and biological properties. Four subtypes of receptors have been distinguished on a functional and/or pharmacological basis. The renal AVP receptor (V_2-type) that mediates the antidiuretic response was among the first membrane receptors for which a functional coupling with adenylate cyclase was demonstrated. AVP receptors of the liver (V_{1a}-type) and adenohypophysis (V_{1b}-type) and OT receptors of the uterus and mammary gland act through increased inositol turnover to mobilize intracellular Ca^{2+} [3]. The immediate transmembrane signaling of V_1-vascular AVP receptors involves ligand–receptor complex formation; receptor lateral mobility and internalization, coupling to a G_q protein; activation of phospholipases A_2, C, and D; translocation and activation of protein kinase C; production of inositol 1,4,5-triphosphate and 1,2-diacylglycerol; mobilization of intracellular Ca^{2+}; alteration of intracellular pH with activation of the Na^+/H^+ exchanger; calmodulin activation; and myosin light-chain phosphorylation. The secondary nuclear signal mechanisms triggered by activation of V_1-vascular AVP receptors include tyrosine phosphorylation, induction of gene expression, and protein synthesis.

AVP and OT have overlapping pharmacological properties (Table 7.2). More specific agonists are therefore useful in determining whether OT or AVP receptors may be involved in mediating a given biological response. Some examples of agonists available for determining whether responses are mediated by OT or by V_1 or V_2 AVP receptors appear

TABLE 7.2   Relative potencies of some analog of AVP and OT

AVP: Cys–Tyr–Phe–Gln–Asn–Cys–Pro–Arg–Gly(NH$_2$)

OT: Cys–Tyr–Ile–Gln–Asn–Cys–Pro–Leu–Gly(NH$_2$)

	Activities, U/mg*		
	VP(V$_1$)	AD(V$_2$)	OT[†]
AVP	380	330	60
OT	4	4	490
dDAVP(1-deamino[D-Arg^8]VP)	0.4	1300	3
[Phe^2,Orn^8]OT	121	1.6	5
[Thr^4,Gly^7]OT	<0.01	0.002	860

*Data from [39].
[†]Oxytocic (OT) activities assayed on isolated rat uteri in a medium containing 0.5 mM Mg^{2+}

in Table 7.2. Regardless of an AVP receptor's pharmacological properties, it can only be definitively classified based on the cellular second messenger its activation evokes. Although many specific antagonists are available, by themselves they are rarely useful for identifying receptor types. Using antagonists, however, one may distinguish differences among receptors that are not clear from studies using agonists alone. For example, one such study showed that V$_{1b}$ receptors on adenohypophysial cells differ pharmacologically from the V$_{1a}$ receptors on hepatocytes or vascular smooth muscle cells, although they have a similar second messenger system [39].

The mechanism of action of AVP has been determined from studies on a variety of epithelia—frog skin, toad bladder, and mammalian nephron. The toad bladder, a storage organ for water, is a useful and simple model system and responds to AVP similarly to the distal tubule of the mammalian nephron. The organ is a relatively large sheet of thin epithelium that survives for long periods in vitro. Exposure of isolated toad bladder to AVP results in an increase in Na$^+$ and water transport from the outer (mucosal or luminal) to the inner (serosal) side. AVP can only affect water permeability if applied to the serosal side of the bladder, and it can only act on the kidney collecting duct when applied to the peritubular (serosal) side. The barrier to water penetration across such membranes is in the mucosal (luminal) side. This barrier is decreased in the presence of AVP, and water is moved across the cells and leaves at the basal (serosal) margins. In the unstimulated state, the apical membranes of these cells have an extremely low permeability to water; the dramatic increase in permeability occurs within minutes of the addition of AVP to the basolateral side of the epithelium. When AVP is withdrawn, the reversal of permeability also occurs within minutes.

Interaction of AVP with toad bladder serosal plasmalemmal receptors activates adenylate cyclase and intracellular levels of cAMP are elevated. The result is that the mucosal membrane then has an increased permeability to water. Cyclic AMP or its analogs, as well as phosphodiesterase inhibitors (e.g., theophylline), enhance water permeability, thus supporting a role for cAMP as the intracellular messenger of AVP. The actions of AVP on frog skin and the mammalian nephron also involve elevations in cAMP levels.

The site of action of these effects is the membrane of the mucosal surface. Structural changes (intramembranous particle aggregation) occur in this barrier to render the membrane more permeable to water. AVP controls renal water retention by inserting water channels into the normally watertight apical membranes of the collecting duct. This allows water flow from the tubule lumen along osmotic gradients between the tubular fluid and the surrounding interstitium. AVP also enhances Na$^+$ reabsorption by the collecting duct and, in some animals, increases transepithelial solute transport in the medullary thick ascending limb, thereby increasing osmotic gradients for water reabsorption. In some amphibia, dilute urine is stored in a large bladder where it can be reabsorbed in response to AVP secreted when body fluid osmolality rises. Since AVP-responsive properties of granular epithelial cells in toad urinary bladder

Figure 7.14 Immunolabeling of AQP2 in kidney collecting ducts. Immunofluorescence microscopy of inner medullary collecting ducts from Brattleboro rats before (−AVP) or after (+AVP) vasopressin-induced change in AQP2 localization and the subapical regions. (From P. Agre, D. Brown, and S. Nielson. "Aquaporin water channels: Unanswered questions and unresolved controversies." *Current Opinion in Cell Biology* 7:472–83, 1995, with permission.)

closely resemble those of principal cells of the mammalian collecting duct, the toad bladder is a useful model of AVP-responsive renal epithelia.

The cloning of water-selective channels has revealed the molecular basis of renal water transport [28, 30, 31, 41, 43, 44]. The water-selective channel (membrane water-transport protein), aquaporin-1 (AQP1), is responsible for the constitutively high water permeability in the proximal tubule and the descending thin limb of the loop of Henle. In mammals, other mechanisms are needed to regulate the delicate water balance in response to the needs of the organism. This is accomplished in kidney collecting ducts where water resorption is regulated by AVP. Binding of this hormone to its V_2 receptor initiates a chain of signaling events that ultimately leads to the transient insertion of water channels in the apical membrane of principal cells and in the inner medullary collecting ducts. The cDNA encoding a second water channel (aquaporin-2, AQP2) was cloned, which, on the basis of its exclusive expression in the collecting duct, is considered to be the AVP-regulated water channel [14].

Immunologically, most AQP2 is localized in small endosomal vesicles in the subapical region of the principal cells of the cortical and outer medullary collecting duct and to the inner medullary cells (Fig. 7.14). In the absence of AVP the apical membrane has a lower permeability for water, but in the presence of AVP there is a rapid increase in water transport. AVP also causes a fusion of the endosomal vesicles with the apical membrane (Fig. 7.15). Removal of AVP results in endocytosis and the restoration of low water permeability of the apical membrane. In Brattleboro rats that lack AVP synthesis, AQP2 is only present in subapical vesicles, but AVP infusion causes a marked redistribution of AQP2 to the apical membrane [43].

Pathophysiology

The control of AVP release and regulation of fluid balance occurs primarily in response to alterations in blood tonicity and blood volume so that a relative constancy of these two parameters is maintained. This finely adjusted homeostatic system can be disrupted by disease states that affect neurohypophysial or renal function and by AVP produced independently of normal regulatory influences. The resulting clinical disturbance of body-water balance will be manifested by hypernatremia or hyponatremia and by excessive water loss or retention.

Diabetes Insipidus. Impairment of the neurohypophysial system to synthesize or release AVP results in a diminished ability of the kidney to conserve water, resulting in pituitary (neurogenic) diabetes insipidus [24]. Failure to synthesize AVP can also occur as a result of disease processes that destroy the hypothalamus or posterior pituitary. Diabetes insipidus can also result from traumatic or surgical injury to the hypothalamus.

In the normal individual, plasma osmolality is maintained in a range of 285 to 290 mOsmol/kg with associated plasma AVP levels of 1 to 3 μU/ml and urinary AVP levels of 11 to 30 μU/24 hours [40, 53]. In patients with severe diabetes insipidus, plasma osmolality may rise to more than 330 mOsmol/kg; under this severe osmotic stress, plasma and urinary AVP remain well below the normal range.

A single base deletion in the AVP gene is the cause of diabetes insipidus in the Brattleboro rat. The mRNA produced by the mutated gene encodes a normal AVP, but an abnormal NPII

Figure 7.15
Distribution of AQP2 and 3 in collecting duct principal cells. Vasopressin binds to AVP receptors (R) and heterotrimeric G protein (Gs) mediate activation of adenylyl cyclase (AC) to produce cAMP, which activates protein kinase A (PK). This presumably results in externalization of AQP2 water channels to the apical plasma membrane, thereby increasing the water permeability. AQP3 is selectively localized to the basolateral plasma membrane. (From S. Nielson and P. Agre [43], with permission.)

moiety, which impairs transport and progression of the AVP-NPII precursor and its retention in the endoplasmic reticulum of the magnocellular neurons where it is produced [56]. Transplantation of vasopressin neurons from normal rat fetuses into the adult Brattleboro rat, which congenitally lacks AVP-producing neurons, alleviates the polydipsia and polyuria that are symptomatic of this genetic defect. Apparently, the axons of the grafted fetal neurons make appropriate and functional connections within the brain of the host. The ability of transplanted neurons to correct a CNS deficiency has important theoretical and clinical implications.

In *nephrogenic* (AVP-resistant) diabetes insipidus (NDI), there is a defect in the urinary concentration mechanism at the level of the kidney. Pituitary diabetes insipidus can be treated by replacement therapy with AVP, but the hormone is without effect in the nephrogenic disease type. In fact, greater than normal circulating levels of AVP are present in this condition. The antidiuretic response of the kidney to AVP is used clinically to diagnose the specific type of defect responsible for the diuresis. Females may have a subclinical form of the disease or the more severe form that is characteristic in males. A dominant sex-linked inheritance with variable penetrance is suggested. The defect involves a failure to generate intracellular levels of cAMP within distal tubular cells of the kidney in response to AVP. The kidney-specific V_2 vasopressin receptor, a G-protein-coupled receptor, is defective in this disorder as both the disease and the receptor map to chromosome Xq28 [14].

In most patients, NDI is caused by mutations in the V_2-receptor Xq28 gene that is inherited as an X-linked recessive trait. In some families, however, NDI revealed an autosomal mode of inheritance. Mutations in the AQP2 gene have been found in such families. Although these patients show the same clinical phenotype, they can be distinguished from patients with a V_2-receptor defect by their normal extrarenal (vascular) response to a V_2-receptor vasopressin agonist [41].

Syndrome of Inappropriate Vasopressin Secretion. The state of continual AVP release without relationship to plasma osmolality or volume is referred to as the syndrome of inappropriate vasopressin secretion. The syndrome is characterized by an inability to excrete a maximally dilute urine, which results in retention of water, an expansion of the extracellular fluid volume, and a resultant dilutional hyponatremia. The most common cause of excessive AVP secretion is malignancy; AVP is secreted from a small cell carcinoma of the lung, and is secreted along with its neurophysin. Although plasma and urinary levels of AVP may be markedly elevated, the amount of hormone in the blood or urine may be similar to that of normal individuals. However, these levels are excessive considering that the hypotonicity should have inhibited AVP secretion.

Evolution of the Neurohypophysial Hormones

Determination of the structure of the neurohypophysial peptides, present within the pars nervosa of different vertebrate classes, provided a remarkable understanding of the evolution of the neurohypophysial hormones [1]. This information has also given insight into the structural requirements for neurohypophysial hormone action. From these studies, a variety of hormone analogs have been designed for detailed analysis of hormone–receptor interaction.

Neurohypophysial hormones have been characterized in representatives of all vertebrate classes [1]. The neurohypophysis of each vertebrate species contains at least two principles, except in the cyclostomes where only a single peptide, arginine vasotocin (AVT), has been detected so far. In the species studied, the same two hormones are usually present in the neurohypophysis of each member of a particular vertebrate group. Only one or two residues differ between the hormones of any two different vertebrate classes. Sequence differences mainly occur at positions 3, 4, and 8 of the nonapeptides (Table 7.1). Structural differences at these positions apparently account for the differing receptor affinities and activities of the neurohypophysial peptides.

Thirteen neurohypophysial hormones have been characterized; nine are regarded as oxytocin-like and the remaining four as vasopressin-like. An early gene duplication led to two lines of neurohypophysial principles. Gene mutation following gene duplication may have resulted in one line originating with isotocin, found in bony fishes, which gave rise by further base mutations to the oxytocin-related structures. The other line, originating directly from AVT, gave rise to the vasopressins much later in evolution. Although the uterotropic and antidiuretic roles of neurohypophysial hormones are well documented in mammals, there is no convincing evidence that the neurohypophysial or related peptides subserve these functions in nonmammalian vertebrates, except for the antidiuretic role of AVT in amphibians, reptiles, and birds. Vasotocin is intermediate in structure between OT and AVP and is considered to be phylogenetically the oldest neurohypophysial hormone. AVT was synthesized and found to have properties identical to the naturally occurring amphibian water-balance principle [29]. Chemical analysis of the amphibian neurohypophysis revealed that the natural peptide was AVT. This provided a unique example where a synthetic hormone was prepared before its natural homologue had been identified.

Some members of the piglike mammals (pigs, wart hogs) contain a vasopressin with a lysine rather than arginine at the 8 position of the molecule (Table 7.1). It has been suggested that lysine vasopressin (LVP) arose as a single-step mutation from AVP. AVP and LVP may both be present in individual members of the pig family according to a Hardy–Weinberg distribution. Homozygotes contain one peptide and the heterozygotes contain both, suggesting the gene for vasopressin is present in two allelic forms. Only LVP is present in the domestic pig, which may be the result of the restrictive and selective force of domestication by humans. Both LVP and AVP are present in individual pituitaries of both Australian macropodian peramelids (bandicoot) and American didelphian marsupials (opossums) [1]. The constant presence of two pressor principles within individual pituitaries suggests that these peptides arose by gene duplication. A new neurohypophysial peptide, phenypressin ([Phe^2, Arg^8]-vasopressin) has been found along with LVP in the pituitary of five marsupials, including the red kangaroo and the tammar wallaby [1].

Other Neurohypophysial Hormones

Hydrins.   Extended forms of vasotocin, called hydrins because of their action on the water permeability of frog skin and urinary bladder, are found in the amphibian neurohypophysis, along with vasotocin. In contrast to other AVT-producing vertebrates such as birds or reptiles, some amphibians have evolved provasotocin processing so that an intermediate vasotocinylglycine (hydrin 2) peptide is present in the neurohypophysis along with AVT. This peptide stimulates water transport through frog skin and frog bladder epithelia as does AVT, but in contrast to AVT it is virtually devoid of antidiuretic activity on the frog kidney. Because hydrin 2 has been identified in frog neurosecretory granules to be a physiological hormone secreted into the blood, it was suggested that the differential processing of provasotocin is important to amphibians, allowing formation of two hormones from a single precursor. Water homeostasis in amphibians involves three organs, namely, skin, bladder, and kidney, and could be under control of both AVT and hydrin 2, the latter acting mainly for external water uptake through the skin.

In contrast to vasotocin, hydrins are virtually devoid of oxytocic, pressor, and antidiuretic activities. It has been suggested that in frogs and toads, hydrin 2 acts specifically on skin in order to rehydrate animals when bathing in freshwater, whereas vasotocin is mainly active on kidney tubules controlling the recovery of water from urine. The finding of hydrin 2 in isolated frog neurosecretory granules supports the assumption that this peptide is secreted in blood as a hormone. Hydrins are detected neither in birds, such as geese, nor in reptiles, such as vipers [55].

The Caudal Neurosecretory System (Urophysis) and the Urotensins.   Within the spinal cord of some teleost and cartilaginous fishes are groups of neurosecretory neurons that possess all the characteristics of a neuroendocrine system, anatomically analogous to the neurohypophysis [5]. This *caudal neurosecretory system* or *urophysis* contains two types of secretory cells based on staining reactions, granule morphology, and response to osmotic or electrophysiological stimuli. Two types of granules have been isolated, and each is associated with its own hormonal-like factor (urotensin I and II). Both aminergic and cholinergic inputs to urophysial secretion are implicated in some species of fishes. The *urotensins* are neuropeptides and, like the neurohypophysial hormones of the pars nervosa, are associated with two or more transport proteins, *urophysins*, which specifically bind either urotensin I or II. There is no evidence for the existence of urotensins in nonpiscine vertebrates, although, as noted presently, structurally related peptides are present, and the urotensins have a variety of actions in tetrapods [5].

Extracts of the urophysis are vasoactive in all vertebrate species studied. In general, a vasopressor response is observed in poikilothermic vertebrates and a vasodepressor effect observed in homeotherms. These differential effects are produced by two distinct peptides: the vasodepressor factor is referred to as urotensin I, whereas urotensin II is the name given to the vasopressor principle of the urophysis. Both urotensins apparently are present in all fish urophyses thus far examined, suggesting that they are indeed peptidergic hormones of this neurosecretory system. The presence of a third urotensin (III) is based solely on experimental data; urotensin IV appears to be arginine vasotocin (AVT).

Urophysectomy in several teleost species results in ionic imbalance, and exposure of euryhaline teleosts to different salinities results in marked histological and ultrastructural changes in the urophysial cells. In addition, injections of urophysial extracts increase plasma ion levels in fishes. Experimental evidence strongly suggests that urotensin II may act directly on the ion-transporting cells of the urinary bladder involved in teleostean seawater osmoregulation.

Urotensin II, isolated from the urophysis of the teleostean fish *Gillichthys mirabilis*, is reported to be a dodecapeptide with an amino acid sequence somewhat similar to somatostatin. The primary structure of urotensin I was determined and found to be strikingly similar to that of a putative corticotropin-releasing hormone of sheep and to sauvagine, a peptide isolated and characterized from frog skin. There is hope that with the elucidation of the structure of urotensin I, synthetic analogs may be produced that are of pharmacological value in the clinical treatment of hypertension in humans.

Endothelin.   Originally characterized as a 21-residue vasoconstrictor peptide from endothelial cells, endothelin (ET) is present in the porcine spinal cord and may act as a neuropeptide. Endothelin-like immunoreactivity was demonstrated by immunohistochemistry in the paraventricular and supraoptic nuclear neurons and their terminals in the posterior pituitary of the pig and the rat. In situ hybridization demonstrated ET messenger RNA in porcine paraventricular nuclear neurons. ET-like immunoreactive products in the posterior pituitary of the rat were depleted by water deprivation, suggesting a release of ET under physiological conditions. These findings indicate that ET is synthesized in the posterior pituitary system and may be involved in neurosecretory functions.

Melanin-Concentrating Hormone (MCH).   This heptadecapeptide is localized to the neurointermediate lobe of teleost fishes (Chap. 8). It is possible that, like the urotensins (Chap. 15), this peptide plays a unique role in certain teleost fishes. MCH is, however, found within the brain of other vertebrates, including mammals (Chap. 8).

MOLECULAR MEDICINE CASE STUDIES

Autosomal dominant neurohypophysial diabetes insipidus (ADNDI) is a rare inherited disorder of free-water conservation. It is characterized by symptoms of AVP deficiency, including polyuria and polydipsia, that are absent at birth but typically develop later in childhood [22]. The cause of ADNDI is a mutation in the single gene that encodes both AVP and its binding protein, neurophysin II. The cellular mechanisms by which these mutations may manifest the symptoms of AVP deficiency with a delayed onset have remained unclear.

A new kindred with ADNDI was identified with a novel mutation in the AVP molecule. A 78-year-old family member was found to have hypotonic polyuria and plasma hyperosmolarity. Treatment with AVP reversed the defect in urinary concentration. The subject and relatives in three generations were found to be heterozygous for a 3-bp deletion in exon 1 of the AVP-NPII gene, predicting a deletion of phenylalanine 3 from the AVP nonapeptide [65]. Previous studies indicated that this residue is critical for binding of AVP to NPII. Studies were conducted to assess the impact of the AVP mutation on the survival of neuronal cells expressing the mutated protein. The neuronal cell line Neuro 2A cells were transfected with the mutant AVP-NP construct and found to show increased rates of apoptosis as measured by flow cytometric methods [65].

These findings indicate that mutations that prevent normal binding, folding, and processing of the AVP and NPII peptides lead to accumulation of mutant proteins in the endoplasmic reticulum, which eventually produces significant cellular toxicity. The dominant transmission of the ADNDI phenotype and the delayed onset of clinically manifested disease are consistent with the idea that cellular toxicity of mutant AVP-NP gene products underlies the pathogenesis of ADNDI.

REVIEW EXERCISES

Compare and contrast each of the following terms:

baroreceptor/osmoreceptor
AVT/AVP
polydipsia/polyuria
paraventricular/
    supraoptic (nuclei)
oviparous/viviparous
myometrium/
    myoepithelial cells
neurogenic/nephrogenic
uterotropic/nephrogenic/
    antidiuretic (actions of
    hormones)

pressophysin/
    oxyphysin
cysteine/cystine
serosal/mucosal
exocytosis/endocytosis
parvocellular/
    magnocellular
urophysin/
    neurophysin
diabetes insipidus/
    diabetes mellitus

Match the animal group(s) with its (their) neurohypophysial hormone(s):

1. Cartilaginous fishes
2. Bony fishes
3. Amphibians
4. Reptiles
5. Birds
6. Mammals except domestic pigs and Macropodidae
7. Domestic pigs and certain marsupials

A. arginine vasopressin
B. lysine vasopressin
C. mesotocin
D. arginine vasotocin
E. oxytocin
F. isotocin
G. valitocin and aspargtocin

Think, analyze and discuss:

1. The Brattleboro rat bears a genetic mutation that renders it incapable of synthesizing and secreting AVP at neurovascular junctions in the posterior pituitary. Would these animals be capable of secreting pressophysin? Why or why not? Would they be capable of secreting oxytocin? Why or why not?

2. Electrophysiological recordings of magnocellular neurons have been made in a variety of settings and in response to a variety of stimuli. If you were conducting such recordings from magnocellular neurons in vivo, how might you determine during the course of the recording which neurons are oxytocinergic and which are vasopressinergic? (Hint: What physiological stimuli might you apply to specifically activate one or the other set of neurons?) Based on previous experimentation, what patterns of activity would you expect to record from each?

3. The osmoregulatory and baroregulatory systems regulate AVP release via separable neural pathways. Design an experiment that could unequivocally demonstrate that this is the case. (Hint: A good strategy would be to demonstrate that signals via route one could be experimentally eliminated while those in the other are left unaffected.)

4. Female mice lacking oxytocin (via a gene knockout) do not eject milk even though they produce milk normally. Can you give a plausible explanation for why this is the case?

5. Arginine vasotocin and oxytocin are similar in structure but have very different affinities for their respective receptors. How might you determine which structural features of the receptors account for this binding specificity?

6. Cyclostomes appear to have only one neurohypophysial hormone. Why does this support the hypothesis that neurohypophysial hormones evolved by gene duplication in more derived vertebrates?

7. In nephrogenic diabetes insipidus, the ability of vasopressin receptors to respond to stimulation by vasopressin is compromised in the renal tubule. Would you expect

vasopressin secretion in this condition to be normal, increased, or decreased? Why?

8. The number of oxytocin receptors in the uterus is relatively low throughout most of pregnancy, but this concentration increases significantly during the later stages of pregnancy, leading up to parturition.
   a. What physiological purpose might this increase in OT receptor number serve?
   b. What are the circulating factors that may be responsible for this increase in OT receptors in late term?
   c. Design an experiment that makes use of a radioligand OT receptor binding assay to test the hypothesis stated in (b). Draw schematic Scatchard plots of the receptor binding data that you would expect to obtain.

References

[1] Archer, R. 1996. Molecular evolution of fish neurohypophysial hormones: Neutral and selective evolutionary mechanisms. *Gen. Comp. Endocrinol.* 102:157–72.

[2] Archer, R., and J. Chavet. 1953. La structure de la vasopressine de boeuf. *Biochem. Biophys. Acta* 12:487.

[3] Barberis, C., et al. 1993. Expression cloning of the human V2 vasopressin receptor. *Regul. Pept.* 45:61–6.

[4] Bargmann, W., and E. Scharrer. 1951. The site of origin of the hormones of the posterior pituitary. *Am. Sci.* 39:255–9.

[5] Bern, H. A., et al. 1985. Neurohormones from fish tails: the caudal neurosecretory system. I. "Urophysiology" and the caudal neurosecretory system of fishes. *Recent Prog. Horm. Res.* 41:533–52.

[6] Bielsky, I. F., et al. 2005. The V1a vasopressin receptor is necessary and sufficient for normal social recognition: a gene replacement study. *Neuron* 47:503–13.

[7] Bielsky, I. F., and L. J. Young. 2004. Oxytocin, vasopressin, and social recognition in mammals. *Peptides* 25:1565–74.

[8] Bisset, G. W. 1974. Milk ejection. In: E. Knobil and W. H. Sawyer, eds. *Handbook of physiology*, Section 7: Endocrinology (Vol. 4, part 1). Washington, DC: American Physiological Society, pp. 493–520.

[9] Bluthe, R. M. and R. Dantzer. 1990. Social recognition does not involve vasopressinergic neurotransmission in female rats. *Brain Res.* 535:301–4.

[10] Carmichael, M. S., et al. 1987. Plasma oxytocin increases in the human sexual response. *J. Clin. Endocrinol. Metab.* 64:27–31.

[11] Carter, C. S. 1992. Oxytocin and sexual behavior. *Neurosci. Biobehav. Rev.* 16:131–44.

[12] Chauvet, J., et al. 1995. A new neurohypophysial peptide, seritocin ([Ser5,Ile8]-oxytocin), identified in a dryness-resistant African toad, *Bufo regularis. Int. J. Pept. Protein Res.* 45:482–7.

[13] Dale, H. H. 1906. On some physiological actions of ergot. *J. Physiol.* 34:163–206.

[14] Deen, P. M., et al. 1994. Requirement of human renal water channel aquaporin-2 for vasopressin-dependent concentration of urine. *Science* 264:92–5.

[15] Engelmann, M., R. Landgraf, and C. T. Wotjak. 2004. The hypothalamic-neurohypophysial system regulates the hypothalamic-pituitary-adrenal axis under stress: an old concept revisited. *Front. Neuroendocrinol.* 25:132–49.

[16] Evans, J. J. 1997. Oxytocin in the human—regulation of derivations and destinations. *Eur. J. Endocrinol.* 137:559–71.

[17] Falke, N. 1989. Oxytocin stimulates oxytocin release from isolated nerve terminals of rat neural lobes. *Neuropeptides* 14:269–74.

[18] Ferguson, J. N., et al. 2001. Oxytocin in the medial amygdala is essential for social recognition in the mouse. *J. Neurosci.* 21:8278–85.

[19] Ferguson, J. N., et al. 2000. Social amnesia in mice lacking the oxytocin gene. *Nat. Genet.* 25:284–8.

[20] Ferguson, J. N., L. J. Young, and T. R. Insel. 2002. The neuroendocrine basis of social recognition. *Front. Neuroendocrinol.* 23:200–24.

[21] Fuchs, A. R., F. Fuchs, and M. S. Soloff. 1985. Oxytocin receptors in nonpregnant human uterus. *J. Clin. Endocrinol. Metab.* 60:37–41.

[22] Gagliardi, P. C., S. Bernasconi, and D. R. Repaske. 1997. Autosomal dominant neurohypophyseal diabetes insipidus associated with a missense mutation encoding Gly23 → Val in neurophysin II. *J. Clin. Endocrinol. Metab.* 82:3643–6.

[23] Goodson, J. L., and A. K. Evans. 2004. Neural responses to territorial challenge and nonsocial stress in male song sparrows: segregation, integration, and modulation by a vasopressin V1 antagonist. *Horm. Behav.* 46:371–81.

[24] Hendy, G. N., and D. G. Bichet. 1995. Diabetes insipidus. *Baillières Clin. Endocrinol. Metab.* 9:509–24.

[25] Higuchi, T. 1995. Oxytocin: a neurohormone, neuroregulator, paracrine substance. *Jpn. J. Physiol.* 45:1–21.

[26] Howell, W. H. 1898. The physiological effects of extracts of the hypophysis cerebri and infundibular body. *J. Exp. Med.* 3:235–58.

[27] Insel, T. R., and L. E. Shapiro. 1992. Oxytocin receptor distribution reflects social organization in monogamous and polygamous voles. *Proc. Natl. Acad. Sci. USA* 89:5981–5.

[28] Jung, J. S., et al. 1994. Molecular structure of the water channel through aquaporin CHIP. The hourglass model. *J. Biol. Chem.* 269:14648–54.

[29] Katsoyannis, P. G., and V. Du Vigneaud. 1958. Arginine-vasotocin, a synthetic analogue of the posterior pituitary hormones containing the ring of oxytocin and the side chain of vasopressin. *J. Biol. Chem.* 233:1352–4.

[30] King, L. S., and P. Agre. 1996. Pathophysiology of the aquaporin water channels. *Annu. Rev. Physiol.* 58:619–48.

[31] Lee, M. D., L. S. King, and P. Agre. 1997. The aquaporin family of water channel proteins in clinical medicine. *Medicine (Baltimore)* 76:141–56.

[32] Lefebvre, D. L., et al. 1994. Uterine oxytocin gene expression. II. Induction by exogenous steroid administration. *Endocrinology* 134:2562–6.

[33] Lefebvre, D. L., et al. 1994. Uterine oxytocin gene expression. I. Induction during pseudopregnancy and the estrous cycle. *Endocrinology* 134:2556–61.

[34] Lim, M. M., I. F. Bielsky, and L. J. Young. 2005. Neuropeptides and the social brain: potential rodent models of autism. *Int. J. Dev. Neurosci.* 23:235–43.

[35] Lim, M. M., and L. J. Young. 2004. Vasopressin-dependent neural circuits underlying pair bond formation in the monogamous prairie vole. *Neuroscience* 125:35–45.

[36] Lincoln, D. W., and J. B. Wakerley. 1974. Electrophysiological evidence for the activation of supraoptic neurones during the release of oxytocin. *J. Physiol.* 242:533–54.

[37] Linzell, J. L. 1961. Recent advances in physiology of the udder. *Vet. Ann.* 2:44–53.

[38] Ludwig, M. 1995. Functional role of intrahypothalamic release of oxytocin and vasopressin: consequences and controversies. *Am. J. Physiol.* 268:E537–45.

[39] Manning, M., and W. H. Sawyer. 1993. Design, synthesis and some uses of receptor-specific agonists and antagonists of vasopressin and oxytocin. *J. Recept. Res.* 13(1–4):195–214.

[40] Mori, M., et al. 1990. Oxytocin is the major prolactin releasing factor in the posterior pituitary. *Endocrinology* 126:1009–13.

[41] Mulders, S. M., et al. 1996. Physiology and pathophysiology of aquaporins. *Eur. J. Clin. Invest.* 26:1041–50.

[42] Murphy, M. R., et al. 1990. Naloxone inhibits oxytocin release at orgasm in man. *J. Clin. Endocrinol. Metab.* 71:1056–8.

[43] Nielsen, S., and P. Agre. 1995. The aquaporin family of water channels in kidney. *Kidney Int.* 48:1057–68.

[44] Nielsen, S., et al. 1995. Vasopressin increases water permeability of kidney collecting duct by inducing translocation of aquaporin-CD water channels to plasma membrane. *Proc. Natl. Acad. Sci. USA* 92:1013–17.

[45] Nishimori, K., et al. 1996. Oxytocin is required for nursing but is not essential for parturition or reproductive behavior. *Proc. Natl. Acad. Sci. USA* 93:11699–704.

[46] Oliver, G., and E. A. Schafer. 1895. On the physiological actions of extracts of the pituitary body and certain other glandular organs. *J. Physiol.* 18:277–79.

[47] Page, S. R., et al. 1990. The effect of oxytocin infusion on adenohypophyseal function in man. *Clin. Endocrinol. (Oxf.)* 32:307–13.

[48] Pedersen, C. A., and A. J. Prange, Jr. 1985. Oxytocin and mothering behavior in the rat. *Pharmacol. Ther.* 28:287–302.

[49] Pickering, B. T. 1978. The neurosecretory neurone: a model system for the study of secretion. *Essays Biochem.* 14:45–81.

[50] Poulain, D. A., J. B. Wakerley, and R. E. Dyball. 1977. Electrophysiological differentiation of oxytocin- and vasopressin-secreting neurones. *Proc. R. Soc. Lond. B Biol. Sci.* 196:367–84.

[51] Richardson, K. C. 1949. Contractile tissues in the mammary gland with special reference to myoepithelium in the goat. *Proc. R. Soc. Lond. B Biol. Sci.* 136:30–45.

[52] Robertson, G. L., S. Athar, and R. L. Shelton. 1977. Osmotic control of vasopressin function. *Disturbances in body fluid osmolality*. Washington, DC: American Physiological Society, pp. 125–48.

[53] Robertson, G. L., R. L. Shelton, and S. Athar. 1976. The osmoregulation of vasopressin. *Kidney Int.* 10:25–37.

[54] Robinson, A. G., and M. D. Fitzsimmons. 1993. Vasopressin homeostasis: coordination of synthesis, storage and release. *Regul. Pept.* 45:225–30.

[55] Rouille, Y., J. Chauvet, and R. Archer. 1991. Heterologue conversion of amphibian hybrin 2 into vasotocin through bovine granule alpha-amidating enzyme. *J. Neuroendocrinol.* 3:15–20.

[56] Rutishauser, J., and E. R. Froesch. 1997. Signal peptide and neurophysin II gene mutations in central hereditary central diabetes insipidus. *News Physiol. Sci.* 12:67–71.

[57] Scharrer, B. 1987. Neurosecretion: beginnings and new directions in neuropeptide research. *Annu. Rev. Neurosci.* 10:1–17.

[58] Schumacher, M., et al. 1993. The oxytocin receptor: a target for steroid hormones. *Regul. Pept.* 45:115–19.

[59] Shimada, K., H. L. Neldon, and T. I. Koike. 1986. Arginine vasotocin (AVT) release in relation to uterine contractility in the hen. *Gen. Comp. Endocrinol.* 64:362–7.

[60] Soloff, M. S., M. Alexandrova, and M. J. Fernstrom. 1979. Oxytocin receptors: triggers for parturition and lactation? *Science* 204:1313–15.

[61] Soloff, M. S., et al. 1975. Autoradiographic localization of radioactivity from [3-H]oxytocin in the rat mammary gland and oviduct. *Endocrinology* 96:1475–7.

[62] Sukhov, R. R., et al. 1993. Vasopressin and oxytocin gene expression in the human hypothalamus. *J. Comp. Neurol.* 337:295–306.

[63] Tindal, J. S., and G. S. Knaggs. 1971. Determination of the detailed hypothalamic route of the milk-ejection reflex in the guinea-pig. *J. Endocrinol.* 50:135–52.

[64] Tuppy, H. 1953. The amino-acid sequence in oxytocin. *Biochim. Biophys. Acta* 11:449–50.

[65] Wahlstrom, J. T., et al. 2004. A novel mutation in the preprovasopressin gene identified in a kindred with autosomal dominant neurohypophyseal diabetes insipidus. *J. Clin. Endocrinol. Metab.* 89:1963–8.

[66] Williams, J. R., et al. 1994. Oxytocin administered centrally facilitates formation of a partner preference in female prairie voles (*Microtus ochrogaster*). *J. Neuroendocrinol.* 6:247–50.

[67] Wray, S. 1993. Uterine contraction and physiological mechanisms of modulation. *Am. J. Physiol.* 264:C1–18.

[68] Yamashita, H. 1977. Effect of baro- and chemoreceptor activation on supraoptic nuclei neurons in the hypothalamus. *Brain Res.* 126:551–6.

[69] Young, L. J., and Z. Wang. 2004. The neurobiology of pair bonding. *Nat. Neurosci.* 7:1048–54.

[70] Zingg, H. H., et al. 1995. Oxytocin and oxytocin receptor gene expression in the uterus. *Recent Prog. Horm. Res.* 50:255–73.

[71] Zoeller, R. T., and F. L. Moore. 1988. Brain arginine vasotocin concentrations related to sexual behaviors and hydromineral balance in an amphibian. *Horm. Behav.* 22:66–75.

CHAPTER

8

Opiomelanocortins

The early studies of Smith and Allen clearly implicated the pituitary gland as the source of a hormone that controlled color changes in amphibians. These color changes were found to be due to the response of certain chromatophores (pigment-bearing cells), particularly melanophores/melanocytes (melanin-containing cells), found within the skin. The melanotropic substance was specifically localized to the neurointermediate lobe (pars intermedia) of the pituitary [1]. This peptide is now referred to as *α-melanocyte-stimulating hormone (α-MSH)* or *α-melanotropin*. MSH and other structurally related peptides found within the pituitary and the brain are referred to generically as *melanocortins (MCs)*. MSH and related MCs regulate skin pigmentation in many vertebrate animals including humans. A more recently discovered hormone, *melanin-concentrating hormone (MCH)*, also regulates integumental color change in some animals. These MCs as well as *endorphins* (opioid peptides) are derived from a multifunctional precursor protein referred to as *proopiomelanocortin (POMC)*. These *opiomelanocortins* regulate a multitude of physiological functions. This chapter will review the interesting story of the MCs and the *opiate peptides* and their suggested roles in vertebrate physiology. Several reviews on the opiomelanocortins are available [14, 24, 25, 36, 49].

Proopiomelanocortin (POMC): A Multifunctional Precursor

The history of research related to the present understanding of the chemistry and proposed roles of the vertebrate MCs began with investigations that established that the pituitary gland contained a number of melanotropic peptides. Indeed, a rather pure MSH (α-MSH) was isolated from the pituitary of a number of mammalian species. Soon after the discovery of α-MSH, another chemically different MSH, β-melanotropin (β-MSH), was also isolated from the pituitary of these same species. A heptapeptide sequence has been conserved within the structures of α-MSH, β-MSH, and corticotropin/ACTH (Fig. 8.1). Unlike the other MCs, the N terminus of α-MSH is acetylated and the C terminus is amidated (Fig. 8.1). The α-MSHs from a number of mammalian pituitaries were chemically characterized and found to be identical in structure. The structure of α-MSH, however, differs slightly in the few poikilotherms that have been studied. Shark (*Squalus acanthias*) and salmon (*Oncorhynchus keta*) α-MSHs are also tridecapeptides, but the N-terminal serine is unacetylated in these species. In addition, in the dogfish shark, the C-terminal amino acid, which is valine in all mammalian α-MSH, is replaced by methionine.

Human pituitaries were said to lack α-MSH, but to contain a β-MSH that was longer (22 amino acids) than the β-MSHs (18 amino acids) isolated from other mammalian pituitaries. It was thought that β-MSH was the principal MC of humans. Radioimmunoassays revealed that in normal humans and in those with certain pathological conditions, the plasma concentrations of β-MSH and ACTH were always correlated. Eventually, it was discovered that pituitaries of a number of species contained an MC that was larger than that of any known pigmentary peptide.

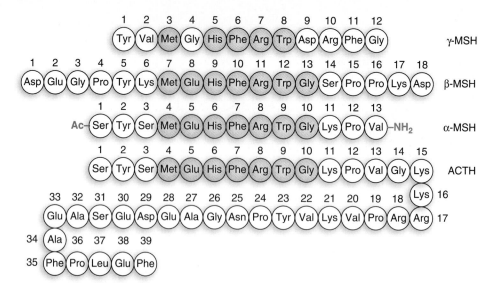

Figure 8.1 Amino acid sequences of bovine γ-, β-, and α-MSH compared to ACTH.

The ovine molecule was shown to contain 91 amino acids and was referred to as β-*lipotropic hormone*, β-*LPH* (Fig. 8.2). The complete structure of β-MSH is contained within the 41–58 sequence of this peptide. Further work revealed that the so-called β-MSH of humans is merely a fragment of β-LPH, artifactually formed during extraction of the tissue. Thus the earlier radioimmunoassay measurements of β-MSH in humans were measurements of the β-LPH present within the plasma. The adult human pituitary, therefore may produce only ACTH and β-LPH, and these peptides are probably not involved, under normal conditions, in the control of integumental melanocyte activity. There is no evidence that β-MSH serves any peripheral physiological function other than as a necessary secretory by-product of other hormones derived from the melanotrophs and corticotrophs.

α-MSH has also been localized to the hypothalamus, where it is found within the perikarya of neurons of the arcuate nucleus. These α-MSH-containing cell bodies in the ventral hypothalamus send multiple projections to numerous extra hypothalamic regions of the brain. Destruction of the arcuate nucleus lowers the α-MSH content of extrahypothalamic regions. Neuronal perikarya of the arcuate region also contain ACTH and β-endorphin, and the reduction in levels of these peptides (including α-MSH) after various treatments suggests that these neuronal peptides are derived from a common precursor. MCs of neural origin are now implicated in numerous physiological functions.

A larger protein (31,000 daltons) was isolated from both the pars distalis and the pars intermedia. This protein, proopiomelanocortin (POMC), contains within its structure the

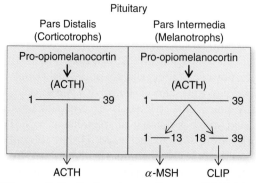

Figure 8.2 Prohormone theory of ACTH and α-MSH biosynthesis. It is unclear whether in the pars intermedia ACTH is first enzymatically released from POMC to yield α-MSH and corticotropin-like-intermediate lobe peptide (CLIP), or whether the latter two peptides are liberated directly from POMC. (Modified from Lowry, P. J., and A. P. Scott. 1975. The evolution of vertebrate corticotropin and melanocyte stimulating hormone. *Gen. Comp. Endocrinol.* 26:16–23, with permission.)

sequences of corticotropin (adrenal cortical stimulating hormone, ACTH) and β-LPH. The first 13 amino acids of ACTH are identical to those of α-MSH. In the pars distalis ACTH is released under certain physiological conditions to regulate adrenocortical function. In the pars intermedia, on the other hand, enzymes are present within the secretory granules and are responsible for the enzymatic cleavage of POMC to α-MSH (Fig. 8.3). Following cleavage from the precursor protein, post-translational amidation and acetylation of the C terminus and N terminus, respectively, of the MSH molecule then occurs. Thus, the precursor protein, POMC, contains within its primary structure the sequences of five MCs: α-MSH, β-MSH, γ-MSH, ACTH, and β-LPH, as well as several opiate peptides (Fig. 8.3).

The Pars Intermedia: A Source of Melanotropins

The pars intermedia develops as a result of contact between the infundibulum and the adeno-hypophysial anlage (Chap. 5). In cyclostomes, amphibians, reptiles, and most mammals, the MSH-secreting cells (melanotrophs) form a well-defined pars intermedia or intermediate lobe (Fig. 8.4). Although the pars intermedia of certain mammals is absent (cetaceans, or whales and dolphins), a zona intermedia does exist in the human fetus, though it subsequently becomes rudimentary (see Fig. 5.1). Birds lack a pars intermedia, but it is claimed, on cytological and bioassay evidence, that MSH-secreting cells are present within the pars distalis. In elasmo-branchs and teleosts the MSH cells are localized caudally but are contiguous with other cells of the pars distalis. The pars nervosa and the pars intermedia of tetrapods are inseparable from each other; this anatomical unit is often referred to as the *neurointermediate lobe*.

The size of the pars intermedia is usually positively correlated with whether or not an animal is able to change color in conformity with the coloration of the substratum. The pars intermedia of the lizard, *Anolis carolinensis* (chameleon), is very large, and this reptile has an outstanding ability for color change, being a bright green or dark brown on light or dark backgrounds, respectively. The pars intermedia is relatively avascular compared to the other components of the pituitary gland and other endocrine tissues. Nevertheless, an extravascu-lar, multibranched transport system penetrates the parenchyma of the pars intermedia and may provide a pathway for the passage of secretory products and regulatory factors to and from the gland. In some species the pars intermedia differs from the pars distalis in that it is penetrated by neurons from the hypothalamus. Neurosecretory and catecholamine-containing neuronal elements may be present; the latter may form a plexus around the secretory cells. These aminergic neurons play a dominant role in the control of melanotroph proliferation and MSH secretion, as will be discussed. Neurons are absent from the neurointermediate lobe of the few lizards that have been studied.

A radioimmunoassay for α-MSH has been successfully used to determine pituitary and plasma levels of α-MSH in frogs adapted to various background (albedo) conditions. The results verified what might be expected (although never confirmed before): plasma levels of MSH were elevated in toads on a black background compared to animals maintained on a gray or a white background. The inverse relationship was observed for α-MSH levels within the neurointermediate lobe of the pituitary [57].

The preferential localization/expression of mRNA for ACTH secretion has been determined by in situ hybridization studies. mRNA for POMC is relatively unaffected by adrenalectomy in the pars intermedia, whereas anterior lobe levels of POMC mRNA are greatly increased. This increase in POMC production is abolished in adrenalectomized animals, however, if the adrenalectomized (ADX) animals are first treated with a synthetic glucocorticoid (dexamethasone). Intermediate lobe levels of POMC mRNA are unaffected by the glucocorticoid (Fig. 8.5). These observations demonstrate the differential control of POMC mRNA synthesis by cells of the pars intermedia and pars distalis.

Control of MSH Secretion

Disruption of the normal anatomical relationships between the pars intermedia and the hypothalamus results in the release of MSH. The endocrine implications of this observation were first appreciated in the early studies of Etkin [1]. Ectopic transplantation of the entire pituitary gland or the isolated neurointermediate lobe usually leads to hypertrophy of the

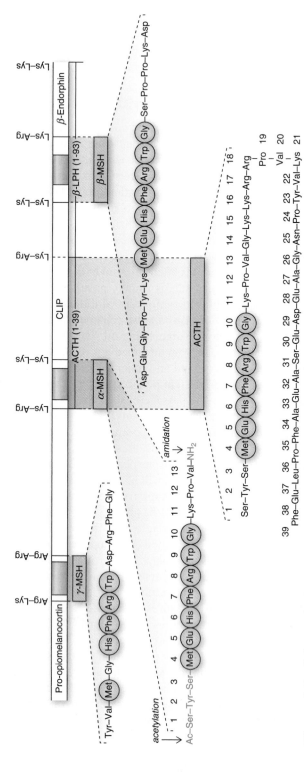

Figure 8.3 Schematic representation of the known, biologically active peptides derived from proopiomelanocortin, which is found in the vertebrate pituitary (corticotrophs and melanotrophs) and hypothalamus. (Reprinted with permission from Sawyer et al. α-Melanocyte stimulating hormone: Chemical nature and mechanisms of action. *Am. Zool.* 23:529–40, 1983. ©1983 by The American Chemical Society.)

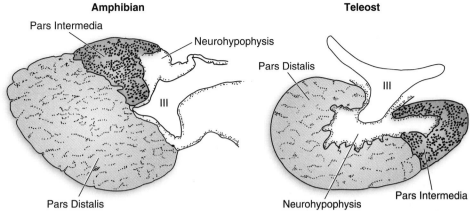

Figure 8.4 Sagittal sections of an amphibian (salamander) pituitary gland (left) and a teleost pituitary gland (right). The three lobular components of the glands are indicated: neurohypophysis, pars intermedia, and pars distalis. The third ventricle (III) is also indicated.

pars intermedia cells and to an increased (uninhibited) release of MSH. These experiments and others involving hypothalamic lesions or pituitary stalk transection yielded similar results in a variety of vertebrates and suggest that the hypothalamus exerts an inhibitory control over MSH release.

Inhibition of pars intermedia MSH secretion is controlled by a catecholamine, most likely dopamine [8]. Catecholamines, such as norepinephrine, epinephrine, and dopamine, are inhibitory to MSH secretion from the isolated neurointermediate lobe of the pituitary [20]. The inhibitory actions of these catecholamines are antagonized by chlorpromazine, a dopaminergic

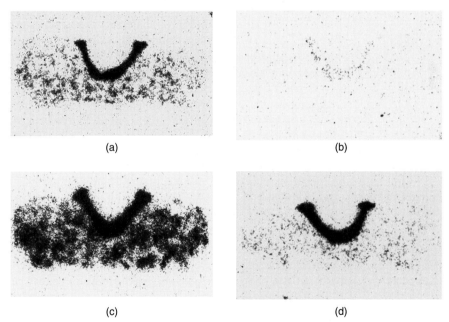

Figure 8.5 Autoradiographs showing hybridization signal in pituitary sections. The intermediate lobe is strongly labeled, whereas a weaker and patchy reaction can be observed in the anterior lobe. (b) Section consecutive to that shown in (a), which has been pretreated with RNAase before prehybridization. No labeling can be observed. (c) Adrenalectomized (ADX) animal. The labeling observed in the anterior lobe is much more intense than that seen in the intact animal. (d) ADX animal treated with dexamethasone (DEX). The intensity of the reaction in the anterior lobe is weaker than that observed in the intact animal. (From Tong et al., with permission. Glucocorticoid regulation of proopiomelanocortin mRNA levels in rat arcuate nucleus. *Mol. Cell. Neurosci.* 1:78–83, 1990.)

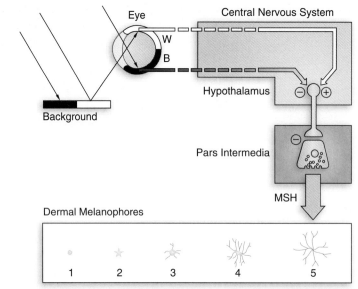

Figure 8.6 The neuroendocrine reflex regulating pigment dispersion in dermal melanophores of amphibians during the process of background adaptation. (Reprinted with permission from B. G. Jenks, V.-V. Kemenade, and G. J. M. Martens, Proopiomelanocortin in the amphibian pars intermedia: A neuroendocrine model system. In *The melanotropic peptides* (pp. 103–126), M. E. Hadley, ed. Boca Raton, FL: 1988 by CRC Press.)

Figure 8.7 Model for the visual control of MSH secretion and the regulation of integumental coloration. (From Fernandez, P. J., Jr., and J. P. Collins. 1988. Effect of environment and ontogeny on color pattern variation in Arizona tiger salamanders (*Ambystoma tigrinum nebulosum* Hallowell). *Copeia* 4:928–38, with permission.)

receptor antagonist. Dopaminergic receptor agonists, such as certain ergot alkaloids, on the other hand, are inhibitory to pars intermedia MSH secretion both in vivo and in vitro [8].

In animals that change color in response to a light- or a dark-colored background, the following model has been proposed from early studies on the frog. The amount of light that is reflected from the background substratum to the dorsal aspect of the retina, relative to the amount that reaches the bottom of the retina from the light source overhead, determines whether MSH will be secreted. On a black background, very little light is reflected to the upper aspect of the retina compared to the amount reflected from a light substratum. In either case the amount reaching the lower part of the retina remains the same (Fig. 8.6). The differential stimulation of the two retinal components therefore determines the chromatic response. On a black background animals turn a dark color due to the release of MSH from the pars intermedia, whereas animals become light on a white background due to an inhibition of MSH secretion (Fig. 8.7).

In the absence of any tonic hypothalamic inhibitory input, melanotrophs and lactotrophs exhibit spontaneous electrical activity in vitro and secrete α-MSH and prolactin, respectively. They both provide informative model systems for determining the relationship between cellular secretion and membrane bioelectrical activity. For example, hormones that affect MSH or PRL secretion do so by mechanisms that modify the membrane electrical activity of the melanotrophs and lactotrophs [8].

Data obtained from a variety of species suggest the following events may be involved in the control of MSH release from the pars intermedia, at least in animals that change color. Environmental photic cues received by the lateral eyes are relayed via neuronal circuits to the hypothalamus. These neurons of inhibitory or stimulatory nature may terminate and synapse with other neurons within the hypothalamus. Aminergic and peptidergic neurons originating in the postoptic nucleus and preoptic nucleus, respectively, have been shown (in the skate) to course through the basal hypothalamus, as a pair of lateral aminergic fiber tracts and a central neurosecretory tract, to penetrate the pars intermedia. The catecholamine-containing neurons make synaptic contact with the individual melanotrophs. The neurosecretory neurons penetrate only to the pars nervosa–pars intermedia border. Other cholinergic neurons of unknown hypothalamic origin may also penetrate into the pars intermedia of some species.

Dopamine released from the aminergic neurons interacts with dopaminergic receptors possessed by the membranes of the pars intermedia cells. The tonic release of the catecholamine maintains the cells in the hyperpolarized state and is inhibitory to MSH secretion.

The cholinergic neurons may antagonize the aminergic neurons by release of acetylcholine at synapses on the aminergic neurons themselves, or by direct synaptic contact with the pars intermedia cells. MSH release would then result from presynaptic inhibition (of dopamine release) or by a direct depolarizing input to the doubly innervated melanotrophs. Release would result if the cholinergic depolarizing input were able to override the aminergic hyper-polarizing inhibitory input. Fine adjustments between the two opposing synaptic events might then modulate the amount of MSH to be secreted.

Physiological Roles of MSH

The role of MSH in the control of color changes in poikilothermic vertebrates is the one clearly documented physiological function of the hormone and one of the earliest described roles for a vertebrate hormone. Numerous other putative functions been also been ascribed to MSH [19, 21].

MSH Regulates Melanin Pigmentation of the Skin

The one unquestionable role of MSH is to control melanin pigmentation of the skin of most vertebrate species [16, 21]. In mammals and many other vertebrates, melanin-containing pigment cells are found in the basal layers of the epidermis. These *melanocytes* (also referred to as melanophores) use the precursor amino acid tyrosine and, through a number of biochemical events controlled by one or more enzymes, produce a colored polymer called *melanin*. This melanin is incorporated into a subcellular structure referred to as a *premelanosome*. When this organelle becomes fully melanized, it is known as a *melanin granule* or *melanosome*. Brown and black melanins are referred to as *eumelanins*, whereas red or lighter-colored melanins are known as *pheomelanins*. Mammals with colored pelage patterns produce one or another of these melanins in different anatomical areas of the skin.

The melanin produced within the melanocytes is released into surrounding cells of the skin by a secretory (cytocrine) mechanism that is not fully understood. The functional unit of epidermal pigmentation, made up of a melanocyte and associated epidermal cells, is referred to as an *epidermal melanin unit* [1]. Melanotropins enhance melanin production within melanocytes, and the melanosomes produced migrate into the dendritic processes of the cells, where they are released into the surrounding cells of the epidermis (Fig. 8.8). The melanocytes in hair-covered parts of the skin are localized to the hair follicles, and synthesis of melanin by these follicular melanocytes is responsible for pigmentation of the hair;

Figure 8.8 Epidermal melanin units of the frog *Rana pipiens*. Melanosomes synthesized by the melanocytes are released into adjacent keratinocytes where they function, at least in humans, as a sunscreen against ultraviolet radiation.

Figure 8.9 Effect of injected α-MSH on melanin pigmentation of the hair of the yellow (C57BL/6JA^y strain) mouse. The yellow control mouse is in the center. (From Geschwind, I. I., R. A. Huseby, and R. Nishioka. 1972. The effect of melanocyte-stimulating hormone on coat color in the mouse. *Recent Prog. Horm. Res.* 28:91–130, with permission.)

a similar process is responsible for melanin pigmentation of feathers. MSH and steroid hormones may sequentially, or in combination, affect the production of eumelanins and pheomelanins within individual follicular melanocytes, which can lead to hairs containing black, brown, or white bands, a so-called "agouti" pattern.

In poikilothermic ("cold-blooded") vertebrates, a variety of *chromatophores* containing a variety of pigments account for variations in color between species [2]. Differences in skin pigmentation in homeotherms ("warm-blooded" vertebrates) can be accounted for by quality (type) and quantity of melanins. As noted earlier, melanins vary in color from yellow-to-brown (pheomelanins) to brown-to-black (eumelanins).

Morphological color changes, which involve alterations in the amount of pigment present within the skin, are generally manifest in response to seasonal changes in background conditions. Seasonal alterations in pigment cell melanogenic activity are an important aspect of the ability of an animal to conform to yearly change in environmental conditions. Rabbits and ptarmigans, for example, develop a white pelage or plumage in conformity with the snow of the winter habitat. During the spring and summer, a dark pelage or feather change accompanies the melting of the snows. MSH is implicated in the white-to-brown pelage changes that occur in the short-tailed weasel and the Siberian hamster, in conformity with the winter to spring change [44]. That mammalian melanocytes of some species can respond to MSH is dramatically demonstrated by the response of the yellow mouse to the hormone (Fig. 8.9). Phenotypically, this genetic strain of mice is normally yellow in color; the response to MSH is unnatural, but does demonstrate the potential for melanogenic activity in the mammal.

Suntanning in humans also results from enhanced melanin pigmentation of the skin [39]. Ontogenic changes in integumental pigmentation occur as in the development of the nuptial coloration of the skin associated with the sexual activity of such vertebrates as birds. The graying of hair due to loss of melanin pigmentation in humans and other mammals is a common phenotypic characteristic of older age, but its physiological significance and etiology are not well understood.

Morphological color changes result from changes in the number and synthetic activity of the integumentary pigment cells. For example, frogs maintained on light- or dark-colored backgrounds for long periods of time become light or dark in color (Fig. 8.10), and the

Figure 8.10 Morphological color change. Effect of long-term (9-week) adaptation of frogs, *Xenopus laevis*, to a white (left) or black (right) background (From Hadley, M. E., and W. C. Quevedo, Jr., with permission. The role of epidermal melanocytes in adaptive color changes in amphibians. *Advan. Biol. Skin* 8:337–59, 1967.)

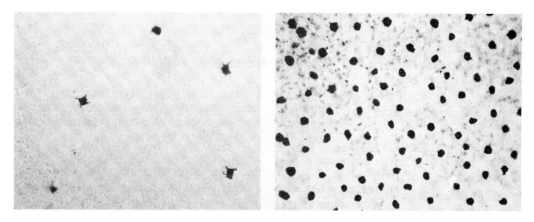

Figure 8.11
Photomicrograph of melanophores in the epidermis of frogs, *Xenopus laevis*, adapted to a white (left) or a black (right) background for a 10-week period.

number of melanocytes found in the epidermis of these animals differs dramatically (Fig. 8.11). This morphological color change is controlled by MSH and clearly demonstrates *hypertrophy* and *hyperplasia* of melanocytes in response to the hormone. In vitro studies demonstrate that melanotropins are clearly stimulatory to melanoblast cytodifferentiation and proliferation, at least in poikilotherms.

During pregnancy the areolae of the nipples in human females may become more darkly pigmented. The darkening of the skin is most pronounced in the last trimester and diminishes slowly after parturition. This increased pigmentation has been considered to be due to elevated levels of an MC. It must be pointed out, however, that gonadal steroid levels are also elevated, and steroid hormones are clearly melanogenic in some species. The MSH-like activity of the blood and urine is increased during pregnancy, and indeed, the frog skin bioassay for MSH was originally designed to measure an elevation of the hormone as an index for predicting pregnancy in the human [48]. The source and nature of the MSH-like activity of the blood and urine during pregnancy are unknown. The activity might be of fetal origin, as the fetal, but not the adult, pituitary is thought to produce a melanotropin.

Melanocortins and Tanning of the Skin in Humans. Because MSH is apparently absent from the pituitary of adult humans, the stimulus for enhanced melanogenic activity during suntanning is not known. Repeated injections of MSH into darkly pigmented individuals, however, increase epidermal pigmentation, which is readily visible after a few days. This demonstrates the capability of the human melanocyte system, at least in dark-skinned individuals, to respond to hormonal activation by MSH [48]. Cholecalciferol (hormonal form of vitamin D) or other vitamin D metabolites and cytokines (Chap. 9) produced within the skin in response to solar radiation may stimulate melanogenesis directly or synergistically in concert with other endogenous hormonal factors. In humans, α-MSH and ACTH are produced locally in the skin and may have a major role in regulating pigmentation [14, 39, 43]. The production of both peptides is up-regulated in the keratinocyte and melanocytes by ultraviolet radiation, and they act as paracrine and autocrine factors that stimulate the melanocyte to produce eumelanin. The contribution of pituitary α-MSH, which circulates at an extremely low level, and serum ACTH, to pigmentation in humans under nonpathological conditions has yet to be determined. In fact, one study failed to support the concept of an involvement of pituitary MCs in tanning of the skin in humans [41]. Loss of the intermediate lobe of the pituitary in humans may have led to the evolution of a cutaneous melanocortin system during vertebrate evolution [24, 33, 43].

Melanocortin Receptors Regulate Animal Pigmentation

The role of melanocortins in the control of integumental pigmentation was documented in the foregoing discussion. It was noted, however, that some animals, birds and humans, for example, lack a pars intermedia and therefore a hormonal source of MC. It is now surprisingly clear that the intrinsic activity of the melanocortin-1 receptor (MC1R) can, in part, account for racial differences in skin coloration in humans, and in pelage and feather pigmentation in some mammals and birds, respectively [11, 24, 35].

The actions of MSH and other MCs are mediated through seven-spanning membrane receptors (Chap. 3). Presently, five melanocortin receptor (MCR) subtypes are recognized [14, 24, 25]. MC1R and MC2R expression is restricted to melanocytes and adrenal cortical

TABLE 8.1   Melanocortin ligands, receptors, responses

Ligand	MSH	ACTH	MC*	MC*	MC*
Receptor	↓	↓	↓	↓	↓
Receptor Subtype	MC1	MC2	MC3	MC4	MC5
Expression	Skin Melanocytes	Adrenal Cortex	Brain	Brain	Exocrine Glands
Response	[1]Melano-genesis	[2]Steroido-genesis	[3]Cardio-vascular?	[4]Weight Homeostasis	[5]Secretion

*Melanocortin (MC): Natural Ligand Unknown.
[1]Tyrosinase activation and melanin production.
[2]Cortisol production in the zone fasciculata.
[3]Variable effects on blood pressure; by modifying sympathetic outflow?
[4]Melanocortins induce satiety (reduce food intake); energy homeostasis.
[5]Lacrimal gland secretion; sebum production/pheromone production.

cells, respectively. Thus, the MC1R and MC2R are targets of a melanotropin (e.g., α-MSH) and corticotropin (ACTH), respectively. The MC3 and MC4 receptors are restricted to the brain, where they are responsive to MCs; the natural ligand for each of these receptors remains to be determined. The MC5R is expressed ubiquitously but the natural MC regulating the receptor is unknown. The known and putative functions of these receptors are shown in Table 8.1.

Mammalian Pelage Pigmentation.   In mammals, pelage coloration is determined by the degree of tyrosinase activity of melanocytes, which are generally relegated to hair follicles and are responsible for the degree of melanization of the individual hairs. The intracellular levels of receptor-generated cAMP determine the nature (color) of the melanin produced (low levels/pheomelanin and higher levels/eumelanin). The intrinsic activity of the MC1R is genetically regulated and therefore generally not regulated by a circulating MC. For example, eumelanin hair pigmentation is preserved in POMC-deficient mice [50]. In addition, there is evidence that the expression of the MC1R gene, but not the POMC gene, plays an important role in the regulation of melanocyte differentiation (in mouse skin) [26]. In mammals, MC1R mutations causing a constitutively active receptor are dominant and associated with black color, whereas loss-of-function mutations are recessive and associated with yellow/red phenotype [4, 14, 24, 49].

The variation (polymorphism) in structure of the MC1R provides an interesting example for "the genetic basis of adaptive melanism in pocket mice" [33]. These mice are usually light colored and live on light-colored soil. Populations of dark (melanic) mice are found on dark lava and this concealing coloration has been shown to provide protection from avian and mammalian predators [16]. Mutations of the MC1R were shown probably to be responsible for adaptive melanism in one population of lava-inhabiting pocket mice [33].

Avian Plumage Pigmentation.   Because birds lack a pars intermedia, it is possible that certain cells of the pars distalis synthesize and secrete an MSH or some other MC. However, MSH has been shown to be without effect on feather pigmentation in the few species of birds studied. Not much is known about the neuroendocrine control of avian pigmentation. One would like to know, for example, what endocrine or other chemical messengers control winter-to-spring and fall-to-winter plumage color changes, particularly in birds such as ptarmigans which are brown in the summer and white in the fall. The findings that MC1R structural variation and plumage coloration in birds are similar to those reported for coat coloration in mammals suggests that the role of the MC system in regulating homeotherm pigmentation has been evolutionarily conserved [24, 33, 43, 53]. The differences between the avian and mammalian melanocortin systems lie in the pattern of expression of melanocortin system peptides and MCRs. There is evidence that the absence of the intermediate lobe from the avian pituitary has resulted in ACTH predominating over α-MSH as an endocrine MC signal, while α-MSH signaling occurs locally in tissues through autocrine/paracrine mechanisms. However, the relative contributions of endocrine (ACTH-mediated) versus autocrine/paracrine (MSH-mediated) melanocortin signaling in birds and their respective physiological effects require further investigation. The predominance of circulating ACTH over MSHs in birds appears to be reflected in the avian MCRs showing a greater relative specificity for ACTH than is the case in mammals [24, 33, 43].

Melanocortin Receptor Polymorphism and Human Skin Pigmentation. As discussed above, polymorphism of the MC1R in mammals and birds can account for pelage and plumage color differences between species. Similarly, racial differences in skin pigmentation in humans are probably associated with MC1R polymorphism [42, 51]. Both gain-of-function and loss-of-function mutations of MC1R have been shown to alter pigmentation in a range of species [4, 24]. MC1R is also highly polymorphic in humans (4, 14, 51). Certain allelic variants of the gene in humans are associated with red hair and pale skin [29, 51]. Although human pigmentation is genetically complex, to date only polymorphism at the MC1R has been associated with phenotypic changes in skin coloration. The relationship of MC1R variants to melanoma and nonmelanoma skin cancer has been the subject of controversy [42].

MSH Directs Color Changes in Nonmammalian Vertebrates

The only known function of MSH in nonmammalian vertebrates is the control of integumental pigmentation [1]. Many poikilothermic vertebrates, for example fishes, amphibians, and reptiles, rapidly adapt to the color of the background over which they reside. The American anole, *Anolis carolinensis*, can change, chameleon like, from a bright green to a darker brown in a matter of minutes after moving from a light- to a dark-colored surface. Rapid *physiological color changes* do not involve changes in the amount of pigment in the skin but, rather, changes in the distribution of melanin within dermal chromatophores (Fig. 8.12). The chromatophores of poikilotherms are the xanthophores, iridophores, and melanophores. The xanthophores may contain carotenoids and pteridines; these pigments may be yellow, orange, or red, and xanthophores may therefore contain combinations of these pigments. The iridophores contain reflecting crystals of purines and related molecules. These three chromatophore types are often grouped together functionally in a *dermal chromatophore unit* (Fig. 8.13). The individual chromatophores of this functional unit respond to MSH by aggregating or dispersing their pigments; in this way the skin becomes light or dark or even yellow or green in color [1, 2, 21].

Other Roles of Melanocortins

Many other physiological roles have been suggested for MSH. A few of these putative functions are discussed, and it is likely that other roles will be discovered for these peptides [6].

Sexual Function. Melanocortins injected into the third ventricle of the brain of rats cause an erectile response. A superpotent analog of α-MSH, Ac-Nle^4-c[Asp^5-His^6-Dphe^7-Arg^8-Trp^9-Lys^{10}]-NH$_2$, injected subcutaneously in men causes erections. Apparently, the peptide crosses the blood–brain barrier to act as a neurotransmitter to activate the erectile center responsible for neurotransmission down the spinal column to the penis. This MC analog may prove particularly important in the treatment of erectile dysfunction of psychogenic

Figure 8.12 A melanophore index is used to evaluate melanosome movements, centrifugal (dispersion) or centripetal (perinuclear aggregation), in response to MSH or other stimuli.

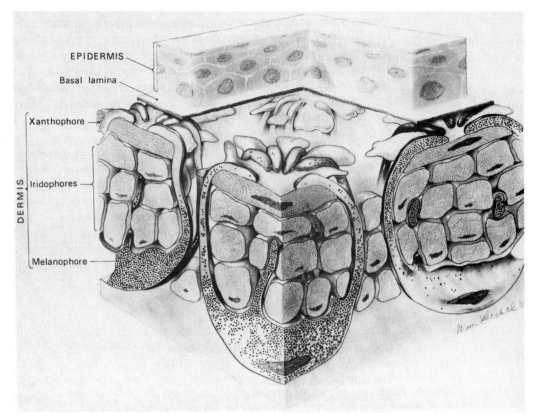

EPIDERMIS

Basal lamina

Xanthophore

DERMIS

Iridophores

Melanophore

Figure 8.13 Dermal chromatophore unit of the lizard *Anolis carolinensis.* (With permission from Taylor, J. D., and M. E. Hadley. 1970. Chromatophores and color change in the lizard *Anolis carolinensis. Z. Zellforsch. Mikroskop. Anat.* 104:282–94.)

origin. Research and development are in progress to develop the drug for clinical use in both males and females [17, 25].

Satiety and Energy Homeostasis.   Leptin, a peptide [7], is a hormonal product of adipose tissue whose expression reflects the body's state of nutritional reserves (fat). Leptin is believed to act as a metabolic signal to the brain to regulate feeding behavior and metabolism to allow the body to maintain normal weight. Mice that are genetically deficient in leptin (ob/ob) are hyperphagic, obese, and infertile; the administration of leptin to these animals reverses these abnormalities. Leptin acts on the central nervous system (CNS) to cause a reduction in food intake and body weight [7]. Melanocortins acting within the brain are also implicated in energy homeostasis since agonists of MC4R reduce food intake [24, 25, 31, 46] and targeted mutation of the MC4R causes obesity [13, 24, 37]. Leptin receptors are on POMC neurons in the arcuate nucleus that synthesize melanocortins [31]. A model for the role of leptin and MCs in energy homeostasis is discussed in Chapter 11.

Thermoregulation.   Certain lizards (e.g., *Sceloporus jarrovi*) orient themselves so that their dorsal surface is maximally exposed to the early morning sun. During this time they are generally dark in color, compared to later in the day when temperatures are elevated. It can be speculated that this adaptive chromatic response is regulated by MSH and that darker skin is able to absorb more radiant energy. Experimental verification is needed as it is possible, at least in some species, that skin darkening could be regulated through direct neural innervation of the melanophores.

An MC may be involved in the central control of body temperature and fever [12, 52]. Both α-MSH and ACTH cause dose-related hypothermia when injected into the cerebral ventricles of the rabbit [see 19]. α-MSH is apparently not involved in the central mechanisms underlying normal thermoregulation, nor does it act as an endogenous antipyretic in the cat, functions that have been postulated in some other species. "Melanocortin agonists act centrally to inhibit fever by acting at receptors, including the melanocortin-4 receptor, which are prominently expressed in key hypothalamic thermoregulatory centers. Furthermore, endogenous melanocortins act centrally as physiological modulators of fever, recruited during the febrile response to restrain its intensity. Functionally, these actions lie at the interface between the anti-inflammatory effects of melanocortins, which involve suppression of the synthesis and actions of proinflammatory cytokines, and the central control of thermoregulation. Considering the extensive neuroanatomic and functional overlaps between central pathways and peripheral effectors involved in thermoregulation and energy balance, it is not surprising that melanocortins have been found to influence the metabolic economy profoundly in pathological as well as normal states. For example, despite suppressing endotoxin-induced fever, endogenous melanocortins appear to mediate the associated anorexia, a classic component of the 'illness syndrome' accompanying acute infections, and promote a negative energy balance. The thermoregulatory actions of melanocortins are in several respects functionally opposed, and are remarkably dependent physiological states, indicating that responsiveness to melanocortins is a physiologically modulated variable" [52].

Melanocortins and Behavior.   Melanocortins have been reported to affect CNS activity in laboratory animals and humans. These effects include arousal, increased motivation, longer attention span, memory retention, and increased learning ability [19]. Immunocytochemical studies have localized MC activity to specific neurons within the brain. The potency of MC action on CNS-related activity is enhanced when administered directly into the ventricles of the brain. It is suggested, therefore, that α-MSH or related MCs may function as a neurotransmitter or neuromodulator within the brain.

Neuroplasticity.   Melanotropic peptides have been shown to alter neurotransmitter synthesis, the electrophysiological parameters of neurotransmission, excitability in the spinal cord and peripheral nerves, and to affect a number of behavioral responses. These neurotropic actions of MSH/ACTH-related peptides may be required for normal functioning of many neuronal processes. There is hope that these peptides may be used to improve the adaptational abilities of the nervous system and to counteract age-related cognitive disorders [19].

Mechanism of MSH Action

Studies on the mechanism of action of MSH have used both in vitro and in vivo methods to monitor responses of integumental melanocytes to the hormone. The frog skin and lizard skin assays monitor the mechanical movements of pigment granules within dermal melanophores and other chromatophores. A few in vitro studies have monitored melanin synthesis within epidermal melanocytes in response to MSH. When melanocytes become cancerous, they are referred to as malignant melanoma. Mouse melanoma cells have been successfully grown in tissue culture and, because these relatively undifferentiated cells respond to MSH, the intracellular biochemical parameters of hormone action have been studied in detail [22, 39].

Melanosome Movements.   Melanophores are found within the dermis of the skin of most poikilothermic vertebrates. Like melanocytes, these specialized pigment cells synthesize melanosomes (melanin granules); instead of being secreted into surrounding cells, these organelles can be rapidly translocated into the dendritic processes of the cell and back toward the cell center. These movements, centrifugal dispersion and centripetal aggregation, result in the skin becoming dark or light in color, respectively. The responses in the skin can be monitored microscopically by using a so-called melanophore index (Fig. 8.12). These changes in skin color can be objectively monitored in response to MSH or other chemical messengers using photoelectric reflectance methods [48]. The endocrine mechanisms controlling melanosome movements are well detailed, but nevertheless incomplete [22].

MSH induces an outward dispersion of melanosomes into the dendritic processes of melanophores. Melanosome dispersion in response to MSH can be mimicked by methylxanthines (caffeine, theophylline) and by (Bu)$_2$cAMP. MSH increases the concentration of cAMP in frog skins concomitant with melanosome dispersion and darkening of the skins. These results implicate cAMP as the intracellular second messenger of MSH action. Epinephrine and norepinephrine also affect melanosome movements within melanophores [22]. Classical pharmacological studies using a variety of adrenergic agonists and antagonists have established that melanosome dispersion in response to these catecholamines is mediated through melanophore β-adrenergic receptors (Chap. 14). These receptors are distinct from MSH receptors, as demonstrated by the preferential blockade of one receptor while the functional response of the other is maintained. Melanosome dispersion in response to MSH or a catecholamine (acting through β-adrenoceptors) is inhibited or reversed by catecholamines acting through α-adrenoceptors possessed by the melanophores. This antagonism of MSH by α-adrenoceptor stimulation involves a decrease in cAMP formation (Chap. 14).

The involvement of adrenergic receptors controlling melanophore responses has been demonstrated in teleosts, amphibians, and reptiles. The melanophores of some amphibians lack α-adrenoceptors but possess β-adrenoceptors [22]. Catecholamines, therefore, fail to inhibit MSH action in these species. Stimulation of β-adrenoceptors in all vertebrate tissues studied results in increased cAMP production, and a similar increase of the cyclic nucleotide probably occurs within melanophores. Melatonin, an indoleamine synthesized within the pineal, antagonizes the action of MSH on melanophores of some animal species. The possible role of the pineal and melatonin in the control of vertebrate pigmentation will be discussed (Chap. 20).

There is a calcium ion requirement for MSH action but not for melanosome movements, per se, because melanosome dispersion proceeds, in the Ca^{2+}-free medium, in response to theophylline or to $(Bu)_2cAMP$. Calcium is the only cation required for MSH action, as the Na^+ and K^+ of the medium can be replaced by lithium, cesium, or rubidium, other monovalent cations. Epinephrine or isoproterenol, acting through melanophore β-adrenoceptors or prostaglandins, do not require Ca^{2+} for activation of melanophore cAMP production. These results demonstrate a receptor-specific Ca^{2+} requirement for MSH action [55]. It is interesting that ACTH and MSH elevate cAMP levels of cells by receptor mechanisms separate from β-adrenergic receptors, which similarly increase the production of this cyclic nucleotide. Adrenocorticotropin and epinephrine, for example, stimulate lipolysis within adipocytes, but through different receptors. As for MSH, ACTH requires Ca^{2+} for its mechanism of action, whereas epinephrine, acting through β-adrenoceptors of adipose cells, does not.

The biochemical events underlying melanophore melanosome dispersion are analogous to those for smooth muscle relaxation: Both processes result from increases in cAMP levels as mediated, for example, by catecholamine stimulation of β-adrenoceptors. An increase in cAMP production results in a transport of Ca^{2+} from the cytoplasm to the endoplasmic reticulum and/or mitochondria or out of the smooth muscle cell. Because melanosome dispersion proceeds in the absence of Ca^{2+} and is enhanced under such conditions [22, 55], a similar Ca^{2+} transport mechanism may also be requisite for melanosome dispersion. Such a model would require the presence of extracellular Ca^{2+} for MSH (but not catecholamine or prostaglandin) action, but the cAMP generated would mediate melanosome dispersion by a subsequent sequestering of cytoplasmic Ca^{2+} [55].

Microtubules, microfilaments, and microtrabeculae are abundant in some, but not all, melanophores. There is no clear consensus for a definitive role of these cytoskeletal organelles within melanophores. The general belief is that they provide the intracellular framework for the translocation of pigment organelles within the cell. A hypothetical model for the control of melanophore melanosome movements is shown (Fig. 8.14).

Figure 8.14
Hypothetical model for a role of MSH and Ca^{2+} ions in the control of melanosome movements within melanophores.

Melanogenesis.   Our understanding of α-MSH action has traditionally been derived from studies on the integumental chromatophores of frogs, lizards, and fishes. Because of the possible malignancy of melanocytes, it is hoped that the results gleaned from these studies may be extrapolated to mammalian melanocytes. Melanocytes and melanoma cells differ from melanophores in that they are undifferentiated cells. Mouse melanocytes, both normal and abnormal (melanoma), possess MSH receptors and also respond to prostaglandins. These agonists activate adenylate cyclase and elevate intracellular levels of cAMP, which results in enhanced tyrosinase activity and increased melanogenesis. MSH action is blocked by actinomycin D and cycloheximide, thus implicating transcriptional and translational effects of the hormone. Although MSH activates cAMP production, and this cyclic nucleotide activates a cAMP-dependent protein kinase, the mechanism by which this cyclic nucleotide activates nuclear transcriptional processes leading to increased enzyme activity is unknown. A model based on present knowledge of the control of melanogenesis by MSH is shown (Fig. 8.15).

Analogs of Melanotropins are Analyzed in Structure–Function Studies

Numerous analogs of α-MSH and related MCs have been synthesized for structure–function studies [20, 22]. The natural melanotropins share a common heptapeptide sequence, -Met-Glu-His-Phe-Arg-Trp-Gly- (Fig. 8.1). Because these peptides (α-MSH, β-MSH, ACTH, β-LPH) possess melanotropic activity, it is believed that this sequence represents the active site of the molecule. Minimal contribution is nevertheless provided by the C-terminal tridecapeptide sequence -Lys-ProVal-NH₂, as well as the N-terminal sequence Ac-Ser-Tyr-Ser-, in some species. The minimal sequence for biological activity in the frog and lizard skin bioassays is the tetrapeptide sequence His-Phe-Arg-Trp [21, 22].

MSH Antagonists.   A number of MC antagonists have been designed and synthesized and their biological actions determined in the frog and lizard bioassays [21, 22]. These peptides differ in their antagonistic activities, pointing out that melanotropin receptors differ between species. Improved efficacy of these antagonists may result in peptides with clinical

Figure 8.15   Model for MSH activation of melanocyte tyrosinase and melanin synthesis. The substrate for cAMP-dependent protein kinase is unknown. The end result of tyrosinase activation, melanosome formation and release into surrounding keratinocytes, is enhanced skin pigmentation (or follicular melanogenesis in some animals).

relevance. Two natural endogenous inhibitors of MC receptors, agouti and agouti-related protein (ARP), have been identified [4, 14, 32]. Agouti probably regulates pelage coloration in some mammals; ARP regulates MC activities in the brain related to food intake and energy metabolism [24].

Melanin-Concentrating Hormone

In 1931, it was postulated that many lower vertebrates exhibit color changes through dual hormonal control by two antagonistic pituitary melanotropic hormones [1]. α-Melanotropin is clearly implicated in regulating darkening of the skin of many animals through stimulation of melanosome dispersion within melanophores. The existence of an antagonist hormone, a *melanin-concentrating hormone* (MCH), in the pituitary gland of teleost fishes was suggested in 1955 [9]. Teleost MCH was then separated from fish pituitary gland extracts in 1958; the highest concentrations of MCH were found in the neurointermediate lobe of the pituitary gland. This hormone induced blanching of the skin (perinuclear aggregation of melanosomes within melanophores) when injected into teleost fishes [9]. MCH was then isolated in pure form from chum salmon pituitaries and was characterized as a cyclic heptadecapeptide [3]. The primary structure of this peptide is shown in Fig. 8.16.

Rat hypothalamic MCH is a nonadecapeptide that differs from salmon MCH by an N-terminal extension of two amino acids and four additional substitutions. Rat MCH has the following primary structure: Asp-Phe-Asp-Met-Leu-Arg-Cys-Met-Leu-Gly-Arg-Val-Tyr-Arg-Pro-Cys-Trp-Gln-Val. The sequence of rMCH found by DNA sequencing confirms the sequence deduced from the purified peptide. rMCH is located at the C terminus of a protein precursor of 165 amino acid residues. Comparison of the amino acid sequence of prepro-MCH and that of the *Aplysia* peptide-A prohormone suggests that these proteins, as well as other precursors, may be evolutionarily related. The human gene for MCH has been isolated and characterized.

MCH and Color Change. Salmon MCH is effective at concentrations as low as 1 nmol, or less, in causing melanosome concentration within teleost melanophores. MCH and several related structural analogs have now been synthesized and characterized for their melanotropic activities in several bioassays [3; see Fig. 8.18]. MCH stimulates melanosome concentration within melanophores of all teleost fishes species studied. Melanosome aggregation in response to MCH is reversible, since removal of the peptide from the bathing medium results in a redispersal of the pigment organelles within the chromatophores. The melanosome-aggregating activity of MCH could also be reversed if MSH was added to teleost skin lightened by MCH. These results clearly reveal that in several species of teleosts, melanophores possess receptors responsive to both MSH and MCH. Melanosome aggregation in response to MCH was not blocked by dibenamine (an α-adrenoceptor antagonist; see Chap. 14), which did block the response to norepinephrine, demonstrating that melanosome-aggregating responses to MCH and norepinephrine are mediated through separate receptors [22].

A most unexpected observation was that MCH, rather than stimulating melanosome aggregation within tetrapod melanophores, instead induced melanosome dispersion. The peptide was about 1/600 as potent as MSH; nevertheless, full melanosome dispersion was effected in melanophores of frogs, toads, and lizards. There are no readily apparent similarities between the primary structures of MCH and α-MSH. To determine the possible structural basis of the opposing actions of MCH, several analogs were synthesized, in addition to the native hormone. These fragment analogs consisted of the central cyclic sequence (MCH$_{5-14}$), as well as the N-terminal (MCH$_{1-14}$) and the C-terminal (MCH$_{5-17}$) extensions of the central sequence of the native peptide (Fig. 8.17). Using skins of the teleost *Synbranchus marmoratus* (an eel) and photoreflectance recordings, it was determined that MCH$_{5-17}$ was at least equipotent to the native hormone, MCH$_{1-17}$. MCH$_{1-14}$ was also quite active, showing about 1/10 the activity of MCH$_{1-17}$. The central cyclic fragment analog, MCH$_{5-14}$, possessed about 1/300 the activity of

```
┌Met–Thr–Asp
│              ┌─────────────────────────────────────────┐
└Arg–Cys–Met–Val–Gly–Arg–Val–Tyr–Arg–Pro–Cys–Trp┐
      5                10                15     │
                                        Val–Glu┘
```

Figure 8.16 Primary structure of melanin-concentrating hormone (MCH).

| | 1 | | 3 | | 5 | | 7 | | 9 | | 11 | | 13 | | 15 | | 17 |

MCH–1–17   Asp–Thr–Met–Arg–Cys–Met–Val–Gly–Arg–Val–Tyr–Arg–Pro–Cys–Trp–Glu–Val

MCH–1–14   Asp–Thr–Met–Arg–Cys–Met–Val–Gly–Arg–Val–Tyr–Arg–Pro–Cys

MCH–5–17   Cys–Met–Val–Gly–Arg–Val–Tyr–Arg–Pro–Cys–Trp–Glu–Val

MCH–5–14   Cys–Met–Val–Gly–Arg–Val–Tyr–Arg–Pro–Cys

Figure 8.17 Primary structures of MCH and related fragment analogs.

the parent peptide. Therefore, the potency ranking of the MCH analogs on teleost melanophores was as follows: $MCH_{1-17} = MCH_{5-17} > MCH_{1-14} > MCH_{5-14}$ (Fig. 8.18). The fragment analogs were full agonists, and their melanosome-aggregating actions were reversible when the skins were transferred to physiological saline in the absence of the peptides. It is interesting to note that this fish-skin bioassay is sensitive to MCH at a minimal effective dose of 10^{-12} M. This assay is therefore 10 and 100 times more sensitive, respectively, than are the classical frog and lizard skin assays to MSH.

It was shown that the fragment analog MCH_{1-14} exhibited MSH-like activity (about 10% of the MCH response) in the frog and lizard skin bioassays. The C-terminal fragment analog, MCH_{5-17}, lacked melanosome-dispersing activity even at the highest concentrations employed (10^{-5} M). It appears, therefore, that tetrapod melanophores lack MCH receptors. These results also suggest that one or more amino acids within the N-terminal 1–4 sequence (Asp-Thr-Met-Arg) are required for the MSH-like activity of MCH, but not for the MCH-like activity of the hormone. These observations suggest that MSH and MCH may be evolutionarily related.

MCH and Energy Homeostasis.   As noted earlier, MCH can reverse/oppose the action of MSH (on skin coloration in some animals). Similarly, MCH injected into discrete hypothalamic nuclei known to express MCH receptors elicited a rapid and significant increase in feeding in satiated rats. Administration of a neuropeptide Y (NPY) antagonist inhibited MCH-stimulated food intake in animals. Incubation of hypothalamic explants in the presence of MCH increased the release of the orexigenic transmitter NPY and decreased the release of the anorectic peptide α-MSH. These studies along with numerous others [45, 47, 56] provide strong evidence for a role of MCH in feeding behavior and energy homeostasis.

Several physiological roles, possibly indirectly related to MCH effects on energy homeostasis, have been suggested: (1) MCH is capable of inhibiting pulsatile LH release in rats. Since fasting also suppresses LH in these animals, it is possible that MCH could play a role in mediating the suppression of LH during periods of reduced nutritional intake [54]. (2) The thyroid axis is important in energy homeostasis and starvation leads to suppression of the hypothalamo-pituitary-thyroid axis. MCH reduces plasma TSH in vivo and reduces from pituitary cell cultures, although basal release of TSH from these cells was unaffected. These

Figure 8.18 In vitro bioassay of MCH and related analogs using skins of the fish *Synbranchus marmoratus* (an eel). (From Castrucci, A. M. L., et al. 1989. Melanotropin structure-activity studies on melanocytes of the teleost fish, *Synbranchus marmoratus. Gen. Comp. Endocrinol.* 4:209–14, with permission.)

observations suggest a possible role for MCH in the control of energy homeostasis by inhibition of the thyroid axis [27, 28].

Pathophysiologies Involving Melanotropic Hormones can Accompany other Endocrinopathies

Because the pituitary of the adult human lacks a pars intermedia, it is not surprising that, unlike most hormones, no pathophysiological states related to overproduction or underproduction of MSH have been described. The discovery that α-MSH is present in the fetal pituitary and may function in the control of fetal growth and development within the uterus should alert the clinician to possible postnatal defects resulting from pars intermedia dysfunction in the fetus. Because α-MSH may function as a neurohormone within the brain, α-MSH or other MCs may eventually be implicated in the etiology of certain behavioral pathologies.

In Addison's disease destruction of the adrenal cortex results in a subsequent failure of adrenal steroid hormone production. Because of an absence of circulating levels of cortisol, there is a lack of negative feedback inhibition to the hypothalamus and pituitary, which results in enhanced pituitary secretion of ACTH (Chap. 15). Hyperpigmentation, a cardinal symptom of Addison's disease, develops because excessive circulating levels of ACTH or other melanotropic sequences are stimulatory to melanogenesis within epidermal melanocytes. In Cushing's syndrome (of pituitary origin), where excessive amounts of ACTH are secreted, hyperpigmentation is often noted and may be due, again, to elevated circulating levels of POMC-derived melanotropic peptides. Hyperpigmentation may also occur in the *ectopic ACTH syndrome* where excessive amounts of ACTH or other melanotropins are secreted by tumors of nonpituitary origin.

Vitiligo is a malady of the skin where melanocytes in certain areas are absent or fail to become pigmentogenic. Areas of the integument are thus unpigmented. There was hope that melanogenesis within these affected areas might be restored by administration of MSH or related melanotropins. Unfortunately, MSH only increases the pigment in the adjacent normal areas, thus, in effect, accentuating the pigmentary problem.

Biomedical Applications of Melanocortins are in Development

A number of unique α-MSH analogs have been synthesized that are superpotent, prolonged acting, and resistant to inactivation by proteolytic enzymes. These peptides provide potential probes for physiological and clinical studies. For example, these analogs can be conjugated to radioisotopes or fluorescent ligands for the cellular- (receptor-) specific delivery to melanoma (cancer). Melanotropins can also be conjugated to anticancer drugs. Melanotropin analogs, therefore, might be utilized for the localization and chemotherapy of melanoma [22, 23].

It was demonstrated that certain melanotropins can be topically applied and transdermally delivered across the skin of mice and humans in vitro, as determined by bioassay and radioimmunoassay (RIA). Studies are under way to determine whether MSH-related analogs may prove useful as a "tanning hormone" for increasing the pigmentation of light-skinned individuals or possibly even for treating people with certain hypopigmentary disorders. It is hoped this "tanning without the sun" may reduce the incidence of skin cancer. The results of initial studies demonstrated that tanning of human skin by a synthetic melanotropic peptide is feasible [18, 30].

The Endorphins

In 1965, C. H. Li discovered a peptide in the pituitary of cattle and named it β-lipotropin. This so-called lipotropic peptide, β-LPH, named for its action on adipose tissue, was considered for many years to be a hormone in search of a function. With the discovery of endogenous morphine-like peptides in the brain, β-LPH may at last have an identified function. Opiate receptors have been discovered in the brain and have been pharmacologically characterized by their interaction with opiate agonists and antagonists such as morphine and naloxone, respectively. Because it is reasonable to conclude that such highly specific receptors have not evolved to interact with exogenous opiate alkaloids, it was suggested that endogenous opiate-like substances might exist as natural ligands for the identified opiate receptors. Two peptides possessing opiate-like activity were isolated from bovine brain tissue as pentapeptides, differing only at the C terminus, possessing either leucine or methionine at that position. These peptides are referred to as enkephalins, and methionine enkephalin was recognized to be identical to an amino acid sequence within a larger peptide of the pituitary, β-LPH [34, 36, 38].

Endorphins are a class of substances isolated from the brain and pituitary gland that exhibit opiate-like activity. It was also discovered that the pituitary contains an endogenous opioid with a molecular weight greater than the enkephalins. This peptide was isolated, sequenced, and found to correspond to the 61–91 sequence of bovine β-LPH. This β-endorphin, as well as the enkephalins and other endorphins, are possible candidates for the body's own anti-pain (analgesic) hormones. Indeed, these peptides do appear to play such a role; therefore, β-LPH might be considered to function as a prohormone for the production of at least some of these endorphins.

Endogenous Opioid Peptides are Derived from POMC, Proenkephalin, and Prodynorphin

Opiate drugs such as morphine affect the perception of pain, consciousness, motor control, and autonomic function by interacting with specific receptors expressed throughout the central and peripheral nervous systems. The endogenous ligands of these opiate receptors have been identified as a family of more than 20 opioid peptides that derive from the three precursor proteins, proopiomelanocortin, proenkephalin, and prodynorphin. Although the opioid peptides belong to a class of molecules distinct from the opiate alkaloids, they share common structural features, including a positive charge juxtaposed with an aromatic ring that is required for interaction with the receptor.

Pituitary β-LPH is found in both the pars distalis and pars intermedia in association with ACTH. Corticotrophs and melanotrophs of the pars distalis and pars intermedia, respectively, of the pituitary produce a large molecular weight (31,000 daltons) protein that contains the sequence of β-LPH and ACTH. The term *proopiomelanocortin* (POMC) was suggested for this protein that appears to be the common precursor for β-endorphin and corticotropin. POMC is found within secretory granules of corticotrophs of the pars distalis and the granules of melanotrophs of the pars intermedia. The precursor protein serves as a prohormone for ACTH production in the pars distalis; in the pars intermedia enzymatic activity results in cleavage of POMC to yield α-MSH (Fig. 8.2). The complete amino acid sequence of bovine POMC has been reported.

Although there is no evidence that β-endorphin of pituitary origin serves any physiologically relevant humoral role, another opioid peptide, dynorphin, has been isolated from the posterior pituitary. This heptadecapeptide contains Leu-enkephalin as its NH_2-terminal sequence. The potency of this peptide is greater than that of any other known endogenous opiate-like peptide, but the peptide's physiological role is undetermined. Cells that stain immunocytochemically for dynorphin are found within specific sites within the hypothalamus and myenteric plexus of the gut. Within the pituitary, the peptide is specifically localized to the neurohypophysis. Dynorphin and vasopressin occur in the same hypothalamic magnocellular neurons of rats; their synthesis, however, appears to be under separate genetic control. Dynorphin is not present within oxytocin-containing neurons.

A number of independent endorphin pathways in the brain have been delineated: a β-endorphin system with a single cell group in the hypothalamus and long axons innervating midbrain and limbic structures, and two enkephalin systems with multiple cell groups throughout the spinal cord and brainstem, which possess relatively short axons. The immunocytochemical mapping of Leu- and Met-enkephalins suggests that the two pentapeptides occur in completely separate nerve cells in neural pathways that differ anatomically. The relative proportions of Met- and Leu-enkephalin vary between different brain regions and also between different species, further demonstrating the existence of separate populations of Met- and Leu-enkephalin nerves. Many areas of the brain that are rich in enkephalins correspond to areas closely associated with dopaminergic, noradrenergic, serotonergic, and substance P-containing neuronal systems. Many enkephalin-containing neurons appear to be short interneurons.

Outside the CNS, there is a rich enkephalinergic innervation of the gastrointestinal tract, and there is evidence that enkephalins may also be contained in various autonomic nerves and ganglion cells and in mucosal cells of the stomach. Present evidence suggests that β-LPH, ACTH, and β-endorphin sequences occur within the same neurons in the brain and that POMC may therefore also function as a prohormone for β-endorphin, α-MSH, or ACTH production within the CNS. The enkephalins, on the other hand, are derived from different, precursors; "big" forms of both Met-enkephalin and Leu-enkephalin have been discovered. The amino acid sequence of these peptides differs from that of β-LPH, suggesting separate precursors for β-endorphin and each of the enkephalins.

The Physiological Roles of Opioid Peptides are Remarkably Diverse

The physiological roles of the identified opioid systems are not fully elucidated [58]. The endorphins are found in high concentrations in brain areas involved in pain transmission, respiration, motor activity, pituitary hormone secretion, and mood. The suggestion of a relationship between the endorphins and ACTH secretion is intriguing as behavioral studies indicate that stress increases the concentrations of endorphins in blood and brain, with parallel changes in pain threshold. Histochemical localization also suggests that the opioid substances may have important relations to noradrenergic and dopaminergic systems.

Analgesic Function. The most clearly understood action of an endorphin is in the spinal cord where small enkephalin-containing neurons impinge on the terminals of peripheral sensory nerve cells that convey pain information to the spinal cord. These primary afferent neurons contain (and release) another peptide known as substance P (SP). Substance P (Arg-Pro-Lys-Pro-Gln-Gln-Phe-Phe-Gly-Leu-Met-NH$_2$) has been immunocytochemically localized to sensory pain fibers of the dorsal root ganglia. The higher concentration of SP in dorsal root neurons compared to ventral root nerves suggests that SP is the neurotransmitter released by the central terminals of primary afferent sensory fibers. SP has an excitatory action on single neural units in the dorsal horn of the spinal cord. The units excited by SP are among those excited by noxious cutaneous simulation; SP causes an enhancement of the responses of these nociceptive (pain-sensing) units to noxious stimulation.

Met-enkephalin blocks the release of SP from nerve terminals of sensory pain fibers, and the effect of the endorphin is antagonized by naloxone (an opiate antagonist). The distribution of opiate receptors closely parallels that of SP neurons, and the SP neurons contain binding sites (receptors) for the enkephalins. Thus, enkephalin-containing neurons within the dorsal horn may inhibit release of SP from dorsal root sensory neurons and thereby inhibit pain transmission to the brain. There is evidence that another major site of enkephalin modulation of the nociceptive information transfer in the dorsal horn is on the projection neurons themselves. The relationship between enkephalins and SP may be the physiological basis for the postulated "pain gate." This gate in the spinal cord permits pain-induced neural impulses to be conveyed from sensory neurons to the brain. Prevention of SP release by enkephalin may be what closes the gate.

One fascinating finding suggests that endorphins and their receptors can affect acupuncture-induced analgesia. For example, the firing rate of cells in the spinal cord is greatly increased in response to painful stimuli. Acupuncture suppressed this increased electrical activity, but this acupuncture effect was completely blocked by the specific opiate antagonist, naloxone. The acupuncture effect was slow in onset and it long outlasted the acupuncture stimulation, suggesting a hormonal rather than a direct neuronal response. Acupuncture and electroacupuncture have also been shown to be reversed by opiate antagonists; experiments suggest that the opioid system may play a role in placebo analgesia, which is effective in about 30% of the population. A study in Beijing, China, indicates that electroacupuncture in rats causes an analgesia that involves release of opioid peptides. By using radioimmunoassays, it was found that low-frequency electroacupuncture led to release of enkephalins into spinal perfusates, whereas high-frequency electroacupuncture resulted in the release of a dynorphin. These results were confirmed by experiments in which the injection of antibodies against enkephalin or dynorphin was shown to block electroacupuncture analgesia.

Several studies have implicated an endogenous opiate system in human behavior specifically related to pain and psychiatric disorders. It was found that stimulation of the periaqueductal gray matter of the brain produces naloxone-reversible analgesia in patients suffering from intractable pain. This response was accompanied by an increase in ventricular endorphin-like activity. These data support the findings that basal levels of endogenous opioids in the cerebrospinal fluid of patients with persistent pain are depressed. These observations suggest, as do the animal studies cited earlier, that analgesic brain stimulation may result in the release of an endogenous opiate-like substance. Preliminary trials have suggested that β-endorphin itself produces significant pain relief when administered to terminal cancer patients. Further well-controlled clinical trials may provide a more detailed understanding of the mechanisms of pain and how pain relief may be achieved.

Endorphins as Possible Adrenomedullary Hormones. Stressful stimuli often elicit marked neurogenic stimulation of the adrenal medulla. Many forms of stress also induce significant analgesia that can be partially blocked by naloxone. A large number of enkephalin-containing peptides are present in mammalian adrenal chromaffin tissue. They are stored within chromaffin granules and are cosecreted in response to the same stimuli that induce catecholamine secretion. Denervation of the rat adrenal increases the amounts of enkephalin and enkephalin-containing polypeptides in the gland. These peptides may all derive from a proenkephalin through proteolysis. One such peptide (peptide E) contains within its structure both the Met- and Leu-enkephalin sequences. This peptide is 30 times more potent than Met-enkephalin. It is suggested that free enkephalins may not be the physiologically relevant end product derived from pro-enkephalin but, rather, that peptide E and other adrenal enkephalin-containing peptides may serve as unique physiological regulatory substances. Specifically, it has been suggested that adrenomedullary enkephalins may contribute to the attenuation of pain during life-threatening stress.

Control of Pituitary Hormone Secretion. There is evidence that opioid peptides may play a physiological role in controlling the release of pituitary hormones [40]. For example, in the pig-tailed monkey the concentration of β-endorphin is more than 100 times greater in the hypophysial blood than in the peripheral plasma. Intravenous injection of opioid peptides causes the release of PRL, GH, AVP, and MSH. These peptides however, are inhibitory to FSH and LH secretion, and these endorphin effects on pituitary hormone release are reversed by naloxone. Opioid peptides and antagonists are without any effect on isolated pituitaries, suggesting that their effects are mediated at the level of the hypothalamus. The simplest interpretation is that endogenous opioid peptides inhibit dopaminergic (or noradrenergic) pathways that normally control some pituitary hormone secretions. Prolactin secretion from the adenohypophysis is normally inhibited by a PRL-inhibiting factor that apparently is dopamine (Chap. 5). Endorphin inhibition of dopamine secretion would therefore result in PRL secretion. The release of PRL under physiological conditions can be reduced by blockade of opiate receptors, which further suggests that endogenous endorphins participate tonically in the regulation of PRL secretion. Likewise, β-endorphin inhibition of dopamine or norepinephrine secretion from median eminence catecholaminergic neurons (which are stimulatory to hypothalamic gonadotropin-releasing hormone neurons) would account for the inhibition of FSH and LH secretion that follows central administration of an endorphin. Opiate receptor antagonists, as expected, stimulate gonadotropin secretion, suggesting that GnRH secretion is under tonic inhibition by an exogenous endorphin.

Role in Reproductive Physiology. A synthetic analog of Met-enkephalin inhibits copulatory behavior in sexually active male rats; its action is prevented by naloxone, a specific inhibitor of opioid receptors. Naloxone itself induces copulatory behavior in inactive male rats, which suggests that endorphins normally exert a tonic inhibition of copulatory behavior. These observations provide strong evidence that endorphins may be important in the regulation of sexual behavior [15].

Opioid Peptides Modulate Neuronal Activity through the δ, μ, and κ Classes of Opioid Receptors

Endorphins modify the excitability of a variety of neurons in the CNS. Microiontophoresis of Met-enkephalin onto single neurons in the rat brainstem shows that endorphins' predominant action is to suppress the firing rate of spontaneously active neurons. Similar effects are obtained with the narcotic agonists morphine and etorphine; their actions and those of Met-enkephalin are blocked by iontophoretically applied naloxone. Endorphins and opiate narcotics inhibit spontaneously responsive cells in the cortex, brainstem, caudate nucleus, and thalamus. In the hippocampus, however, pyramidal cells are usually excited and are also naloxone sensitive. Opiate receptors are apparently localized presynaptically on some nerve fibers, and endorphins may reduce the release of dopamine and other neurotransmitters by an action on these receptors. A major function of an endorphin, therefore, may be to mediate presynaptic inhibition on a variety of neuronal systems in the CNS. The presynaptic effects of endorphins or opiate narcotics on neuronal activity would depress or excite neurons depending on whether the presynaptic neurons are excitatory or inhibitory to the neurons being monitored electrophysiologically. Thus *disinhibition* of an active neuron that is inhibitory to a quiescent neuron would result in excitation of this latter neuron.

Endorphins interact with opiate receptors, as shown by their ability to displace radiolabeled narcotic agonists and antagonists from the receptors. Opiate receptors fall into a number of distinct classes as characterized by pharmacological and biochemical methods. Classical pharmacological studies have defined three classes of opioid receptors, delta receptors (δ), mu receptors (μ) and kappa receptors (κ), which differ in their affinity for various opioid ligands and in their anatomical distribution. The δ receptors bind with the greatest affinity to enkephalins and have a more discrete distribution in the brain than either μ or κ receptors, with high concentrations in the basal ganglia and limbic regions. Although morphine interacts principally with μ receptors, peripheral administration of this opiate induces release of enkephalins. Thus enkephalins may mediate part of the physiological response to morphine, presumably by interaction with δ receptors. The specific anatomical localizations suggest that the different types of receptors mediate different physiological functions [38]. The μ receptors may mediate analgesic actions, whereas δ receptors may preferentially regulate emotional behavior. The μ and δ receptors are regulated by Met- and Leu-enkephalins, respectively. Dynorphin appears to be a specific endogenous ligand for the κ subclass of opioid receptor. Thus, the opiates, like adrenergic, cholinergic, and dopaminergic agonists, initiate their broad spectrum of diverse physiological actions by interaction with multiple receptor types. This provides some hope that opiate drugs might be developed that possess morphine-like analgesic actions but lack addictive effects. Despite pharmacological and physiological heterogeneity, the three types of opioid receptors inhibit adenylyl cyclase, increase K^+ conductance, and inactivate Ca^{2+} channels through a pertussis toxin-sensitive mechanism (Chap. 3). Opioid receptors belong to the large family of seven-spanning membrane receptors (see Fig. 3.3) that signal through G proteins [38].

Opioid Peptide Systems are Involved in the Pathophysiology of Drug Addiction

In studies on a neuroblastoma hybrid cell line grown in tissue culture, it was found that continuous exposure to opiates resulted initially in decreased cAMP production. With time, more of the opiate agonist was required to decrease cAMP production to the original levels produced by the opiate; the cells had apparently become *tolerant* to the actions of the drug. It was found that the cells synthesized more adenylate cyclase and, on removal of the opiate from the cells, cAMP levels rose dramatically and responded excessively to other hormonal stimulation. This excessive production of cAMP may represent the biochemical correlate of withdrawal symptoms noted in humans taken off opiate drugs. There is evidence that opiate drugs and peptides also mediate their actions on nervous tissue through stimulation of cGMP production.

Classical *tolerance* and *dependence* develop in rodents continuously infused with endorphins. The animals are also cross dependent on morphine. This might be expected, as the receptors for opiate drugs and peptides are identical. It has been suggested that heroin addicts, at some stage in their addiction, may suffer from an endorphin deficiency. Excess target tissue hormones (e.g., cortisol) are known to exert a negative feedback to hypothalamic production of releasing hormones (i.e., CRH). Possibly the production of brain or pituitary endorphins is shut off in a similar manner due to feedback inhibition by opiate drugs. Addicts then might be suffering from a true hormone (endorphin) deficiency.

According to the catecholamine theory of schizophrenia, psychosis results from the overproduction of dopamine and therefore overstimulation of dopaminergic receptors. There is evidence that endorphins affect certain CNS dopaminergic pathways. The opiate antagonist, naloxone, alters some schizophrenic symptoms. This observation might support the hypothesis that endorphins may be involved in some schizophrenic symptomatology.

Neurohormonal/Neuroanatomical Correlates of Addictive Drugs. The mesolimbic system of the brain appears to be a neural center responsible for receiving signals that lead to euphoric (pleasant) feelings that can become addictive. When the mesolimbic system is stimulated, certain neurons release dopamine (DA) [34]. This neurotransmitter stimulates postsynaptic neuronal membranes, and a signal is generated that leads to a feeling of euphoria, conditioning an animal to seek out substances causing the sensation again. Cocaine and related addictive drugs block the reuptake of DA at the nerve terminals, thus prolonging its action and enhancing its euphoric effects. Nicotine also works on these same dopaminergic neurons. Nicotine, however, acts by stimulating the release of DA rather than by inhibiting its reuptake. But the effects are the same: a pleasant, euphoric sensation, a pleasurable habit hard to kick [10].

REVIEW EXERCISES

Match the hormone/receptor/cell with its anatomical location:

1. Melanocortin receptor MC1-R
2. α-Melanotropin
3. Melanocortin receptor MC2-R
4. Adrenocorticotropin
5. Chromatophores
6. Melanocortin receptor MC3-R
7. Melanin-concentrating hormone
8. β-Endorphin

A. hypothalamus/limbic system
B. pituitary/hypothalamus
C. pars distalis
D. adrenal cortex
E. melanocytes
F. pars intermedia/arcuate nucleus
G. dermis

Think, analyze and discuss:

1. Early studies demonstrated that the pituitary gland, specifically the intermediate lobe of the pituitary, is the source of a hormone that controls color changes in amphibians. Which experimental strategies may have been adopted to make these original discoveries? Design a set of experiments that might have been used by these early investigators to (a) demonstrate the existence of a melanotropic hormone, (b) specifically localize the source of this hormone to the intermediate lobe, and (c) purify and characterize the molecular structure of the hormone. (Hint: You may wish to first devise a simple in vitro bioassay to monitor melanotropic activity.)

2. Do all vertebrate species possess a pars intermedia? If not, then what is the possible significance of these species differences? Have differing mechanisms evolved in some species to mediate melanotropic activity?

3. In chemical terms, how might one improve upon the biological (clinical) value of a peptide hormone such as α-MSH or dynorphin?

4. Five melanocortins and several opiate peptides are derived from proteolytic processing of the POMC prohormone. To determine the concentrations of each of these peptides in various tissues, would you use radioimmunoassays, bioassays, or radioreceptor assays? Why? Consider the different anatomical locations in which POMC is expressed. What would be the relative concentrations of the different POMC-derived melanotropic and opioid peptides at these different anatomical loci?

5. Using a radioimmunoassay, levels of α-MSH can be measured in the plasma of toads. Would you expect these levels to be higher, lower, or unchanged in toads on a black background as compared to a gray or white background? Why? Draw a hypothetical standard curve for an α-MSH RIA. Where on this standard curve would you expect to find values of the samples from the toads on black and white backgrounds, relative to each other?

6. In recent work, mice have been developed that bear a null mutation in the POMC gene. Can you predict what the physiological consequences of POMC gene deletion might be? Which physiological phenotypes might be evident in these animals?

7. Describe in detail the mechanisms of action of α-MSH and of ACTH. Identify the specific target cells of each of the hormones, and the physiological response that they elicit. If each of these hormones is radiolabeled and used in radioligand receptor binding assays, in which tissues would you expect to find the highest concentration of binding sites for each, respectively? Which receptor subtype would most likely be reflected in each of the two radioligand binding assays?

8. What are the factors affecting secretion of the melanocortins (α-MSH, ACTH)? Do feedback mechanisms operate the control of their secretion? If so, how do they work?

9. There is currently widespread interest in the development of pharmacological agents that might be useful in reducing food intake to treat obesity. Which melanocortin receptor might be a useful target for the development of such a drug? Would an agonist or an antagonist be the likely goal of this research effort?

10. What is the endocrine basis for the pigmentation associated with Addison's disease?

11. Given the gene structure of POMC, how might this gene have evolved? How could you test theories about the evolution of the POMC gene?

12. Suppose you found an albino with a mutation in his or her melanotropin genes, but not in any of the other genes involved in the regulation of melanin synthesis. What might this finding suggest about the hormonal control of skin color?

References

[1] Bagnara, J. T., and M. E. Hadley. 1972. *Chromatophores and color change: Comparative physiology of animal pigmentation.* Englewood Cliffs, NJ: Prentice Hall Publishing.

[2] Bagnara, J. T., J. D. Taylor, and M. E. Hadley. 1968. The dermal chromatophore unit. *J. Cell Biol.* 38:67–79.

[3] Baker, B. I. 1991. Melanin concentrating hormones: A general vertebrate neuropeptide. *Int. Rev. Cytol.* 126:1–47.

[4] Barsch, G. S., et al. 2000. Biochemical and genetic studies of pigment-type switching. *Pigment Cell Res.* 13 (Suppl. 8):48–53.

[5] Branson, R. 2003. Binge eating as a major phenotype of melanocortin 4 receptor gene mutations. *N. Engl. J. Med.* 348:1096–103.

[6] Cooper, A., et al. 2005. Alpha-melanocyte-stimulating hormone suppresses antigen-induced lymphocyte proliferation in humans independently of melanocortin 1 receptor status. *J. Immunol.* 175:4806–13.

[7] Cowley, M. A., et al. 2001. Leptin activates anorexigenic neurons through a neural return in the arcuate nucleus. *Nature* 411:430–4.

[8] Davis, M. D., and M. E. Hadley. 1978. Pars intermedia electrical potentials: changes in spike frequency induced by regulatory factors of melanocyte stimulating hormone (MSH) secretion. *Neuroendocrinology* 26:277–82.

[9] Enami, M. 1955. Melanophore-concentrating hormone (MCH) of possible hypothalamic origin in the catfish *Parasilurus. Science* 121:36–7.

[10] Evans, C. J. 2004. Secrets of the poppy revealed. *Neuropharmacology* 47 (Suppl.):293–9.

[11] Everets, R. E., J. Rothuizen, and B. A. van Oost. 2000. Identification of a premature stop codon in the melanocyte-stimulating hormone receptor gene (MC1R) in Labrador and golden retrievers with yellow coat colour. *Anim. Genet.* 31:194–9.

[12] Fan, W., et al. 2005. Regulation of thermogenesis by the central melanocortin system. *Peptides* 24:1800–13.

[13] Farooqi, I. S., et al. 2003. Clinical spectrum of obesity and mutations in the melanocortin receptor gene. *N. Engl. J. Med.* 348:1085–95.

[14] Gantz, I., and T. M. Fong. 2003. The melanocortin system. *Am. J. Physiol. Endocrinol. Metab.* 284:E468–74.

[15] Gessa, G. L., E. Paglietti, and B. Pelligrini Quarantotti. 1979. Induction of copulatory behavior in sexually inactive rats by naloxone. *Science* 204:203–4.

[16] Hadley, M. E. 1972. The significance of vertebrate integumental pigmentation. *Am. Zool.* 12:63–76.

[17] Hadley, M. E. 2005. Discovery that melanocortin regulates sexual function in male and female humans. *Peptides* 26:1687–9.

[18] Hadley, M. E., and R. T. Dorr. 2006. Melanocortin peptide therapeutics: Historical milestones, clinical studies and commercialization. *Peptides* 27(4):9921–30.

[19] Hadley, M. E., and C. Haskell-Luevano. 1999. The proopiomelanocortin system. *Ann. N. Y. Acad. Sci.* 885:1–21.

[20] Hadley, M. E. (ed.) 1988a. *The melanotropic peptides, Vol. I, Source, synthesis, chemistry, secretion, and metabolism.* Boca Raton, FL: CRC Press.

[21] Hadley, M. E. (ed.). 1988b. *The melanotropic peptides, Vol. II, Biological roles.* Boca Raton, FL: CRC Press.

[22] Hadley, M. E. (ed.). 1988c. *The melanotropic peptides, Vol. III, Mechanisms of action and biomedical applications.* Boca Raton, FL: CRC Press.

[23] Hadley, M. E., et al. 1996. Melanocortin receptors: Identification and characterization by melanotropic peptide agonists and antagonists. *Pigment Cell Res.* 9:213–34.

[24] Haskell-Luevano, C. (ed.). 2005. The melanocortin pathway 2005. *Peptides* 26(10):1971–2036.

[25] Haskell-Luevano, C. (ed.). 2005. The melanocortin pathway 2005. *Peptides* 26(11):2294–301.

[26] Hirobe, T., S. Takeuchi, and E. Hotta. 2004. The melanocortin-1 gene but not the proopiomelanocortin gene is expressed in melanoblasts and contributes to this differentiation in the mouse skin. *Pigment Cell Res.* 17:627–35.

[27] Kennedy, A. R., et al. 2001. Melanin-concentrating hormone (MCH) suppresses thyroid stimulating hormone (TSH) release, in vivo and in vitro, via the hypothalamus and the pituitary. *Endocrinology* 142:3265–8.

[28] Kennedy, A. R., et al. 2003. Effect of direct injection of melanin-concentrating hormone into the paraventricular nucleus: further evidence for a stimulatory role in the adrenal axis via SLC-1. *J. Neuroendocrinol.* 15:268–72.

[29] Krude, H., and A. Gruters. 2000. Implications of proopiomelanocortin (POMC) mutations in humans: the POMC deficiency. *Trends Endocrinol. Metab.* 11:15–22.

[30] Levine, N., et al. 1991. Induction of skin tanning by the subcutaneous administration of a potent synthetic melanotropin. *J. Am. Med. Assoc.* 266:2730–36.

[31] Low, M. J. 2004. Role of proopiomelanocortin neurons and peptides in the regulation of energy homeostasis. *J. Endocrinol. Invest.* 27(6 Suppl.):95–100.

[32] Millhauser, G. L., et al. 2003. Loops and links: structural insights into the remarkable function of the agouti-related protein. *Ann. N. Y. Acad. Sci.* 994:27–35.

[33] Nachman, M. W., H. E. Hoekstra, and S. L. D'Agostino. 2003. The genetic basis of adaptive melanism in pocket mice. *Proc. Natl. Acad. Sci.* 100:5268–73.

[34] Nestler, E. J., and G. H. Aghajanian. 1997. Molecular and cellular basis of addiction. *Science* 278:58–63.

[35] Newton, J. J., et al. 2000. Melanocortin 1 receptor variation in the domestic dog. *Mamm. Genome* 11:24–30.

[36] Okada, Y., Y. Tsuda, S. D. Bryant, and L. H. Lazarus. 2002. Endomorphins and related opioid peptides. *Vitam. Horm.* 65:257–79.

[37] Online Mendelian Inheritance in Man. 2005. Melanocortin 4 receptor; MC4R. Johns Hopkins University.

[38] Pasternak, G. W. 2004. Multiple opiate receptors: déjà vu all over again. *Neuropharmacology* 47 (Suppl):312–23.

[39] Pawelek, J. M., et al. 1992. Molecular cascades in UV-induced melanogenesis: A central role for melanotropins? *Pigment Cell Res.* 5:348–56.

[40] Pechnick, R. N. 1993. Effects of opioids on the hypothalamo-pituitary-adrenal axis. *Annu. Rev. Pharmacol. Toxicol.* 32:353–82.

[41] Pichler, R., et al. 2004. Plasma levels of alpha-melanotropin and ACTH-like immunoreactivities do not vary by season or skin types in women from southern or central Europe. *Neuropeptides* 38:325–30.

[42] Rees, J. L. 2004. The genetics of sun sensitivity in humans. *Am. J. Hum. Genet.* 75:539–51.

[43] Rouzaud, F., et al. 2005. MC1R and the response of melanocytes to ultraviolet radiation. *Mutat. Res.* 571:133–52.

[44] Rust, C. C., and R. K. Meyer. 1969. Hair color, molt, and testis size in male, short-tailed weasels treated with melatonin. *Science* 165:921–2.

[45] Sakamaki, R., et al. 2005. Melanin concentrating hormone enhances sucrose intake. *Int. J. Mol. Med.* 15:1033–9.

[46] Seeley, R. J., D. L. Drazen, and D. J. Clegg. 2004. The critical role of the melanocortin system in the control of energy balance. *Annu. Rev. Nutr.* 24:133–49.

[47] Shi, Y. 2004. Beyond skin color: emerging roles of melanin-concentrating hormone in energy homeostasis and other physiological functions. *Peptides* 10:1605–11.

[48] Shizume, K., A. B. Lerner, and T. B. Fitzpatrick. 1954. In vitro bioassay for the melanocyte stimulating hormone. *Endocrinology* 54:553–60.

[49] Slominski, A., et al. 2004. Melanin pigmentation in mammalian skin and its hormonal regulation. *Physiol. Rev.* 84:1155–228.

[50] Slominski, A., et al. 2005. Preservation of eumelanin hair pigmentation in proopiomelanocortin-deficient mice on a nonagouti (a/a) genetic background. *Endocrinology* 146:1245–53.

[51] Sturm, R. A., R. D. Teasdale, and N. F. Box. 2001. Human pigmentation genes: identification, structure and consequences of polymorphic variation. *Gene* 277:49–62.

[52] Tatro, J. B., and P. S. Sinha. 2003. The central melanocortin system and fever. *Ann. N. Y. Acad. Sci.* 994:246–57.

[53] Theron, E., et al. 2001. The molecular basis for avian plumage polymorphism in the wild. A melanocortin-1-receptor point mutation is perfectly associated with the melanic plumage morph of the bananaquit, *Coereba flaveola. Curr. Biol.* 11:550.

[54] Tsukamura, H., et al. 2000. Intracerebroventricular administration of melanin-concentrating hormone represses pulsatile luteinizing hormone release in the female rat. *J. Neuroendocrinol.* 12:529–34.

[55] Vesley, D. L., and M. E. Hadley. 1979. Ionic requirements for melanophore stimulating hormone (MSH) action on melanophores. *Comp. Biochem. Physiol.* 62A:501–8.

[56] Whitlock, B. K., et al. 2005. Intracerebroventricular melanin-concentrating hormone stimulates food intake in sheep. *Domest. Anim. Endocrinol.* 28:224–32.

[57] Wilson, J. F., and M. A. Morgan. 1979. α-Melanotropin-like substances in the pituitary and plasma of *Xenopus laevis* in relation to colour change responses. *Gen. Comp. Endocrinol.* 38:172–82.

[58] Wollemann, M., and S. Benyhe. 2004. Non-opioid actions of opioid peptides. *Life Sci.* 75:257–70.

Hormonal Control of Calcium Homeostasis

The calcium ion (Ca^{2+}) is a key element in numerous physiological functions. Derived from the diet or from the structural component of bone, this divalent cation is important in bone structure, and it is readily available to serve in a variety of intracellular and extracellular roles. Ca^{2+} is necessary for normal blood clotting, and, with Na^+ and K^+, it aids in maintaining the transmembrane potential of cells and is involved in mechanisms of cell replication. Ca^{2+} may be necessary for the transduction of signal between hormone receptor and second messenger formation and action in some cells. Stimulus-secretion and stimulus-contraction coupling also require the participation of Ca^{2+}.

Three hormones are of prime importance in the control of Ca^{2+} homeostasis, and a number of other hormones also directly or indirectly affect the availability of this cation. **Parathyroid hormone**, or **parathormone (PTH)**, derived from the parathyroid glands, increases circulating levels of Ca^{2+}, whereas **calcitonin (CT)**, derived from the parafollicular cells of the mammalian thyroid, lowers the circulating levels of the ion. A metabolite of vitamin D, **1,25-dihydroxyvitamin D₃**, also increases serum levels of Ca^{2+}. These three hormones interact to maintain normal plasma Ca^{2+} levels. **PTH-related peptide (PTHrP)** is now also implicated in the control of Ca^{2+} homeostasis. Because of the importance of Ca^{2+} to normal bodily function and because of the complex number of interactions between the hormones regulating Ca^{2+} homeostasis, it is not surprising that a large number of endocrinopathies related to Ca^{2+} homeostasis and bone mineral metabolism have been described.

Calcium and Bone Physiology

Cytosolic and extracellular fluid concentrations of Ca^{2+} must be maintained within narrow limits despite the wide fluctuations in Ca^{2+} intake. In humans, the Ca^{2+} level of plasma is maintained at about 10 mg/100 ml. Ca^{2+} derived from the diet is delivered to the blood after being actively transported across the intestinal mucosa. Urinary Ca^{2+} loss is partially prevented by active transport of the cation back across the renal tubular epithelium. Bone serves as the immediate source of Ca^{2+} to maintain serum Ca^{2+} homeostasis. Half of the Ca^{2+} present in blood is in the free ionized form and half is bound to albumin. The free ionized form of Ca^{2+} is readily available and important in physiological processes. Three factors can alter the distribution of Ca^{2+} in plasma: albumin concentration, acid–base disturbances, and protein abnormalities. Calcium metabolism consists of relationships between a large skeletal pool, a smaller soft tissue pool, and a much smaller extracellular fluid pool, modified by input from intestinal absorption and loss via renal and fecal excretion. The placenta and the mammary glands represent other routes of Ca^{2+} loss.

To understand the actions of hormones on skeletal formation and resorption, it is necessary to review the cellular processes involved in the mineralization and demineralization of bone. Bone is covered by the periosteum, which consists of connective tissue fibers. A layer of *osteoblasts* within the deeper layer of the fibrous periosteum synthesizes and releases molecules of collagen. The individual collagen molecules become oriented in a specific molecular architecture to form an extracellular matrix around the osteoblasts. Calcium and phosphate ions are stereochemically bound to specific sites on the collagen matrix where they are precipitated as $Ca_{10}(PO_4)_6(OH)_2$, hydroxyapatite. Precipitation of calcium phosphate depends on the product of the concentrations of Ca^{2+} and PO_4^{-3}. Whenever the concentration of $[Ca^{2+}] \times [PO_4^{-3}]$ exceeds the solubility product at the local site of ossification, calcium phosphate precipitates. Precipitation of bone mineral may be enhanced under conditions of local alkalinization resulting from osteoblastic activity. After calcification of the collagen matrix, the embedded cells are referred to as *osteocytes*. Demineralization of bone is effected by large multinucleate cells, *osteoclasts*, which release acid phosphatase and hyaluronic acid. Local decreases in pH caused by the osteoclasts favor the solubilization of hydroxyapatite with the resulting release of Ca^{2+} and PO_4^{-3} from the collagen matrix.

Bone remodeling is the process by which the catabolic effects (bone resorption) of one cell type of bone, osteoclasts, are balanced by the anabolic effects (bone formation) of a second cell type, osteoblasts. Normal bone remodeling proceeds in a highly regulated cycle in which osteoclasts adhere to bone and subsequently remove it by acidification and proteolytic digestion. Once osteoclasts leave the removal site, osteoblasts enter and secrete osteoid (a matrix of collagen and other proteins), which is then calcified into new bone. Osteoclast-mediated resorption is influenced by two processes: activation, in which the resorptive function of mature osteoclasts is increased, and recruitment, in which osteoclast progenitors are stimulated to yield more mature cells [18].

The processes of bone formation and bone resorption are largely balanced to maintain bone mass. In certain physiological and pathophysiological circumstances, the actions of certain hormones, as discussed in this chapter, can produce an imbalance in bone formation and bone resorption, producing a net change in bone mass. Mechanical strain on bone can also influence bone mass, by mechanisms that have yet to be elucidated. Thus, a loss of bone mineral density occurs under conditions of low mechanical strain, such as in astronauts who experience prolonged weightlessness, or in paralyzed subjects. Weight-bearing exercise, on the other hand, has been shown to reduce the rate of bone loss in osteoporotic individuals.

Bone serves as a reservoir for the rapid uptake and release of Ca^{2+} during daily plasma Ca^{2+} fluctuations. A layer of osteoblasts is separated from the underlying layers of osteocytes by a *bone fluid compartment*, a so-called bone-lining cell/osteocyte unit. Calcium stored in the bone fluid compartment is present in a labile, metastable form, which is kept from being transferred to hydroxyapatite crystals.

Parathormone

Historically, parathormone (PTH) was the first of the trio of calcitropic hormones controlling Ca^{2+} homeostasis to be discovered. Because Ca^{2+} is essential in cellular function, PTH is necessary for life. Although other hormones may be required for normal body function, with the exception of aldosterone (Chap. 15), they are not essential for survival.

The "Chief Cells" of the Parathyroid Glands Secrete Parathormone

Parathormone is derived from the parathyroids, which in most mammals are embedded on the surface of the thyroid gland. In humans four parathyroid glands are present; they are located on the back side of the thyroid gland, one near each pole of the two lobes of the gland (Fig. 9.1). The parathyroid glands are derived from the third and fourth pharyngeal pouches, the two superior glands from the fourth, and the two inferior glands from the third. Removal of the thyroid gland usually leads to death in animals; it was subsequently discovered, however, that the lethal effects of thyroidectomy could be duplicated solely by removal of the parathyroids, rather than the thyroid itself. In mammals other than humans, there may be one or two pairs of parathyroids that may or may not be associated with thyroid tissue. The parathyroids are composed of two cell types, the *chief* cells, which are the source of PTH, and the *oxyphil* cells, of unknown function. The chief cells

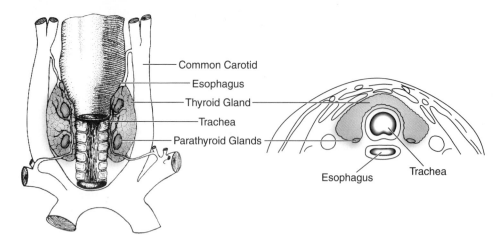

Figure 9.1 Posterior (left) and transverse (right) views of the human thyroid with attached parathyroids.

are most numerous and in some mammals may be the only cells present. Oxyphil cells in humans appear around puberty and increase in number with age; they contain many mitochondria and an eosinophilic granular cytoplasm.

Removal of the parathyroids results in a drop in plasma Ca^{2+} levels, which usually results in tetanic convulsions and death. In 1925, Collip isolated a biologically active fraction from bovine parathyroid glands that could restore Ca^{2+} levels in parathyroidectomized dogs. This active substance of the parathyroid glands was appropriately named parathyroid hormone, or, as it is more commonly known, parathormone (PTH).

Synthesis, Chemistry, and Metabolism of PTH. Parathormone, a polypeptide 84 amino acids long, is derived from a precursor molecule of 115 amino acid residues. This so-called preproparathyroid hormone (PreProPTH) then undergoes proteolytic cleavages to yield a proPTH of 90 amino acids, from which six residues are then removed to yield the definitive hormonal product. In an in vitro translation system (for the production of protein from messenger RNA), PreProPTH has been biosynthesized and shown to be converted to PTH in the Golgi zone of the chief cells by a trypsin-like protease. The hormone is then packaged into secretory vesicles that migrate to the periphery of the cell where the hormone is secreted by a mechanism of vesicular exocytosis. The primary structures of human PTH, as well as those of the pig, cow, and other mammals, have been determined (Fig. 9.2).

Control of PTH Secretion. The release of PTH from the parathyroid glands is controlled by circulating levels of Ca^{2+}. Parathyroid cells possess recognition sites (receptors) for Ca^{2+}, as incubation of parathyroid slices in a low concentration of Ca^{2+} increases PTH release, and high concentrations of the cation decrease PTH release. The molecular mechanisms of extracellular Ca^{2+} sensing by PTH-secreting cells has been elegantly demonstrated by Brown and his colleagues [6, 9, 16, 25, 31]. They cloned and characterized an extracellular Ca^{2+}-sensing receptor from bovine parathyroid cells. The cloned cDNA encodes a typical seven-spanning membrane G-protein-coupled receptor (Chap. 3).

Figure 9.2 Comparative structures of parathormone.

The human parathyroid cell Ca^{2+} receptor is composed of 1,018 amino acids with a 93% sequence similarity to the bovine receptor. The very large extracellular domain contains a number of acidic amino acid residues that are likely Ca^{2+}-binding sites. A simplified model of the regulation of parathyroid cell PTH secretion is as follows: Elevated extracellular Ca^{2+} would interact with the acidic residues of the extracellular domain of the seven-spanning membrane receptor. Binding of Ca^{2+} to the receptor results in a conformational change in the receptor such that coupling to the G protein results in lowered cAMP levels and decreased PTH secretion. Below normal levels of Ca^{2+} would result in diminished binding of the cation to receptor binding sites, and under this state of receptor conformation there would be an increased intracellular production of cAMP leading to enhanced PTH secretion (see Fig. 9.13).

Theophylline stimulates PTH release as does $(Bu)_2$ cAMP, demonstrating that cAMP is involved in the mechanism of PTH release. As discussed later, vitamin D is inhibitory to PTH secretion; its action is on PTH gene expression since short-term incubations with the hormone have no effect on PTH release [46].

Parathormone Acts to Raise Plasma Ca^{2+} Levels

Parathormone acts on a number of tissues, in most cases elevating, directly or indirectly, plasma levels of Ca^{2+} and decreasing circulating concentrations of PO_4^{-3}. Parathormone receptors are particularly abundant in kidney, gut, and bone, indicating sites of obvious importance in Ca^{2+} homeostasis. The distribution of these receptors to a multitude of other tissues suggest others as yet to be defined roles of the hormone.

Bone Mineral Metabolism. A major target tissue of PTH is bone, specifically stromal osteoblast cells of the bone marrow [23]. In response to PTH, these cells secrete one or more cytokines (growth regulatory factors) that then stimulate osteoclastic activity leading to the resorption of bone. In this way, demineralization of bone results in elevated levels of Ca^{2+}. More specific details of PTH action on bone will be discussed later (see Fig. 9.12).

Renal Reabsorption of Calcium. A major physiological role of PTH is to increase renal tubular reabsorption of Ca^{2+}. Parathyroidectomy, for example, leads to calciuria, which can be corrected immediately by injections of PTH.

Renal Excretion of Phosphate. Parathyroidectomy leads to a decrease in urinary phosphate levels and elevated serum PO_4^{-3} levels (phosphatemia). Injections of PTH, on the other hand, cause a rapid increase in urinary PO_4^{-3} concentration (phosphaturia). Increased renal excretion of PO_4^{-3}, in response to PTH (phosphaturic action of PTH), enhances the ionization of plasma Ca^{2+} through a lowering of the $[Ca^{2+}] \times [PO_4^{-3}]$ solubility product. Other renal effects of PTH include enhanced Mg^{2+} reabsorption and inhibition of exchange of hydrogen ions for Na^+ ions by the tubules. The resulting metabolic acidosis favors removal of Ca^{2+} from plasma proteins and bone, thereby increasing circulating levels of Ca^{2+}.

Intestinal Absorption of Calcium. Parathormone enhances intestinal uptake of Ca^{2+}, but this action may be mediated indirectly through its effect on vitamin D metabolism.

Control of Vitamin D Synthesis. A major role of PTH in Ca^{2+} homeostasis is to stimulate the biosynthesis of 1,25-dihydroxyvitamin D_3 from vitamin D precursors by the kidney. Thus, some of the actions of PTH are mediated indirectly through the action of this steroid hormone.

Other Possible Actions of PTH. Parathormone increases the mitotic rate of red cell progenitors (reticulocytes) and thymic lymphocytes. Mitotic activity is also increased in regenerating rat liver following partial hepatectomy in response to PTH. The physiological significance, if any, of these observations on the mitogenic actions of PTH is unknown. PTH and related fragments produce vasodilation in coronary and other vascular beds in the dog. The blood-pressure lowering effect of bPTH is not blocked by α- or β-adrenergic, cholinergic, or histaminergic blocking agents, thus suggesting direct effects of the peptide on vascular smooth muscle receptors. This vasodepressor response has been demonstrated in a variety of species.

Parathormone-Related Peptide (PTHrP)

PTH-related peptide (PTHrP) originally was isolated from human tumor cells or tissues obtained from patients with humoral hypercalcemia of malignancy. PTHrP consists of 139–173 residues, depending upon the species [7]. Both the PTH-like and the non-PTH-like regions of the peptide are highly conserved across species. PTHrP shows a high degree of N-terminal homology with PTH (Fig. 9.3) and appears to interact with the same receptor as PTH in renal and osseous tissues, thereby accounting for its hypercalcemic activity in certain cancer patients (due to tumor secretion of PTHrP). Unique biological actions also have been attributed to peptide sequences in the midportion and C-terminal region of the molecule. Unlike PTH, PTHrP and its mRNA have been detected in a wide variety of normal tissues, prompting considerable interest in potential physiological roles for the peptide. Although no physiological roles have been established unequivocally, the widespread expression of the PTHrP gene and its organizational similarity to that of certain growth factor genes have led to the suggestion that PTHrP may play a paracrine or autocrine role in growth and development. Both developmental and Ca^{2+} regulatory roles have been suggested in the developing fetus [20, 39].

The lactating rat mammary gland contains high levels of PTHrP mRNA that decrease rapidly when suckling is interrupted by removal of pups and reappear within 2 hours of the resumption of suckling or prolactin (PRL) injection. In addition, large quantities of PTHrP or fragments of PTHrP have been found in the milk of a number of species and in the blood of suckling calves. Other recent studies have indicated that mammary gland derived PTHrP may reach the maternal circulation and influence Ca^{2+} homeostasis in the mother. PTHrP might play some role in development of the lactating breast, milk Ca^{2+} transport, maternal or fetal Ca^{2+} homeostasis, or neonatal gut function. PTHrP modulates the delivery of milk to the nipple during suckling, and myoepithelial cell-derived PTHrP could contribute to the large pool of PTHrP found in milk. Alternatively, myoepithelial cell-derived PTHrP could act on neighboring secretory epithelial cells in a paracrine fashion to alter growth and differentiation, or to affect milk formation [39].

The elevated levels of fetal serum Ca^{2+} may be due to PTHrP of fetal parathyroid origin. PTHrP may be expressed by fetal tissue during pregnancy to maintain the Ca^{2+} gradient across the placenta, which is required for normal skeletal development. In studies with sheep, thyroparathyroidectomy of fetuses *in utero* results in substantial fetal hypocalcemia. However, serum Ca^{2+} levels return to normal on infusion of a partially purified preparation obtained from cell culture medium containing PTHrP. Parathormone infusion is ineffective, suggesting a unique role for PTHrP in fetal physiology [22].

Figure 9.3 Aligned sequences of the 1–34 region of PTH and PTHrP from various species. Conserved residues are outlined in black. Note the lack of substantial sequence identity between PTH and PTHrP from amino acid residue 14 through the C terminus. (From Cohen et al., *Journal of Biological Chemistry* 266:1997–2004, 1991.)

Calcitonin

Although Ca^{2+} is directly inhibitory to PTH release from the parathyroids, this is not the only means of protecting an animal against the elevated Ca^{2+} levels that occur, for example, after a meal. If plasma Ca^{2+} levels are elevated by injecting Ca^{2+} salts, Ca^{2+} concentrations rapidly return to normal. Infusion of a Ca^{2+} chelator, on the other hand, effectively lowers Ca^{2+} levels, which soon return to normal after cessation of the infusion. It was discovered, however, that depressed or elevated Ca^{2+} levels fail to return to normal in thyroidectomized animals. This failure could be partly explained by the absence of PTH, due to the removal of the parathyroids along with the thyroid glands. The solution, however, was not so simple. It was concluded that the thyroid might also produce a hormone whose role is to lower Ca^{2+} levels under conditions where the cation is elevated. Although this hypocalcemic factor, referred to as calcitonin (CT), was initially believed to be derived from the parathyroids, other experimental evidence pointed toward the thyroid [24].

The Parafollicular Cells of the Thyroid Secrete Calcitonin

The thyroid gland is mainly composed of follicular cells (see Fig. 13.2), which synthesize and store thyroid hormones (Chap. 13). Another cell nestled among the follicular cells of the thyroid is referred to as a C (clear) cell. Immunohistochemical staining techniques reveal that these C cells synthesize and secrete CT. In mammals, including humans, these cells are derived from the ultimobranchial bodies that develop from the most posterior branchial pouch. Cells of the neural crest migrate to the posterior branchial pouch to form the *ultimobranchial glands* early in development. In nonmammalian vertebrates (cartilaginous and bony fishes, amphibians, reptiles, birds) the ultimobranchial glands persist and are the source of CT in the adult animal. In the human fetus the appearance of functional activity of parafollicular cells at the onset of skeletal calcification suggests a role for CT in fetal bone growth.

Synthesis, Chemistry, and Metabolism. Calcitonin was purified in 1967 and its amino acid sequence determined in 1968 [10]. Human CT (Fig. 9.4) was isolated from medullary carcinoma (composed of C cells) of the thyroid and found to be structurally similar to circulating CT. The primary sequences of CT from a number of species are structurally similar (Fig. 9.5). All contain 32 residues, have a 1–7 intrachain disulfide ring, and have a prolinamide carboxy-terminal group. As are many peptide hormones, CT is derived from a larger precursor molecule. Analysis of CT from four separate species of salmon reveals that each species produces two forms of the molecule, a salmon I plus a salmon II or salmon III variant of the molecule. These molecular varieties of CT represent *isohormonal* forms of the hormone; that is, the primary structure of these forms varies slightly from one molecule to another. Human and salmon CT share only 16 of 32 amino acids in common. Surprisingly, eel and salmon CT are more potent in mammalian species (particularly well tested in humans) than are the corresponding human and other mammalian calcitonins. This potency may be due to resistance of the peptides to degradation and may also have to do with greater receptor affinity [34].

A second peptide also related to CT has been discovered. This *calcitonin gene-related peptide* (CGRP) is mainly found in the nervous system. The homology between CGRP and CT reflects their common evolutionary origin. Human CGRP shares a greater structural homology with salmon than with human CT. Both peptides are derived from the CT/CGRP gene. Alternate splicing of the primary RNA transcript leads to the translation of CT and CGRP peptides in a tissue-specific manner [47]. Human CT and CGRP exert their actions on separate receptors that are distributed differently throughout the body.

Control of Secretion. Perfusion of hypercalcemic blood through the thyroid is a stimulus to CT secretion, and incubation of thyroid tissue in a hypercalcemic medium also results in secretion of the hormone. Is there evidence that elevated levels of Ca^{2+} are also a stimulus to CT secretion in humans? Changes in plasma Ca^{2+} (caused by oral ingestion of Ca^{2+})

```
  ┌S──────────S┐
Cys-Gly-Asn-Leu-Ser-Thr-Cys-Met-Leu-Gly-Thr-Tyr-Thr-Gln-Asp-Phe-Asn-
  1   2   3   4   5   6   7   8   9  10  11  12  13  14  15  16  17

Lys-Phe-His-Thr-Phe-Pro-Gln-Thr-Ala-Ile-Gly-Val-Gly-Ala-Pro-NH2
 18  19  20  21  22  23  24  25  26  27  28  29  30  31  32
```

Figure 9.4 Primary structure of human calcitonin.

	1	2	3	4	5	6	7	8	9	10	11	12	13	14	15	16
Human	Cys	Gly	Asn	Leu	Ser	Thr	Cys	Met	Leu	Gly	Thr	Tyr	Thr	Gln	Asp	Phe
Salmon	Cys	Ser	Asn	Leu	Ser	Thr	Cys	Val	Leu	Gly	Lys	Leu	Ser	Gln	Glu	Leu
Ovine	Cys	Ser	Asn	Leu	Ser	Thr	Cys	Val	Leu	Ser	Ala	Tyr	Trp	Lys	Asp	Leu
Bovine	Cys	Ser	Asn	Leu	Ser	Thr	Cys	Val	Leu	Ser	Ala	Tyr	Trp	Lys	Asp	Leu
Porcine	Cys	Ser	Asn	Leu	Ser	Thr	Cys	Val	Leu	Ser	Ala	Tyr	Trp	Arg	Asn	Leu

	17	18	19	20	21	22	23	24	25	26	27	28	29	30	31	32	
	Asn	Lys	Phe	His	Thr	Phe	Pro	Gln	Thr	Ala	Ile	Gly	Val	Gly	Ala	Pro	NH$_2$
	His	Lys	Leu	Gln	Thr	Tyr	Pro	Arg	Thr	Asn	Thr	Gly	Ser	Gly	Thr	Pro	NH$_2$
	Asn	Asn	Tyr	His	Arg	Tyr	Ser	Gly	Met	Gly	Phe	Gly	Pro	Glu	Thr	Pro	NH$_2$
	Asn	Asn	Tyr	His	Arg	Phe	Ser	Gly	Met	Gly	Phe	Gly	Pro	Glu	Thr	Pro	NH$_2$
	Asn	Asn	Phe	His	Arg	Phe	Ser	Gly	Met	Gly	Phe	Gly	Pro	Glu	Thr	Pro	NH$_2$

Figure 9.5 Comparative structures of some calcitonins. Three molecular species (isoforms) of salmon CT exist; the structure of salmon I calcitonin is shown, which differs from eel CT at only three residues (eel: 26, Asp; 27, Val; 29, Ala).

within the physiological range are indeed associated with parallel changes in circulating levels of CT in humans. The increase in CT release in response to Ca^{2+} infusion is greater in males than in females, and the basal levels of CT and the response to Ca^{2+} wane with age in both sexes. Animal studies indicate that estrogens and androgens enhance CT secretion, and the progressive decreases in gonadal function may therefore contribute to the age- and sex-related decline in CT secretion in humans [4].

If a very small amount of Ca^{2+} is delivered to the stomach (of the pig) so as not to produce a detectable hypercalcemia, plasma CT still increases severalfold. It was hypothesized that some gastrointestinal factor in addition to Ca^{2+} might be a CT secretogogue. Gastrin is a potent stimulator of CT secretion, and analogs of gastrin (Chap. 10) exhibit a potency profile similar to their effectiveness in stimulating gastric acid secretion. Cholecystokinin is also effective, due most likely to its partial structural similarity to gastrin. Physiological stimuli that increase gastrin levels in the blood cause a parallel increase in CT secretion. In some patients with Zollinger–Ellison syndrome (hypergastrinemia), there is an elevation in circulating CT.

Like parathyroid cells, C cells express an identical Ca^{2+}-sensing receptor whose function is to regulate CT secretion in response to extracellular Ca^{2+} levels [36]. In contrast to parathyroid cells, however, they show stimulation rather than inhibition of secretion in response to increases in extracellular Ca^{2+}.

Because it is composed almost entirely of CT-secreting cells, the ultimobranchial gland of nonmammalian vertebrates is a rich source of CT. Isolated cells from the fish ultimobranchial gland have been used in vitro for studies on CT secretion. Secretin, glucagon, and pentagastrin are stimulatory to CT secretion and, in combination, secretin and pentagastrin or secretin and glucagon have a synergistic effect on CT secretion from isolated teleost ultimobranchial cells. cAMP is the second messenger controlling CT secretion.

Calcitonin Acts to Lower Plasma Ca^{2+} Levels

Bone Mineral Metabolism.   Because CT is released from the parafollicular cells in direct relation to the circulating level of Ca^{2+}, it has been suggested that CT functions in the prevention of hypercalcemia. In particular, CT may prevent the postprandial hypercalcemia that results from the absorption of Ca^{2+} from foods during a meal. Calcitonin might also promote mineralization of skeletal bone via Ca^{2+} absorbed from milk in preweanling animals. In addition, CT may protect against Ca^{2+} loss from the skeleton during such periods of Ca^{2+} stress as pregnancy, lactation, and prolonged Ca^{2+} deprivation.

The CT secreted in response to food entering the digestive tract causes the movement of serum Ca^{2+} into the bone mineral compartment. This labile Ca^{2+} then returns to the extracellular compartment as postprandial plasma Ca^{2+} levels decline. By this process Ca^{2+} levels are maintained during periods of fasting. The return of Ca^{2+} to the extracellular fluid would be inhibitory to PTH release, and this might be an effective safeguard against bone resorptive activity during fasting. High circulating levels of CT have been observed during gestation and lactation. At least in ruminants (goats and ewes), CT may protect the maternal skeleton against excessive demineralization.

Calcitonin as a Satiety Hormone. Subcutaneous injections of CT inhibit the 24-hour food intake of rats and rhesus monkeys. Intracerebroventricular injections of CT in the rat are also inhibitory to feeding. In humans, significant reduction in body weight is observed 24 to 36 hours following a single subcutaneous injection of CT. These results suggest that CT may have a physiologically relevant action on the central nervous system. It is speculated that CT is involved in the regulation of feeding and appetite, possibly under specialized circumstances such as infancy, lactation, or Ca^{2+}-specific hunger.

Vitamin D Regulation. Calcitonin directly stimulates vitamin D metabolism and indirectly stimulates it by lowering plasma Ca^{2+} levels, resulting in the release of PTH, which activates renal vitamin D synthesis and secretion.

Vitamin D

Historically, vitamin D is the name applied to two fat-soluble substances, cholecalciferol and ergocalciferol, that possess the common ability to prevent or cure rickets [28]. Rickets (osteomalacia in adults) develops from a failure of the bones to ossify properly in the child, and it was originally believed that the disease was due to a lack of sunshine or to some dietary factor. There is some truth in both these early theories. Vitamins are defined as organic dietary constituents necessary for life and development, but that do not act as dietary energy sources. In that respect, it has been argued that the term vitamin D is a misnomer because normally the active hormonal form of vitamin D is produced within the body from dietary substrates or endogenous substances [22]. It is now accepted that vitamin D is not a vitamin but rather a precursor of one or more steroid-like hormones produced by specific tissues within the body. These vitamin D metabolites mediate their actions on a number of target tissues, and in the absence of the hormones, bones fail to mineralize.

Vitamin D is Produced by a Pathway that Involves the Skin, Liver, and Kidneys

In 1924, it was discovered that, in animals, prior irradiation of certain dietary foodstuffs was as effective in curing rickets as direct irradiation of the animal itself. Vitamin D_3 (cholecalciferol) is actually produced in the skin of humans by the action of ultraviolet light on a precursor molecule, 7-dehydrocholesterol (an intermediate in the biosynthesis of cholesterol). Actually, 7-dehydrocholesterol is first converted to a so-called previtamin D_3, which subsequently equilibrates in the skin to form cholecalciferol through a temperature-dependent thermal isomerization (Fig. 9.6). From the skin, cholecalciferol is transported by a binding protein

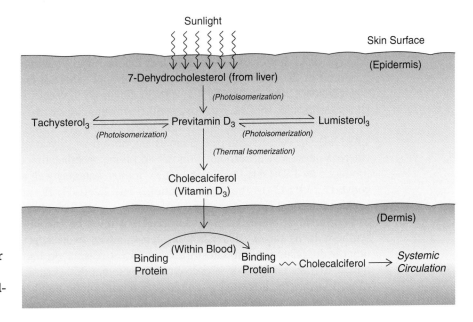

Figure 9.6 Photic stimulation of integumental cholecalciferol (vitamin D_3) formation and subsequent transfer to the general circulation by a cholecalciferol-binding protein.

Figure 9.7 Production of ergosterol and ergocalciferol from their precursors.

(transcalciferin) present in the general circulation. Under continuous exposure to the sun, previtamin D_3 also photoisomerizes to lumisterol and tachysterol, which are biologically inert. Because transcalciferin has no strong affinity for these isomers, they are not translocated into the circulation but instead remain in the skin. Within the skin, these photoisomers are in a quasi-stationary state and may serve as reserve substrates for photoconversion back to previtamin D_3 when the latter substance is converted to vitamin D_3 [17].

Rickets, a vitamin D deficiency disease, may therefore develop if the skin does not receive adequate irradiation. The disease is now a rarity in most countries because irradiated foods provide an adequate supply of the vitamin. Ergosterol is a provitamin for vitamin D_2 (ergocalciferol), and both differ from cholecalciferol and vitamin D_3, respectively, because they possess a double bond between C22 and C23 and a methyl group at the C24 position (Figs 9.7 and 9.8). Vitamin D_2 is the antirachitic principle of irradiated foodstuffs. Although vitamin D_3 is the normal physiologically relevant antirachitic substrate, vitamin D_2 is equally effective as vitamin D_3 in some species, including humans.

Actually, cholecalciferol is without biological activity at physiological concentrations. Cholecalciferol must first be converted to 25-hydroxyvitamin D_3 (25-OH-D_3, 25-hydroxycholecalciferol) in the liver (Fig. 9.8). The liver appears to be the major site of 25-hydroxylation in mammals. In the chicken, however, the 25-hydroxylase enzyme exists in extrahepatic sites such as the intestine and kidney. Although this steroid is the major circulating metabolite of cholecalciferol, it must undergo one other chemical modification before it can function as a hormone. The 25-OH-D_3 produced in the liver then circulates to the kidney where it is converted by a mitochondrial 1α-hydroxylase to $1\alpha,25(OH)_2D_3$ ($1\alpha,25$-dihydroxycholecalciferol), the hormonal form of cholecalciferol [5, 16]. The exclusive synthesis in the kidney of $1,25(OH)_2D_3$ was demonstrated by the failure of nephrectomized rats given radioactive 25-OH-D_3 to produce radiolabeled $1,25(OH)_2D_3$. Nephrectomized animals do not show physiological responses to 25-OH-D_3, whereas physiological responses on gut and bone, whether the kidneys are present or not, are produced by $1,25(OH)_2D_3$. Chick kidney homogenates, as well as isolated renal mitochondria, convert 25-OH-D_3 to the active hormone. The $1,25(OH)_2D_3$ product was originally detected in chick intestinal chromatin, one of its now recognized sites of action. $1,25(OH)_2D_3$ functions as a hormone in the classical sense because it must be carried by the blood from its site of synthesis to its target cells. Cholecalciferol and its hydroxylated metabolite, 25-OH-D_3, and other hydroxylated metabolites are bound to a plasma protein, originally referred to in the human as transcalciferin or calciferol-binding protein. Although $1,25(OH)_2D_3$ is the active antirachitic principle, the literature often refers to this hormone simply as vitamin D, or, more recently, as calcitriol.

Figure 9.8   Sequential steps in the biosynthesis of vitamin D.

Another enzyme present in kidney mitochondria and possibly other extrarenal sites, 25-hydroxyvitamin D_3-24 hydroxylase, produces $24,25(OH)_2D_3$ (Fig. 9.8), which is inactive biologically in mammals. A trihydroxylated derivative of vitamin D_3, 1,24,25-trihydroxyvitamin D_3 ($1,24,25(OH)_3D_3$), has also been isolated from the plasma, but it too is biologically inactive (Fig. 9.8). 25,26-Dihydroxyvitamin D_3 has also been isolated from the blood of humans and some animals receiving pharmacological doses of cholecalciferol. The origin and possible significance of this metabolite are unknown, and the physiological importance, if any, of the other cholecalciferol metabolites is also unclear. Pregnant anephric female rats synthesize $1,25(OH)_2D_3$, and conversion of 25-OH-D_3 to $1,25(OH)_2D_3$ apparently takes place in the fetal placental unit of the rat. The physiological significance, if any, of the placental synthesis of $1,25(OH)_3D_3$ is unknown.

Regulation of Vitamin D Metabolism.   If a kidney 1α-hydroxylase is the key enzyme in $1,25(OH)_2D_3$ biosynthesis, it might be expected to be tightly regulated by endocrine or other factors under conditions of hypocalcemia. Indeed, the production of $1,25(OH)_2D_3$ is markedly stimulated in animals on low Ca^{2+} diets and is suppressed in animals given high

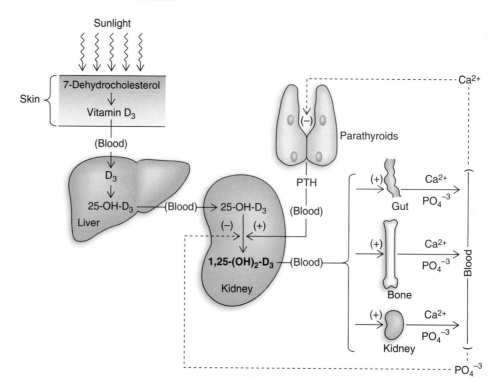

Figure 9.9   Feedback control of vitamin D biosynthesis.

Ca^{2+} diets. Thus, there is a strict inverse relationship between the serum Ca^{2+} level and the ability of animals to produce $1,25(OH)_2D_3$. Conversely, whenever $1,25(OH)_2D_3$ synthesis is suppressed, $24,25(OH)_2D_3$ synthesis is stimulated. There is no evidence, however, that hepatic 25-OHase activity is regulated by a feedback control mechanism. Removal of the parathyroid glands eliminates the hypocalcemic stimulation of $1,25(OH)_2D_3$ production, and $24,25(OH)_2D_3$ is produced. Conversely, PTH restores the ability of hypocalcemic animals to make $1,25(OH)_2D_3$ and suppresses the production of $24,25(OH)_2D_3$. In vitamin D deficient animals there is an increase in renal 1α-OHase activity, whereas administration of vitamin D causes a dramatic disappearance of this enzyme. A direct effect of PTH on renal tubular production of $1,25(OH)_2D_3$ has been demonstrated. Suppression of renal 1α-OHase activity is correlated with increased 24-OHase activity. PTH alters 25-OH-D_3 metabolism through a cAMP-mediated mechanism. The metabolic tendency of the kidney to produce primarily $1,25(OH)_2D_3$ or $24,25(OH)_2D_3$ is subject to dynamic modulation by the opposing effects of $1,25(OH)_2D_3$ and PTH either directly or indirectly.

The feedback mechanism regulating $1,25(OH)_2D_3$ production can be summarized as follows (see also Fig. 9.9): Hypocalcemia is stimulatory to PTH secretion from the parathyroids; PTH stimulates renal cortical 1α-OHase activity and $1,25(OH)_2D_3$ biosynthesis; $1,25(OH)_2D_3$ then stimulates Ca^{2+} absorption from the gut, increases release of Ca^{2+} from the bone, and stimulates Ca^{2+} reabsorption from the kidney. The increasing levels of Ca^{2+} then feed back to inhibit further synthesis of PTH. In the absence of further stimulation of 1α-OHase production, 24-OHase activity is increased and any available $25-(OH)_2D_3$ is converted to the inactive metabolite, $24,25(OH)_2D_3$ (Fig. 9.8). Parathyroid gland cells possess $1,25(OH)_2D_3$ receptors, and there is evidence that $1,25(OH)_2D_3$ may exert a negative feedback on this gland to inhibit PTH production.

Besides its effect on renal $1,25(OH)_2D_3$ production, PTH stimulates renal excretion of phosphate. Low plasma levels of PO_4^{-3} are directly stimulatory to renal 1α-OHase activity and $1,25(OH)_2D_3$ production, whereas elevated levels of PO_4^{-3} are inhibitory to production of the hormone. Thyroparathyroidectomized rats maintained on a low phosphate, high Ca^{2+} diet also synthesize $1,25(OH)_2D_3$ from 25-OH-D_3. The plasma concentration of PO_4^{-3} may therefore be an important local regulator of renal $1,25(OH)_2D_3$ biosynthesis. Although the synthesis of $1,25(OH)_2D_3$ can be stimulated directly by low plasma PO_4^{-3} concentration, this hypophosphatemia does not stimulate PTH secretion. Without stimulation by PTH, resorption of Ca^{2+} from bone, renal reabsorption of Ca^{2+}, and renal excretion of PO_4^{-3} is minimal. The net change is predominantly an increase in plasma PO_4^{-3} concentration.

Vitamin D Promotes Ca^{2+} Absorption in the Gut and Ca^{2+} Reabsorption in the Kidney

Intestine. Ca^{2+} absorption from the intestine is the best-documented action of vitamin D. The hormone also causes translocation of PO_4^{-3} across the gut epithelium. Both processes require metabolic energy and are therefore active transport processes. 1,25 $(OH)_2D_3$ stimulates transepithelial Ca^{2+} transport in the intestine by stimulating: Ca^{2+} entry, Ca^{2+} buffering by fixed cellular sites, and Ca^{2+} extrusion at the basolateral pole of the cell. Each of these steps is important, but the major effect of 1,25$(OH)_2D_3$ is to facilitate intracellular diffusion from mucosa to serosa via a cytosolic Ca^{2+}-binding protein.

Bone.   In the absence of sunlight or a dietary source of vitamin D precursors, rickets (bone demineralization) develops. Although vitamin D is necessary for proper bone growth, it seems a paradox that vitamin D also causes demineralization to provide Ca^{2+}, and possibly PO_4^{-3}, to maintain the critical plasma levels of these ions. The demineralization process may, however, be necessary to provide Ca^{2+} and PO_4^{-3} for accretion of new bone.

Kidney.   There is evidence to suggest that 1,25$(OH)_2D_3$ stimulates tubular reabsorption of Ca^{2+} in the kidney. In addition, data support a direct role of the hormone on proximal tubular retention of PO_4^{-3}. Because PTH causes phosphaturia and 1,25$(OH)_2D_3$ production, feedback inhibition of parathyroid PTH release by the steroid might favor PO_4^{-3} retention. A specific 1,25$(OH)_2D_3$ receptor has been isolated from rat kidney cytosol. A renal Ca^{2+}-binding protein has also been demonstrated and may facilitate tubular uptake of Ca^{2+} by the kidney, as it does in the intestine.

Other Putative Roles.   A number of tissues possess specific 1,25$(OH)_2D_3$ receptors: skin, mammary gland, placenta, avian shell gland, and such peptide-secreting endocrine tissues as the parathyroids, pituitary, pancreas, and even the brain. The parathyroid glands might be expected to represent a site for 1,25$(OH)_2D_3$ feedback inhibition of parathormone secretion. Elevated serum levels of 1,25$(OH)_2D_3$ are known to lead to a decrease in the release of PTH through two different mechanisms. A long feedback loop is established by means of increased serum concentrations of Ca^{2+}, which represent an inhibitory signal for the secretion and production of PTH. In a short feedback loop, 1,25$(OH)_2D_3$ directly inhibits the synthesis of PTH through an interaction with the preproparathyroid hormone gene [46]. There is evidence that insulin is required for optimal 1,25$(OH)_2D_3$ production, and PRL and growth hormone (GH) also appear to stimulate production of the hormone. These endocrine glands may therefore represent additional sites for negative feedback inhibition by 1,25$(OH)_2D_3$. Nuclear receptors for 1,25$(OH)_2D_3$ are also present in cells of the pars distalis, and it has been reported that the hormone may regulate PRL production.

The hormone is also known to play essential roles in more basic cellular responses, such as those involved in proliferation and differentiation. Examples include the differentiation and maturation of hematopoietic stem cells, myoblasts, and dermal keratinocytes. In addition, actions on mature B and T cells of the immune system clearly support a physiological role for 1,25$(OH)_2D_3$ in immunoregulation. The hormone also appears to induce a family of catabolic enzymes in all target cells, which metabolize it through a discrete pathway to calcitroic acid. Evidence from autoradiographic studies with [^{3}H]-1,25$(OH)_2D_3$ about its many sites of nuclear binding and multiple actions suggests that the traditional view of vitamin D and Ca^{2+} is too limited and requires modification. It has been proposed that the skin-derived hormone of sunshine, "soltriol" (1,25$(OH)_2D_3$), is a somatotrophic activator and modulator that affects all vital systems. Regulation of Ca^{2+} homeostasis may be only one of its many actions [40, 44].

Although the role of 1,25$(OH)_2D_3$ in mammals and birds is well documented, the role of the hormone or related metabolites in other vertebrates is less understood. Apparently, teleost fishes synthesize cholecalciferol without the aid of sunlight, and the livers of such animals are a well-known source of precursor metabolites for 1,25$(OH)_2D_3$ production in humans. Frogs and other amphibians are reported to be susceptible to vitamin D deficiency. The availability of Ca^{2+} and PO_4^{-3} in aquatic environments could eliminate the need for vitamin D in some aquatic vertebrates.

Hormone Mechanisms of Action in Calcium Homeostasis

The mechanisms of action of the calcitropic hormones are being very precisely delineated, thus providing a clearer understanding of the molecular basis of disease states related to Ca^{2+} homeostasis.

Parathormone, Calcitonin, and Vitamin D Activate their Cognate Receptors in Multiple Tissues

Prothormone.   Because the renal cortex is a major site of PTH action, this tissue has provided the main source of information on the mechanism of action of PTH. $[^3H]$-labeled PTH is localized preferentially to the proximal tubule cells of the kidney cortex. Renal cortical membranes bind PTH and respond by increasing the production of cAMP. Human PTH^{1-34} is a full agonist in that it can produce a maximal effect, but has approximately 1/10 the potency of the parent molecule (hPTH 1–84). Deletion of the two amino-terminal residues completely abolishes the activity of PTH, thus demonstrating the importance of the N terminus for biological activity of the hormone. The mechanism of action of PTH is unique in that interaction of PTH with its receptor results in activation of two different transduction pathways, one leading to cAMP formation and one to IP_3/DAG production. Different G proteins are involved in these separate pathways (Fig. 9.10).

PTH depends to a remarkable degree on vitamin D for mobilization of Ca^{2+} from bone in vivo. In rats on a vitamin D deficient, low Ca^{2+} diet, serum Ca^{2+} levels drop to very low values in spite of secondary hyperparathyroidism, and there is no histological evidence of enhanced bone resorption. It appears, therefore, that PTH and vitamin D act in concert to effect mobilization of bone mineral. PTH stimulates adenylate cyclase activity in particulate bone cell fractions from vitamin D deficient and normal rats. The data suggest that the cause of skeletal refractoriness to PTH in vitamin D deficient animals is not a defective activation of adenylate cyclase. Most likely the vitamin D requirement for PTH action is related to later steps in the biochemical events leading to bone cell activation. In addition, vitamin D may be necessary for recruitment of new (additional) osteoblasts (see Fig. 9.12). Vitamin D

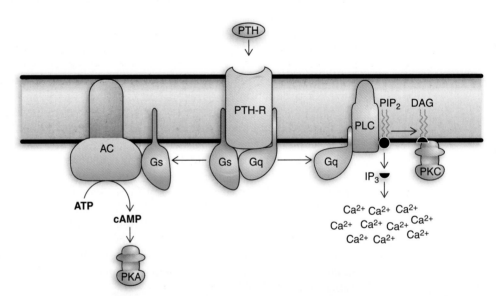

Figure 9.10   Cell-surface receptors for PTH are coupled to two classes of G proteins. G_s mediates stimulation of adenylyl cyclase (AC) and the production of cAMP, which in turn activates protein kinase A (PKA). G_q stimulates phospholipase C (PLC) to form the second messengers inositol-(1,4,5)-triphosphate (IP_3) and diacylglycerol (DAG) from membrane-bound phosphatidyl-inositol-(4,5)-biphosphate. IP_3 increases intracellular calcium (Ca^{2+}) and DAG stimulates protein kinase C (PKC) activity. Each G protein consists of a unique α chain and a βγ dimer.

appears to be permissive to the actions of PTH, possibly by one or more mechanisms described for steroid hormone actions (see Fig. 3.15).

Calcitonin.   The entire 32-amino-acid sequence of CT appears to be required for biological activity. Seven of the nine common residues of the salmon CTs are at the N-terminal end of the molecule and are probably intimately involved in biological activity. Cleavage of the 1–7 disulfide bond in the hormone causes considerable loss of biological activity. The C-terminal prolinamide is also essential for activity. When studied in the rat, piscine (salmon, eel) CTs show markedly enhanced biological activities compared to human and other mammalian CTs. The high biological effectiveness of salmon CT relative to that of mammals may be due to a longer half-life in vivo, due to resistance of the hormone to degradation by plasma or tissue enzymes.

Receptors for CT are present in skeletal tissue, kidney, and testicular Leydig cells. The affinities of several CT analogs for specific receptors in vitro parallel closely the biological activity of those analogs in vivo. Human CT has no greater relative potency when tested against receptors from human tissue than for receptors from rat tissues. Thus, in contrast to the marked evolutionary changes in CT structure, there is no evidence suggesting phylogenetic modification in the nature of the CT receptor. CT receptor complementary DNA (cDNA) has been cloned [47]. The receptor has high affinity for CT and is functionally coupled to adenylate cyclase activation. The receptor is homologous to the PTH/PTHrP receptor, suggesting these Ca^{2+} regulatory G protein-coupled receptors are evolutionarily related [22]. The CT receptor may be coupled to different G proteins, G_s, G_i, and possibly G_q (a G protein coupled to PKC) in a cell cycle-dependent fashion. Coupling of the CT receptor to one pathway leads to an opposite biological response from that induced by activation of the other receptor. The basis for cell cycle-regulated coupling of different G proteins to the CT receptor (or subtypes thereof) is unknown. It might be speculated that cell cycle-related changes in phosphorylating and dephosphorylating enzyme activities may affect the particular transduction pathway and the biological responses associated with activation of the receptors. Therefore, CT may induce different biological responses in target cells, depending on their position in the cell cycle [8].

PTH-Related Peptide.   The cDNA encoding a 585-amino-acid PTH/PTHrP receptor with seven potential membrane-spanning domains was cloned from a cDNA library. The expressed receptor binds PTH and PTHrP with equal affinity, and both ligands stimulate adenylate cyclase. Striking homology with the CT receptor and lack of homology with other G-protein-linked receptors indicate that receptors for these Ca^{2+}-regulating hormones are related and represent a new family of peptide hormone receptors. The surprising structural similarity between the PTH/PTHrP receptor and the CT receptor suggests that these novel receptors may share functional features distinguishing them from other G-protein-linked receptors. This family of receptors also includes the rat secretin receptor, which is similar in sequence to both the CT and PTH/PTHrP receptors, with 30% and 42% identity, respectively [19].

Most surprising is the observation that stimulation of placental Ca^{2+} transport requires the 75–85 region of PTHrP and is unresponsive to PTH 1–84. The possibility exists that PTHrP possesses the potential for different biological actions depending on the molecular species present, which may be regulated by tissue-specific processing by target tissues [35]. The term *polyhormone* has been suggested to describe the plural potential of these peptides [22].

Vitamin D.   As for other steroid hormones, $1,25(OH)_2D_3$ interacts with target-tissue nuclear receptors to activate transcriptional and translational processes [14, 15, 26, 30, 32]. In this regard the action of the hormone on the intestine has been well characterized, whereas the effects of $1,25(OH)_2D_3$ on bone, kidney, and other tissues is less well understood (Fig. 9.11). There is a lag period of some 2 hours before the effects of the hormone can be noted, suggesting that the induction of new proteins is a prerequisite for the actions of the hormone. One of these is a Ca^{2+}-binding (transport) protein (CaBP). This protein may enhance the movement of Ca^{2+} from the brush border into the cytoplasm. An early event in the action of $1,25(OH)_2D_3$ in intestinal cells is a rapid, apparently nongenomic, activation of Ca^{2+} channels (called *trans-caltachia*), which has recently been linked to PKC activity [44].

The sequence of the avian, rat, and human vitamin D receptor has been deduced from molecular cloning data, revealing that the receptor belongs to a family of related proteins, including several other steroid hormone receptors. The members of this family all have a ligand-binding domain at the carboxy terminus, a DNA-binding domain in the middle, and

Figure 9.11
Mechanism of action and general functions of 1,25(OH)$_2$D$_3$ in target cells. (From M. R. Haussler et al. [14] with permission. Reproduced by permission of the Society for Endocrinology.)

a less evolutionary conserved amino terminus that may have domains that help select among potentially responsive genes. After binding to the specific ligand, these receptor proteins influence gene expression via association with specific DNA elements known as hormone-responsive elements (HREs). 1,25(OH)$_2$D$_3$ exerts its effects through a vitamin D-responsive element (VDRE) [5].

The gene that produces osteocalcin, the major noncollagenous bone protein, is stimulated by vitamin D but inhibited by glucocorticoids. The DNA sequence of the vitamin D response element, which is within the promoter gene for osteocalcin, was shown to be unresponsive to other steroid hormones. On the other hand, a DNA domain of this promoter, distinct from the element, controls the potent glucocorticoid repression of vitamin D's induction of osteocalcin. Thus, the low circulating serum osteocalcin levels associated with glucocorticoid excess could be explained by a direct influence of the hormone on the osteocalcin gene promoter, resulting in antagonism of the gene.

Receptors for 1,25(OH)$_2$D$_3$ are present in bone, and vitamin D causes a large (100-fold) increase in immunoreactive CaBP in chick bone. 1,25(OH)$_2$D$_3$ stimulates alkaline phosphatase activity of osteoblast-like bone tumor cells in tissue culture. In view of the postulated role of the enzyme in calcification, these observations suggest a direct involvement of vitamin D in bone mineralization. There is also evidence that the action of vitamin D on the kidney may involve synthesis of a Ca^{2+}-binding protein; a vitamin D dependent CaBP has been localized immunohistochemically in distal tubules of avian and mammalian kidneys. Autoradiographic studies with 1,25(OH)$_2$D$_3$ also reveal that the hormone is preferentially localized to cells of the distal tubules.

Hormone Integration in Calcium Homeostasis

Isolated bone cell populations of osteoblasts and osteoclasts have been obtained and the effects of PTH, CT, and vitamin D on these cells studied. CT inhibits the actions of the two hormones on osteoclasts but not on osteoblasts. PTH, but not vitamin D, mediates its effects through cAMP production. Although vitamin D and PTH activate similar cellular processes, they do so through separate receptors, plasma membrane, and cytosolic, respectively. The actions of PTH and vitamin D elevate serum Ca^{2+} levels by enhancing the bone-resorbing activities of the osteoclasts, while inhibiting concomitantly the bone-building activities of the osteoblasts. CT mediates its serum Ca^{2+}-lowering effect by preferentially inhibiting osteoclastic (bone-resorbing) activity without disturbing the mineralization (bone-building) activity of osteoblasts. The fact that both PTH and CT increase cAMP production in bone has been explained by the PTH effect taking place in osteoblasts and the CT effect in osteoclasts.

The multinucleate osteoclast has long been recognized as the principal cell involved in bone resorption; its characteristic resorbing apparatus consists of a ruffled border. CT inhibits bone resorption by altering the morphology and activity of the osteoclast. CT-treated osteoclasts separate from bone surface, lose their ruffled borders, and demonstrate decreased release of lysosomal enzymes. All CTs possess an anti-osteoclastic activity. Osteoclasts possess specific receptors that bind CT. Administration of CT causes the brush borders of the osteoclasts to disappear and the osteoclasts to move away from the bone resorption surface. CT radically alters the internal structure of isolated osteoclasts, inhibiting cytoplasmic motility, which is essential for bone resorption. Finally, CT reduces the lifespan and number of osteoclasts that are known to possess CT receptors. An assessment of the relative potencies of the various CTs reveals that CTs from teleostean fish are 50–100 times more potent than those from mammals.

Strong evidence indicates that the osteoblast is the main target cell for PTH action, regulating indirectly, via cell–cell communication, osteoclastic bone resorption. Precursor cells of mesenchymal origin give rise to cells that can differentiate under the influence of $(1,25(OH)_2D_3)$ to a mature phenotype, the osteocyte, which synthesizes and secretes a number of matrix proteins, including collagen and osteocalcin. Some precursor cells follow another path of differentiation to become mature osteoblasts. Osteoclasts also derive from precursor cells of the macrophage/monocyte cell lineage which fuse to become multinucleate osteoclasts. Under the influence of either parathormone (PTH) or vitamin D hormone, or cytokines [44] such as interleukin-1 (IL-1) and tumor necrosis factor alpha (TNFα), osteoblasts secrete one or more "osteoclast differentiation-inducing" factors such as interleukin-6 (IL-6), macrophage colony stimulating factor (M-CSF), and "receptor activator of NFκB ligand" (RANKL). They also stimulate osteoclasts to undergo morphological (shape) changes and to secrete hydrogen ions and acid proteases of lysosomal origin. Under these acidic conditions, proteolysis of osteocyte matrix proteins takes place. This results in the release of Ca^{2+} and PO_4^{-3} to enter the general circulation. Calcitonin is inhibitory to osteoclastogenesis and osteoclastic activity and therefore prevents bone demineralization.

Estrogen is also inhibitory to osteoclastogenesis and osteoclastic activity, and therefore the loss of estrogen in some menopausal women is accompanied by the development of osteoporosis. The molecular mechanisms that mediate estrogen's actions in bone have thus been the subject of intense research. The RANKL protein has now been recognized as a particularly important, if not essential molecule in the regulation of osteoclast development and activation [42]. It is expressed on the surface of osteoblast precursor cells, and when released it can bind its cognate receptor, RANK, on osteoclast precursor cells, and thereby activate differentiation and proliferation of osteoclasts. This process can be blocked by the binding of RANKL to a soluble "decoy" receptor, also produced by the osteoblast, called osteoprotegerin (OPG). Many studies have now convincingly demonstrated that estrogen suppresses RANKL production and increases OPG production; through these actions estrogen may exert its major suppressive effects on osteoclastic activity and bone loss. In addition, estrogen may also regulate the production of other cytokines in osteoblasts or bone marrow cells, such as IL-1, IL-6, TNFα, M-CSF, and prostaglandins. In the absence of estrogens, in postmenopausal women, the decreased production of OPG and enhanced release of RANKL and other cytokines result in increased osteoclastic activity and increased likelihood of osteoporosis. Under other pathological states (e.g., Paget's disease) the actions of these cytokines may also increase osteoclastic activity by their stimulation of osteoblasts. An even more complex cytokine circuitry than depicted here is undoubtedly involved in the reciprocal regulatory interactions between osteoblasts, osteoclasts, and osteocytes (Fig. 9.12) [18, 29, 41, 42].

Brown [31] has succinctly summarized the integrated roles of hormones in Ca^{2+} homeostasis: "In health, the extracellular Ca^{2+} ion concentration (Ca^{2+}) is maintained within strict limits by the actions of the major calciotropic hormones, PTH and 1,25-dihydroxyvitamin D_3 $(1,25(OH)_2D_3)$. The latter has long-term effects, regulating both intestinal Ca^{2+} absorption and skeletal calcium turnover over days to weeks. In contrast, it is the circulating PTH that has the predominant role in the regulation of Ca^{2+} on a minute-to-minute basis. A decrease in the extracellular Ca^{2+} concentration of the order of 10–20 μmol/L leads to an increase in the rate of PTH release from the parathyroid chief cells within seconds. Circulating PTH then acts via the PTH receptor to increase the distal tubular reabsorption of Ca^{2+} and decrease tubular phosphate reabsorption within minutes. PTH also enhances osteoclast activity causing skeletal Ca^{2+} release within 1 to 2 hours, and more prolonged PTH release produces an increase in renal 1α-hydroxylase activity and subsequent $1,25(OH)_2D_3$ production. Thus, the

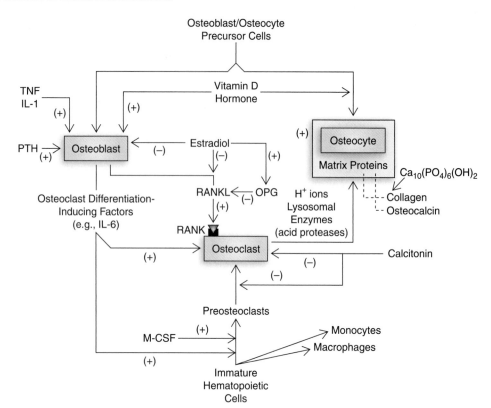

Figure 9.12
Generalized model of the role of hormones controlling bone mineralization and demineralization.

two cornerstones of normal extracellular Ca^{2+} homeostasis are the ability of the parathyroid glands to secrete PTH at a rate that is rapidly responsive to changes in Ca^{2+} and the capacity of the effector tissues, namely the renal tubule, skeleton, and intestine, to respond appropriately to changes in the circulating concentrations of PTH and $1,25(OH)_2D_3$."

Bone mineral density of the forearm, hip, and lumbar spine is greater in African-American than Caucasian men and women. This racial difference begins in childhood, and African-Americans have a lower incidence of osteoporosis and fractures than Caucasians. It was found that African-American males had significantly higher serum levels of both estrogen and GH. Insulin-like growth factor I (IGF-I) binding protein levels were also lower. As estrogens increase GH secretion and GH increases bone mass, it was postulated that circulating estradiol may contribute to the higher GH secretion and bone mass in African-American men [48]. Estrogens acting singularly or in combination with GH may also affect bone mass directly. The systemic hormone differences noted between African-Americans and Caucasians, however, may not be sufficient to explain bone mineral density (BMD) differences between the races.

Hormonal Regulation of Intracellular Calcium

Most membrane-mediated hormone actions involve changes in the transmembrane potential. Because of the unequal distribution of ions between the extracellular and intracellular environments of a cell, a cell is generally 60 to 90 mV (millivolts) negative on the inside. The unequal charge distribution across the plasmalemma causes the cell to be electrically excitable. Muscle and nerve cells are particularly excitable, as are some secretory cells. The excitability of certain cells is of pivotal importance in hormonal control of cellular function. In response to hormonal stimuli, cells may become *depolarized* or *hyperpolarized*. Acetylcholine, for example, depolarizes skeletal muscle cells, which leads to contraction. Interaction of acetylcholine with membrane receptors causes Na^+ flow into the cell, thus depolarizing the muscle. Sodium ion flux into the cell is linked to an increase in cytosolic Ca^{2+}; Ca^{2+} interacts with the contractile proteins of the muscle and contraction ensues. This event is referred to as *stimulus-contraction coupling*. A similar *stimulus-secretion coupling* is responsible for hormone-induced cellular secretion. These phenomena are collectively termed *stimulus-response coupling*.

Substitution of Na^+ by other monovalent cations, such as Li^+ (lithium), provides information on the specificity of the cation requirement for hormone action. Magnesium (Mg^{2+}) or barium (Ba^{2+}) ions are often substituted for Ca^{2+} to determine the divalent cation specificity for hormone action. Their failure to substitute is considered to mean that Ca^{2+} is the specific divalent cation required for hormone action. Although Ca^{2+} is of prime importance to stimulus-response coupling, this ion undoubtedly plays other more subtle roles in cellular responses to hormones. Calcium modulates adenylate cyclase and cyclic nucleotide phosphodiesterase activities. Ca^{2+} is also required in some cellular systems for coupling between hormone receptors and nucleotide cyclase activity. Melanocyte-stimulating hormone (MSH) action, for example, requires Ca^{2+} for activation of adenylate cyclase; this is a receptor-specific requirement, as prostaglandin and epinephrine stimulation of melanocyte adenylate cyclase is without such a requirement. In a number of cellular systems Ca^{2+} may also be specifically required for hormone activation of guanylate cyclase.

Calmodulin is an Intracellular Calcium Receptor

Calcium, a divalent cation, is required for the actions of many hormones. Calcium may be essential for hormone activation of phospholipase A_2 and thus prostaglandin biosynthesis. Calcium may be directly required for transduction of a signal between a hormone receptor and adenylate or guanylate cyclase. Hormones may translocate Ca^{2+} into the cytosol to function in such processes as enzyme activation or cellular contraction. However, the precise mechanism of action of Ca^{2+} was for a long time an enigma. Ca^{2+} is now known to interact with its own cellular receptor, a protein referred to as *calmodulin* (*CaM*), or calcium-dependent regulatory protein. This ubiquitous protein is found in all eukaryotic cells and therefore in plants.

Calmodulin exists as a monomer of 148 amino acid residues. The primary sequence of CaM has been stringently conserved throughout phylogeny; for example, there are only seven conservative amino acid substitutions between vertebrate CaM and that of a marine coelenterate. A distinctive feature of the protein is that the amino group of lysine 115 is post-translationally trimethylated. CaM possesses four Ca^{2+}-binding sites, and the amino acid sequences within each domain contain a high degree of homology (Fig. 9.13). CaM may have

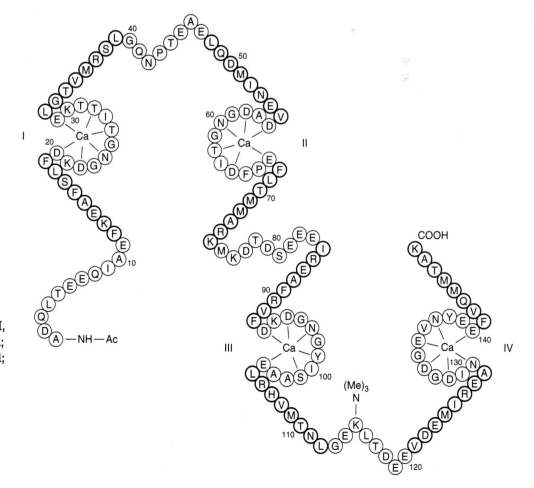

Figure 9.13 Primary structure of calmodulin (CaM), an intracellular calcium receptor. The following are one-letter codes for amino acid residues: A, Ala; D, Asp; E, Glu; F, Phe; G, Gly; H, His; I, Ile; K, Lys; L, Leu; M, Met; N, Asn; P, Pro; Q, Gln; R, Arg; S, Ser; T, Thr; V, Val; Y, Tyr. (Reproduced with permission, from the *Annual Review of Biochemistry*, Klee et al., "Calmodulin." Vol. 49, pp. 480–515. © 1980 by Annual Reviews, Inc.)

evolved from a smaller precursor (which bound a single Ca^{2+}) by gene duplication. The homology is greatest between domains 1 and 3, and 2 and 4; it is possible that CaM may have arisen by two successive doublings or a primordial gene coding for a Ca^{2+}-binding domain. CaM is structurally related to troponin C, found in skeletal and cardiac muscle.

The binding of Ca^{2+} to CaM results in a conformational change of the protein that may be required for the interaction of CaM with its substrate. It has been concluded that at physiological ionic strength, the Ca^{2+}-binding sites on CaM are not filled in a sequentially ordered fashion. CaM needs only three atoms of Ca^{2+} per molecule of protein for activation; the binding of the fourth atom of Ca^{2+} is apparently neither necessary nor inhibitory. Activation of CaM by Ca^{2+} is apparently an all-or-none process. When CaM has three or four Ca^{2+} ions bound, it is active; when it has fewer than three it is inactive.

Three major roles of CaM are regulation of intracellular Ca^{2+} levels, enzyme activation, and control of cellular filamentous organelle activity. The actions of CaM are direct and indirect; for example, CaM may activate an enzyme directly or indirectly through prior activation of another enzyme. A number of peptide and steroid hormones are without effect on cellular levels of CaM; levels of the Ca^{2+} regulatory protein apparently remain constant, regardless of the hormonal environment.

As an intracellular Ca^{2+} receptor, CaM may play a pivotal role in cellular Ca^{2+} homeostasis. The levels of Ca^{2+} within cells fluctuate due to fluxes of Ca^{2+} across the plasma membrane from or into storage depots within mitochondria and smooth endoplasmic reticulum, each of these pathways being of more or less importance, depending on the cell type. In each case, CaM stimulates a Ca^{2+}-Mg^{2+}-dependent ATPase (Ca^{2+} pump) in the membranes of these organelles. In the presence of excessive cytosolic Ca^{2+}, CaM would become activated and would subsequently stimulate one or more of these membrane Ca^{2+} pumps, which would bring Ca^{2+} levels back to normal.

Calmodulin may play an important role in the control of cyclic nucleotide levels. CaM is stimulatory to adenylate cyclase and phosphodiesterase. Although these two actions of CaM may first appear to be opposed, the sensitivities of the two enzymes to CaM may differ considerably. In fact, cAMP increases the affinity of phosphodiesterase for CaM, which may provide a cellular homeostatic mechanism involving an initial activation of cAMP production, followed by a mechanism for the degradation of the cyclic nucleotide. In addition to a role for a cytosolic CaM in the control of adenylate cyclase activity, CaM may function by a Ca^{2+}-dependent mechanism in the transduction of signal between receptor and adenylate cyclase. Thus, CaM can be envisioned to function at a number of sites in the control of cAMP levels.

Calmodulin regulates a variety of cellular contractile or motile processes. Actin and myosin are the major proteins responsible for cell motility, and they are present in both muscle and nonmuscle cells. Calcium is required for muscle contraction, and in smooth muscle it is now known that Ca^{2+} activates CaM that then binds to a regulatory subunit of an enzyme, myosin light-chain kinase, whose catalytic domain phosphorylates the light-chain protein of myosin (see Fig. 7.13). Activation of myosin ATPase provides the stimulus for formation of the actomyosin complex leading to the contractile process. In skeletal muscle, an elevation of cytosolic Ca^{2+} is the stimulus to the contractile process resulting from actin and myosin interaction. Binding of Ca^{2+} to troponin C (which is structurally related to CaM) results in a conformational change in the troponin–tropomyosin–actin complex that causes actomyosin formation.

Microtubules are filamentous components of cells and are involved in cellular activities involving motile processes, such as chromosome movement, axoplasmic flow, and neurite extension. Most interesting is the apparent role of CaM in chromosomal movement during mitosis. There is a major shift of CaM from a diffuse distribution within the cell during interphase to high local concentrations within the mitotic apparatus during mitosis. In this process, CaM may perform such roles as regulating the concentration of Ca^{2+} in the microenvironment and thus affect microtubular assembly/disassembly. In addition, CaM may activate other proteins or enzymes that may be involved in the mitotic machinery.

In skeletal muscle, CaM regulates the activity of the enzyme phosphorylase kinase, which causes glycogen degradation to provide the glucose substrate necessary for mitochondrial ATP production. CaM is an integral regulatory subunit of phosphorylase, as the enzyme is completely dependent on Ca^{2+} for activity. Phosphorylase kinase is composed of four different subunits, α, β, γ, δ, and the δ subunit is CaM. In liver, skeletal, and cardiac muscle, phosphorylase kinase plays a dual role in the control of glycogen metabolism. It activates the

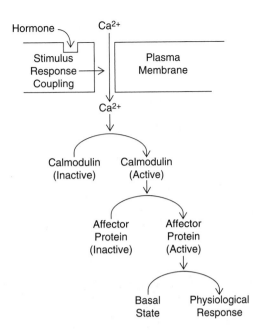

Figure 9.14 Model for the mechanism of action of calmodulin.

enzyme phosphorylase, which splits glycogen into its glucose subunits, and it may function as glycogen synthetase kinase, an enzyme that inactivates glycogen synthetase through phosphorylation of the enzyme.

A general model for the action of CaM is shown in Figure 9.14. Interaction of Ca^{2+} with CaM results in a conformational change in an associated effector protein, which then induces a physiological response. The effector protein would differ in each cell type. For example, one of the subunits of skeletal muscle phosphorylase kinase would be considered to function as the effector protein. The effector molecule associated with troponin, for example, might be tropomyosin.

Pathophysiology

Decreased or increased production of PTH leads to hypocalcemic or hypercalcemic states, respectively. Because an important role of PTH is to enhance production of $1,25(OH)_2D_3$, the etiology of either calcemic state is most directly related to decreased or increased levels of this steroid hormone. Calcium ions play a critical role in nerve and muscle excitability. Alterations in extracellular Ca^{2+} concentrations, therefore, may affect neural transmission and contractility of cardiac and skeletal muscle, thus leading to serious clinical problems.

Hypoparathyroidism Results in Hypocalcemia

Hypoparathyroid patients display hypocalcemia as their major clinical symptom. This hypocalcemia is caused, in part, by a partial deficiency of $1,25(OH)_2D_3$. The hyperphosphatemia resulting from PTH deficiency might also suppress $1,25(OH)_2D_3$ production. Restoration of normocalcemia may be attained by treatment with $1,25(OH)_2D_3$ or related metabolites. Tetany and convulsions are the most serious complications of the hypoparathyroid state. Latent tetany may be detected by tapping over the facial nerves, which results in a contraction of the facial muscles (Chvostek's sign), or by producing carpal (wrist) spasm (Trousseau's sign) following occlusion of arterial blood supply to the forearm, as often happens when applying a sphygmomanometer to the arm. In some disorders, although Ca^{2+} levels are depressed, suggestive of PTH deficiency, the levels of the hormone may actually be increased above normal. The defect responsible in one type of *pseudohypoparathyroidism* is related to a failure to generate cAMP. In an inherited pseudohypoparathyroidism, type Ia (PHP-Ia), patients inherit a defect in one of the two autosomal alleles of the gene for α_s, the α subunit of G_s, the stimulatory regulator of adenylyl cyclase. Although G_s mediates effects of many hormones, the ~50% decrease in G_s activity produced by loss of an autosomal allele causes clinically evident impairments of receptor responsiveness to PTH [13].

Hyperparathyroidism Results in Hypercalcemia

Patients with primary hyperparathyroidism have moderate to severe hypercalcemia and elevated plasma $1,25(OH)_2D_3$ levels; the pathology may involve *neoplasia* or *hyperplasia*. Primary hyperparathyroidism usually results from a benign adenoma of one of the parathyroids. Hyperparathyroidism due to primary hyperplasia, on the other hand, involves overactivity of all the parathyroid glands usually due to an unknown (idiopathic) etiology. Secondary hyperparathyroidism often results from a peripheral defect of PTH action; the resulting hypocalcemia is the stimulus to enhanced parathyroid chief cell activity. Secondary hyperparathyroidism is a frequent consequence of chronic renal failure. Retention of phosphate depresses serum Ca^{2+}

Figure 9.15   Proposed structural model for the predicted BoPCaR1 Ca^{2+}-sensing receptor protein. The large N-terminal domain is located extracellularly and contains nine potential N-linked glycosylation sites (shown as branched chains). Amino acids are indicated at intervals of 50 in the N-terminal domain. Amino-acid segments forming each of the seven putative membrane-spanning helices are numbered. Potential phosphorylation sites for PKC are shown. Symbols represent individual amino acids. The hydrophilic signal protein (SP) and hydrophobic A-segment (HS) are indicated. (With permission from Edward M. Brown et al., *Nature Lond.* 366:575–80, 1993.)

levels, and reduced synthesis of $1,25(OH)_2D_3$ by the kidney impairs intestinal Ca^{2+} absorption. Excessive levels of PTH are then secreted in response to lowered levels of Ca^{2+}.

The structure of the Ca^{2+}-sensing receptor has been cloned and biologically characterized (Fig. 9.15). Defects in this receptor (CaR) that cause "familial hypocalciuric hypercalcemia and neonatal severe hyperparathyroidism" have now been described [1, 6, 9, 16, 25, 31, 33]. Defective Ca^{2+}-sensing receptors cause chief (PTH) cell hypertrophy and hyperplasia; the resulting hyperparathyroidism causes excessive bone resorption and elevated serum Ca^{2+} levels (hypercalcemia) and excessive renal tubular Ca^{2+} reabsorption causes decreased urinary Ca^{2+} concentrations (hypocalciuria).

As for other seven-spanning membrane receptors, mutations can lead to constitutively active receptors resulting in decreased PTH secretion and hypocalcemia. It is thought that mutations within the extracellular domain enhance the affinity of receptors for extracellular Ca^{2+} or mimic the ligand-bound state of the extracellular domain. Cell surface Ca^{2+} receptors provide novel and discrete molecular targets for designer drugs that mimic or antagonize the action of extracellular Ca^{2+} at these receptors. These so-called "calcimimetics" could either depress parathyroid cell PTH secretion or stimulate calcitonin secretion from thyroid C cells [31].

Hypercalcemia can Accompany Some Malignancies

One mechanism considered responsible for the hypercalcemia that frequently accompanies malignancy is secretion of a circulating factor that alters Ca^{2+} metabolism by the tumor (see earlier discussion). The structure of a tumor-secreted peptide was determined and found to be partially homologous to PTH. The amino-terminal 1–34 region of the factor, PTHrP, was synthesized and evaluated biologically. In vivo, it produced hypercalcemia, acted on bone and kidney, and stimulated $1,25(OH)_2D_3$ formation. In vitro, it interacted with PTH receptors and, in some systems, was more potent than PTH. These observations support a long-standing hypothesis regarding pathogenesis of malignancy-associated hypercalcemia.

An immunometric assay that measures intact PTH is replacing the traditional radioimmunoassay, because it provides for the differential diagnosis of hypercalcemic disorders. These assays take advantage of saturation kinetics, rather than competitive binding [48], and use two affinity-purified antisera (or monoclonal antibodies), both of which can simultaneously bind to the ligand with little, if any, steric interference. One of the antisera also binds to a solid-phase matrix, and the other is labeled with radioiodine or with a chemiluminescent compound. Immunoradiometric and immunochemiluminometric assays for iPTH measure intact hormone by "capturing" iPTH with immobilized affinity-purified antisera by epitopes with PTH's middle and carboxyl-terminal sequence and reacting the serum iPTH with soluble, labeled, affinity-purified amino-terminal antisera. The concentration of hormone is determined by quantifying the amount of labeled amino-terminal antisera bound to the solid phase by gamma counting or with a luminometer (Figs 9.16 and 9.17).

Figure 9.16 A schematic illustration of an immunoradiometric assay for iPTH. (Reprinted by permission of the publisher from "Advances in techniques for measurement of parathyroid hormone. Current applications in clinical medicine and directions for future research," Segre, *Trends in Endocrinology and Metabolism* 1:243–247, 1990. © 1990 by Elsevier Science Inc.)

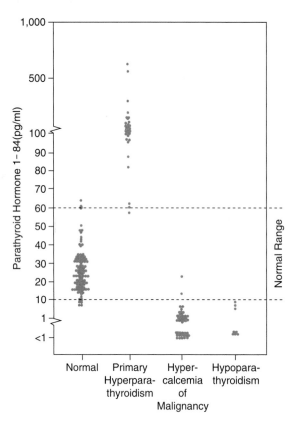

Figure 9.17 Intact iPTH measured by an immunoradiometric assay in sera of normal subjects, and patients with hyperparathyroidism, hypercalcemia of malignancy, and hypoparathyroidism. (Reprinted by permission of the publisher from "Advances in techniques for measurement of parathyroid hormone. Current applications in clinical medicine and directions for future research," Segre, *Trends in Endocrinology and Metabolism* 1:243–47, 1990. © 1990 by Elsevier Science Inc.)

Osteomalacia is a Condition of Inadequate Bone Mineralization

This disorder is characterized by a failure of normal mineralization of bone in the adult. (In children, the disease is referred to as rickets.) This undermineralization of cartilage and bone results in retardation of growth and in development of characteristic skeletal deformities [28]. Rickets and adult osteomalacia encompass a group of diseases that have similar skeletal defects but diverse causes. An historical perspective on the socioeconomic and ecological factors predisposing to rickets in earlier times is well characterized by Gibbs [13] and Loomis [21].

Osteomalacia is classified as vitamin D responsive or vitamin D resistant. The vitamin-D-responsive disorders may be due to a deficiency in dietary intake of vitamin D precursors (vitamin D deficiency rickets), inadequate exposure to sunlight, or intestinal malabsorption of Ca^{2+}. The vitamin-D-resistant disorders result from diverse etiologies, such as familial or acquired renal-tubular phosphate wasting, defective collagen matrix formation, and specific hereditary defects in the metabolic transformation of vitamin D to its active form, probably due to failure of 1α-hydroxylation. Several unusual forms of vitamin-D-resistant rickets have been described, which involve end-organ hyposensitivity (pseudovitamin D deficiency) to biologically active vitamin D. Hypocalcemic vitamin-D-resistant rickets is a human genetic disease resulting from target organ resistance to the action of $1,25(OH)_2D_3$. Two families with affected children homozygous for this autosomal recessive disorder were studied for abnormalities in the intracellular vitamin D receptor (VDR) and its gene. Although the receptor displayed normal binding of $1,25(OH)_2D_3$, VDR from affected family members had a decreased affinity for DNA. Genomic DNA isolated from these families was subjected to oligonucleotide-primed DNA amplification, and each of the exons encoding the receptor protein was sequenced for a genetic mutation. In each family, a different single nucleotide mutation was found in the DNA-binding domain of the protein (Fig. 9.18).

Paget's Disease is Characterized by Excess Osteoclastic Activity

This focal disorder, which is often familial and is fairly common in England and certain northern European countries, is characterized by the presence of excessive numbers of osteoclasts, which leads to structurally weakened bone tissue [12]. Although susceptibility to Paget's disease is believed to be transmitted by a simple autosomal Mendelian dominant gene, the etiology

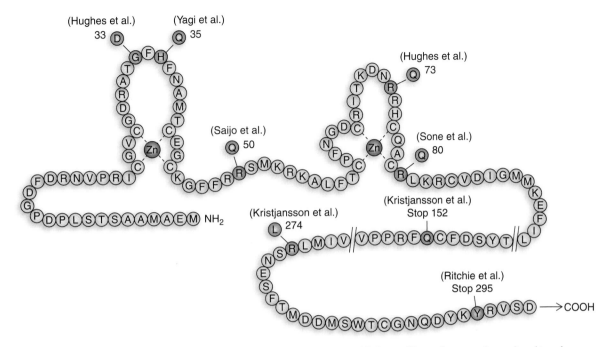

Figure 9.18 Natural mutations in the VDR from patients with hereditary hypocalcemic vitamin-D-resistant rickets. The amino acid residues are indicated in the diagram by the single letter abbreviations: A, Ala; C, Cys; D, Asp; E, Glu; F, Phe; G, Gly; H, His; I, Ile; K, Lys; L, Leu; M, Met; N, Asn; P, Pro; Q, Gln; R, Arg; S, Ser; T, Thr; V, Val; W, Trp; and Y, Tyr. (From MacDonald, Dowd, and Haussler, "New insights into the structure and functions of the vitamin D receptor," in *Seminars in Nephrology* 14:101–118, 1994. Used by permission.)

remains elusive. Osteoclasts from Pagetic bone may be enlarged and contain greatly increased numbers of nuclei. Virus-like inclusions have been noted in the nuclei of some Pagetic osteo-clasts. Certain individuals may be born with the genetic susceptibility to osteoclastic invasion by a virus organism. The expression of the abnormality is, however, usually only manifested later in life. Calcitonin is a powerful pain suppressant, stimulating the secretion of the natural opiate, β-endorphin, and reducing the evoked potentials in central pain pathways. Because CT inhibits bone resorption and relieves pain, it is now widely used in the treatment of bone disease (e.g., Paget's disease). Worldwide sales of CT approach $1 billion a year, ranking it second only to insulin as a peptide used in clinical medicine [10].

Osteoporosis is a Condition of Decreased Bone Mineral Density

This disease is manifested as a decrease in bone density, with demineralization being attributable to several possible etiologies [27, 43].

Postmenopausal (Type I) Osteoporosis. In the United States nearly 1.2 million women begin menopause each year. During her expected remaining lifetime of about 30 years, the average woman will lose approximately 30–50% of her bone mass. After age 65, the incidence of spine and hip fractures rises almost exponentially. The pathogenesis of osteoporosis that occurs after menopause is related to a decrease in gonadal steroids (Chap. 19). Common sites of fracture among postmenopausal females are the vertebrae, forearm, and hip. The incidence of such fractures among males of similar age is much less, whereas in younger adults, there is little difference in incidence between the sexes. On this basis, the prevention of such fractures might be realized if estrogen treatment is continued after menopause. Virtually all the available evidence indicates that the use of estrogens lowers the risk of postmenopausal fractures, and therefore some women may benefit from long-term estrogen use (see also Chap. 19). Hormone replacement therapy (HRT) consisting of estrogen alone, or estrogen and progesterone, has clearly been found to be useful in reducing menopausal vasomotor symptoms, viz. "hot flashes," and in reducing the incidence of skeletal fractures. However, the risk/benefit ratio of HRT has recently been the subject of debate, as the results of the Women's Health Initiative trials, a large National Institutes of Health (NIH) sponsored study, have suggested that HRT may be associated with increased risk for breast cancer in women with a uterus, and increased rate of thromboembolic events and stroke (Chap. 19). The role of estradiol in bone physiology and its relationship to postmenopausal osteoporosis is depicted in Fig. 9.12.

Postmenopausal osteoporosis appears not to be associated with (or be) the result of CT deficiency. CT alone or in combination with $1,25(OH)_2D_3$ is effective in enhancing the bone mineral content of postmenopausal and elderly osteoporotic patients. Three years of $1,25(OH)_2D_3$ therapy in women with postmenopausal osteoporosis significantly reduced the incidence of new vertebral fractures, as compared with Ca^{2+} gluconate supplementation. When administered in a dose of 0.25 μg twice a day, $1,25(OH)_2D_3$ had no important side effects. The results suggest that $1,25(OH)_2D_3$ may be an important therapeutic option in the treatment of women with postmenopausal osteoporosis [43].

Senile (Type II) Osteoporosis. In elderly people with osteoporosis, not only is there reduced $1,25(OH)_2D_3$ secretion, but PTH plasma levels are also diminished [4]. Whether these phenomena are specific characteristics of osteoporosis or are just endocrine changes common to all aging persons is unclear. Deficiency of vitamin D is uncommon in the general population of the North American continent because of the availability of sunlight, vitamin D fortified milk, and over-the-counter preparations containing the vitamin. There are elderly individuals who are, however, at risk of developing a deficiency of the vitamin because of lack of exposure to sunlight and failure to ingest milk or vitamin supplements containing vitamin D. Vitamin D deficiency is a real risk in old age. It may be preceded by a period of active bone disease, which can be mistaken clinically for osteoporosis. If aging patients are to be maintained in an optimal state of health, "it is important to evaluate their exposure to sunlight and their vitamin D intake, and recommend vitamin D prophylaxis to patients at risk" [2].

Winter decreases $1,25(OH)_2D_3$ and increases PTH plasma levels; these changes are well documented. It has been postulated that these hormonal changes in the winter could have deleterious effects on the skeleton because $1,25(OH)_2D_3$ is required to maintain Ca^{2+} absorption, and PTH is a potent stimulator of bone resorption. Serum PTH and plasma 25-hydroxyvitamin D levels vary inversely with one another, and the concentration of each changes with the season in the temperate zone. There is indirect evidence that seasonal increases in PTH may affect bone mass adversely. Patients with hip fractures have been shown to have wintertime increases in PTH and lower levels of $1,25(OH)_2D_3$ than controls. At latitude 42°, healthy postmenopausal women with vitamin D intake of 100 IU daily can significantly reduce late wintertime bone loss and improve net bone density of the spine over one year by increasing their intake of vitamin D to 500 IU daily [11].

In elderly men and women, administration of biosynthetic (recombinant) human growth hormone (rhGH) induces dose-related elevations in circulating IGF-I, indicating that older subjects retain the capacity to respond to exogenous rhGH. Growth hormone activates osteoblasts to increase local synthesis of IGF-I, which acts in an autocrine or paracrine way to enhance bone matrix apposition, suggesting a role in the preservation of bone mass. GH deficiency in the elderly therefore may be of pathogenetic significance in senile osteoporosis. However, critical evidence does not yet support the concept that the decreased activity of the growth hormone–IGF-I axis alters bone remodeling, and the extent to which geriatric hyposomatotropism contributes to the age-related femoral bone loss remains to be elucidated. Despite the fact that biochemical estimates of bone turnover indicate that (short-term) administration of rhGH and IGF-I stimulates bone metabolism in nonosteoporotic older people, no significant changes have been observed in bone mineral density at the proximal femur. Additional studies are needed to assess the therapeutic potential for rhGH in attenuating or reversing bone loss in elderly people. Moreover, data on long-term adverse side effects of rhGH therapy are not yet available. Because of the known mitogenic action of IGF-I, the neoplastic potential of long-term rhGH therapy needs to be considered [4].

Since vitamin D is produced by the action of sunlight on the skin, gloomy winter skies may be a causative factor in the etiology of rickets in some individuals. It has been reported that infants that breast-feed exclusively are at risk for rickets in the cloudy northwest. Children of color who breast-feed may be at greatest risk since vitamin D production is decreased in dark-skinned people. Since breast milk does not contain sufficient vitamin D, a young child needs exposure several hours a week to full sunlight if they continue to breast-feed rather than take vitamin D fortified milk (or formula). Elderly individuals who often remain confined indoors may also be at risk for the development of osteopenia (bone demineralization) [47].

New Pharmacological Therapies for Diseases of Ca^{2+} Homeostasis are Available

Bisphosphonates.   These are drugs that bind to bone mineral and are then taken up by osteoclasts during bone resorption. In the osteoclast, they deactivate it and trigger apoptosis. As a result, bone turnover is reduced and bone mass is increased.

Selective Estrogen Receptor Modulators (SERMs).   The SERMs have been developed in an attempt to provide the benefits of HRT therapy without the unwanted side effects. These ligands for the ER have been utilized because they appear to exert agonistic effects in bone, while acting as an antagonist of ERs in breast and uterus. The SERMs are therefore effective in reducing bone turnover, although they are less potent in this regard than estrogens.

Pharmaceutical Preparations of Vitamin D.   The oral administration of $1,25(OH)_2D_3$, although effective in the treatment of some vitamin D deficiency syndromes, may cause hypercalcemia due to the high transient local concentrations of the hormone in the serum. A novel alternative method of providing vitamin D to the patient may be through the topical application of $1,25(OH)_2$-7-dehydrocholesterol, combined with phototherapy. Cutaneous generation of $1,25(OH)_2D_3$ results (see Fig. 9.6), which may provide a more prolonged release and sustained stimulation of intestinal Ca^{2+} absorption [17].

A number of plant species throughout the world cause severe calcinosis in domestic animals when ingested as part of their forage. A calcinogenic factor extracted from the leaves of *Solanum malacoxylon* has been found to be $1,25(OH)_2D_3$ glycoside. After ingestion, endogenous glycosidases or intestinal microbes hydrolyze the glycoside to the hormonally active form. The reason for the existence of such a calcinogenic factor is unclear, but it and other related substances may function in mineral metabolism in plants [45]. The controlled administration of powdered leaves of *S. malacoxylon* has been used therapeutically in both humans and farm animals and improves eggshell quality when given to hens [3].

Dietary Calcium and Osteoporosis.   Lifestyle modifications that can reduce the risk of osteoporosis include weight-bearing exercise and the maintenance of an adequate intake of Ca^{2+} in the diet. It has been reported that, contrary to popular belief, excess Ca^{2+} intake in adulthood may not reduce any further the risk of osteoporosis. A high Ca^{2+} intake can lead to kidney stones in susceptible people, and Ca^{2+} supplements may cut off vitamin D production, which is necessary for the cellular activation of bone cells (but see [37]).

MOLECULAR MEDICINE CASE STUDIES

Familial hypocalciuric hypercalcemia associated with mutation in the human Ca^{2+}-sensing receptor gene (K. Aida, S. Kioshi, M. Inoue, M. Nakazato, M. Tawata, and T. Onaya. *J. Clin. Endocrinol. Metab.* 80:2594–8, 1995). "Familial hypocalciuric hypercalcemia (FHH) is generally characterized by lifelong hypercalcemia without hypercalciuria and is inherited in an autosomal dominant manner. Affected individuals show abnormal parathyroid and renal responses to changes in the extracellular calcium concentration. A Japanese FHH family was screened for mutations in the Ca^{2+}-sensing receptor gene by the polymerase chain reaction and single strand conformation polymorphism. The proband with hypercalcemia showed an abnormal pattern in exon 1 of the gene, whereas her two sisters with normocalcemia showed a normal pattern. The consanguineous parents with borderline serum calcium concentrations showed both

patterns. Nucleotide sequence analysis identified a G→C point mutation at nucleotide 118 that resulted in the conversion of the normal codon for proline into a codon for alanine at amino acid 40 (numbered according to the bovine complementary DNA). The proband was homozygous for the mutation, and the parents were heterozygous. These results imply that this mutation in the human Ca^{2+}-sensing receptor gene causes FHH and that the dosage of the gene defect determines disease phenotype" (Fig. 9.19).

A novel parathyroid hormone (PTH)/PTH-related peptide receptor mutation in Jansen's Metaphyseal Chondrodysplasia (E. Schipani, C. Langman, J. Hunzelman, M. Le Merrer, K. Y. Loke, M. J. Dillon, C. Silve, and H. Juppner. *J. Clin. Endocrinol. Metab.* 84:3052–7, 1999). "Two heterozygous PTH/PTH-related peptide (PTHrP) receptor missense mutations were previously identified in

(Continued)

(Continued)

Figure 9.19 Polymerase chain reaction/single strand conformation polymorphism (PCR-SSCP) analysis of the first exon of the human Ca^{2+}-sensing receptor gene from the family and a normal subject. The genomic DNAs were amplified by PCR with end-labeled primers and analyzed by SSCP. An abnormal pattern was detected in the proband. Her parents showed both the abnormal and normal patterns, whereas the proband's sisters showed the normal pattern. (From K. Aida et al. [1], with permission.)

patients with Jansen's metaphyseal chondrodysplasia (JMC), a rare form of short limb dwarfism associated with hypercalcemia and normal or undetectable levels of PTH and PTHrP [38]. Both mutations, H223R and T410P, resulted in constitutive activation of the cAMP signaling pathway and provided a plausible explanation for the abnormalities in skeletal development and mineral ion homeostasis. In the present study we analyzed genomic DNA from four additional sporadic cases with JMC to search for novel activating mutations in the PTH/PTHrP receptor, to determine the frequency of the two previously identified missense mutations, H223R and T410P, and to determine whether different mutations present with different severity of the disease. The H223R mutation was identified in three novel JMC patients and is, therefore, to date the most frequent cause of JMC. In the fourth patient, a novel heterozygous missense mutation was found that changes isoleucine 458 in the receptor's seventh membrane-spanning region to arginine (I458R). In COS-7 cells expressing the human PTH/PTHrP receptor with the I458R mutation, basal cAMP accumulation was approximately 8 times higher than that in cells expressing the wild-type receptor despite impaired surface expression of the mutant receptor. Furthermore, the I458R mutant showed higher responsiveness to PTH than the wild-type receptor in its ability to activate both downstream effectors, adenylyl cyclase and phospholipase C. Like the H223R and the T410P mutants, the I458R mutant had no detectable effect on basal inositol phosphate accumulation. Overall, the patient with the I458R mutation exhibited clinical and biochemical abnormalities similar to those in patients with the previously identified H223R and T410P mutations."

REVIEW EXERCISES

Match the disease/defect with its primary effect on plasma hormone levels:

1. Hypoparathyroidism
2. Paget's disease
3. Defective calcium sensing receptor
4. Parathyroid cancer (neoplasia or hyperplasia)
5. Vitamin-D-responsive osteomalacia
6. Secondary hyperparathyroidism
7. Senile osteoporosis

A. lowered parathormone
B. elevated parathormone
C. lowered vitamin D
D. elevated vitamin D

Think, analyze and discuss:

1. Secretions of both PTH and calcitonin are controlled by the level of Ca^{2+} in blood.
   a. In which specific cell types are PTH and calcitonin produced?
   b. Describe the common receptor that mediates the Ca^{2+}-sensing process in both PTH- and calcitonin-producing cells. Does elevated blood Ca^{2+} stimulate or inhibit PTH secretion through this receptor? Does it stimulate or inhibit calcitonin secretion through this receptor?
   c. If PTH and calcitonin secretions are affected in opposite ways by elevated blood Ca^{2+}, then how

might this occur, given that the same receptor mediates both processes? Propose a hypothesis that might account for the differential effects of Ca^{2+} in PTH and calcitonin-secreting cells. How might you test your hypothesis?

2. The Ca^{2+}-sensing process can be considered as an important feature of a homeostatic control system in which the secretion of both PTH and calcitonin are subject to feedback regulation by the very factor that they both regulate, i.e. Ca^{2+}. Construct separate schematic diagrams which depict the homeostatic control systems for the regulation of blood Ca^{2+} by PTH and calcitonin, respectively. Include the hormone-secreting cells, target tissues, and the effects of the hormone at each tissue on Ca^{2+} levels. For both hormone control systems, predict the sequence of events that would follow an increase or decrease in blood Ca^{2+} levels.

3. Osteopenia is a major concern for patients who require treatment with high doses of glucocorticoids. Propose a molecular mechanism by which glucocorticoids may exert this undesirable and potentially serious side effect.

4. Describe the consequences of vitamin D deficiency that lead to the developments of rickets. Why is this condition relatively rare in developed countries?

5. A patient is seen by a physician and presents with latent tetany and other signs of hypocalemia. His plasma Ca^{2+} levels are measured and found to be quite low. Measurement of serum PTH levels, however, reveal that they are elevated, ruling out hypoparathyroidism. What do you think is the most likely explanation for this patient's symptoms? How would you confirm your diagnosis? What treatment would you prescribe?

6. Compare and contrast the effects of PTH and vitamin D on plasma Ca^{2+} levels.
   a. What would be the relative time courses of their actions?
   b. How might the time courses of their actions be predicted from the respective types of receptors that they activate?
   c. In which ways do these hormones affect the secretion and/or actions of each other? Where possible, describe the specific molecular mechanism by which one hormone may exert a "permissive" effect on the actions elicited by the other.

7. Describe a putative physiological role of a PTH-related peptide. What is the evidence that it plays an especially important role in fetal physiology?

8. The primary sequence of PTH is highly conserved in mammals. Why might this be so?

9. Frogs "breathe" and exchange some ions through their skin while under water. Would you predict that calcium exchange could also occur through their skin? Explain your answer.

10. Describe the metabolic conversions that are required to produce the active form of vitamin D. In which tissues do each of these reactions takes place?

References

[1] Aida, K., et al. 1995. Familial hypocalciuric hypercalcemia associated with mutation in the human Ca(2+)-sensing receptor gene. *J. Clin. Endocrinol. Metab.* 80:2594–8.

[2] Barzel, U. S. 1983. Vitamin D deficiency: a risk factor for osteomalacia in the aged. *J. Am. Geriatr. Soc.* 31:598–601.

[3] Boland, R. L. 1986. Plants as a source of vitamin D3 metabolites. *Nutr. Rev.* 44:1–8.

[4] Boonen, S., J. Aerssens, and J. Dequeker. 1996. Age-related endocrine deficiencies and fractures of the proximal femur. I implications of growth hormone deficiency in the elderly. *J. Endocrinol.* 149:7–12.

[5] Bouillon, R., W. H. Okamura, and A. W. Norman. 1995. Structure-function relationships in the vitamin D endocrine system. *Endocr. Rev.* 16:200–57.

[6] Brown, E. M., and S. C. Hebert. 1997. Calcium-receptor-regulated parathyroid and renal function. *Bone* 20:303–9.

[7] Burtis, W. J. 1992. Parathyroid hormone-related protein: structure, function, and measurement. *Clin. Chem.* 38:2171–83.

[8] Chakraborty, M., et al. 1991. Cell cycle-dependent coupling of the calcitonin receptor to different G proteins. *Science* 251:1078–82.

[9] Chattopadhyay, N., A. Mithal, and E. M. Brown. 1996. The calcium-sensing receptor: a window into the physiology and pathophysiology of mineral ion metabolism. *Endocr. Rev.* 17:289–307.

[10] Copp, D. H. 1992. Remembrance: calcitonin: discovery and early development. *Endocrinology* 131:1007–8.

[11] Dawson-Hughes, B., et al. 1991. Effect of vitamin D supplementation on wintertime and overall bone loss in healthy postmenopausal women. *Ann. Intern. Med.* 115:505–12.

[12] Delmas, P. D., and P. J. Meunier. 1997. The management of Paget's disease of bone. *N. Engl. J. Med.* 336:558–66.

[13] Gibbs, D. 1994. Rickets and the crippled child: an historical perspective. *J. R. Soc. Med.* 87:729–32.

[14] Haussler, M. R., et al. 1997. The vitamin D hormone and its nuclear receptor: molecular actions and disease states. *J. Endocrinol.* 154:S57–73.

[15] Haussler, M. R., et al. 1995. New understanding of the molecular mechanism of receptor-mediated genomic actions of the vitamin D hormone. *Bone* 17:33S–38S.

[16] Hebert, S. C., E. M. Brown, and H. W. Harris. 1997. Role of the Ca(2+)-sensing receptor in divalent mineral ion homeostasis. *J. Exp. Biol.* 200:295–302.

[17] Holick, M. F., et al. 1980. The photoproduction of 1 alpha,25-dihydroxyvitamin D3 in skin: an approach to the therapy of vitamin-D-resistant syndromes. *N. Engl. J. Med.* 303:349–54.

[18] Horowitz, M. C. 1993. Cytokines and estrogen in bone: anti-osteoporotic effects. *Science* 260:626–7.

[19] Juppner, H., et al. 1991. A G protein-linked receptor for parathyroid hormone and parathyroid hormone-related peptide. *Science* 254:1024–6.

[20] Lippuner, K., et al. 1996. PTH-related protein is released into the mother's bloodstream during location: evidence for beneficial effects on maternal calcium-phosphate metabolism. *J. Bone Miner. Res.* 11:1394–9.

[21] Loomis, W. F. 1970. Rickets. *Sci. Am.* 223:76–82 passim.

[22] Mallette, L. E. 1991. The parathyroid polyhormones: new concepts in the spectrum of peptide hormone action. *Endocr. Rev.* 12:110–17.

[23] Morley, P., J. Whitfield, and G. Willick. 1997. Anabolic effects of parathyroid hormone on bone. *TEM* 8:225–231.

[24] Munson, P. L., and P. F. Hirsch. 1966. Thyrocalcitonin: newly recognized thyroid hormone concerned with metabolism of bone. *Clin. Orthop. Relat. Res.* 49:209–32.

[25] Nemeth, E. 1995. Ca^{2+} receptor-dependent regulation of cellular function. *News Physiol. Sci.* 10:1–5.

[26] Norman, A. W., et al. 1993. Selective biological response by target organs (intestine, kidney, and bone) to 1,25-dihydroxyvitamin D3 and two analogues. *Cancer Res.* 53:3935–42.

[27] Ooms, M. E., et al. 1995. Prevention of bone loss by vitamin D supplementation in elderly women: a randomized double-blind trial. *J. Clin. Endocrinol. Metab.* 80:1052–8.

[28] O'Riordan, J. L. 1997. Rickets, from history to molecular biology, from monkeys to YACS. *J. Endocrinol.* 154:S3–13.

[29] Oursler, M. J., et al. 1993. Oestrogen effects on osteoblasts and osteoclasts. *Ann. Med.* 25:361–71.

[30] Ozono, K., T. Sone, and J. W. Pike. 1991. The genomic mechanism of action of 1,25-dihydroxyvitamin D3. *J. Bone Miner. Res.* 6:1021–7.

[31] Pearce, S., and E. Brown. 1996. The genetic basis of endrocrine disease: Disorders of calcium ion sensing. *J. Clin. Endocrinol. Metab.* 81:2030–5.

[32] Pike, J. W. 1991. Vitamin D3 receptors: structure and function in transcription. *Annu. Rev. Nutr.* 11:189–216.

[33] Pollak, M. R., et al. 1993. Mutations in the human Ca(2+)-sensing receptor gene cause familial hypocalciuric hypercalcemia and neonatal severe hyperparathyroidism. *Cell* 75:1297–303.

[34] Potts, J. T., Jr. 1992. Chemistry of the calcitonins. *Bone Miner.* 16:169–73.

[35] Ratcliffe, W. A. 1992. Role of parathyroid hormone-related protein in lactation. *Clin. Endocrinol. (Oxf.)* 37:402–4.

[36] Raue, F., and H. Scherubl. 1995. Extracellular calcium sensitivity and voltage-dependent calcium channels in C cells. *Endocr. Rev.* 16:752–64.

[37] Reid, I. R., et al. 1993. Effect of calcium supplementation on bone loss in postmenopausal women. *N. Engl. J. Med.* 328:460–4.

[38] Schipani, E., et al. 1999. A novel parathyroid hormone (PTH)/PTH-related peptide receptor mutation in Jansen's metaphyseal chondrodysplasia. *J. Clin. Endocrinol. Metab.* 84:3052–7.

[39] Seitz, P. K., et al. 1993. Parathyroid hormone-related peptide production and action in a myoepithelial cell line derived from normal human breast. *Endocrinology* 133:1116–24.

[40] Stumpf, W. E. 1988. The endocrinology of sunlight and darkness. Complementary roles of vitamin D and pineal hormones. *Naturwissenschaften* 75:247–51.

[41] Suda, T., N. Takahashi, and T. J. Martin. 1992. Modulation of osteoclast differentiation. *Endocr. Rev.* 13:66–80.

[42] Syed, F., and S. Khosla. 2005. Mechanisms of sex steroid effects on bone. *Biochem. Biophys. Res. Commun.* 328:688–96.

[43] Tilyard, M. W., et al. 1992. Treatment of postmenopausal osteoporosis with calcitriol or calcium. *N. Engl. J. Med.* 326:357–62.

[44] Walters, M. R. 1992. Newly identified actions of the vitamin D endocrine system. *Endocr. Rev.* 13:719–64.

[45] Wasserman, R. H., et al. 1976. Calcinogenic factor in *Solanum malacoxylon*: evidence that it is 1,25-dihydroxyvitamin D3-glycoside. *Science* 194:853–5.

[46] Watson, P. H., and D. A. Hanley. 1993. Parathyroid hormone: regulation of synthesis and secretion. *Clin. Invest. Med.* 16:58–77.

[47] Wimalawansa, S. J. 1996. Calcitonin gene-related peptide and its receptors: molecular genetics, physiology, pathophysiology, and therapeutic potentials. *Endocr. Rev.* 17:533–85.

[48] Wood, P. J. 1992. The measurement of parathyroid hormone. *Ann. Clin. Biochem.* 29:11–21.

Gastrointestinal Hormones

*T*he *first hormone to be discovered was **secretin**, a chemical messenger released from the epithelium of the small intestine in response to acid released from the stomach [2]. The gut is the source of many hormones; in fact, the gastrointestinal mucosa may be considered the largest endocrine organ. Elucidation of the chemical nature of the gut hormones has been difficult because the endocrine-secreting cells are distributed individually throughout the gut epithelium. Thus, an easy source of the hormones is not readily available for chemical identification. Their specific cellular distribution has, however, been determined precisely in a number of animal species by immunocytochemical methods.*

Of the known gastrointestinal (GI) peptides, four clearly function as hormones: gastrin, secretin, cholecystokinin (CCK), and gastric inhibitory peptide (GIP). Other candidate hormones, such as the recently discovered peptide ghrelin, will probably derive full hormonal status after further studies. One of the major problems confronting the endocrinologist is to determine whether the experimentally determined biological effects of the hormones are indeed indicative of such a physiological function. Many GI hormones fall into families of related hormones that share overlapping structures. Thus, members of the same hormonal family evoke similar target tissue responses, which confuses any issue relating to their individual putative physiological roles.

The actions of the GI hormones are primarily concerned with the digestion and movement of food products along the GI tract. They release the enzymes necessary to split specific food substrates, such as proteins, carbohydrates, and fats, into their simpler components, amino acids, sugars, and fatty acids, respectively. The GI hormones also enhance the activity of enzymes by stimulating the secretion of acid, which provides the pH optimum for enzymatic action. Hormonal stimulation of bile salt secretion provides the medium in which fat globules can become emulsified, thus increasing the surface area for enzyme activity. Thus, a major role of the GI hormones is to facilitate the conversion of food substrates into molecular forms that then can gain access into the bloodstream [14].

Gastrointestinal Tract Structure and Function

In order to appreciate the roles and actions of hormones on digestive processes it is necessary to review briefly the structure and function of the GI tract. Food enters the mouth, is mixed with saliva, passes down the esophagus, and enters the stomach through the lower esophageal sphincter. The emulsified, partly digested food is then released as a bolus of chyme through the pyloric sphincter into the duodenum, the initial segment of the small intestine (small bowel). The food continues through the jejunal (jejunum) and ileal (ileum) segments of the small intestine to enter the large intestine (colon), where the undigested components of the food making up the stool are dehydrated before defecation from the anus.

Food is propelled distally along the GI tract because of peristaltic contractions. Peristalsis results from the rhythmic contractions and relaxations of the longitudinal and circular layers of muscle that comprise part of the gut wall. Muscle contraction and relaxation are controlled by neurons of the parasympathetic and sympathetic components of the autonomic nervous system. These *extrinsic nerve fibers* innervate *intrinsic neurons* of the *myenteric plexus of Auerbach*, which are found between the circular and longitudinal muscle layers. Other intrinsic neurons of the gut form the *submucosal plexus of Meissner*, which regulates the activity of muscles responsible for movements of the villi.

The pancreas plays an important role in GI function. The islets of Langerhans (the endocrine pancreas) are the source of insulin and glucagon, two hormones important in the control of carbohydrate metabolism (Chap. 11). The exocrine pancreas is composed of the *acinar cells* that are the source of a variety of enzymes essential to digestion of foodstuffs arriving in the small intestine. The pancreatic duct provides an exit for the release and delivery of these enzymes to the small intestine. Certain ductule cells lining this excretory passageway provide water and electrolytes (i.e., bicarbonate ion), which are also important to digestive processes.

The gallbladder is a pear-shaped hollow organ that serves as a reservoir for *bile salts* excreted by the liver. Contraction of the smooth muscles of the walls of the gallbladder discharges the bile salts into the common bile duct, which then connects with the pancreatic duct leading to the opening into the small intestine. Bile salts are necessary for emulsification of fats within the intestine.

In the mouth, starch is acted on by ptyalin, an α-amylase present within the saliva. The saliva is secreted from the salivary (parotid, sublingual, submaxillary) glands. Because the optimal pH for α-amylase activity is 6.7, the action of the enzyme is subsequently inhibited by the acidic environment of the stomach. In the small intestine, an α-amylase secreted by the *exocrine pancreas* acts on the various polysaccharides present in the partly digested food. Other enzymes localized within the luminal surface of the mucosa further hydrolyze sugars to glucose. Glucose and other hexoses and pentoses are rapidly absorbed across the wall of the duodenum and ileum to enter the bloodstream.

Protein digestion begins in the stomach where enzymes, the pepsins, cleave particular peptide linkages. The pepsins are released from the chief cells of the body of the stomach as precursor (proenzyme) molecules, pepsinogens, which are activated by gastric hydrochloric acid (HCl) released from *parietal* or *oxyntic* (from the Greek to make sour or acid) cells of the gastric glands. The actions of the pepsins are terminated in the alkaline pancreatic juice of the duodenum. In the small intestine, the shorter peptides are formed by the action of protein-splitting enzymes, trypsin and chymotrypsin, released from the pancreas. Other enzymes, pancreatic carboxypeptidases, intestinal aminopeptidases, and dipeptidases, split the smaller peptides into free amino acids. These amino acids are actively transported across the intestinal lumen and enter the bloodstream.

The digestion of fats begins in the intestine. Free fatty acids (FFAs) are liberated by the enzymatic actions of *pancreatic lipase* on dietary triglycerides. This enzyme acts on fats that have been emulsified by the detergent action of bile salts released into the intestinal lumen following contraction of the gallbladder. Small micelles consisting of lipids and bile salts provide the reactive surface for lipase activity. The FFAs and monoglycerides within the micelles are released by enzymatic action to enter the mucosal cells by passive diffusion; they may then pass directly into the portal blood or they may become reesterified to triglycerides within the mucosal cells and then enter into the lymphatics.

Source and Chemistry of the Gastrointestinal Hormones

The GI hormones are synthesized within a system of clear cells (enterochromaffin, argyrophil, or argentaffin cells), so called because they are selectively stained by certain silver salts. These clear cells, scattered within the GI tract mucosa from the stomach through the colon, are often referred to as the diffuse or dispersed endocrine system, or, along with the pancreatic hormones, as the gastroenteropancreatic hormones [30]. This diffuse distribution of enterochromaffin-like (ECL) cells [12] prevents the endocrinologist from surgically removing the source of any one hormone as is done for many other endocrine glands. It is suggested that the distribution of ECL cells throughout extensive areas of mucosa "ensures

| | 1 | 2 | 3 | 4 | 5 | 6 | 7 | 8 | 9 | 10 | 11 | 12 | 13 | 14 | 15 | 16 | 17 |

Gastrin (G-17)   (pyro)Glu–Gly–Pro–Trp–Leu–Glu–Glu–Glu–Glu–Glu–Ala–Tyr–Gly–Trp–Met–Asp–Phe–NH₂

Cholecystokinin   Lys–Ala–Pro–Ser–Gly–Arg–Val–Ser–Met–Ile–Lys–Asn–Leu–Gln–Ser–Leu–Asp–
Pro–Ser–His–Arg–Ile–Ser–Asp–Arg–Asp–Tyr–Met–Gly–Trp–Met–Asp–Phe–NH₂

Figure 10.1 Amino acid sequences of human G-17 gastrin and cholecystokinin (CCK). Identical C-terminal pentapeptide sequences are indicated.

that hormone release is regulated by an integrated sampling of mixed luminal contents rather than by a specific stimulus that might exist transiently at only one point" [11]. One surface of each of the ECL cells often reaches the lumen, thus providing a receptive surface for metabolite recognition.

The ECL cells of the gut and pancreas have been classified as deriving from certain cell types, designated, for example, as D (somatostatin), G (gastrin), or S (secretin). A tenet of neuroendocrinology has been the "one-hormone, one-cell" concept. However, in the gut and elsewhere, a peptide hormone (e.g., substance P) and the biogenic amine serotonin (5-HT) are often found within the same cell. The physiological significance of two biologically active moieties within the same cell is unclear.

Based on their homology of structure, the gut hormones can be conveniently grouped into two families. The *gastrin family* comprises the gastrins and the cholecystokinins. The *secretin family* consists of secretin, glucagon, vasoactive intestinal polypeptide (VIP), and gastric inhibitory peptide (GIP). There may be molecular heterogeneity (isoforms) of a particular hormone; the hormone may exist in a number of molecular forms of variable length with differing biological potencies. Only one of these peptides is generally considered to be the physiological messenger, and it usually constitutes the principal form stored within the secretory granules of the cell. Molecular forms larger than the principal form may be viewed as biosynthetic precursors (prohormones), which may escape and be detected in the circulation. Molecular forms smaller than the principal form probably represent postsecretory degradation products.

Gastrin Hormone Family Members Contain a Biologically Active C-Terminal Pentapeptide Sequence

The C-terminal five-amino-acid sequences of gastrin and CCK are identical (Fig. 10.1). Because the biologically active site of these peptides is this pentapeptide sequence, the overlapping actions of one hormone on the physiologically relevant target tissues of the other hormone are explained. The minimal active fragment of these peptides is actually the C-terminal tetrapeptide. Pentagastrin, which exhibits full agonistic activity, is often used in physiological and clinical studies where the actions of gastrin are to be determined (Fig. 10.2). The NH₂-terminal component of gastrin and CCK influences the potency of the hormones, and may also be responsible in part for providing target cell specificity. Note that there are sulfated tyrosyl residues at the 6 and 7 (numbering from the C-terminal end) positions of gastrin and CCK, respectively. Approximately half the gastrin isolated from the gastric mucosa is sulfated on tyrosine. In the case of CCK, where tyrosine is always

Figure 10.2 Structure of pentagastrin.

TABLE 10.1 Amino acid sequences of human gastrin isoforms

Component[a]	Sequence
I Gastrin (big-big gastrin)	Preprogastrin (95 amino acid residues)
II Gastrin$_{34}$ (big gastrin)	(pyro)Glu–Leu–Gly–Pro–Gln–Gly–His–Pro–Ser–Leu–Val–Ala–Asp–Pro–Ser–Lys–Lys– Glu–Gly–Pro–Trp–Leu–Glu–Glu–Glu–Glu–Glu–Ala–Tyr–Gly–Trp–Met–Asp–Phe–NH$_2$ $\quad\quad\quad\quad\quad\quad\quad\quad\quad\quad\quad\quad\quad\quad\quad\quad\quad\quad\quad\quad\quad\mid$ $\quad\quad\quad\quad\quad\quad\quad\quad\quad\quad\quad\quad\quad\quad\quad\quad\quad\quad\quad$SO$_3$H
III Gastrin$_{17}$ (little gastrin)	(pyro)Glu–Gly–Pro–Trp–Leu–Glu–Glu–Glu–Glu–Glu–Ala–Tyr–Gly–Trp–Met–Asp–Phe–NH$_2$ $\quad\quad\quad\quad\quad\quad\quad\quad\quad\quad\quad\quad\quad\quad\quad\quad\quad\mid$ $\quad\quad\quad\quad\quad\quad\quad\quad\quad\quad\quad\quad\quad\quad\quad\quad$SO$_3$H
IV Gastrin$_{14}$ (mini-gastrin)	Trp–Leu–Glu–Glu–Glu–Glu–Glu–Ala–Tyr–Gly–Trp–Met–Asp–Phe–NH$_2$ $\quad\quad\quad\quad\quad\quad\quad\quad\quad\quad\quad\quad\quad\mid$ $\quad\quad\quad\quad\quad\quad\quad\quad\quad\quad\quad\quad$SO$_3$H

[a]Gastrin-34, G-17, and G-14 also exist without a sulfate ester at their tyrosyl residue.

sulfated, however, the sulfated form of the hormone is about 160-fold more potent than the nonsulfated form in binding to CCK$_A$ receptors on pancreatic acini and in promoting gallbladder contraction [16]. CCK$_B$ receptors are less specific and sulfation is not required for receptor activation. The CCK$_B$ receptor is, in fact, the gastrin receptor through which acid secretion is stimulated [28].

Gastrin circulates in most mammalian species in at least three molecular forms (Table 10.1). A macromolecular form of gastrin called big-big gastrin (component I) apparently does not circulate, but could exist as an early intracellular biosynthetic precursor for one or more of the gastrins. It is believed that component I serves as a preprogastrin for gastrin-34 (big gastrin, component II), which may in some cells function as a hormone or as a progastrin. Component III, gastrin-17, may be the physiologically relevant form of the hormone secreted by some cells, and component IV (mini-gastrin, gastrin-14) is considered to be an extracellular degradation product of component III.

Secretin Shares Partial Sequence Identity with Glucagon, GIP, and VIP

Secretin is similar to glucagon in structure: 14 of the 27 amino acids of secretin are similar to those found in glucagon, which is 29 amino acids long. The structures of GIP and VIP possess many amino acids in common with those found in glucagon and secretin (Fig. 10.3). A glucagon-like peptide is also found in the small intestine; this enteroglucagon (glucagon-like peptide 1, GLP-1) regulates, in concert with other hormones, pancreatic

Figure 10.3 Amino acid sequences of porcine peptides of the secretin family. Boxed areas indicate identical amino acid sequences between peptides.

TABLE 10.2   Candidate hormones of the gut

Hormone	
Substance P	Arg–Pro–Lys–Pro–Gln–Gln–Phe–Phe–Gly–Leu–Met–NH$_2$
Somatostatin	Ala–Gly–Cys–Lys–Asn–Phe–Phe–Trp–Lys–Thr–Phe–Thr–Ser–Cys
Motlin	Phe–Val–Pro–Ile–Phe–Thr–Tyr–Gly–Glu–Leu–Glu–Arg–Met–Glu–Gly–Lys–Glu–Arg–Asn–Lys–Gly–Glu
Neurotensin	(pryo)Glu–Leu–Tyr–Glu–Asn–Lys–Pro–Arg–Arg–Pro–Tyr–Ile–Leu

insulin secretion. Most of the entire sequences of each of the peptides is required for their biological actions on their respective target tissues. The hormones of the secretin family lack a well-defined function site where, as in the melanotropins, a particular amino acid sequence has been conserved within the individual peptides (see Fig. 8.1).

The GI Tract Produces other Biologically Active Peptides that are Putative Hormones

The other putative hormones of the GI tract are ghrelin and motilin, which bear some structural similarities with each other, and somatostatin, substance P, neurotensin, and gastrin-releasing peptide, which bear no structural similarity to each other or to the other GI hormones. The formulae of some of these peptides are provided (Table 10. 2). These peptides are variably localized to immunocytochemically characterized cells of the GI mucosa. Other physiologically active peptides are also present within the GI tract and, in time, may also obtain hormone status. These include urogastrone, villikinin, calcitonin gene-related peptide, and one or more endorphins.

Physiological Roles of the Gastrointestinal Hormones

A major role of the GI hormones is to stimulate the secretion of enzymes necessary to degrade complex food substrates into their simpler molecular components so that these smaller molecules can cross the luminal mucosal cells into the bloodstream. GI hormones also stimulate the secretion of acid or base to provide the optimal pH conditions for enzyme activity. By their actions on smooth muscle, the GI hormones move the food distally down the GI tract to the colon. They stimulate release of hormones from the pancreatic islets, which then aid in cellular utilization of metabolic substrates after reaching the bloodstream. The GI hormones may even provide satiety signals to the brain to affect eating behavior (Chap. 11).

Each of the GI hormones has a number of known biological actions of questionable physiological significance. Because many of the hormones are related in structure, they can exhibit overlapping actions when studied experimentally. Gastrin and CCK are partially similar in structure; they both stimulate gastric acid and pancreatic enzyme secretion. It is likely, however, that each hormone is delivered by specific circulatory routes to its own target tissues. This would then provide the mechanism for the necessary specificity of its actions. The release of each of the GI hormones is in response to chemical stimuli, such as hydrogen ions, certain amino acids, FFAs, and sugars. Nutrient receptors are apparently present on the surface of the hormone-secreting cells, which are in open communication with the lumen of the GI tract (Fig. 10.4).

Gastrin Stimulates Acid Secretion in the Stomach

Although the existence of an antral hormone controlling gastric acid secretion was postulated as early as 1905, the hormone gastrin was not isolated until 1964. The antral mucosa of the stomach is the richest source of gastrin in all investigated species, although the peptide is also present in G cells of the duodenal mucosa, particularly in humans. In the antrum and small intestine, the apical pole of the cell, which possesses numerous villi, is in contact with the lumen. Gastrin is present in the gastric juice, which has aroused speculation that gastrin

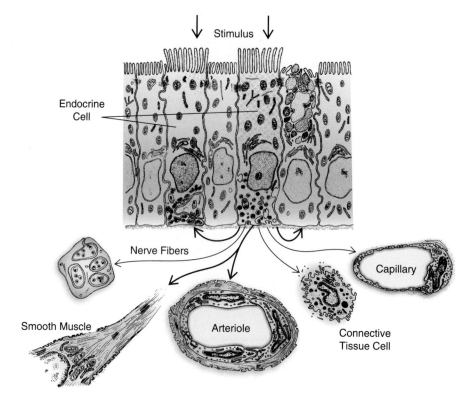

Figure 10.4 Schematic drawing indicating the possible actions of enteroendocrine cells. The stimulus from the intestinal lumen acts on the receptors of the brush-border membrane, resulting in a release of hormones by exocytosis. The peptide hormones may exert their effect on the following: (a) adjacent epithelial cells, nerve fibers, nerve cells, smooth muscle, and connective tissue cells of the lamina propria; (b) cells of the whole organism following delivery to the systematic circulation. Method (a) is described as paracrine; method (b) is referred to as endocrine. (From Grube, D., and W. G. Forssmann. 1979. Morphology and function of the entero-endocrine cells. *Horm. Metab. Res.* 11:589–606, with permission.)

might be released from the luminal surface (as a lumone), as well as from the basal surface into the blood. Electrical stimulation of the vagus nerve of the cat causes a minor increase in circulating gastrin, whereas a much greater amount can be detected in the gastric juice.

Food is the primary physiological stimulus of gastrin secretion. Peptide fragments, amino acids, and to a lesser extent FFAs are stimulatory to gastrin secretion, but sugars are without such an effect. Gastrin secretion is under autonomic nervous system control. For example, in some species, the vagus nerve stimulates gastrin secretion in anticipation of the ingestion of food or through activation of local neural reflexes following distension of the stomach after food intake. Somatostatin- and VIP-secreting cells are found in close association with antral gastrin-secreting cells and may function in an inhibitory role by a paracrine mechanism.

One physiological function of gastrin is to stimulate hydrochloric acid and pepsinogen secretion within the fundus of the stomach; the activated enzyme then initiates the digestion of proteins. The known targets for gastrin mediating these responses are (a) histamine-releasing ECL cells, and (b) acid-secreting parietal cells [26]. Both cell types have been shown to possess a gastrin-CCK$_B$ receptor [3]. The CCK$_B$ receptor is a CCK receptor subtype mainly found in the brain, and possesses pharmacological characteristics similar to those of the gastrin receptor. Gastrin may also stimulate acid secretion indirectly, and gastrin receptors are present on cells other than parietal cells. More recent evidence suggests that gastrin (and agents used to treat ulcers) may act on ECL cells in the lamina propria and not on parietal cells as previously thought. The actions of gastrin may be indirectly transmitted to the epithelial (parietal) cells via the ECL cells [26]. Gastrin does not stimulate pepsinogen secretion directly, but rather indirectly, through release of HCl. In other words, hydrogen ions from the acid are stimulatory to pepsinogen secretion from the chief cells (Fig. 10.5).

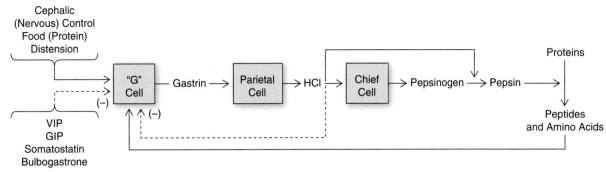

Figure 10.5   Neuroendocrine integration of gastric acid secretion. (See also Fig. 10.14.)

The gastrin present within the antrum is the small (G-17) form of the molecule. The cell responsible for gastrin production in the duodenum contains the larger (G-34) form of the peptide. It is only in humans, where high concentrations of duodenal gastrin occur, that a significant proportion of G-34 appears in the circulation. These two cells, therefore, contain different molecular forms of the peptide, which supports the observation that the two cells are ultrastructurally distinguishable. It is possible that these two circulating forms of gastrin have selective actions on different target cells. It is also possible that a particular molecular form of gastrin may be less susceptible to enzyme degradation.

Starvation or total parenteral (venous) nutrition dramatically reduces the levels of both antral and serum gastrin. This suggests that hormone secretion is acutely dependent on the presence of food in the gut. If rats are fed totally by vein, tissue sensitivity to the trophic action of gastrin becomes diminished. This loss of sensitivity can be prevented by the concomitant infusion of pentagastrin. The pancreatic and colonic mucosa, as well as the duodenal and oxyntic gland mucosa, undergo atrophy in the antrectomized rat, but these deleterious effects can be reversed by supplying gastrin exogenously. These observations suggest that gastrin is an important regulator of gastromucosal cellular growth [4].

The following biological effects are also ascribed to gastrin: stimulation of lower esophageal sphincter pressure; relaxation of the pyloric sphincter; stimulation of pancreatic enzyme secretion; enhancement of motor activity in the intestine; and moderate stimulation of pancreatic bicarbonate and water secretion.

Secretin Stimulates Pancreatic Bicarbonate and Enzyme Secretions

Secretin is one of many peptide hormones of the small intestine. The tissue concentration of secretin diminishes from duodenum to ileum. Secretin-like immunoreactivity is localized to the granular S cells, which are present between the crypts and villi of the mucosa of the small intestine, where maximum concentrations of the hormone have also been extracted. Acidification of the duodenal mucosa, resulting from HCl arriving in the duodenum from the stomach, is the normal stimulus for secretin secretion. At a pH above 4.5, secretin is not released in sufficient amounts to stimulate pancreatic bicarbonate secretion and continued release of secretin is pH-dependent. Nevertheless, it has been difficult to demonstrate increases in plasma secretin levels after a meal. Because a secretin response (increased pancreatic secretion of water and bicarbonate) is observed in humans and dogs after ingestion of meat, a small amount of secretin (insufficiently large to be detected by radioimmunoassay) may be released from the duodenum and may interact with CCK to stimulate bicarbonate secretion. There is an endocrine closed-loop type of relationship governing secretin and HCO_3^- release. Secretin stimulates pancreatic secretion of HCO_3^- into the duodenum; the HCO_3^- neutralizes the H^+ from the stomach, which raises the pH, hence decreasing the release of secretin, which removes any further stimulus to bicarbonate secretion (Fig. 10.6).

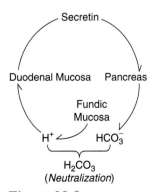

Figure 10.6
Homeostatic closed-loop endocrine mechanism of small intestine pH control.

The clearly defined roles of secretin are to stimulate pancreatic bicarbonate secretion and to potentiate CCK-stimulated pancreatic enzyme secretion. The numerous other physiological actions of secretin may only be pharmacological in nature and may relate to similarities in structure to glucagon, VIP, and GIP, the other members of the secretin family of hormones.

Cholecystokinin (CCK) Stimulates Gallbladder Contraction and Pancreatic Enzyme Secretions

The presence of a hormone in the duodenal mucosa that is liberated by food (particularly lipids) and causes contraction and emptying of the gallbladder was discovered by Ivy and Oldberg in 1928 and named *cholecystokinin* (CCK). Another hormone from the same source that stimulated the release of pancreatic enzymes and also contracted the gallbladder was named *pancreozymin* (PZ). It was subsequently established that CCK and PZ were the same hormone. CCK is a polypeptide hormone of 33-amino-acid residues, but the peptide also exists in a number of other (isohormonal) forms. The carboxy-terminal five amino acids of CCK are identical to those in gastrin (Fig. 10.1). The seventh amino acid from the carboxy terminus is sulfated, which is necessary for the normal physiological activity of the molecule. All C-terminal forms of CCK that exceed seven residues are virtually equipotent in stimulating pancreatic enzyme secretion and gallbladder contraction [16].

The physiological significance of the tissue-specific distribution of CCK variants may be related to the fact that small forms of CCK, such as the octapeptide (CCK-8), are efficiently cleared by the liver and thus could not subserve an effective endocrine role in the GI tract, whereas larger forms more readily survive hepatic transit. This constraint is not present in the central nervous system (CNS), and the majority of C-terminal CCK-like immunoreactivity in the brain comprises CCK-8. It may also be that using shorter forms as central neurotransmitters or neuromodulators promotes delivery to target receptors and subsequent rapid deactivation.

CCK is immunocytochemically localized to the I cells of the duodenal, jejunal, and ileal mucosa. CCK is released by L-isomers of amino acids, hydrochloric acid, and certain fatty acids. One or more "monitor" or "CCK-releasing factor" peptides may also regulate CCK secretion [23]. Entry of high levels of hydrogen ion into the duodenum results in gallbladder contraction, a specific biological response attributed to circulating CCK. CCK plays a major role in gallbladder regulation, although other neural or hormonal factors may also participate [9, 29]. CCK in physiological concentrations has been shown to correlate with postprandial gallbladder contraction in humans.

The other recognized physiological roles of CCK are stimulation of pancreatic enzyme secretion, inhibition of gastric emptying, and potentiation of secretin-induced pancreatic bicarbonate secretion. CCK also appears to be a physiological regulator of the growth of the exocrine pancreas. Although the peptide shares structural similarity with gastrin, which has a trophic growth effect on the GI mucosa, CCK is without such an effect, its trophic actions being specific to the acinar cells of the pancreas.

Depending on the region of the gut, the effect of CCK may be neurally mediated, direct, or both. Neurally mediated effects may be relaxant or contractile depending on the transmitter released by CCK. Based on mimicry by infusion of CCK to postprandial levels and the ability of specific CCK receptor antagonists to abolish effects of endogenous CCK released in response to a meal, three physiological effects of CCK, all of which are neurally mediated, have been identified: (1) contraction of the gallbladder mediated by CCK-induced release of acetylcholine, (2) relaxation of the sphincter of Oddi mediated by CCK-induced release of VIP, and (3) inhibition of gastric emptying mediated by CCK-induced activation of an inhibitory vago-vagal reflex involving vasoactive intestinal peptide-induced relaxation of the gastric fundus. Gallbladder contraction and relaxation of the sphincter of Oddi regulate the flow of bile, and inhibition of gastric emptying regulates the flow of chyme into the duodenum. Combined with the potent stimulation of pancreatic enzyme secretion by CCK, these effects ensure optimal conditions for digestion and absorption of nutrients by the intestine. [9]

As discussed in more detail in Chapter 11, CCK as well as other gut peptides appear to function as satiety hormones [8, 39]. Satiety hormones are generated within the GI tract during the consumption of a meal. They convey signals to integrative centers in the hindbrain, either via the bloodstream or through activation of sensory vagal and sympathetic afferents in the gut, and thereby provide continuous information on the amount of nutrients ingested during the meal. This information is used by the nervous system to determine the appropriate point at which the meal should be terminated. Administration of CCK or other satiety factors thus reduces meal size. Along with CCK, gastrin-releasing peptide (GRP), glucagon, GLP-1, amylin, somatostatin, and peptide YY have similarly been implicated as satiety signals to the brain. By contrast, only one GI peptide, ghrelin (see below) is known to function as an appetite stimulant that increases meal size.

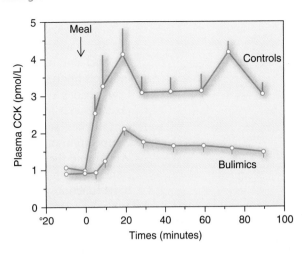

Figure 10.7 Plasma cholecystokinin (CCK) responses to a meal in normal subjects and patients with bulimia. After an overnight fast, 14 patients with bulimia and 10 age- and sex-matched normal volunteers were fed a 400 ml mixed-liquid meal. Plasma was collected and extracted at the indicated times and assayed for CCK bioactivity, expressed as cholecystokinin-8 equivalents. Values are means ± SEM. The arrow indicates the beginning of the meal. (From J. Geracioti and R. A. Liddle. Reprinted by permission of the *New England Journal of Medicine* 319:683–89, 1988.)

Bulimia nervosa is a prevalent disorder of unknown cause, characterized by recurrent episodes of uncontrollable eating. Since CCK induces satiety and reduces food intake in laboratory animals and humans, it has been hypothesized that abnormalities in CCK secretion and satiety may occur in patients with bulimia and contribute to their disturbed eating patterns [8]. Individuals with bulimia may not have normal satiety and may have an impaired secretion of CCK in response to a meal. Abnormally low plasma CCK secretion in response to a mixed-liquid meal in patients with bulimia nervosa has been noted. These patients had lower peak levels of CCK immediately after a meal and also had a low total integrated secretion of the hormone. An impaired satiety response to food was also noted. Impaired satiety after a normal-sized meal is consistent with the histories provided by patients with bulimia (Fig. 10.7).

Disturbances in appetite and food intake are often associated with certain states of depression. Patients with melancholic depression frequently have anorexia, whereas atypically depressed patients have hyperphagia. Similarly, it has been proposed that in the anorexia of aging, elevated CCK levels or increased sensitivity to CCK may contribute to decreased appetite by inducing early satiety. There has been great interest in CCK and related analogs as "satiety hormones" that might prove useful for the control of obesity. These hopes have been complicated by the observations in animals that intermittent CCK administration, while tending to reduce meal size, results in a compensatory increase in the number of meals eaten per day. It remains to be seen if long-acting CCK analogs can be developed that may nevertheless be of therapeutic value.

Gastric Inhibitory Peptide (GIP) Inhibits Gastric Emptying and Gastric Acid Secretion

As early as 1886, it was demonstrated that the presence of fats in a meal inhibited gastric emptying in humans. Fat ingestion was later shown to inhibit gastric acid secretion. Crude intestinal extracts duplicated the actions of fat on gastric acid secretion and motility. The active substance was referred to as enterogastrone. Although a number of gut hormones exhibit enterogastrone-like activity, only one, gastric inhibitory peptide (GIP), is considered to play such a physiological role. This 43-amino-acid peptide, which bears structural similarity to other members of the secretin family of hormones (Fig. 10.3), is localized to certain K cells of the duodenum and jejunum of humans and dogs.

In addition to its inhibitory effects on gastric acid secretion, GIP is insulinotropic, potentiating insulin release in response to an intravenous infusion of glucose, a response that in humans improves glucose tolerance. GIP has therefore been referred to as the *glucose-dependent insulinotropic peptide*. Both GIP and GLP-1 (see below) are also defined as *incretins*—intestinal hormones released in response to nutrient ingestion, which potentiate glucose-induced insulin secretion. Oral glucose ingestion in humans produces a sustained increase in serum GIP levels capable of stimulating insulin release. Indeed, glucose ingestion induces a greater insulin release than intravenous administration of the same amount of glucose. The insulinotropic action of GIP appears to be specifically dependent on concomitant glucose administration as fat ingestion increases serum GIP levels but not serum insulin concentrations. Like glucagon and VIP, GIP is a potent stimulator of pancreatic water and electrolyte secretion from the duodenal glands of Brunner (Brunner's glands, located in the vicinity of the pyloric sphincter).

Besides these well-described effects on gastric secretion and pancreatic β cells, GIP also has direct metabolic effects on other tissues and organs, such as adipose tissue, liver, muscle, GI tract, and brain. In adipose tissue, it activates lipoprotein lipase; it also inhibits glucagon-induced lipolysis and potentiates the effect of insulin on incorporation of fatty acids into triglycerides. It may play a role in the development of obesity because in obese animals adipose tissue is hypersensitive to some of these actions. It may increase glucose use in peripheral tissues such as muscle. GIP also has an effect on the volume and/or electrolyte composition of intestinal secretion and saliva. The relationship of GIP with insulin is integrated, and the presence of both insulin and GIP is sometimes necessary for the greater efficiency of both hormones. GIP can be considered to be a true metabolic hormone with most of its functions, like insulin, tending to increase anabolism.

Glucagon-Like Peptide-1 (GLP-1) Stimulates Insulin Secretion and Inhibits Glucagon Secretion

The structure and biological actions of pancreatic glucagon are well-documented (Chap. 11). In addition, glucagon-like substances are present within the GI mucosa. Glucagon-like peptide 1 (GLP-1) is an intestinal peptide encoded in the proglucagon gene. Its primary structure is highly conserved from ancient species to humans. The proglucagon gene is expressed in the intestinal L cells, pancreatic α cells, and some neurons in the brainstem. The majority of L cells are located in the distal jejunum and ileum. The L-cell number increases from the proximal colon to the rectum [5, 6]. GLP-1 is released into the circulation after oral ingestion of nutrients. GLP-1 is released rapidly (15 minutes) after the oral ingestion of glucose, fat, and amino acids, and after mixed meals. The nutrient-dependent signal responsible for triggering GLP-1 release is still unknown, but there is some evidence that neural and probably hormonal (e.g., GIP) factors are involved. The GLP-1 peptide is considered to be the second major incretin, along with GIP. It stimulates insulin secretion in the presence of elevated glucose levels; it also stimulates proinsulin gene expression and inhibits glucagon secretion. Since GLP-1 can lower glucose levels in noninsulin-dependent diabetes mellitus when administered in pharmacological doses, there is hope that GLP-1 agonists may prove to be useful in managing glycemic control in type 2 diabetic patients. Another glucagon-like peptide, GLP-2, is also derived from the preproglucagon precursor and may have some effects on nutrient absorption and GI tract function. Unlike GLP-1, however, it exhibits minimal effects on glucose levels. The GLP-2 peptide does appear to exert potent trophic actions on the intestinal epithelia [6].

Vasoactive Intestinal Peptide (VIP) Inhibits Gastric Acid Secretion and Stimulates Pancreatic Electrolyte and Water Secretion

This peptide, first isolated from the pig intestine, contains 28 amino acid residues and is structurally related to secretin, glucagon, and GIP. Like other members of the secretin family the entire primary structure of VIP is important for biological activity. The structure of VIP is relatively well conserved throughout the animal kingdom. The amino acid sequence of human VIP is identical to that of pigs, cows, and rats, but is slightly different in guinea pigs and chickens. Immunohistochemical studies reveal that the peptide is diffusely distributed throughout the entire length of the mammalian and avian intestinal tract (esophagus through the colon). VIP was named for its potent vasodilator and hypotensive effects [14]. It relaxes a variety of smooth muscles and antagonizes the effects of smooth muscle constrictor agents. VIP inhibits histamine and pentagastrin-stimulated gastric acid secretion. Electrolyte and water secretion by the pancreas are stimulated and bile flow is increased. VIP stimulates lipolysis, glycogenolysis, and insulin secretion, but because these actions are shared by some other members of the secretin family of hormones, these observed effects of VIP may be pharmacological rather than physiological in nature. In addition, the presence of this peptide in nerve cells and the absence of a meal-induced change in VIP plasma concentrations further argue against its role as a humoral gastroenteropancreatic hormone. The selective localization of VIP within neurons in the CNS and autonomic nervous system, especially in the superior and inferior mesenteric ganglia, the submucosal (Meissner's) and myenteric (Auerbach's) plexuses of the intestinal wall, the cerebrovascular nerves, and nerves in the female and male genitourinary tracts, suggests that its role may be restricted to that of a neurohormone acting by a neurocrine or paracrine mechanism in a variety of organs including the GI tract (Fig. 10.8).

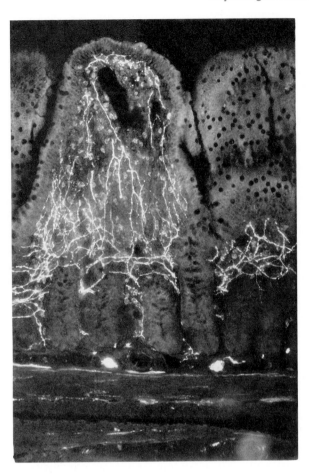

Figure 10.8 Immunoreactive VIP nerve plexus in small intestine of the rat. (Reprinted with permission from T. Hökfelt, R. Elde, O. Johansson, A. Ljungdahl, M. Schulzberg, K. Fuxe, M. Goldstein, G. Nilsson, B. Pernow, L. Terenius, D. Ganten, S. L. Jeffcoate, J. Rehfeld, and S. I. Said. 1978. "Distribution of peptide-containing neurons." In *Psychopharmacology: A generation of progress*. (pp. 39–66) M. A. Lipton, A. DiMascio, and K. F. Killam (eds.). New York: Raven Press.)

There is strong evidence that in humans and other species, the descending relaxation component of the peristaltic reflex is mediated by VIP. This transmitter is released during descending relaxation only, and its neutralization with VIP antiserum or blockade of its effect with VIP antagonists inhibits descending relaxation. Although VIP appears to be the only relaxant transmitter acting at neuromuscular junctions, its release is modulated by two other types of myenteric neurons, somatostatin neurons and opioid neurons.

Neurotensin Stimulates Pancreatic Secretion and Inhibits Gastric Motility

The tridecapeptide neurotensin (NT) was discovered and isolated from the bovine hypothalamus and subsequently found by radioimmunoassay also to be present in the GI tract (Table 10.2). Neurotensin (or a neurotensin-like peptide) is present in the discrete (N) cells rather specifically localized in the ileal mucosa of various birds and mammals. The NT-immunoreactive cells are situated in the upper two-thirds of the villi and appear to communicate with the intestinal lumen by means of microvilli. The morphological features of the NT-containing cells, which have microvilli and secretory granules located at the vascular pole, suggest that they may be sensitive to nutrient or other changes in the gut lumen. This sensitivity may provide the stimulus for the release of the peptide into the circulation.

Peptide YY Inhibits Pancreatic Bicarbonate Secretion, Gallbladder Contraction, and Gastric Emptying

Peptide YY (PYY), neuropeptide Y (NPY), and pancreatic polypeptide (PP) are three members of a family of regulatory peptides that exhibit considerable sequence homology [33, 34, 36, 37]. In pigs, there are 18 sequence identities (50% homology) between PP and PYY or NPY and 25 sequence identities (70% homology) between PYY and NPY. PYY and NPY are evolutionarily highly conserved peptides, with very similar sequences in most mammalian species.

PYY is localized in endocrine cells of the intestinal mucosa from various species. PYY-immunoreactive cells are numerous in the terminal ileum, colon, and rectum, whereas only a few such cells are found in the duodenum and jejunum. PYY cells extend from the basal lamina to the gut lumen. PYY is an intestinal hormone released into the blood in response to a meal or after intestinal perfusion with oleic acid. In contrast to PYY, NPY is strictly a neuropeptide. NPY is expressed in central neurons located in the hypothalamus and caudal brainstem, where the peptide plays a key role in neuroendocrine mechanisms governing food intake and body weight regulation, as well as reproductive hormone secretions (Chap. 11). NPY nerve fibers are also found throughout the intestinal tract, with the largest number in the upper small intestine. In the small intestine the presence of NPY-containing nerve cell bodies in the submucosal and myenteric ganglia indicates an intrinsic origin of NPY fibers. The distribution of NPY fibers in all layers of the gut wall suggests multiple functions of NPY, including a role in the regulation of intramural neuronal activities, smooth muscle tone, local blood flow, and epithelial transport. PYY and NPY have potent antisecretory effects in the small intestine. There is evidence that the hormone PPY and the neurotransmitter NPY are involved in the regulation of fluid and electrolyte secretion, motility, and blood flow in the intestine. There is preferential localization of PYY-preferring receptors negatively coupled to adenylate cyclase and cAMP production in small intestinal crypt cells. Because PYY and NPY are the most potent physiological agents thus far identified as inhibitors of intestinal electrolyte secretion, the cryptic PYY receptor represents a promising target for antidiarrheal drugs [33, 34].

Substance P (SP) May Serve as a Physiological Modulator of Intestinal Smooth Muscle Contractility

Stimulation of the abdominal vagal nerve releases a substance whose actions on smooth muscle motor activity are not blocked by atropine. This substance, therefore, is not acetylcholine (Chap. 14). This peptide consists of 11 amino acid residues (Table 10.2) and is called substance P (SP) in reference to an early preparation of active gut extract. This was the first neuropeptide to be found in both the brain and gut. SP is found localized within nerve fibers in all areas of the gut wall, including the two muscle layers (the myenteric and submucosal plexuses), the mucosa, and the submucosa. Substance P is also distributed widely but selectively within the brain and spinal column; it is structurally related to a number of peptides present within the skin of anuran (frogs, toads) amphibians (see Fig. 10.17). Substance P is a member of a family of structurally related peptides (neurokinin A, neurokinin B), called tachykinins, that are involved in the regulation of many biologic processes. Diversity in the generation of tachykinin peptides arises due to encoding of these peptides from multiple genes as well as by mechanisms of alternative mRNA processing and differential post-translational processing. These peptides are neurotransmitters and/or neuromodulator substances, and they bring about their actions mainly by activating three primary types of neurokinin receptors, NK-1, NK-2, and NK-3 [36, 37].

The peripheral action site of SP outside the CNS seems to be mainly on smooth muscle. SP lowers arterial blood pressure and is recognized as one of the most potent vasodilators. Almost all peripheral tissues contain SP-positive nerves, often in close association with blood vessels and secretory cells. The high potency of SP, together with its presence in intrinsic nerves in the gut, suggests that SP may function as a physiological modulator of smooth muscle activity in gut tissue. Intestinal peristalsis changes from bidirectional to unidirectional shortly after birth, concomitant with the appearance in the myenteric plexus of peptidergic nerve fibers. A role for SP in the regulation of intestinal peristalsis has been suggested, and SP may be involved in the postnatal induction of propulsive motility. Intraventricular injections of SP have a marked antidipsogenic effect without depressing food intake or producing other behavioral modifications. It has been suggested that because SP is found in the brain, it may be a natural satiator of thirst.

Somatostatin Inhibits Gastrin and Hydrochloric Acid Release

This tetradecapeptide (Table 10.2), referred to as somatostatin to describe its role as a GH release-inhibiting hormone, is also localized to specialized D cells of the GI mucosa. Highest concentrations are localized to the gastric antrum with progressively decreasing levels found within the small intestine and colon. Somatostatin-producing cells of the stomach have long cytoplasmic processes that terminate on other cell types (Fig. 10.9), including the gastrin-producing and HCl-producing cells [18]. The release of gastrin and hydrochloric

Figure 10.9 Schematic drawing showing a three-dimensional arrangement of the somatostatin cells and their processes in an antral gland. (From Larsson, L. I., et al. 1979. Somatostatin cell processes or pathways for paracrine secretion. *Science* 205:1393–4, with permission. ©1979 by the American Association for the Advancement of Science.)

acid, respectively, from these cells is tonically inhibited by somatostatin. Somatostatin is also localized to D cells of the pancreatic islets and may regulate glucagon and insulin secretion (Chap. 11). The observation that long processes may emanate from other endocrine cells of the gut epithelium suggests that other GI hormones may function by a paracrine mode of control [22].

There are two naturally-occurring bioactive forms of somatostatin (SST) (Figs 6.7 and 6.8), the tetradecapeptide SST-14 (S14) and the N-terminally extended form SST-28 (S28). S14 is the predominant SST present in the D cells of the pancreatic islets and the gastric antrum, whereas S28 is the predominant form in the epithelial D cells of the duodenal, jejunal, ileal, and colonic mucosa. After a mixed meal, SST-like immunoreactivity increases in the peripheral circulation. Changes in peripheral SST have been shown to arise mainly from gut SST, and, indeed, in humans the postprandial rise in SST consists predominantly of SST-28.

Gastrin-Releasing Peptide (GRP) Stimulates Release of Several GI Hormones, Pancreatic Secretion, and Motility

Bombesin is a tetradecapeptide originally isolated from frog (*Bombina*) skin. Bombesin-like immunoreactivity was subsequently localized to both the mammalian brain and GI tract. A 27-amino-acid gastrin-releasing peptide (GRP) was isolated from the porcine gut that has a C-terminal decapeptide sequence identical to the C-terminal decapeptide of frog skin bombesin, except for a Gln/His interchange at position 20 (Fig. 10.10). The C-terminal

	1	2	3	4	5	6	7	8	9	10	11	12	13	14
Bombesin	pGlu–	Gln–	Arg–	Leu–	Gly–	Asn–	Gln–	Trp–	Ala–	Val–	Gly–	His–	Leu–	Met–NH$_2$

	1	2	3	4	5	6	7	8	9	10	11	12	13
Gastrin-Releasing Peptide	Ala–	Pro–	Val–	Ser–	Val–	Gly–	Gly–	Gly–	Thr–	Val–	Leu–	Ala–	Lys–

	14	15	16	17	18	19	20	21	22	23	24	25	26	27
	Met–	Tyr–	Pro–	Arg–	Gly–	Asn–	His–	Trp–	Ala–	Val–	Gly–	His–	Leu–	Met–NH$_2$

Figure 10.10 Primary structures of bombesin and porcine gastrin-releasing peptide (GRP).

octapeptide fragment of GRP retains full biological activity, as does the C-terminal bombesin octapeptide, suggesting that the previously demonstrated effects of bombesin in the mammal might mediate through a GRP receptor. However, it has been shown that frogs have both bombesin and GRP. Frogs express distinctly different GRP and bombesin mRNAs in stomach extracts. The homology between frog GRP and mammalian GRP pro-hormones is significantly higher than between frog GRP and frog bombesin prohormones. The relatively high levels of bombesin mRNA in frog brain might suggest that mammals, like frogs, will have a bombesin mRNA expressed in the CNS that is distinct from GRP mRNA [33]. GRP exerts a variety of stimulatory effects, including release of gastrin and several other GI hormones, intestinal and pancreatic secretions, and intestinal motility.

GRP is present in nerve fibers in the antral mucosa. Bombesin produces atropine-resistant stimulation of gastrin release from isolated rat stomach. This stimulation of gastrin release is not accompanied by a reciprocal decrease in SST release; therefore it clearly differs from the pattern produced by cholinergic stimulation of gastrin secretion. Electrical stimulation of the vagus nerve causes release of immunoreactive GRP from the stomach of anesthetized pigs or sheep. GRP can therefore be added to the growing list of peptides (substance P, neurotensin, CCK, VIP, SST, endorphins) that are present in ECL cells and in central and peripheral neurons.

Motilin Stimulates GI Motility and Emptying of Chyme into the Small Intestine

Motilin is a candidate peptide hormone containing 22 amino acid residues which bears structural similarity to ghrelin [21] but not to any other known GI hormone [17]. The peptide is present in highest concentration in the duodenum, where it is present in ECL cells of the mucosa, and in lesser amounts throughout the remainder of the small intestine. The peptide was named for its ability to stimulate gastric motor activity. The potent actions of motilin on GI motility and emptying of chyme into the small intestine suggest possible physiological roles for the peptide. Motilin regulates contractions that occur in 2-hour cycles after meals and that serve to empty the intestine of residual contents. The start of each cycle, which begins in the stomach and travels caudally throughout the intestine, coincides with a peak of circulating motilin. Infusion of motilin can initiate a premature cycle, whereas infusion of motilin antiserum disrupts the phase of maximal contraction. The stimulus for secretion of motilin remains unclear but may be in response to duodenal alkalinization.

Ghrelin is a Multifunctional Peptide that Stimulates Gastric Acid Secretion and Gastric Motility

Ghrelin is a 28-amino-acid peptide with a fatty acid chain (8-carbon acyl group, or octanoyl group) on the N-terminal third amino acid. The peptide was originally isolated from the stomach [7]. It is now known to be expressed primarily in the fundus of the stomach in the oxyntic gland. These ghrelin-producing cells are located close to capillaries rather than the lumen of the stomach, and they appear to be the source of the majority of circulating ghrelin [1]. Ghrelin increases gastric acid secretion and gastric motility, probably by exerting both local and central effects. Ghrelin's prokinetic actions in the gut are similar to those of motilin, as described above. Its central actions appear to be exerted in the brainstem and mediated by the vagal innervation of the GI tract [7]. The ghrelin molecule was discovered on the basis of its GH-stimulating properties, as a ligand [19] for the GH-secretotogue receptor (GHS-R) [15] (Chap. 12). It has since been found to be a potent appetite stimulant, and it is likely that it plays this physiological role, as well as several others, in the control of energy homeostasis [21]. Ghrelin's involvement in the control of food intake and GH secretion is discussed in more detail in Chapters 11 and 12, respectively.

Other Putative Gut Hormones Exert Specific Actions in the GI Tract

A number of other biologically active peptides are also distributed throughout the GI mucosa. They too can be considered candidate hormones. Considering the size of the GI tract, it is not surprising that such a large a number of hormones are distributed throughout this complex organ.

Urogastrone/EGF. Pregnancy causes an improvement in the symptoms of duodenal ulceration. Extracts of urine from pregnant and nonpregnant women, as well as those from

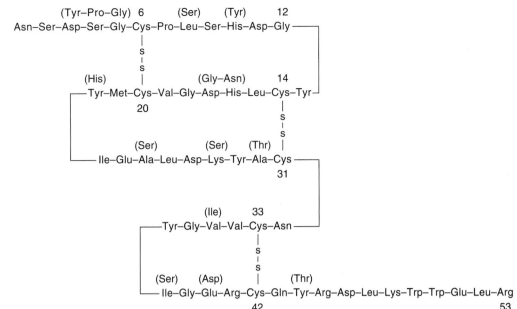

(Tyr–Pro–Gly) 6   (Ser)   (Tyr)   12
Asn–Ser–Asp–Ser–Gly–Cys–Pro–Leu–Ser–His–Asp–Gly
                            |
                            s
                            |
         (His)   s   (Gly–Asn)   14
         ─Tyr–Met–Cys–Val–Gly–Asp–His–Leu–Cys–Tyr─
                    20 |
                                                    s
                                                    |
         (Ser)   (Ser)   (Thr) | s
         ─Ile–Glu–Ala–Leu–Asp–Lys–Tyr–Ala–Cys ─
                                            31

                        (Ile)   33
               ─Tyr–Gly–Val–Val–Cys–Asn ─
                            |
                            s
                            |
         (Ser)   (Asp)   s   (Thr)
         ─Ile–Gly–Glu–Arg–Cys–Gln–Tyr–Arg–Asp–Leu–Lys–Trp–Trp–Glu–Leu–Arg
                        42   53

Figure 10.11 Amino acid sequence of human β-urogastrone. Positional amino acid differences between β-urogastrone and mouse EGF are shown in parentheses.

men, afford protection against experimentally induced ulceration in dogs. These extracts cause inhibition of gastric acid secretion and also promote fibroblastic proliferation and epithelialization of the mucosa. Purification of urine led to the isolation of two fractions, the *beta* and *gamma* urogastrones, which had different physical properties but the same biological potency. The structure of β-urogastrone consists of a single polypeptide chain of 53 residues with three internal disulfide bonds, whereas γ-urogastrone lacks the C-terminal arginine residue. Although urogastrone is structurally different from other known GI peptides, it is strikingly similar to mouse epidermal growth factor, EGF (Fig. 10.11). Mouse EGF (see Fig. 12.17) is a powerful epithelial mitogen, and urogastrone is equipotent in activity; both peptides are also equally potent in suppressing gastric acid secretion in a number of animals. Urogastrone is considered the human hormonal equivalent of mEGF.

Immunochemical studies have localized urogastrone-like activity to the submaxillary glands, to Brunner's glands of the small intestine, and to saliva and gastric juice. Studies in ulcer patients confirmed the ability of urogastrone to suppress basal gastric acid secretion, and acid secretion in response to pentagastrin also could be partially blocked. The action of the peptide was specific as salivary, pancreatic, and bile secretions were not affected similarly by any doses of the peptide. Mouse EGF has a trophic effect on the oxyntic gland mucosa, but, unlike the effects of gastrin, has no such trophic effects on duodenal or colonic mucosa. Secretin inhibits the trophic effects of pentagastrin on the oxyntic mucosa, but not that of mEGF; the trophic action of mEGF is thus not mediated through increased serum gastrin levels. EGF appears to play an important role in the development of the neonatal intestinal epithelium. Administration of EGF in mature animals with a normal intestinal tract results in increased mucosal DNA content and proliferative activity and increased substrate absorption from the intestine. Continuous intravenous infusion of EGF reduces mucosal atrophy and maintains disaccharidase activity during parenteral alimentation. Numerous other studies have supported the concept that EGF is an important trophic hormone of the intestinal mucosa [4].

Villikinin.   Villi are a characteristic cellular feature of the mucosa of the small intestine. The fingerlike villi exhibit a number of peculiar movements, such as contraction and relaxation and a pendular swaying, and each villus moves independently of its neighbors. It is believed that lymph flow within these structures is hastened by their movements. Villous movement is affected by mechanical and chemical stimuli, nervous stimulation, and extracts of intestinal mucosa. Villous motility of an isolated jejunal loop transplanted into the carotid-jugular circulation was shown to be stimulated by intraduodenal administration of HCl. This observation suggested that villous activity might be regulated by a humoral factor. In cross-circulation experiments involving carotid-jugular anastomoses between two animals, administration of HCl into the stomach of one animal caused a substantial increase in villus activity in both animals. Other experiments provide evidence that acid chyme releases a substance that enters the bloodstream to stimulate villous movement. A substance that stimulates villous motility was extracted from the intestinal mucosa and named villikinin to describe its physiological action. Villikinin activity is found only in mucosa of the small intestine, with highest concentrations occurring in the duodenal mucosa of a number of mammalian species, including humans. Villikinin activity increases in human urine after a meal and after intraduodenal acid administration. The substance does not exhibit actions characteristic of the other GI hormones, therefore ruling any of them out as the putative humoral messenger. Villikinin appears to be a polypeptide, but little is known about its chemistry.

Enkephalins.   Endorphins, so-called opiate peptides, which include the enkephalins and β-endorphin, play important roles in CNS function. Enkephalins have been demonstrated in the ECL cells and nerves of the digestive tract. Opiate drugs, well known for their powerful actions on the GI tract, exhibit pronounced effects on GI motility and secretion. The opiate peptides also profoundly affect activity of the GI tract, by mechanisms identical to opiate drugs. They act as presynaptic or postsynaptic inhibitors and suppress the firing of most neurons tested. For example, opiate peptides specifically inhibit electrically induced contractions of the ileal smooth muscle by inhibiting neurotransmitter (acetylcholine) release. Opiate peptides are potent inhibitors of bicarbonate and protein secretion from the pancreas, suggesting that they affect the secretory mechanisms common to CCK and secretin on pancreatic secretion.

Enkephalins stimulate gastric acid secretion in dogs and also enhance histamine-stimulated acid secretion by isolated rat parietal cells. There are opioid receptors in the gastric muscle layers and in the mucosa. Naloxone and other opiate receptor antagonists inhibit acid secretory responses to food in humans. Large doses of naloxone also inhibit feeding-induced acid secretion in humans. These results suggest that endogenous opioid peptides have some physiological stimulatory role in the regulation of acid secretion in the stomach. However, morphine and some opioid peptides inhibit acid secretion. Both stimulatory and inhibitory opiate receptors may exist in the stomach. The major roles of endorphins in the GI tract may be to act as neurotransmitters and neuromodulators of autonomic nervous system actions on GI motility and secretion.

Hormones in Milk.   Besides the numerous hormones derived from the mucosal lining of the gut and the enteric neurons, hormones are also delivered to the lumen by the way of milk [20]; the low proteolytic activity of the newborn may enhance the availability of peptide hormones found in milk so that they can act locally (as hormones) or be taken up by the gut to enter the systemic circulation [20].

Autonomic Nervous System Control of GI Function

Although hormones play a dominant role in the control of GI function, the autonomic nervous system subserves a similar function [10, 25]. "Acting singly and in concert, neural and hormonal mechanisms control the transverse flow of materials across the mucosa and the axial flow of digesta within the lumen" [24]. In addition, "The overlap of neural and endocrine segments, and the continuously changing character and location of intraluminal stimuli, engender the simultaneous release of several hormones whose interplay on digestive target tissues may be augmentary or inhibitory. The infusion of their effects determines the orderly progress and digestion of food."

The initial phase of neural control of GI function is regulated centrally by the anticipation of food, the so-called cephalic phase. Subsequently, local neural and hormonal mechanisms are activated within the GI tract by mechanical and chemical stimuli derived from ingested foods. The stomach and small intestine are richly innervated by intrinsic and extrinsic nerves. The intrinsic nerves comprise various plexuses that lie between the longitudinal and circular smooth muscle layers of the gut (Auerbach's plexus) and beneath the submucosal muscle layer (Meissner's plexus). These plexuses are innervated by extrinsic nerves derived mainly from the vagus nerve. Axons from neurons within the plexuses synapse with muscle fibers and glandular elements of the gut. Parasympathetic cholinergic (acetylcholine) and sympathetic adrenergic (norepinephrine) neurons affect smooth muscle motor activity and mucosal glandular secretion. Acetylcholine, for example, is a potent stimulus to gastric acid secretion. The intrinsic neurons of the gut contain a number of neurohormones such as VIP, substance P, SST, NPY, and one or more endorphins.

Gastrointestinal Hormone Mechanisms of Action

Like other peptide hormones, the GI hormones interact with cell membrane receptors to stimulate or inhibit second messenger production [31]. Members of the secretin family of hormones (secretin, glucagon, VIP, and GIP) activate adenylate cyclase, which results in an elevation of intracellular levels of target tissue cAMP. Several models of GI hormone-action mechanisms are provided.

Integrated Actions of Gastrin, Acetylcholine and Histamine Control Gastric Acid Secretion

The regulation of gastric acid secretion by the parietal cell involves complex interactions between a number of humoral or neurohormonal factors [25]. Stimulation of GI secretions (e.g., HCl, pepsinogen, secretion from Brunner's glands) is, as for most secretory processes, regulated by intracellular increases in cAMP. Although gastrin is a potent secretogogue of gastric acid secretion, acetylcholine and histamine are also stimulatory to HCl secretion. The cholinergic neural pathways involved in gastrin and HCl secretion are unresolved. Histamine (see Fig. 6.12) is present in large amounts in the oxyntic mucosa of humans and other mammals. In addition to gastrin and acetylcholine receptors, parietal cells possess histamine (H_2) receptors. The actions of histamine are mediated through cAMP. Although gastrin and acetylcholine also stimulate parietal cell HCl secretion and potentiate the actions of each other and histamine, their actions do not involve cAMP, but rather an activation of phospholipase C and the production of inositol triphosphate and diacylglycerol as second messengers. Somatostatin and prostaglandins of the E series are inhibitory to HCl secretion by a mechanism involving inhibition of adenylate cyclase activation [27, 34]. A hypothetical model depicting the control of parietal cell HCl secretion is provided (Fig. 10.12).

Synergistic Actions of Secretin and CCK Control Exocrine Pancreatic Secretion

Pancreatic acinar cells possess two distinct classes of receptors coupled to the production of different second messengers. Secretin (and VIP in some species) elevates pancreatic cAMP levels and stimulates amylase secretion. Cholecystokinin (and related structures) also stimulates

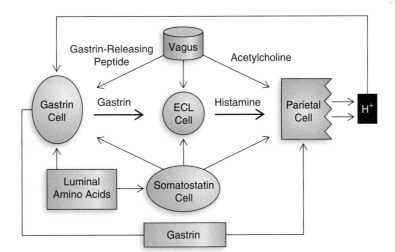

Figure 10.12 This diagram represents the interaction of the gastrin, enterochromaffin-like (ECL), parietal, and somatostatin cells. Both antral and fundic somatostatin cells appear to exert inhibitory influences on gastrin, ECL, and parietal cells, respectively. Neurotransmitter substances from either the vagus or the intrinsic gastric neural system are responsible for modulation of each of the cells and their secretory activity. Luminal amino acids stimulate gastrin release, whereas luminal protons inhibit gastrin release. Systemic secretion of gastrin primarily drives ECL cells to secrete histamine but may play some part in parietal cell secretion, although a trophic regulatory effect is more likely. The ECL cells release histamine, which presumably functions in a paracrine fashion to stimulate parietal cell secretion. Inhibitory actions of hormones are noted (–). (Reprinted by permission of the publisher from "A new look at an old hormone: Gastrin," Modlin and Tang. *Trends in Endocrinology and Metabolism* 4:51–57.©1993 by Elsevier Science Inc.)

Figure 10.13
Hypothetical model for the synergistic actions of CCK and secretin (S) and second messengers on pancreatic enzyme and bicarbonate secretion.

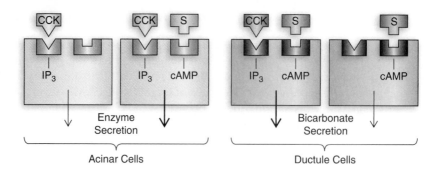

pancreatic amylase secretion and appears to do so by mobilizing cellular Ca^{2+}. Secretogogues that increase Ca^{2+} efflux and cAMP also cause depolarization of acinar cells. Acinar cells within the same acinus are electrically coupled; this coupling may provide a mechanism for amplifying the response of acinar cells to low concentrations of secretogogues. The result may be the potentiation of the CCK action by secretin on acinar enzyme secretion, because the action mechanism of each secretogogue is different and not funneled through the same transduction/second messenger system. Synergism between CCK and secretin probably reflects their coupling to different signal transduction pathways: adenylate cyclase in the case of secretin, and phospholipase C, phosphoinositide turnover, and Ca^{2+} mobilization in the case of CCK (Fig. 10.13).

The GI Hormones can also Exert Trophic Actions

The GI mucosa is sensitive to the trophic effects of several peptides. Although gastrin increases RNA, DNA, and protein synthesis in the stomach and duodenum, it does not appear to be trophic to the jejunoileum. The mucosal gastrin receptor has been characterized. Specific gastrin binding is present in the oxyntic gland and duodenal mucosa, but is absent from the antral mucosa, liver, spleen, and kidney. Fasting decreases the circulating level of gastrin and the number of gastrin binding sites, whereas refeeding increases the plasma gastrin levels and restores the receptor number to normal. Treatment of fasted animals with pentagastrin prevents the decrease in receptor number. Thus, gastric mucosal receptors are autoregulated, that is, their number is influenced by the availability of gastrin; they exhibit up-regulation in response to the hormone (Chap. 4).

Gastrin stimulates RNA, DNA, and protein synthesis along the entire length of the gut, with the exception of the esophagus and antrum. The pancreas is also a target for the trophic action of gastrin. These trophic effects are direct actions of gastrin and are not mediated through the action of another hormone. These observations suggest that increased food intake increases circulating levels of gastrin, which then increases gastrointestinal receptor numbers. This allows an enhanced trophic response to the hormone, which enables the GI tract to better use the increased metabolic substrates available.

By gene targeting, G-protein-coupled CCK-B/gastrin-receptor deficient mice were generated. These mice showed remarkable atrophy of the gastric mucosa, even in the presence of severe gastrinema. Both parietal cells and ECL cells were severely decreased in number. These results clearly demonstrate the CCK-B/gastrin receptor to be essential for the physiological as well as the pathological proliferation of gastric mucosal cells [28].

EGF appears to play an important role in the development of neonatal intestinal epithelium. Administration of EGF in mature animals with normal intestines results in increased mucosal DNA content and proliferative activity, and increased substrate absorption from the intestine. Continuous intravenous infusion of EGF reduces mucosal atrophy and maintains disaccharidase activity during parenteral alimentation. Numerous other studies support the concept that EGF is an important trophic hormone of the intestinal mucosa [4].

Summary of the Neuroendocrine Control of GI Function

At the close of the nineteenth century, the digestive system was assumed to be solely under nervous control. The discovery of secretin introduced the concept of hormones in the control of GI functions. In recent years, a complex system of regulation of these functions has been revealed. In addition to the generally accepted influence of the autonomic nervous system (sympathetic and parasympathetic) and of hormones (peptides), a system of peptide-containing nerves and local-acting peptide-releasing cells has been found to be important. Therefore, regulatory peptides can exert a general humoral control via the blood supply, a local paracrine action, or a neurotransmitter/neuromodulator action when released from nerves [10].

Food is taken into the mouth where ptyalin (salivary α-amylase) initiates digestion of starch. Food in the mouth is responsible for a reflex (cephalic) stimulation of gastric acid secretion. The food then transverses the esophagus to enter into the stomach through the gastroesophageal junction. Local reflex stimuli, resulting from distension of the stomach and from partially digested food products, particularly peptides and amino acids, are stimulatory to gastric acid secretion. Gastrin is the major humoral stimulus to hydrochloric acid secretion from the parietal cells of the gastric mucosa. Gastrin is also indirectly stimulatory to pepsinogen secretion from the chief cells of the mucosa of the body of the stomach. The pepsinogen is acted on by HCl and split into the active enzyme pepsin. Increased gastric acid secretion then becomes inhibitory to further gastrin secretion. Gastrin and local reflex stimulation may then relax the pyloric sphincter and allow a bolus of food (chyme) to enter the first segment of the small intestine, the duodenum. The acid present in the chyme is stimulatory to secretin release from cells present within the duodenal mucosa. This bloodborne messenger then travels to the exocrine pancreas to cause water and bicarbonate release. These secretory products neutralize the acid present within the small intestine. Fats and proteins in the chyme stimulate the secretion of CCK from cells within the duodenal, jejunal, and ileal mucosa. CCK is carried by the blood to the exocrine pancreas and stimulates the acinar cells to release pancreatic enzymes: α-amylase, trypsin, chymotrypsin, and pancreatic lipase. Proteases split proteins and partially degraded proteins into their constituent amino acids. CCK also contracts the gallbladder, thus releasing bile salts into the intestinal lumen. These salts emulsify the fats into smaller globules and the fats are enzymatically degraded by pancreatic lipase into FFAs and monoglycerides. Starch and its partially degraded components, oligopolysaccharides, are further degraded by pancreatic α-amylase into glucose. Glucose is stimulatory to GIP secretion and possibly GLP-1 secretion from cells of the intestinal mucosa. These humoral messengers may then stimulate the release of insulin from beta cells of the pancreatic islets. By the action of insulin on the liver, the glucose now within the portal vein is taken up into the liver cells where it may be formed into starch and stored (Fig. 10.14).

GIP and possibly other hormones of the small intestine, released in response to gastric acid, glucose, fats, and protein products, may provide feedback to the stomach to inhibit further secretion of gastric acid. Certain intrinsic neurons and other neuron-like cells within the intestinal lining contain peptide hormones such as SST, VIP, substance P, and others. These neuropeptides, acting by neurocrine or paracrine mechanisms, control local secretory events and smooth muscle activity. The autonomic nervous system, particularly through its cholinergic component, plays an equally important augmentary role in the movement and digestion of foods within the GI tract. A summary of the roles of chemical messengers in the control of GI function is provided (Table 10.3).

Pathophysiology

There are two well-documented examples of direct involvement by GI hormones in abnormal clinical conditions [32]. Most endocrine tumors of the GI system originate in the pancreatic islets. Although these tumors secrete hormones that are normally produced there (e.g., glucagon and insulin), these tumors may also secrete VIP or gastrin. Vasoactive intestinal peptide stimulates intestinal water secretion, and tumors consisting of VIP-secreting cells (VIPomas) are responsible for *pancreatic cholera* or the *watery diarrhea syndrome* (or syndrome of profuse watery diarrhea). Patients with the Zollinger–Ellison syndrome (gastrinoma) have high circulating gastrin levels (hypergastrinemia) of tumor origin. The overproduction of gastric acid usually results in severe duodenal ulcer formation. Two different types of the Zollinger–Ellison syndrome may exist, type I, due to a hyperplasia of the antral G cells, and type II, due to gastrinoma of the pancreatic islets.

Regulation of the lower esophageal sphincter (LES), which is important in preventing the reflux of gastric contents, may be regulated by one or more GI hormones. Gastrin and motilin can contract the LES, whereas VIP is particularly potent as an inhibitor of LES tone. *Achalasia* is a condition where food accumulates in the esophagus because the gastroesophageal junction fails to relax. There is evidence that the smooth muscle of this junction is hypersensitive to normal circulating levels of gastrin, which could account for the prolonged contraction characteristic of this condition. Gastroesophageal reflux, on the other hand, is due to abnormal

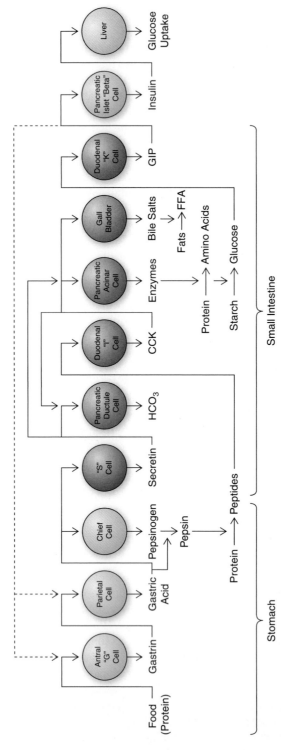

Figure 10.14 Summary scheme of hormone-metabolite control of GI function. Solid lines indicate stimulatory influences; dashed lines represent inhibitory stimuli.

TABLE 10.3 Physiological roles or effects of the GI hormones and candidate hormones within the GI tract

Hormone	Physiological roles*
Gastrin	↑ gastric acid selection, gastrointestinal growth, and antral motility
Secretin	↑ pancreatic and biliary bicarbonate secretion; ↑ CCK-stimulated pancreatic enzyme secretion
CCK	↑ gallbladder contraction and pancreatic enzyme secretion; ↓ gastric emptying; ↑ growth of the exocrine pancreas, satiety signal
GIP	↓ gastric acid secretion; ↑ glucose-mediated insulin release
Ghrelin	gastric acid secretion; GI motility
Somatostatin	↓ antral gastrin secretion
VIP	↑ smooth muscle relaxation; ↑ blood flow and intestinal secretion
Gastrin-releasing peptide (GRP)	↑ gastrin secretion, gallbladder contraction, pancreatic enzyme secretion, and gastrointestinal motility; ↓ gastric acid secretion (when delivered intracisternally)
Bulbogastrone	↓ gastric acid secretion
Urogastrone	↓ gastric acid secretion; ↑ oxyntic gland growth
Enteroglucagon	Unknown
Villikinin	↑ villous movement and lymph flow
Enkephalins	Unknown (neuromodulator?) ↑ or ↓ gastric acid secretion
Neurotensin	Unknown (neuromodulator?)
Substance P	Unknown, possibly modulates gut motility and mucosal secretions
Motilin	↑ gastrointestinal motility
Histamine	↑ gastric acid secretion by parietal cells
Prostaglandins	↑ mucus production by the stomach

*Arrows indicate increased/stimulated (↑) or decreased/inhibited (↓) activity in response to the hormone.

relaxation of the sphincter, and it is claimed that in some patients with this condition gastrin levels are low. The available data, however, are controversial.

GIP-containing cells are reported to be most numerous in duodenal samples from patients with low gastric secretory activity and less numerous in patients with duodenal ulcer disease. These observations correlate well with the proposed role of this hormone in the inhibition of gastric acid secretion.

Pernicious anemia is the result of an autoimmune process in which the gastric fundus undergoes atrophy and parietal cells are destroyed. As a result of ablation of the parietal cell mass, varying degrees of hypochlorhydria result. During this process, unregulated hypergastrinemia appears to reflect the lack of an acid feedback effect on the G cell and culminates in a profound trophic effect, predominantly evident in ECL (enterochromaffin-like) cell hyperplasia. Under physiologic conditions, ECL cells multiply by self-replication, and replication is greatly increased under the influence of gastrin. Consequent to sustained elevation of circulating gastrin levels, ECL cells initially undergo hyperplasia, followed by development of micronodules and finally carcinoids [27].

A number of GI hormones have proven useful in clinical practice. Gastrin is used for testing the potential for gastric acid secretion. Pentagastrin (Fig. 10.2), which is commercially inexpensive, is usually used in these studies. CCK is used in the evaluation of gallbladder function; this hormone is also used to test for pancreatic exocrine function. Secretin has been used in the treatment of duodenal ulcer because it is inhibitory to gastric acid secretion and stimulatory to pancreatic bicarbonate ion secretion. Secretin and glucagon stimulate tumor gastrin release (in contrast to their inhibitory effects on antral release of the hormone) and are used in the diagnosis of the Zollinger–Ellison syndrome. A summary of pathophysiological states associated with G1 tract dysfunction is provided (Table 10.4).

Evolutionary Relationships of the Gut Hormones

The gut hormones are localized to specific cells distributed throughout the GI tract. Most interesting, however, is that many of the gut hormones are also found in a variety of other tissues, including in the pancreas, pituitary, in neurons of the central and peripheral nervous systems, and in the skin of some vertebrates. Within each of these tissues, they regulate specific functions. In the hypothalamus of the brain, SST regulates pituitary release of GH; in the pancreas this peptide may regulate insulin and glucagon secretion; in the antrum of the stomach, SST controls gastrin secretion.

TABLE 10.4 Endocrine pathophysiology of GI disorders

Achalasia
Failure of gastroesophageal sphincter to relax (and food accumulates in the esophagus). May be due to smooth muscle hypersensitivity to gastrin.

Anorexia nervosa
Decreased desire to eat. Possibly due to increased CCK secretion or increased sensitivity to CCK. May also relate to decreased appetite in aging individuals.

Bulimia nervosa
Recurrent episodes of uncontrolled eating. Possibly due to lowered CCK secretion.

Cholera
Cholera toxin irreversibly activates intestinal cell adenylate cyclase. This results in enhanced intestinal fluid secretion leading to dehydration and death if not corrected.

Chronic idiopathic* constipation
Possibly due to elevated circulating levels of motilin.

Disordered gastric emptying
Possibly due to hypopyloric valve dysfunction.

Gastric (peptic) ulcers
Multiple causes: enhanced HCl secretion resulting from increased parietal cell stimulation (e.g., by gastrin as in gastrinemia); decreased PGE_2 secretion resulting in: (a) increased HCl secretion, (b) decreased mucus production (e.g., as induced by aspirin) resulting in epithelial-cell damage by HCl; enhanced vagal (cholinergic stimulation; enhanced histamine secretion; etc.).

Gastrin and cancer
Gastrin may be a trophic factor for several cancer cells, and gastrin receptors have been identified in colonic mucosa, adenocarcinoid, and pancreatic tumor cells.

Gastroesophageal reflux
Possibly due to hypogastrinemia and low pressure.

Hypergastrinemia (Zollinger–Ellison syndrome)
Type I: G-cell hyperplasia (may be due to hypochlorhydria/achlorhydria due to pernicious anemia).
Type II: Gastrinoma (gastrinoma syndrome).

Hypochlorhydric disease states
Pernicious anemia is the result of an autoimmune process in which the gastric fundus undergoes atrophy and parietal cells are destroyed. (Achlorhydric anemia: lowered levels of gastric acid result in enhanced, uninhibited, gastrin secretion. This results in hypertrophy and hyperplasia of ECL cells, often resulting in neoplasia.)

Idiopathic delay in gastric emptying
Possibly as directly above.

Pancreatic cholera (watery diarrhea syndrome)
Due to excess VIP secretion (VIPoma syndrome).

* Idiopathic: "Without clear pathogenesis or disease without recognizable cause, as if of spontaneous origin."

The skin of anuran amphibians contains a number of biologically active peptides. Two of these peptides, cerulein and phyllocerulein, from related species of frogs (Fig. 10.15), contain the C-terminal pentapeptide sequence found in gastrin and CCK [5, 8]. A peptide containing the C-terminal octapeptide of CCK has been found within the brain of sheep. These structurally related peptides would be expected to have been derived from

$$SO_3H$$
Gastrin$_{(17)}$ (pyro)Glu–Gly–Pro–Trp–Leu–Glu–Glu–Glu–Glu–Glu–Ala–Tyr–Gly–Trp–Met–Asp–Phe–NH$_2$

$$SO_3H$$
CCK$_{(17-33)}$ –Asp–Pro–Ser–His–Arg–Ile–Ser–Asp–Arg–Asp–Tyr–Met–Gly–Trp–Met–Asp–Phe–NH$_2$

$$SO_3H$$
Cerulein   (pyro)Glu–Gln–Asp–Tyr–Thr–Gly–Trp–Met–Asp–Phe–NH$_2$

$$SO_3H$$
Phyllocerulein   (pyro)Glu–Glu–Tyr–Thr–Gly–Trp–Met–Asp–Phe–NH$_2$

Figure 10.15
CCK-gastrin family of peptides.

```
                  SO₃ SO₃
                   |   |
Cionin       Asn–Tyr–Tyr–Gly–Trp–Met–Asp–Phe–NH₂


                  SO₃
                   |
CCK          –Asp–Tyr–Met–Gly–Trp–Met–Asp–Phe–NH₂


                 (SO₃)
                   |
Gastrin      –Glu–Ala–Tyr–Gly–Trp–Met–Asp–Phe–NH₂
```

Figure 10.16 Structure of cionin isolated from the protochordate *Ciona intestinalis* compared to the C-terminal sequences of gastrin and CCK. Note that cionin is a perfect hybrid of gastrin and CCK with sulfated Tyr in both positions 6 and 7 from the C terminus. (Modified from Johnson and Rehfeld [18].)

a common ancestral molecule by gene duplication and divergence. A CCK-related peptide has been found in the brain and gut of cyclostomes and representatives of the agnathans, the oldest of the vertebrates. Immunoreactive gastrin has even been discovered in gut extracts of certain molluscan species and also in ganglia of an insect. Other hormones of the gut and brain are also related to peptides found in the skin of amphibians and in glands of mollusks.

Gastrin, CCK, and cerulein have been proposed to originate from a common ancestor during evolution. An evaluation of the evolutionary tree at a point near the stem of the vertebrate branch has revealed the existence of a novel neuropeptide, cionin, in the prochordate *Ciona intestinalis*, which is a possible common ancestor for both CCK and gastrin (Fig. 10.16). Evidence thus exists that a common C-terminal pentapeptide has been preserved over a long period of evolution.

Members of the secretin family of peptides are similar in structure, again suggesting that they are related by a common ancestry. The genes that coded for the ancestral member of this group of peptides probably underwent duplication, thus producing one or more daughter genes. These genes, through independent mutations, diverged to yield distinct, but related, peptide hormones.

Substance P is structurally similar to certain peptides found in frog skin (Fig. 10.17). These substances are referred to as *tachykinins* (from the Greek *takus* for fast) because of their rapid actions on smooth muscle. Physalaemin is found in the skin of a South American frog, *Physalaemus bigilonigerus*, and other species of this genus. The shorter peptide, phyllomedusin, is found in the skin of the Amazonian hylid frog, *Phyllomedusa bicolor*, and several related species. Eledoisin, a peptide similar in structure to SP and other tachykinins, is found in the posterior salivary glands of the Mediterranean octopus of the genus *Eledone*.

A most amazing discovery relative to gastric acid secretion has been made in frogs, the implications of which have relevance to clinical medicine [35]. In the frog *Rheobatrachus silus*, the female broods its young (tadpoles) in its stomach. Apparently, the young secrete a substance that inhibits gastric acid secretion. This substance has been identified as prostaglandin E_2. Inhibition of acid secretion presumably commences when the eggs or early stage larvae are swallowed and lasts until the young emerge from the mother's mouth as frogs (Fig. 10.18). Thus, this species of frog has apparently evolved a unique hormonal control of the environment in which the young develop. Prostaglandins are known to inhibit gastric acid secretion and also to stimulate gastric mucin secretion to form a protective barrier. It is known that nonsteroidal anti-inflammatory drugs inhibit the synthesis of prostaglandins. These drugs, therefore, can induce peptic ulcers by removing the normal protective covering of the mucosal surface normally protected by prostaglandins [35, 38].

```
Substance P      Arg–Pro–Lys–Pro–Gln–Gln–Phe–Phe–Gly–Leu–Met–NH₂
Physalaemin      pGlu–Ala–Asp–Pro–Asn–Lys–Phe–Tyr–Gly–Leu–Met–NH₂
Phyllomedusin        pGlu–Asn–Pro–Asn–Arg–Phe–Ile–Gly–Leu–Met–NH₂
Eledoisin        pGlu–Pro–Ser–Lys–Asp–Ala–Phe–Ile–Gly–Leu–Met–NH₂
```

Figure 10.17 Comparative primary structures of peptides related to substance P. Amino acid residues within the peptides located at identical positions to substance P are enclosed.

Figure 10.18 Role of a prostaglandin in protecting growth of tadpoles within the stomach of a female frog. (Adapted from "No frogs in Berlin," Nancy Lou Makris, and used by permission. *Hospital Practice* 19(2):33–46, 1984.)

Perspectives

The cellular and molecular basis for chemoreception in the gut may now have been resolved [13]. Previously unknown were the mechanisms by which cellular elements of the gut were able to detect specific species of foodstuff (amino acids, FFAs, sugars, etc.) and then respond by releasing a particular GI hormone to then regulate an effector organ/tissue (e.g., gallbladder). Taste detection is mediated by sensory cells of the tongue. Certain (brush/brush border) cells of the gut lining are also able to detect metabolic substrates (taste molecules/tastants). Ligand– (tastant–) receptor interaction results in the production of an intracellular second messenger, which then causes the release of a chemical messenger, which stimulates nearby gut ECL cells to release a hormone (e.g., gastrin, etc.).

REVIEW EXERCISES

Match the GI hormone with its cellular/anatomic source:

1. GIP   **A.** Meissner's and Auerbach's plexuses
2. CCK   **B.** D cells
3. Gastrin   **C.** K cells
4. Secretin   **D.** G cells
5. VIP   **E.** I cells
6. Somatostatin **F.** S cells

Think, analyze and discuss:

1. Pentagastrin is often used in physiological and clinical studies where the actions of gastrin are to be determined
   a. Which of the 17 amino acid residues in gastrin-17 are included in the pentagastrin molecule? Which of the 33 amino acid residues in CCK are included in the pentagastrin molecule?
   b. Would you predict that pentagastrin has the same potency as gastrin-17 at the gastrin receptor? Why or why not?
   c. Would you predict the pentagastrin would activate CCK receptors? Why or why not?
2. Secretin shares sequence identity with glucagon at 14 or 27 amino acids within the secretin molecule. Other members of the peptide family, GIP, VIP, GLP-1 and GLP-2, also possess many amino acids in common with glucagon and secretin. Would you predict that any of these peptides would exhibit any significant affinity for the receptor of another peptide in this same family? Why or why not?
3. Would antral and serum gastrin levels be high, low, or normal in a starving person? What would these levels be in a person receiving total parenteral (venous) nutrition? In both conditions, would the sensitivity to gastrin's trophic effects be increased, decreased, or unchanged?

Would the number of gastrin receptors expressed in the mucosa be increased, decreased, or unchanged? Justify your answers in terms of what you know about the control of gastrin secretion.

4. The multiplicity of CCK actions ensures optimal conditions for digestion and absorption of nutrients by the intestine. Can you name the three major actions of this peptide, including the location in the GI tract where they are exerted? Are these effects direct, or neurally mediated? Design an experiment with which you could distinguish which, if any of these effects are neurally mediated. Predict the results that you would obtain in this experiment.

5. The gastrointestinal tract is innervated by nerve fibers of the sympathetic and parasympathetic nervous systems. In general, what effects do these two divisions of the autonomic nervous system have on gastrointestinal function?

6. Secretin and CCK appear to act synergistically in stimulating pancreatic amylase release. Can you propose a cellular basis for this synergy, taking into account the signaling pathways activated by each, and the features of the acinar cells that they stimulate?

7. Nonsteroidal anti-inflammatory drugs inhibit the synthesis of prostaglandins, and can induce peptic ulcers. What function is normally ascribed to endogenous prostaglandins in the gut? Why is it that prostaglandin synthesis inhibition can lead to the development of gastric ulcers?

8. Many peptides function as chemical messengers in several different tissues, often exerting very specific and very different effects at each target organ. Somatostatin is one such hormone, as injection of relatively high concentrations of SST into an individual would be expected to have actions at three or more organs or tissues. Name three consequences of SST administration, indicating the identity of the specific target cells of SST, and describing the specific cellular effects evoked by the peptide in the different cells.

9. Pernicious anemia is an autoimmune disease that leads to the destruction of parietal cells. How does the loss of these cells lead to ECL cell hyperplasia? Describe the likely steps involved in this pathophysiological process.

References

[1] Ariyasu, H., et al. 2001. Stomach is a major source of circulating ghrelin, and feeding state determines plasma ghrelin-like immunoreactivity levels in humans. *J. Clin. Endocrinol. Metab.* 86:4753–8.

[2] Bayliss, W. M., and E. H. Starling. 1902. The mechanism of pancreatic secretion. *J. Physiol.* 28:325–53.

[3] Boden, P., M. D. Hall, and J. Hughes. 1995. Cholecystokinin receptors. *Cell. Mol. Neurobiol.* 15:545–59.

[4] Bragg, L. E., J. S. Thompson, and L. F. Rikkers. 1991. Influence of nutrient delivery on gut structure and function. *Nutrition* 7:237–43.

[5] Dimaline, R., and G. J. Dockray. 1994. Evolution of the gastrointestinal endocrine system (with special reference to gastrin and CCK). *Baillieres Clin. Endocrinol. Metab.* 8:1–24.

[6] Drucker, D. J. 2002. Biological actions and therapeutic potential of the glucagon-like peptides. *Gastroenterology* 122:531–44.

[7] Fujino, K., et al. 2003. Ghrelin induces fasted motor activity of the gastrointestinal tract in conscious fed rats. *J. Physiol.* 550:227–40.

[8] Garlicki, J., et al. 1990. Cholecystokinin receptors and vagal nerves in control of food intake in rats. *Am. J. Physiol.* 258:E40–5.

[9] Grider, J. R. 1994. Role of cholecystokinin in the regulation of gastrointestinal motility. *J. Nutr.* 124:1334S–1339S.

[10] Grossman, M. I. 1979. Neural and hormonal regulation of gastrointestinal function: an overview. *Annu. Rev. Physiol.* 41:27–33.

[11] Grube, D., and W. G. Forssmann. 1979. Morphology and function of the entero-endocrine cells. *Horm. Metab. Res.* 11:589–606.

[12] Hakanson, R., et al. 1994. The biology and physiology of the ECL cell. *Yale J. Biol. Med.* 67:123–34.

[13] Hofer, D., B. Puschel, and D. Drenckhahn. 1996. Taste receptor-like cells in the rat gut identified by expression of alpha-gustducin. *Proc. Natl. Acad. Sci. USA* 93:6631–4.

[14] Holst, J. J., and P. Schmidt. 1994. Gut hormones and intestinal function. *Baillieres Clin. Endocrinol. Metab.* 8:137–64.

[15] Howard, A. D., et al. 1996. A receptor in pituitary and hypothalamus that functions in growth hormone release. *Science* 273:974–7.

[16] Huang, S. C., et al. 1989. Importance of sulfation of gastrin or cholecystokinin (CCK) on affinity for gastrin and CCK receptors. *Peptides* 10:785–9.

[17] Itoh, Z. 1997. Motilin and clinical application. *Peptides* 18:593–608.

[18] Johnsen, A., and J. Rehfeld. 1993. Phylogeny of gastrin. In: J. W. Wals, ed. *Gastrin*, pp. 15–27.

[19] Kojima, M., et al. 1999. Ghrelin is a growth-hormone-releasing acylated peptide from stomach. *Nature* 402:656–60.

[20] Koldovsky, O. 1995. Hormones in milk. *Vitam. Horm.* 50:77–149.

[21] Korbonits, M., et al. 2004. Ghrelin—a hormone with multiple functions. *Front. Neuroendocrinol.* 25:27–68.

[22] Larsson, L. I., et al. 1979. Somatostatin cell processes as pathways for paracrine secretion. *Science* 205:1393–5.

[23] Liddle, R. A. 1995. Regulation of cholecystokinin secretion by intraluminal releasing factors. *Am. J. Physiol.* 269:G319–27.

[24] Makhlouf, G. M. 1974. The neuroendocrine design of the gut. The play of chemicals in a chemical playground. *Gastroenterology* 67:159–84.

[25] Makhlouf, G. M. 1990. Neural and hormonal regulation of function in the gut. *Hosp. Pract.* 25:79–87, 90–5, 98.

[26] Mezey, E., and M. Palkovits. 1992. Localization of targets for anti-ulcer drugs in cells of the immune system. *Science* 258:1662–5.

[27] Modlin, I. M., and L. H. Tang. 1993. A new look at old hormones: Gastrin. *TEM* 4:51–7.

[28] Nagata, A., et al. 1996. G protein-coupled cholecystokinin-B/gastrin receptors are responsible for physiological cell growth of the stomach mucosa in vivo. *Proc. Natl. Acad. Sci. USA* 93:11825–30.

[29] Niebergall-Roth, E., S. Teyssen, and M. V. Singer. 1997. Neurohormonal control of gallbladder motility. *Scand. J. Gastroenterol.* 32:737–50.

[30] Pearse, A. G. E. 1981. The diffuse neuroendocrine system: Falsification and verification of a concept. In: M. I. Grossman, M. A. B. Brazier, and J. Lechago, eds. *Cellular basis of chemical messengers in the digestive system.* New York: Academic Press, pp. 13–19.

[31] Roettger, B. F., et al. 1997. Antagonist-stimulated internalization of the G protein-coupled cholecystokinin receptor. *Mol. Pharmacol.* 51:357–62.

[32] Silen, M., and J. Gardner. 1993. Gastrointestinal peptides and cancer. *TEM* 4:131–5.

[33] Spindel, E. R., et al. 1993. Bombesin-like peptides: Of ligands and receptors. *Recent Prog. Horm. Res.* 48:365–91.

[34] Tsunoda, Y., and I. Modlin. 1996. Signal transduction machinery of the parietal cell secretory system. *Biochem. Res.* 17:403–28.

[35] Tyler, M. J., et al. 1983. Inhibition of gastric acid secretion in the gastric brooding frog. *Rheobatrachus silus. Science* 220:609–10.

[36] Voisin, T., C. Rouyer-Fessard, and M. Laburthe. 1990. Distribution of common peptide YY-neuropeptide Y receptor along rat intestinal villus-crypt axis. *Am. J. Physiol.* 258:G753–9.

[37] Wahlestedt, C., and D. J. Reis. 1993. Neuropeptide Y-related peptides and their receptors—are the receptors potential therapeutic drug targets? *Annu. Rev. Pharmacol. Toxicol.* 33:309–52.

[38] Weissmann, G. 1984. No frogs in Berlin. *Hosp. Pract.* 19:33–46.

[39] Woods, S. C. 2004 Gastrointestinal satiety signals: I. An overview of the gastrointestinal signals that influence food intake. *Am. J. Physiol.* 286:G7–G13.

Pancreatic Hormones and Metabolic Regulation

I n 1889, Von Mering and Minkowski noted that total pancreatectomy in dogs resulted in severe and fatal diabetes [35]. Subsequent experimenters using a variety of animal species also observed that polyuria and glycosuria (characteristic symptoms of diabetes mellitus) and death always followed removal of the pancreas. It was then noted that after ligation of the pancreatic ducts in rabbits, the acinar component of the gland atrophied, but the islets remained normal; the animals did not become hyperglycemic as they did after total pancreatectomy. From these and other observations, it was concluded that the islets of Langerhans, rather than the pancreatic acinar cells, are essential in the control of carbohydrate metabolism.

Two mechanisms of control were suggested: the blood was modified while passing through the islet tissue or the islets produced an internal secretion. Extracts from the ligated pancreases of dogs, which consisted mainly of islet tissue, were shown to reduce blood sugar levels of diabetic dogs. Canadians Banting and Best [5, 8] provided convincing evidence that, indeed, the pancreatic islets produced an internal secretion, a hormone, that was responsible for the control of blood glucose levels. In 1926, **insulin** was obtained in crystalline form, and in 1954, Sanger determined the primary structure of this hormone, and received a Nobel Prize for his discovery [43]. The physiological roles and chemistry of the other major pancreatic hormone concerned with carbohydrate metabolism, glucagon, also have been elucidated. More recently, it has been discovered that the pancreas is the source of other hormones (e.g., somatostatin and pancreatic polypeptide) also concerned with nutrient homeostasis. Moreover, hormones produced by adipocytes (e.g., leptin and adiponectin) and the gastrointestinal tract (e.g., ghrelin and cholecystokinin) have also been shown to play important roles in nutrient intake and metabolic regulation.

The endocrine roles of the pancreas are to maintain a constant blood glucose level and to facilitate cellular storage of foodstuffs following a meal, and to provide for the mobilization of these depot metabolic substrates during periods of fasting. The underproduction or overproduction of insulin or glucagon therefore can profoundly affect the storage and use of carbohydrates, fats, and proteins within the liver, adipose tissue, and muscle, thus severely affecting cellular metabolic processes. Of all the described endocrinopathies, **diabetes mellitus** is by far the most common.

The Endocrine Pancreas

The endocrine pancreas, which consists of islets of tissue (Fig. 11.1) dispersed among the much larger mass of the exocrine pancreas [36], was first described by Langerhans in 1869 in his doctoral dissertation. There are approximately 1 to 2 million islets in a normal human pancreas, but they represent only about 1 to 2% of pancreatic tissue. Two main cell types can be visualized by histological methods; the α cells are the source of glucagon and the more

Figure 11.1
Photomicrograph of a
human pancreatic islet.

prevalent β cells are the source of insulin. The following cells are present in much smaller numbers: D cells, the source of pancreatic somatostatin (SST), and F cells, the source of pancreatic polypeptide (PP). Several lines of evidence point to the β cell as the source of insulin. Fluorescent-labeled antibodies to insulin localize to the β cells, and alloxan, a drug that specifically destroys the β cells, causes diabetes mellitus. In addition, stimuli that excessively increase insulin secretion cause β-cell degranulation.

In humans the pancreas develops during the fifth week of gestation from two diverticula of the duodenum close to the hepatic diverticulum [45]. The two primordia then fuse and the duct of the ventral diverticulum becomes the main pancreatic duct leading to the opening into the duodenum. Initially, each primordium consists of a network of anastomosing tubules lined by a single layer of cells. These cells differentiate into the individual acini that constitute the functional units of pancreatic enzyme secretion. It is believed that the islet cells derive from the embryonic pancreatic ducts, which are endodermal in origin [31].

It is not clear why the pancreatic cells are disseminated as discrete clusters within the exocrine gland in most higher vertebrates. There is evidence, however, that the *peri-insular acini* differ from the remaining exocrine pancreas, both in their cytological features and secretory activity. There is also evidence for the preferential release of certain enzymes from the exocrine pancreas in response to certain intragastroduodenal nutrients. Therefore, the coordination of particular exocrine gland enzyme secretions may be regulated by hormones deriving from the pancreatic islets. Acinar amylase mRNA levels progressively decrease in rats rendered diabetic. Insulin reverses this effect in the pancreatic acinar cells by inducing a selective increase in amylase mRNA synthesis [29]. Through a paracrine action on amylase production within adjacent acinar cells, insulin may indirectly control the degradation of starch within the gut and thus control the availability of glucose for absorption into the animal.

Glucose homeostasis involves a push–pull system that controls glucose flux into and out of the extracellular space. By their actions on the liver, adipose tissue, and muscle, insulin and glucagon maintain a balance of glucose production and utilization that requires "a coordinated relationship of the glucagon-producing α (A) cells and the insulin-secreting β (B) cells under the guidance of a perceptive glucose sensor" [52]. The individual insulin cells, glucagon cells, and somatostatin cells are believed to be arranged within the pancreas in such a manner as to accomplish that feat. In humans and rats the generalized arrangement of the cellular subtypes of the pancreatic islets is shown (Fig. 11.2). Endocrine cells are arranged as cords among the capillary channels within the islets [52]. Gap junctions have been demonstrated between β cells, as well as between α and β cells. These plasma-membrane specializations are known to permit electrical conductivity between cells, as well as the passage of low-molecular-weight substances from one cell to another. There is evidence that depolarization of one islet cell may lead to the concomitant depolarization of other islet cells. Thus, it is possible that hormone secretion from the pancreatic islets may involve the functional integration of a number of secretory

(a)

(b)

Glucagon

Somatostatin

Insulin

Figure 11.2 (a) Schematic representation of the number and distribution of insulin-, glucagon-, and somatostatin-containing cells in the normal rat islet. Note the characteristic position of most glucagon- and somatostatin-containing cells at the periphery of the islet, surrounding the centrally located insulin-containing cells. (b) Schematic representation of the number and distribution of insulin-, glucagon-, and somatostatin-containing cells in the normal human islet. This pattern divides the total islet mass into smaller subunits, each of which contains a center formed mainly of insulin cells and surrounded by glucagon and somatostatin cells. Cell types for which a definite function and morphology have not been determined are intentionally omitted. (From Unger et al. [50], with permission of Academic Press, Inc., New York.)

units. It may be significant that the α and D cells contact other cell types, whereas the β cells mainly contact other β cells. The peripheral tricellular zone of the islets is innervated by autonomic afferent nerves and is particularly well vascularized.

Intermediary Metabolism

To appreciate fully the physiological roles of the pancreatic hormones and the consequences of their underproduction or overproduction, one should review the general outline of carbohydrate metabolism and the relationships of lipid and protein metabolism to glucose production. The consequences of an excess or deficiency of insulin, for example, are hypoglycemia or hyperglycemia, respectively, which result from metabolic defects in glucose metabolism.

As discussed earlier (Chap. 10), the gastrointestinal hormones promote the movement of foodstuffs through the GI tract and provide the chemical environment and enzymes necessary for their degradation into less complex metabolic substrates. These molecular products (e.g., monosaccharides, free fatty acids, and amino acids) then traverse the luminal lining of the gut and enter the hepatic portal vein and/or the lymphatic system. Most venous outflow of the abdominal GI organs passes through the liver before reaching the hepatic veins to be carried to other parts of the body.

The normal fasting level of glucose in the peripheral venous blood of humans is 60 to 80 mg/dl. The movement of glucose into hepatic cells is by facilitated diffusion in response to insulin. Once within the hepatocyte, glucose may move in a pathway toward glycogen formation (glycogenesis), or it may be catabolized through the glycolytic (Embden–Meyerhof) pathway to pyruvic acid. An alternate pathway for glucose catabolism prominent in certain cells (e.g., adrenal steroidogenic cells) is the *direct oxidative pathway*, or *hexose monophosphate shunt* (HMP). The HMP pathway provides pentoses, which are essential components of nucleic acids and nucleotides. This pathway also provides $NADPH_2$, which is important in many reductive biosynthetic processes such as fatty acid and steroid hormone biosynthesis.

Intracellular glucose is first converted to glucose-6-PO_4 by the enzyme *glucokinase* (Fig. 11.3). Depending on the particular hormonal status of the hepatocyte, the glucose-6-PO_4 may be converted to glucose-1-PO_4 by phosphoglucomutase and then combined with uridine

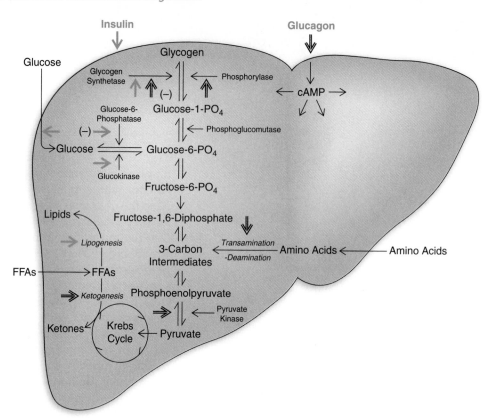

Figure 11.3 General scheme of hormonal regulation of hepatic carbohydrate metabolism. The more prominent actions of insulin (solid arrows) and glucagon (open arrows) are indicated.

diphosphate to form uridine diphosphoglucose (UDPG). Through the action of the enzyme *glycogen synthetase*, a glucose moiety is transferred to existing glycogen polymers through a glycosidic linkage. Hormonal stimulation of hepatic *phosphorylase* may subsequently cleave the glycogen polymer into monomeric glucose-1-PO_4 units. The glucose-1-PO_4 produced through *glycogenolysis* is converted to glucose-6-PO_4, which can then follow one of two pathways: it may be converted to glucose through the action of glucose-6-phosphatase (an enzyme specific to liver and kidney) and be released from the cell, or it may be metabolized through a number of enzymatic steps to pyruvate [32]. Pyruvic acid is then converted to acetyl-CoA, which can enter into the *Krebs (citric acid) cycle* or be utilized in fat biosynthesis (lipogenesis).

Glycogen formation and deposition within hepatic cells provides an important storage form of readily utilizable carbohydrate for energy production through the glycolytic pathway and the citric acid cycle. Similar depositions of glycogen are found within skeletal muscle cells and other cells that require immediate sources of this substrate for energy production. Hormones play key roles in the conversion of these metabolites into more readily available and usable energy substrates.

Molecular interconversion between carbohydrates, proteins, and fats provides metabolic intermediates for use within the Embden–Meyerhof pathway and the citric acid cycle. For example, glycerol derived from the breakdown of fats (lipolysis) can enter the glycolytic pathway. *Deamination* of amino acids or *transamination* between certain amino acids and keto acids may provide intermediates, such as pyruvic acid or α-ketoglutaric acid, that can be used within the glycolytic pathway or citric acid cycle, respectively (Fig. 11.4). Lactate (and pyruvate) released from muscle is transported to the liver, where it serves as a gluconeogenic precursor (Cori cycle). Alanine can flow from muscle to liver where it, too, serves as a gluconeogenic precursor (glucose-alanine cycle). Use of noncarbohydrate substrates, such as amino acids, provides a glucose-sparing action, and the molecules may also be employed directly in glucose formation (*gluconeogenesis*).

Free fatty acids (FFAs) absorbed from the gut may be reformed within mucosal cells into monoglycerides, diglycerides, or triglycerides and complexed with phospholipids and proteins within these cells into small micelles referred to as *chylomicrons*. These particles circulate initially within the lymphatic ducts and are then delivered to the blood vascular system. Through the action of the enzyme *lipoprotein lipase*, localized within the endothelium of the capillaries, the chylomicrons are cleared from the circulation. The released

R_1
|
H – C – NH_2   +   C = O   ⇌ (Transaminase) ⇌   C = O   +   H – C – NH_2
| | | |
COOH   COOH   COOH   COOH
Amino Acid   Keto Acid   Keto Acid   Amino Acid

(with R_2 on the C=O keto acid, and R_1 / R_2 as shown)

$$
\begin{array}{lll}
\text{R}_1 & & \text{R}_2 \\
\text{H}-\text{C}-\text{NH}_2 + \text{C}=\text{O} & \underset{\text{Transaminase}}{\rightleftharpoons} & \text{C}=\text{O} + \text{H}-\text{C}-\text{NH}_2 \\
\text{COOH} \quad \text{COOH} & & \text{COOH} \quad \text{COOH}
\end{array}
$$

Amino Acid + Keto Acid ⇌ Keto Acid + Amino Acid

$$
\begin{array}{lll}
& \text{CH}_2-\text{COOH} & \text{CH}_2-\text{COOH} \\
\text{CH}_3 \quad \text{CH}_2 & & \text{CH}_3 \quad \text{CH}_2 \\
\text{H}-\text{C}-\text{NH}_2 + \text{C}=\text{O} & \underset{\substack{\text{Alanine}\\\text{Transaminase}}}{\rightleftharpoons} & \text{C}=\text{O} + \text{H}-\text{C}-\text{NH}_2 \\
\text{COOH} \quad \text{COOH} & & \text{COOH} \quad \text{COOH}
\end{array}
$$

Alanine + α-Ketoglutaric Acid ⇌ Pyruvic Acid + Glutamic Acid

Figure 11.4 General (top) and specific (bottom) scheme of amino acid–keto acid transamination.

FFAs are then taken up by adipose cells to be reesterified into triglycerides. Most of the glycerol required for fat synthesis is derived from the glycolytic metabolism of glucose within adipocytes. Within these cells, the fats are stored in the form of one or more large fat globules. Through the initial action of *triglyceride lipases* and the subsequent action of diglyceride and monoglyceride lipases, these fats are converted back to FFAs and glycerol and released into the bloodstream.

Within the liver the glycerol liberated by fat breakdown within adipocytes is converted to phosphoglyceraldehyde and used within the glycolytic pathway by catabolism to pyruvic acid or by conversion through glucogenic processes to glucose. The FFAs are broken down by β-oxidation within mitochondria to acetyl-CoA. The acetyl-CoA is then used within the Krebs cycle, another example of a glucose-sparing mechanism. Free fatty acids are also derived de novo from acetyl-CoA through a lipogenic pathway present in many cells. Fatty acid synthesis stops in most cells when the chain is 16-carbon atoms long. Within fat cells the FFAs are combined with glycerol to form neutral fats. Fatty acids are also combined with phosphoric acid and other cellular components to form phospholipids, which may comprise important structural elements of cell membranes or other organelles.

Amino acids derived from the breakdown of proteins within the digestive tract are actively transported across the intestinal mucosal cells and delivered to the liver, where they are used after deamination or transamination processes in carbohydrate metabolism (Fig. 11.4). They also pass through the liver to the general circulation to be used by other cells as energy substrates, or they can be employed as building blocks in protein synthesis, particularly in muscle cells. The entrance of amino acids into cells involves an active transport mechanism that is stimulated by insulin and other growth hormones.

Insulin

Insulin is one of a number of hormones that is required for normal growth and development (Chap. 12). In addition, it is the only hormone that directly lowers blood glucose levels. Most other hormones, if they have an effect on glucose metabolism, tend to elevate blood levels of the sugar. Insulin is a dominant metabolic regulatory factor. Absolute insulin deficiency results in unrestrained glucose production, lipolysis, ketogenesis, proteolysis and, ultimately, death. Insulin excess results in hypoglycemia with consequent brain failure and again, ultimately, death. Clearly, insulin is a potent and critically important hormone [10]. An understanding of the chemistry and biological actions of insulin is necessary, therefore, before the normal and abnormal physiology of carbohydrate metabolism can be understood.

Insulin Consists of Two Polypeptide Chains Derived from a Single Preprohormone

Insulin is a polypeptide consisting of an A and a B chain of 21 and 30 amino acids, respectively [10]. The two chains of the dimer are linked through a pair of disulfide bonds; an intrachain disulfide bond connects the sixth and eleventh amino acids within the A chain. There are minor differences in the primary structure of insulin from different vertebrate species. In mammals these differences most often are restricted to the 8, 9, and 10 positions within the intrachain disulfide bond of the A chain and to position 30 of the B chain (Fig. 11.5). Although these differences do not alter considerably the biological potency of the mammalian insulins used in replacement therapy for diabetes mellitus, they are sufficient to make

Figure 11.5
Comparative primary structures of the vertebrate insulins.

insulin antigenic in some patients. Individuals who become resistant to insulin from one species of animal usually respond to insulin from another source.

Insulin is synthesized from a *proinsulin* molecule where the two chains are united by a connecting peptide, in the human usually consisting of 31 amino acids, not counting the pair of basic residues at the sites of cleavage (Fig. 11.6). Studies on the translation of insulin mRNA have demonstrated that proinsulin is itself derived from a *preproinsulin* precursor. After removal of a C-terminal 23-amino-acid sequence, the proinsulin structure folds onto itself to provide disulfide linkage between the two presumptive individual chains [39]. Enzymatic action then cleaves the connecting peptide to yield the definitive hormonal product (Fig. 11.6). Under conditions of excessive stimulation, proinsulin is also secreted by vesicular exocytosis, along with insulin from the β cells. Because of its slower disappearance rate, proinsulin may constitute up to 50% of the insulin-like material in the blood in the basal state.

Proinsulins and C peptides have been isolated and sequenced from several mammalian species. The high interspecies variability of mammalian C peptides is considered to be the

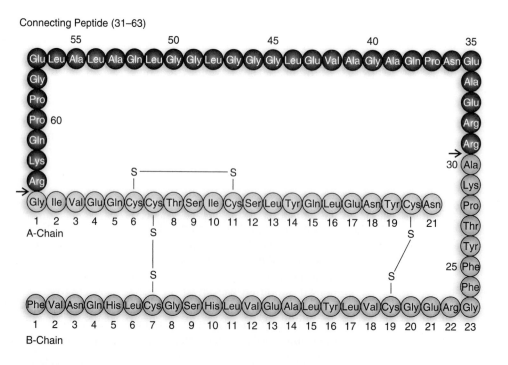

Figure 11.6   Primary structure of porcine proinsulin.

result of an evolutionary rate many times that of insulin. Such structural variation might be expected since this portion of the molecule is a by-product of insulin production. Nevertheless, this structural heterogeneity has allowed for the evolution of the insulin-like growth factors (Chap. 12). There is some evidence that the C peptide may subserve some function(s), along with insulin, in glucose homeostasis [46].

Insulin is complexed with zinc within the β cells of the pancreas and, in some species, in the form of rhombic crystals within the secretory vesicles. Insulin is normally degraded within the liver and kidneys, having a half-life of about 5 minutes in the human. The major enzyme responsible for insulin degradation is *hepatic glutathione insulin dehydrogenase*, which disrupts the hormone into its individual A and B chains. The transhydrogenase acts in conjunction with *glutathione*, a cysteine-containing tripeptide, that acts as a cofactor for the transhydrogenase and reduces the individual half-cysteine moieties of the interchain disulfide bonds.

Insulin Regulates Carbohydrate, Fat, and Protein Metabolism in Many Target Tissues

In response to elevated glucose levels, insulin is promptly released from the pancreatic islets. Insulin interacts with plasmalemmal receptors of a number of different cell types. Most important are the actions of insulin on hepatic cells, muscle cells, and adipose tissue cells. In each case, the effect of insulin is to enhance the uptake of glucose into the cells, where it is metabolized and stored as glycogen or used as an energy substrate in the synthesis of proteins or fats.

Within the liver, insulin activates glycogen synthetase, which produces a direct flow of glucose toward glycogen formation. Glucokinase activity is enhanced, which provides a pool of glucose-6-PO_4 that is then converted to glucose-1-PO_4 and to uridine diphosphoglucose. Conversion of intracellular glucose to glucose-6-PO_4 prevents glucose release from hepatocytes.

In fat cells, insulin-stimulated glucose uptake results in enhanced catabolism of the sugar to glycerol [13]. Insulin activation of endothelial cell lipoprotein lipase results in the release of FFAs from chylomicrons. These fatty acids are then transported into fat cells where they combine with glycerol to form triglycerides and are added to the lipid droplets within the fat cells. Lipid synthesis is stimulated by insulin via an activation of citrate lipase, acetyl-CoA carboxylase, fatty acid synthase, and glycerol-3-phosphate dehydrogenase.

Insulin stimulates the active transport of glucose and amino acids into muscle cells and, subsequently, protein synthesis is enhanced. Glycolysis and oxidative phosphorylation of glucose derivatives provide the energy required for such metabolic activity.

Insulin plays an important role in potassium homeostasis. Insulin is stimulatory to K^+ uptake by cells and, at excessively high concentrations, causes extracellular hypokalemia. Low levels of insulin appear to have a permissive effect on the cellular uptake of K^+. Infusion of somatostatin, which reduces fasting insulin levels, is associated with an increase in basal serum K^+ concentration in the human.

Insulin's Actions are Mediated by a Receptor Tyrosine Kinase

Insulin, like other growth factors (Chap. 12), mediates its action through novel plasma membrane receptors that possess tyrosine kinase activity. Some of the post-receptor intracellular signals that may mediate insulin's actions are now known. Nevertheless, the details of the mechanisms leading to cellular responses remain ill-defined.

Insulin Receptor.   The insulin receptor consists of an α subunit that contains the insulin-binding domain and a β subunit that contains a tyrosine kinase domain [40]. The insulin receptor is composed of two α and two β subunits held together covalently by both inter- and intrasubunit disulfide bridges (Fig. 11.7). Both subunits are derived from a common polypeptide precursor, and both are glycosylated in their native forms. The α subunits provide the binding sites for insulin and are wholly extracellular, being anchored by virtue of covalent attachment to the β subunit. The β subunit is a transmembrane protein with globular domains at both the extracellular and cytosolic surfaces. Insulin binding to the α subunit causes a conformational change in the receptor complex which activates autophosphorylation of the β subunit. Once phosphorylated, the β subunit is an activated tyrosine kinase, which then phosphorylates multiple intracellular proteins, including insulin-receptor substrate-1 (IRS-1). Phosphorylation of

Figure 11.7
Diagrammatic structure of the insulin receptor, and schematic representation of insulin receptor stimulation, activation of insulin receptor substrate 1 (IRS-1), and binding and activation of PI-3 kinase by IRS-1. PIP3 is generated as a result of PI-3-kinase activity and mediates activation of several downstream effectors.

IRS-1 generates secondary signals that couple the insulin pathway to transmembrane glucose transport. One of the signaling molecules, growth receptor-binding protein 2, further couples IRS-1 to glycogen synthesis in some cells.

When insulin binds to cell-surface receptors on cultured or freshly isolated cells, the hormone–receptor complex is internalized. Subsequently, a series of intracellular events ensue that can dissociate the hormone from its receptor. Internalization is the major mechanism by which cell-surface insulin receptors are down-regulated. The structures involved in endocytosis appear to be relatively nonspecific and similar for many other peptide hormones. Insulin is initially localized in coated pits on the cell surface, which invaginate, fuse, and then fission to form coated vesicles. These vesicles progressively become larger noncoated structures called endosomes. The acidification of endosomes promotes dissociation of the ligand–receptor complex, permitting the ligand and receptor to be processed independently.

The receptor appears to be recycled predominantly from this endosomal compartment. The receptor can also be recycled from other vesicular structures such as lysosomes. Certain types of receptors, such as the LDL receptor (Chap. 15), recycle continuously, whereas internalization and recycling of the insulin receptor predominantly requires ligand binding. Thus, down-regulation of the receptor is determined primarily by the rate of receptor endocytosis and the rate of receptor recycling. In the short term, binding of insulin therefore may cause some reversible redistribution of receptor between plasma membrane and subcellular pools, which is manifested as a decrease in the number of cell-surface binding sites. If a substantial fraction of receptors is occupied, this may (in the longer term) lead to accelerated degradation of the internalized receptor pool, resulting in a net loss of receptors from the cell surface.

Second Messengers of Insulin Receptor Activation. The mechanisms by which insulin elicits its various intracellular effects have been the focus of much research, yet these mechanisms remain incompletely understood. The intrinsic tyrosine kinase activity of the insulin receptor is implicated in the initiation of all of the diverse biological responses to insulin. The activated insulin receptor phosphorylates tyrosine residues in several intracellular proteins, including insulin receptor substrate (IRS) protein family members IRS-1–4, as well as signaling molecules such as *Shc* (Fig. 11.8). Once phosphorylated, these substrate proteins interact with a series of adaptor and effector molecules that contain "Src homology" (SH2) domains, which specifically recognize and bind to the phosphotyrosine-containing amino acid sequences within the insulin receptor substrates. The phosphorylation of these molecules initiates signaling through several complex pathways. In general, there are two major routes by which insulin signals are transmitted: (1) the IRS proteins phosphorylate a multifunctional enzyme called phosphatidylinositol-3-kinase (PI-3-kinase), which in turn activates signaling pathways leading to glycogen synthesis, fatty acid synthesis and transport, and glucose transport into cells, and (2) phosphorylated Shc

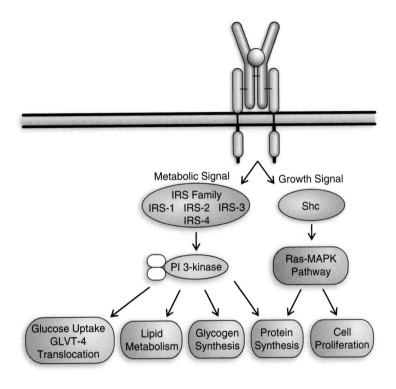

Figure 11.8
Insulin-activated
intracellular signal
transduction pathways.

and activates a cascade of kinases that ultimately stimulate gene transcription, protein synthesis, and mitotic activity.

Glycogen Synthesis. A major physiological role of insulin is formation of glycogen from glucose in a number of tissues. Glycogen formation is controlled by the activity of a glycogen synthetase. This enzyme is active in the dephosphorylated state and inactive in the phosphorylated state. Hepatic phosphorylase, the enzyme responsible for activating glycogenolysis, is, on the other hand, activated on phosphorylation by action of a cAMP-dependent protein kinase (Fig. 11.9). An attractive hypothesis has been that insulin mediates its action by an inhibition of the phosphorylated state of these two enzymes. In both muscle and liver, it has been shown that insulin acts to regulate glycogen synthetase by a mechanism not directly related to tissue cAMP concentration. It is now known that insulin does indeed stimulate glycogen synthesis via PI-3-kinase-mediated activation of protein phosphatase 1 (PPtase1), a phosphatase that dephosphorylates (and activates) glycogen synthetase [11, 20].

Lipoprotein lipase (LPL) is an enzyme that is synthesized within parenchymal cells of a tissue and is then transported to capillary endothelial cells where it hydrolyzes triglycerides from circulating chylomicrons and very low-density lipoproteins (VLDLs). The fatty acids are then transported into the adjacent parenchymal cells. Insulin activates LPL and thus facilitates local transport of FFAs into tissues. Severe uncontrolled diabetes is associated with hypertriglyceridemia and low plasma LPL activity, both of which revert to normal levels on insulin treatment. Insulin appears to stimulate both the transcription and translation of the enzyme by a PI-3-kinase-mediated mechanism. In addition, insulin induces rapid

Figure 11.9 General scheme for the control of glycogen synthesis and degradation.

release of LPL from cells by the activation of a specific phospholipase that hydrolyzes a glycosyl phosphatidylinositol (PI) molecule. The insulin-sensitive glycosyl-PI is structurally similar to the glycolipid membrane anchor of a number of proteins. LPL appears to be anchored to the cell surface by glycosyl-PI, and its rapid release by insulin may be due to activation of a glycosyl-PI-specific phospholipase C.

Glucose Transporter Systems.   A key element in the regulation of blood glucose levels is the detection of ambient glucose by α and β cells of pancreatic islets and the consequent secretion of either glucagon, which stimulates glucose release from the liver, or insulin, which induces glucose storage in the liver and stimulates glucose uptake by muscle cells and adipocytes. These mechanisms of glucose uptake, release, and sensing require the presence of membrane proteins known as facilitated-diffusion glucose transporters (GTs), which transport D-glucose and closely related sugars down a chemical concentration gradient. Isoforms of this transporter are expressed in a tissue-specific manner and comprise a family of structurally and functionally related molecules. Their tissue distribution, differences in kinetic properties, and differential regulation by ambient glucose and insulin levels indicate they play specific roles in the control of glucose homeostasis.

All cells express at least one transporter isoform in a constitutive fashion, because a certain level of glucose uptake is an absolute necessity, regardless of influences by various regulatory factors. The level of the constitutive transporter, usually the erythroid glucose-transporter isoform, can be regulated by environmental factors, for example, nutrition. Certain cells express unique transporter isoforms, the quantitatively most important of which is the muscle–liver–adipocyte glucose-transporter isoform that functions in response to insulin to clear most of the blood glucose after a meal. Most commonly, insulin causes a modest (50%) to dramatic (>30-fold) increase in the rate of glucose uptake, depending on the cell type. The most physiologically important aspect of glucose-transport regulation occurs in muscle cells and adipocytes and involves an acute 20- to 40-fold stimulation of transport rates by circulating insulin. This response does not require new protein synthesis and is fully manifest in 10 to 20 minutes. The major insulin target tissues appear to be uniquely able to produce this transporter isoform, sequester it in a unique intracellular organelle, and bring it to the cell surface, where it is inserted by an exocytotic process in response to insulin (Fig. 11.10) [48]. Insulin stimulates the translocation of GLUT4 through at least two parallel signal transduction mechanisms [11]. The first is PI-3-kinase dependent, in which PI-3-kinase activity leads to the activation of protein kinases such as PDK1, which in turn activates a series of additional downstream protein kinases. Insulin also activates a second set of signals though a PI-3-kinase-independent mechanism, via kinases that

Figure 11.10 Insulin activation of glucose transporters.

are localized to membrane microdomains called "lipid rafts." It is not known how the signals conveyed by these parallel pathways are integrated, and how they may prompt insertion of the transporter into the membrane. Given the importance of this process in understanding the pathophysiology of diabetes, however, it is not surprising that it is a subject of intense research.

The diversity of glucose transporters expressed in mammalian tissues presumably reflects the importance of glucose as a source of metabolic energy, and different glucose transporters have evolved to allow its dietary uptake and tissue-specific utilization. For example, the Na$^+$-glucose cotransporter is able to actively absorb glucose from the lumen of the small intestine and proximal nephron; the glucose is then passively transferred across the antiluminal surface of the cell. Glucose uptake by other tissues and cells is mediated by transporters whose properties are suited to the specific requirements of the tissues and their cells for glucose and their role in the maintenance of glucose homeostasis.

Somatic Cell Growth.   In addition to its metabolic functions, insulin also acts as a mitogen under certain developmental and physiological circumstances. (The structurally related insulin-like growth factors, IGF-I and IGF-II, also exert mitogenic effects through a closely related receptor, as discussed in Chap. 12.) Insulin's mitogenic actions are mediated by phosphorylation of the insulin receptor substrate Shc, which in turn activates the proto-oncogene *ras* (Fig. 11.8), a GTP-binding protein; with the exchange of GTP for GDP, ras activates a related protein called raf, which in turn activates a series of other kinases including mitogen-activated protein kinase kinase (MAPK-K) and mitogen-activated protein kinase (MAPK). MAPK activation leads to the regulation of gene transcription, protein synthesis, and mitogenesis.

Glucagon

A second important pancreatic hormone that regulates glucose homeostasis was discovered by Kimball and Murlin [27]. Numerous workers had noted that injections of pancreatic extracts into diabetic animals produced a transient hyperglycemia before the hypoglycemic effects of the extracts were observed. Collins and Murlin [12] suggested that besides insulin, the extracts might contain a physiologically relevant hyperglycemic factor, which they named glucagon. Glucagon is essential for the complete metabolic syndrome of severe diabetes, previously attributed entirely to the direct consequences of insulin deficiency.

Glucagon is Structurally Related to Secretin, GIP, and VIP

Mammalian pancreatic glucagon is a single-chain polypeptide of 29 amino acid residues, which bears a striking structural similarity to secretin, gastric inhibitory peptide (GIP), and vasoactive intestinal peptide (VIP) (see Fig. 10.3). Glucagon is derived from a large precursor (preprohormone) that then undergoes a number of post-translational modifications to yield the definitive hormone. The amino acid sequences of glucagons derived from a number of mammalian species (bovine, ovine, rabbit, rat), including the human, are identical (Fig. 11.11). Glucagons from turkeys and chickens are identical and differ from mammalian glucagons by substitution of the penultimate asparagine (position 28) by serine. Duck glucagon differs from human glucagon by two residues: The asparagine at position 28 is again replaced by serine and the serine at position 16 is replaced by threonine. Such a high degree of structural conservation within the glucagons from these diverse animal species suggests that the integrity of most of the molecule is necessary for its biological activity.

Figure 11.11 Primary structure of mammalian glucagon and related structures of avian glucagons.

Glucagon Stimulates Glycogenolysis, Gluconeogenesis, and Lipolysis

The classical experiments of Foa demonstrated conclusively the role of glucagon in glucose homeostasis [18]. In cross-circulation experiments, the pancreatoduodenal vein of one dog (A) was anastomosed to a femoral vein of a second dog (B) and a return flow was established between a femoral artery of dog B and a femoral vein of dog A. Reduction of plasma blood glucose levels in dog A by insulin resulted in an elevation of blood glucose levels in dog B. Conversely, when hyperglycemia was induced in dog A by administration of glucagon or glucose, a rapid hypoglycemia developed in dog B. These results demonstrated that a reduction or an elevation of blood glucose in dog A was the stimulus to glucagon or insulin secretion, respectively, in dog B. From these experiments, the importance of pancreatic glucagon, along with insulin, in the control of blood glucose levels was elucidated. Subsequent experiments showed that glucagon had a direct effect on glycogenolysis and gluconeogenesis in the isolated perfused liver.

The biological actions of glucagon are essentially the opposite of those of insulin (Fig. 11.3). Glucagon stimulates hepatic glucose synthesis and release through a glycogenolytic action or through gluconeogenesis. The glycogenolytic action is particularly important in maintaining the short-term levels of blood glucose in well-fed animals that have available stores of liver glycogen. Under conditions of prolonged fasting, exercise, or during neonatal life, the gluconeogenic actions of glucagon are crucial to the maintenance of glucose homeostasis.

Glucagon at physiological levels stimulates the conversion of amino acids to glucose within the liver. Glucagon also promotes the conversion of amino acids and glycerol into glucose by affecting the enzymes in the gluconeogenic and glycolytic pathways in the liver (Figs 11.3 and 11.9). Glucagon has a lipolytic action on adipose tissue. The FFAs and glycerol liberated from fat cells are used to a minor extent within the hepatocyte in gluconeogenesis. Insulin is such a potent inhibitor of fat cell lipolysis that the actions of glucagon may be manifested only when insulin concentrations are low. The ability of administered glucagon to stimulate lipolysis has nevertheless been demonstrated in the human diabetic.

During fasting, the prevention of hypoglycemia is not due solely to decreased insulin secretion; decrements in insulin are probably important, but insulin is not the only relevant glucoregulatory hormone. Glucagon plays a primary counterregulatory role. Adrenal catecholamines compensate and become critical when glucagon is deficient. Adrenomedullary epinephrine is probably the relevant catecholamine [13].

Glucagon Activates Receptors Coupled to cAMP Formation in Hepatocytes and Adipocytes

The major target tissues of glucagon are liver and adipose tissue and also cardiac muscle under certain conditions. The actions of the hormone are at the level of the plasma membrane to stimulate adenylate cyclase production of cAMP; this initial action of the hormone is followed by activation of protein kinase A and subsequent substrate phosphorylation. The actions of glucagon on the hepatocyte are similar to those of epinephrine, but each hormone mediates its effects through separate receptors. In the hepatocyte, a cascade of protein (enzyme) phosphorylations eventually results in the release of individual glucose-1-PO_4 units from the glycogen polymer (Fig. 11.12). Conversion of inactive (dephosphophosphorylase) phosphorylase to the active enzyme is the final, key step in this cascade phenomenon. At the same time, phosphorylation of glycogen synthetase inactivates this enzyme (Fig. 11.9).

Glucagon also stimulates gluconeogenesis within the hepatocyte; again its action is mediated through the intracellular messenger cAMP. The actions of the cyclic nucleotide block the flow of carbohydrate substrates from glucose-6-PO_4 to pyruvate, specifically by inhibiting enzyme activities between pyruvate and phosphoenolpyruvate and between fructose-6-PO_4 and fructose 1,6-diphosphate. The cytosolic form of P-enolpyruvate carboxykinase (PEPCK) is a regulatory enzyme of gluconeogenesis. PEPCK activity is regulated by the transcription rate of its gene. Glucagon activates while insulin inhibits PEPCK gene transcription (Fig. 11.3). Within the hepatocyte, glucagon also prevents the conversion of FFAs to ketone bodies. The control site of hepatic ketogenesis is at the level of the enzyme carnitine fatty acid transferase. This enzyme promotes the reversible coupling of long-chain fatty acids to carnitine, which is required for the translocation of fatty acids into mitochondria for

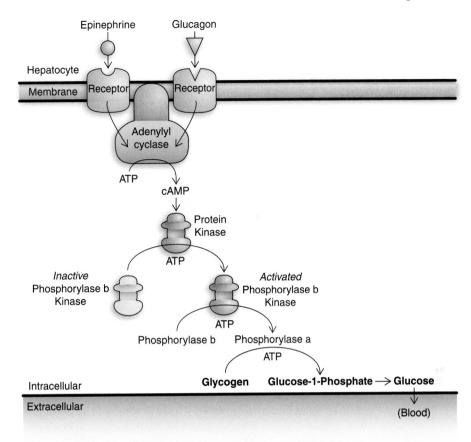

Figure 11.12
Glucagon activation of hepatic adenylate cyclase and the subsequent events in glucose formation.

oxidation. The use of ketones for production of ATP by oxidative phosphorylation within mitochondria provides a glucose-sparing action. Figure 11.3 summarizes the actions of glucagon on a hepatocyte.

Although glucagon is a potent lipolytic hormone, there is great species variation with respect to the sensitivity of adipose tissue to the hormone. Here, as for the hepatocyte, cAMP formation is increased in response to glucagon. In the adipocyte, activation of one or more *hormone-sensitive* lipases (triglyceride, diglyceride, and monoglyceride lipases) results in the release of fatty acids and glycerol from fats. These metabolic products of lipolysis circulate to the liver where they subserve substrate roles in gluconeogenic processes. By the actions of glucagon on adipocytes and hepatocytes, plasma glucose levels are elevated; thus under pathological conditions of pancreatic function, the actions of the hormone are diabetogenic.

Other Pancreatic Peptide Hormones

The α and β cells are the predominant cell types within the pancreas. Nevertheless, using immunocytochemical methods, at least two other peptide hormone-containing cells have been demonstrated to be present within the islets. The control of insulin and glucagon secretion from the islets is much more complicated than described and may be regulated or modulated by these more recently discovered pancreatic peptide hormones.

Somatostatin (SST) is Secreted by Pancreatic D Cells

Immunoreactive SST was shown by immunofluorescence to be localized to a discrete population of cells (D cells) of the endocrine pancreas. The juxtaposition of SST-containing D cells to the α and β cells of the islets (Fig. 11.2) is consistent with a local or paracrine role for the hormone. SST is a tetradecapeptide containing a disulfide bond (see Fig. 6.7); in the pancreas, the hormone is derived, as for insulin and glucagon, from a preprohormone.

```
                      5                    10                  15
     Ala–Pro–Leu–Glu–Pro–Val–Tyr–Pro–Gly–Asp–Asn–Ala–Thr–Pro–Glu–Gln–Met–Ala ─┐
                                                                               │
       20                25                 30                 35              │
 ┌─ Gln–Tyr–Ala–Ala–Asp–Leu–Arg–Arg–Tyr–Ile–Asn–Met–Leu–Thr–Arg–Pro–Arg–Tyr–NH₂
```

Figure 11.13 Primary structure of human pancreatic polypeptide. Variations within ovine, porcine, and bovine PP sequences are shown.

		2	6	11	23
Ovine	(oPP)	Ser			
Porcine	(pPP)		Asp		
Bovine	(bPP)		Gln	Asp	Glu

SST-like immunoreactivity is elevated in the arterial plasma of dogs that have received a protein meal, suggesting that SST may function as a humoral messenger in the control of GI function. Infusions of SST, at a rate approximating the postprandial increase in endogenous plasma SST-like activity, markedly lower postprandial triglyceride levels. In addition, neutralization of circulating SST by antibodies to the peptide is accompanied by higher levels of plasma triglycerides. SST, therefore, may function as a splanchnic (visceral) humoral hormone that regulates the movement of nutrients from the gut to the internal environment.

Pancreatic Polypeptide (PP) is Secreted by Pancreatic F Cells

A linear polypeptide has been isolated from the human, pig, cow, sheep, and chicken pancreas (Fig. 11.13) [21, 22]. Avian and beef pancreatic polypeptide (PP) exhibit homology at 16 of 36 amino acid residues, whereas some of the mammalian polypeptides differ by only 2 to 3 residues. Rat PP also contains 36 amino acids; however, there are 8 amino acid substitutions compared with human PP.

The physiological functions of these pancreatic polypeptides are not clearly delineated, but some of the hormone actions in the chicken have been described [22]. In chickens, avian PP decreases liver glycogen, apparently by stimulating hepatic lipogenesis. Avian PP decreases plasma glycerol and FFAs in chickens by inhibiting adipose tissue lipolysis, apparently by reducing fat cell cAMP levels [21]. In humans, PP suppresses secretion of SST from the gut and pancreas. Similarly, there is a postprandial rise in plasma PP in humans, which can be suppressed by infusions of SST. Administration of antisera to SST in dogs increases plasma PP levels, suggesting that an inhibitory control of PP secretion by SST takes place under physiologic conditions. It was suggested, therefore, that the SST-containing D cells and PP-containing F cells control the secretory activity of each other (and probably of insulin and glucagon) within the pancreatic islets by a paracrine mechanism.

Ingestion of a protein meal is a stimulus to PP secretion in humans. Because intravenous infusions of amino acids only modestly elevate plasma PP levels, protein digestion within the GI tract is most likely the stimulus to PP secretion from the pancreatic islets. Acute hypoglycemia is a stimulus to PP secretion, whereas hyperglycemia is associated with a decrease in plasma PP levels. Vagal cholinergic innervation of the pancreas is important in the regulation of PP release. For example, secretion of PP in response to insulin-induced hypoglycemia in humans is abolished by cholinergic (atropine) blockade. Electrical stimulation of the vagus nerve increases portal levels of PP in pigs, a response that is partially inhibited by cholinergic blockage. Protein-rich meals may activate the release of some factor, possibly cholecystokinin, that enhances the release of PP, possibly in concert with vagal activation of pancreatic F cells. Despite the very dramatic effects of meal ingestion on circulating levels of PP, a biological role for PP has not been clearly established. The only clearly documented physiologic effects of PP in humans are inhibition of gallbladder contraction and pancreatic enzyme secretion.

Adipocytokines

Like the endocrine pancreas, adipose tissue is capable of responding to certain metabolic and neural signals, and secreting hormones into the circulation. There is now considerable evidence that many of these adipocyte-derived hormones, called adipokines or adipocytokines, are critically important in regulating energy and glucose homeostasis [28]. The most intensely studied of these hormones is leptin, a catabolic hormone that decreases food intake and increases energy expenditure. Less is known about the functions of the more recently discovered adipokines, adiponectin, and resistin [41].

Leptin is an Adiposity Signal that Suppresses Food Intake

Discovered in 1994 [55], leptin is a 167-amino-acid peptide hormone that is produced mainly by white adipose tissue. It is usually secreted in proportion to fat mass, and thereby conveys a signal to target tissues reflecting the prevailing degree of body adiposity. The best characterized target tissue for leptin is the central nervous system, where it exerts inhibitory effects on food intake. Thus, low doses of leptin administered into the brain ventricles reduce food intake and body weight, while the absence of leptin or leptin receptors in mice, rats, and humans results in morbid obesity. Leptin receptors (ObRs) belong to the cytokine receptor superfamily that signal via "Janus kinases" (JAKs) and "signal transducers and activators of transcription" (STAT). Five different ObRs are produced by alternative splicing of the ObR mRNA. A short form of the leptin receptor, ObRa, is expressed in high levels in brain microvasculature, and is thought to function in receptor-mediated transport of leptin across the blood–brain barrier, into the brain. The long form of the receptor is expressed in nuclear groups within the basal hypothalamus, including the arcuate nucleus, ventromedial nucleus, and dorsomedial nucleus. It is at these sites that leptin receptors appear to mediate the suppressive effects leptin on food intake, as well as its activating effects on the descending autonomic pathways that control of energy expenditure [7]. Although leptin is best known for its weight-reducing properties, like other structurally related cytokines, leptin is a remarkably pleiotropic hormone that can regulate a variety of other physiological processes, including reproductive function, brain development, angiogenesis, hematopoiesis, and immune cell function. It was originally hoped that leptin would prove useful in the treatment of obesity. However, clinical studies have confirmed that the vast majority of obese subjects have normal or high serum leptin levels, indicating that the obese state is a consequence of resistance to leptin's actions, and not a leptin deficiency.

Adiponectin is an Endogenous Insulin-Sensitizing Factor

Adiponectin is a protein hormone that appears to be solely produced by adipocytes. Experiments in rodents have demonstrated that adiponectin has pronounced insulin-sensitizing effects. In animal models of obesity, adiponectin can reverse insulin resistance. When adiponectin expression is experimentally induced in the livers of rats, insulin sensitivity is significantly enhanced, indicating that the hepatocyte is a major site of adiponectin's insulin-sensitizing actions. Adiponectin also appears to exert central catabolic effects, as cerebroventricular injection of the hormone causes weight loss and reduced glucose and lipid levels. Unlike leptin, these effects do not appear to be mediated by changes in food intake, but are instead likely manifest as increased energy utilization via activation of descending autonomic pathways. Adiponectin levels in the circulation have been found to be reduced in individuals with obesity and insulin resistance, suggesting that adiponectin deficiency contributes to these pathological states. Therefore, adiponectin replacement in humans may ultimately be found to be an effective approach in preventing or treating obesity, insulin resistance, and non-insulin-dependent diabetes mellitus.

Resistin can Induce Hepatic Insulin Resistance

Resistin is a polypeptide adipocytokine that is synthesized as oligomeric high-molecular-weight isoforms, and as a monomeric low-molecular-weight isoform that is thought possess greatest bioactivity. In animal studies, the major action of resistin has been found to be exerted in the liver, where it causes hepatic resistance to insulin's actions [34]. Since resistin appears to be present at increased levels in animal models of obesity and insulin resistance, it has been suggested that resistin may play a role in the development of hepatic insulin resistance that accompanies human obesity and type II diabetes mellitus. Its physiological and pathophysiological roles in humans, however, remain to be clarified.

Control of Pancreatic Islet Function

Although insulin secretion from the pancreatic islets is controlled by endocrine, neural, and metabolic factors, blood glucose is the most important regulator [2]. The temporal hyperglycemia, which develops after an exogenous carbohydrate source, is stimulatory to insulin and inhibitory to glucagon secretion (Fig. 11.14a). The fuel hypothesis model for nutrient-stimulated insulin release proposes that the metabolism of glucose is responsible for generating a signal for insulin secretion and that the glycolytic enzyme glucokinase is the β-cell glucose sensor [25].

The amino acids arginine and leucine, as well as such keto acids as acetoacetic acid, are also stimulatory to insulin secretion. Insulin is important in the use of these substrates in protein and fat synthesis, respectively. Most amino acids stimulate (aminogenic action) the secretion of insulin and glucagon (Fig. 11.14b). The enormous structural differences within the R(side)-chain of the active amino acids argue against a structure–activity relationship involving a specific receptor activation. Aminogenic insulin secretion is important, at least from a teleological viewpoint, in that the secreted insulin is available to stimulate incorporation of amino acids into proteins in muscle and other tissues. The concomitant release of glucagon may serve to prevent hypoglycemia as a consequence of the insulin secretion. Aminogenic glucagon secretion is abolished whenever exogenous glucose accompanies the influx of amino acids, such as occurs when carbohydrate is ingested with protein during a meal. In carnivores, the release of glucagon as well as insulin in response to a protein meal would be of obvious adaptive value.

Orally administered glucose is a greater stimulus to insulin secretion than intravenously injected glucose. Glucose is stimulatory to gastric inhibitory peptide (GIP) secretion from the GI tract, which, through circulation to the pancreatic islets, is then stimulatory in conjunction with glucose to insulin secretion (Chap. 10). Glucagon-like peptide 1 (GLP-1) is another member of a class of circulating hormones that subserve humoral communication between the GI tract and the pancreas (the entero-insular axis) [16]. The timing of the secretion of GLP-1 is such that circulating levels of the hormone rise coincident with the postprandial increase in the concentration of blood glucose. By binding to specific β-cell receptors and stimulating cAMP production, GLP-1 synergizes with glucose to induce insulin secretion, thereby increasing the concentration of circulating insulin to a level above

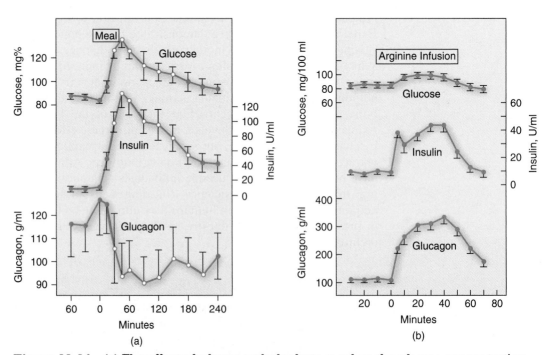

Figure 11.14 (a) The effect of a large carbohydrate meal on the plasma concentration of pancreatic glucagon, insulin, and glucose in 11 normal humans. (b) The effect of an infusion of arginine on the peripheral venous plasma levels of pancreatic glucagon, insulin, and glucose in normal humans. (From Müller-Wieland et al. [37]. Reprinted by permission of the *New England Journal of Medicine*, vol. 283, pp. 109–15, 1970.)

and beyond that attributable to glucose alone. β cells secrete insulin in response to glucose only when they are "glucose-competent" [23, 49]. Glucose competence is proposed to result from the conditioning influences of circulating insulinotropic hormones, or incretins (e.g., GLP-1 and GIP) that render the β-cell glucose-signaling system capable of responding to glucose. Of special significance to the "glucose-competence concept" is the existence of a reciprocal relationship between the concentrations of glucagon and GLP-1 in the bloodstream. This is a consequence of the inhibition of glucagon secretion from the α cells of the islets when blood concentrations of glucose and insulin rise. Such a fall in circulating glucagon levels would ultimately lead to diminished β-cell glucose competence if it were not for the compensatory ability of GLP-1 to maintain the glucose-signaling system in a fully functional state. The action of GLP-1, therefore, contrasts with that of glucagon in that GLP-1 confers glucose competence to β cells during the feeding state [23].

The pancreas receives neural innervation from the sympathetic and parasympathetic divisions of the autonomic nervous system [2, 42]. Secretions from the exocrine and endocrine components of the pancreas can be increased by parasympathetic vagal stimulation or by sympathetic stimulation. Neurotransmitters of cholinergic (acetylcholine) and adrenergic (norepinephrine) neurons directly affect pancreatic insulin secretion. Both cholinergic and adrenergic neuronal fibers can be detected in the endocrine and exocrine pancreas. Electron microscopic histochemical studies reveal that both types of neurons innervate the α and β cells of the islets. Transplantation experiments reveal, however, that the pancreatic β cells do not require an intact innervation for functioning. Similarly, unilateral or bilateral vagotomy does not result in observable effects on depression of insulin secretion due to an intravenous glucose load. Nevertheless, cholinergic drugs potentiate glucose-induced insulin release, and the insulin-releasing effect of electrical vagus stimulation increases with the blood glucose concentration. Probably, the vagal nerve modulates the responsiveness of β cells to blood sugar variations in vivo. Furthermore, nervous input to the pancreas may represent a trophic influence of importance for islet cell growth and function over an extended period, and there are data to support such an hypothesis.

Catecholamines of neural (ANS) or endocrine (adrenal) origin play a major role in the control of pancreatic islet cell secretion (Chap. 14). Pancreatic α and β cells possess different adrenergic receptors that produce opposite effects on cellular cAMP levels and that are thus primarily responsible for the divergence in the rate of glucagon and insulin release known to occur in several physiological and pathological conditions.

Epinephrine of adrenal origin inhibits insulin secretion under physiological states such as stress. The effects of the catecholamine are mediated through α-adrenergic receptors of the islet β cells. During stress, insulin secretion is depressed so that glucose, rather than being converted and stored as glycogen or fat, is more readily available to tissues, such as the liver, muscle, and brain, that are particularly active under such conditions. Glucagon secretion, on the other hand, is stimulated by epinephrine and norepinephrine activation of β receptors of pancreatic α cells; this response provides a mechanism of activating hepatic glucose production and release.

Islet α and β cells have been purified from the rat pancreas and examined for their respective sensitivity to somatostatin. Both SST-14 and SST-28 inhibited glucagon and insulin release through direct interactions with the corresponding cell types. A dose-dependent suppression of pancreatic secretory activities was paralleled by a reduction in cellular cAMP formation.

Galanin is a 29-amino-acid glucagon-like peptide that is widely distributed within the body and exerts a variety of effects. Immunocytochemistry has revealed that galanin occurs in intrapancreatic nerves in the dog. The nerves were found in the endocrine as well as in the exocrine portion of the pancreas and around blood vessels. The strongest fluorescence was observed in close association with nerves innervating the pancreatic islets. This finding supports an earlier observation of galanin-like immunoreactivity in the rat and pig pancreas, as determined by radioimmunoassay. Galanin may have a major influence on islet hormone secretion.

The discovery that glucagon stimulates insulin (β-cell) secretion and conversely that insulin suppresses glucagon (α-cell) secretion has led to the hypothesis of an intra-islet, negative–positive, insulin–glucagon feedback. It was originally proposed that, because of their anatomical juxtaposition, the β and α cells might interact with one another via diffusion through intercellular spaces (Fig. 11.2). This concept was bolstered by the observations that SST (D cell) is a potent inhibitor of α-cell and β-cell secretion; thus, the extended "paracrine" hypothesis proposed that α, β, and D cells mutually regulate the secretion of each other via the interstitium in order to facilitate metabolic homeostasis. A physiologically functional "directed" microvascular circulation within the islets has been conclusively established with a strict sequence of perfusion of β cells, then α cells, then D cells. Abnormalities in glucagon secretion in diabetes mellitus might be explained by a deficiency in intra-islet microvascular insulin. This intra-islet "sequenced" microcirculation plays a major role in islet regulation and, therefore, metabolic homeostasis [50].

There is evidence that the pancreatic glucose sensor may be solely a component of the β cell. The "liver-type" glucose transporter is present in the insulin-producing β cells of rat pancreatic islets but not in other islet endocrine cells. These results support a possible role for this glucose transporter in glucose sensing by β cells [47]. In response to glucose, information may be conveyed to the α cells directly by way of tight junctions or through the release of insulin, which may then interact with receptors on the α cells. In either case, glucose release would be lowered by the action of insulin on its target tissues, such as liver, adipose tissue, and muscle, and additionally through its inhibition of glucagon secretion. In the absence of β cells, as in certain types of diabetes, both these effects of insulin would be lacking. Indeed, the α cell may then be hyperactive; in the juvenile diabetic (who lacks insulin), glucagon levels are elevated even in the presence of hyperglycemia. The observation that glucagon is increased relative to insulin levels in all known forms of endogenous hyperglycemia supports the view that glucagon participates in the marked hepatic overproduction of glucose that is characteristic of the insulin-deficient state.

A number of neural or endocrine influences affect glucose homeostasis and glucose intolerance in the diabetic. Growth hormone, in particular, is diabetogenic, but its exact mode of action is undetermined. GH is stimulatory to insulin secretion, but at the same time this hormone reduces the sensitivity of peripheral tissues (e.g., muscle and adipose tissues) to insulin. Acromegalics have increased circulating levels of GH and exhibit abnormal glucose tolerance due to severe insulin resistance. GH-induced insulin release may be indirect because of the developing hyperglycemia resulting from inhibition of glucose uptake by peripheral tissues. Elevated plasma glucose levels would then be stimulatory to insulin secretion; elevated insulin levels, however, would lead to down-regulation of peripheral tissue insulin receptors (insulin resistance) and the vicious cycle would continue.

Glucocorticoid secretion is increased in Cushing's syndrome (Chap. 15); the effect of these adrenal steroids is generally to increase gluconeogenesis in the liver. In addition, glucocorticoids have a catabolic action on muscle and adipose tissues. The liberated amino acids and FFAs provide substrates for increased gluconeogenesis within the liver. Glucocorticoids also enhance the actions of adrenal catecholamines on their target tissues; for example, the lipolytic actions of catecholamines on adipose tissue are enhanced. All these glucocorticoid actions are hyperglycemic in nature and, therefore, are potentially diabetogenic over a prolonged period. Diabetes mellitus is thus a usual sequelae of hypercortisolism (Cushing's syndrome).

Glucose Counterregulation is Mediated by Several Different Hormones

Glucose is the major metabolic substrate for the brain, and since the brain cannot synthesize or store glucose or increase its capacity to take up glucose from the circulation, the prevention or correction of hypoglycemia is critical to survival. Therefore physiological mechanisms have evolved to effectively prevent or correct the hypoglycemic state [13]. Most important is the decline in insulin secretion in the absence of the β-cell stimulatory actions of glucose. Concomitantly, low levels of glucose are stimulatory to α-cell secretion of glucagon. Under more extreme conditions of hypoglycemia, adrenal medullary release of epinephrine is crucial. Epinephrine is both stimulatory to α-cell glucagon secretion and inhibitory to β-cell insulin secretion. Both glucagon and epinephrine are stimulatory to hepatic glycogenolysis and glucose output. In addition, both hormones are stimulatory to adipose cell lipolytic mechanisms that release glycerol and FFAs for hepatic use (glucogenesis). Other hormones such as GH and cortisol also play roles in defense against prolonged hypoglycemia.

Neuroendocrine Regulation of Food Intake and Body Weight

Humans and other animals maintain a relatively constant body weight when fed an ad libitum diet. When animals are maintained on a food-restricted diet, they lose weight; however, upon reintroduction of an ad libitum diet, they exhibit "catch-up" feeding behavior, eventually reaching body weights equivalent to their fed counterparts. On the other hand, if animals are forced to gain weight through hyperalimentation, their food intake upon resumption of ad libitum diet is reduced, and their body weights eventually return to those of the untreated animals. Thus, under normal conditions, animals possess the ability to precisely match caloric intake with energy expenditure, rendering them in neutral energy balance. Excess caloric intake and/or insufficient energy expenditure produces a state of positive energy balance, while reduced caloric intake and/or excess energy expenditure produces a state of negative energy balance. Physiological signals are generated in both states that tend to return an animal to neutral energy balance.

It is clear that the central nervous system (CNS) controls energy balance by regulating both feeding behavior and energy expenditure. Certain neuropeptidergic cell groups in the mediobasal hypothalamus have been demonstrated to function as effectors of this control system. Neurons producing neuropeptide transmitters that stimulate appetite and feeding behavior are referred to as anabolic effector systems; the best known of these are cells in the arcuate nucleus of the hypothalamus that express neuropeptide Y (NPY). Thus, injections of NPY into the cerebroventricles can rapidly induce a robust feeding response, and eventually increase body weight. On the other hand, neurons producing transmitters that suppress appetite and food intake are referred to as catabolic effector systems. The melanocortin system of the hypothalamus is a major catabolic effector system, and intracerebroventricular injection of α-melanocyte-stimulating hormone (Chap. 8) accordingly inhibits food intake and reduces body weight. The relative activity of these and other anabolic and catabolic effector systems determines the appetitive state of the animal, amount of food ingested over time, and thus body weight.

The ability of the CNS to control food intake and body weight is dependent, in turn, on the transmission of two different types of signals from the periphery to the brain. Short-term "satiety" signals are those that reflect gastric fullness before, during, and after meals, and can thereby influence feeding behavior in the short-term [53]. Most of these satiety signals, such as cholecystokinin (CCK), are released by cells of the GI tract in proportion to the amount of calories consumed during the course of a meal. The released peptides stimulate sensory nerves in the gut, which then convey signals to the hindbrain that prompt termination of the meal. Only one gut peptide, ghrelin (Chap. 10), is known to initiate feeding behavior, rather than terminate it. The second type of signal is produced in proportion to body fat stores, and includes both leptin from adipose tissue and insulin from the pancreatic islets [7]. These adiposity signals are conveyed via the circulation to the brain, where they are transported across the blood–brain barrier and thereafter can bind specific leptin and insulin receptors on central neurons, such as those in the mediobasal hypothalamus. By stimulating these receptors, leptin and insulin can reduce appetite and decrease feeding behavior. Together, leptin and insulin provide the brain with continuous feedback information on the content of body fat depots, and they act to adjust the rate of food intake to maintain a relatively constant level of body adiposity. Both hormones probably exert their inhibitory effects on feeding by stimulating the activity of proopiomelanocortin neurons, as well as by suppressing NPY neuronal activity in the arcuate nucleus of the hypothalamus. It is not known how short-term satiety signals and homeostatic adiposity signals are integrated within the CNS. It is possible that leptin and insulin may enhance the sensitivity of central neurons to the actions of satiety signals, increasing their potency in terminating individual meals.

Pancreatic Islet Pathophysiology

Diabetes mellitus was first described about 1500 BC in Egypt [33]. *Mellitus*, the Latin word for honey, characterizes the high sugar content of the urine of diabetics. The word *diabetes*, derived from the Greek for siphon, refers to the copious excretion of water that characterizes the disease. For centuries the disease was known as "the pissing evil" in England, an epithet that appropriately characterizes its most observable symptom. Although diabetes mellitus is generally thought to result from a lack of insulin, it can, however, be considered a heterogeneous group of diseases (Table 11.1).

Insulin-Dependent and Non-insulin-Dependent Diabetes Mellitus Have Different Etiologies

In patients with *insulin-dependent diabetes mellitus* there is a marked decrease in the number of insulin-containing β cells. The pathogenesis may result from the development of islet cell-surface antibodies [15, 24]. The cues responsible for the production of cytotoxic antibodies are not known. Autoantibodies play a role in the pathogenesis of several other endocrine-based disease states. Juvenile-onset diabetes develops in youth; the symptoms begin rather abruptly, and control of the disease almost always requires insulin replacement therapy. There is evidence that juvenile-onset diabetes may also be caused by a virus, but initiation may require more than a single virus infection. The symptoms may only be manifested when sufficient damage has been caused by a number of infections such as mumps and rubella.

There are about 10 million people with diabetes mellitus in the United States. About 80% of these people have non-insulin-dependent diabetes. Non-insulin-dependent diabetes mellitus (NIDDM) is readily distinguishable from insulin-dependent diabetes mellitus (IDDM), as it is not characterized by a lack of insulin production, but instead arises from a reduced

TABLE 11.1 Pathology of the endocrine pancreas

Type I (insulin-dependent diabetes mellitus, IDDM) [15]
Juvenile-onset diabetes. Viral-induced β-cell destruction
Cytotoxic autoantibodies to β cells lead to β-cell destruction [24]

Type II (non-insulin-dependent diabetes mellitus, NIDDM; previously called adult (maturity) onset diabetes)
Insulin resistance [1, 3, 14, 51]
Pre-receptor resistance
Antibodies against insulin
Mutant insulin structures
Defect in primary structure of insulin β chain at one or more positions
Familial hyperproinsulinemia
B-C proinsulin: mutation at the cleavage site between the B chain and the connecting (C) peptide
A-C proinsulin: mutation at the cleavage site between the A chain and the connecting (C) peptide
Receptor resistance
Type A. Decrease in insulin receptor number and/or affinity for the hormone
Point mutation in insulin receptor gene prevents processing of the receptor precursor
Impaired expression of receptor tyrosine kinase activity [47]
Point mutation blocks insertion of mature receptor into plasma membrane
Type B. Receptor blocked by circulatory antibodies to the receptor
Leprechaunism
An autosomal recessively inherited disorder of insulin function that leads to severe intrauterine growth retardation, characteristic dysmorphic features and a disturbed glucose homeostasis. The process underlying this disease is a structural defect in the insulin receptor
Post-receptor resistance
Decreased capacity of pancreatic β cells to compensate for the underlying insulin resistance by increased secretion of insulin [51]
Possible underexpression (down-regulation) of β-cell glucose transporters (therefore failure to recognize and respond to hyperglycemia)
Autoantibodies to the GLUT2 glucose transporter of β cells [24]
Mutation of the glucokinase gene may prevent uptake and metabolism of glucose necessary for the mechanism of insulin secretion. May be responsible for a young onset type II diabetes (MODY) [6, 25]

Islet cell tumors
Insulinoma. Excess insulin secretion from a β-cell pancreatic tumor (severe hypoglycemia)
Glucagonoma syndrome. Excess glucagon secretion from an α-cell pancreatic tumor
Somatostatinoma. Excess somatostatin secretion from D-cell pancreatic tumor

Hypoglycemic disorders
Hypoglucagonemia (isolated glucagon deficiency). Possibly due to autosomal recessive inheritance
Hyperinsulinemia (β-cell tumor)
Antibodies (stimulatory) to the insulin receptor (increased glucose uptake by cells)

sensitivity of target tissues to insulin's actions. This phenomenon referred to as insulin resistance, may be due to multiple causes [1, 3, 37]. NIDDM patients thus often exhibit hyperinsulinemia, which occurs as a compensatory response by the pancreas to the elevated blood glucose. NIDDM is also referred to as type II diabetes mellitus. NIDDM used to be called adult- or mature-onset diabetes mellitus, because NIDDM used to occur almost exclusively in overweight or obese middle-aged to elderly adults. However, increased rates of overweight and obesity in children in recent years has been accompanied by an increase in the incidence of NIDDM in juveniles, and thus the characterization of this disease as "mature onset" has become outmoded. NIDDM is much more prevalent among Native Americans than among American Caucasians, African Americans, or Hispanic Americans [9, 19, 54]. In particular, the Pima Indians of Arizona have the highest reported prevalence of the disease of any ethnic population in the world [9]. More than half of these Native Americans over 35 years of age have the disease.

Understanding of the mechanisms of insulin actions allows the division of the mechanisms of insulin resistance into three groups: receptor, prereceptor, and post-receptor insulin resistance. The receptor type insulin resistance is due to a decrease in the number or receptivity of insulin receptors, whereas patients with prereceptor insulin resistance have circulating antibodies against some portion of their insulin receptors, and this results in impaired binding of insulin to target cells. The majority of insulin resistance is of the post-receptor type that is due to the failure of signaling by some intracellular effector of insulin's actions [3, 11].

Patients with NIDDM, in contrast to patients with IDDM, may retain the ability to normally synthesize, store, and release insulin. In the insulin resistant state, however, the continued hyperglycemia may eventually overwhelm and exhaust the capacity of the cell to secrete insulin. Thus, abnormal pancreatic secretion of insulin in response to glucose may also develop as a defect in NIDDM [51].

The phosphorylation of glucose in mammalian tissues is mediated by a family of hexose phosphotransferases, which includes glucokinase and hexokinases [25]. Glucokinase is expressed only in the insulin-secreting pancreatic β cells and in hepatocytes. Glucokinase catalyzes the phosphorylation of glucose and plays a key role in the regulation of insulin secretion by pancreatic β cells and glucose metabolism in hepatocytes [6]. The secretion of insulin by the pancreatic β cell is highly regulated by extracellular glucose. The mechanisms by which β cells sense and respond to physiological changes in blood glucose levels has been the subject of intense investigation, especially since the mechanism involved may be responsible in some cases in the etiology of diabetes mellitus. Glucose metabolism is essential for glucose sensing, and both the high-Km glucose transporter GLUT2 and the high-Km glucose phosphorylating enzyme glucokinase have been implicated in coupling insulin secretion to extracellular glucose levels (Fig. 11.15). Mutations in the gene encoding of this key regulatory enzyme of glycolysis are a common cause of an autosomal dominant form of NIDDM that often has an onset during childhood. The association of mutations in the glucokinase gene with impaired pancreatic β-cell function underscores the importance of glycolysis in the regulation of insulin secretion. The demonstration that mutations in the glucokinase gene can cause diabetes suggests that NIDDM may be, at least in part, a disorder of glucose metabolism, which implies that genes encoding other glycolytic and gluconeogenic enzymes, especially those enzymes that control rate-limiting steps in these pathways, are candidates for contributing to the development of this genetically heterogenous disorder [6].

The circulating levels of insulin rise in individuals who have insulin resistance and in pancreatic islets that function normally. Some patients treated with exogenous insulin develop antibodies to the hormone, and these proteins inhibit access of the active hormone to its receptors. Insulin resistance may also develop in individuals who produce an abnormal hormone that has decreased receptor affinity. In the abnormality of *familial hyperproinsulinemia*, for example, individuals possess elevated circulating levels of a partially cleaved proinsulin. This abnormality is inherited as an autosomal dominant and probably involves a mutation of arginine 32 at the cleavage site connecting the B chain to the C peptide. Another defect resulting in hyperproinsulinemia involves a mutation at the cleavage site connecting the C peptide to the A chain (Fig. 11.6). A biologically defective insulin molecule was produced in another hyperinsulinemic patient, most likely by a single-point mutation (probably a single base change in the DNA), resulting in substitution of leucine for phenylalanine at position 24 or 25 of the insulin B chain. These positions are known to compose part of the active receptor-binding region of insulin that is responsible for its biological activity.

Figure 11.15 Cellular events in glucose-induced insulin secretion in pancreatic β cells. Glucose is transported into the cell by the glucose transporter GLUT2. It is then phosphorylated by glucokinase. Further glucose metabolism generates signals that inhibit the ATP-sensitive K^+ channels, resulting in membrane depolarization. This activates the voltage-gated Ca^{2+} channels and increases intracellular Ca^{2+} levels. Ca^{2+} in turn triggers the fusion of prestored insulin vesicles with the plasma membrane. (Modified from S. Efrat, M. Tal, and H. F. Lodish, "The pancreatic β-cell glucose sensor." *Trends in Biochemical Sciences* 19:535–8, 1994).

In the absence of insulin, most activities described relating to the actions of insulin are reversed. Failure to activate hepatic glycogen synthetase increases the levels of glucose-6-PO_4, and this substrate is now available for dephosphorylation by glucose-6-phosphatase to glucose. The concomitant decreased activity of glucokinase results in the loss of glucose from the hepatocytes and, more important, impedes the flow of glucose into the cells, thus failing to provide substrates for glycolysis and ATP production by way of the Krebs cycle. This sets up a situation within hepatocytes and all other cells where, although there are increased circulating levels of glucose, there is little intracellular glucose for ATP production. Thus, cellular famine exists in the midst of plenty. Indeed, polyphagia is a characteristic behavioral trait of these energy-starved individuals. The resulting excess of sugar in the blood leads to the excretion of large amounts of urine (polyuria), which in turn leads to dehydration and intense thirst (polydipsia).

The unavailability of glucose for lipogenesis within fat cells results in increased lipolysis; the released FFAs and glycerol are now available to liver cells as substrates for glucogenesis, which enhances the hyperglycemia, the cardinal symptom of diabetes mellitus [33]. The FFAs released from the fats stored within adipocytes undergo β-oxidation within hepatocytes with resultant production of acetyl-CoA. Although this high-energy compound is available for entry into the Krebs cycle, the increased levels of this substrate may result in condensation of acetyl-CoA moieties into acetoacetyl-CoA. Subsequent condensation of acetoacetyl-CoA with another molecule of acetyl-CoA results in formation of β-hydroxyl-β-methylglutaryl-CoA. In the liver, deacylase activity converts acetoacetyl-CoA to acetoacetic acid. This β-keto acid then can be converted to β-hydroxybutyric acid and to acetone (Fig. 11.16). These ketones, acetoacetate and β-hydroxybutyrate, are normally used as energy substrates. If, however, the entry of acetyl-CoA into the citric acid cycle is depressed, the rate of ketone formation may exceed the tissue oxidation of these substrates. They then accumulate within the bloodstream, which is followed by an elevation of ketone

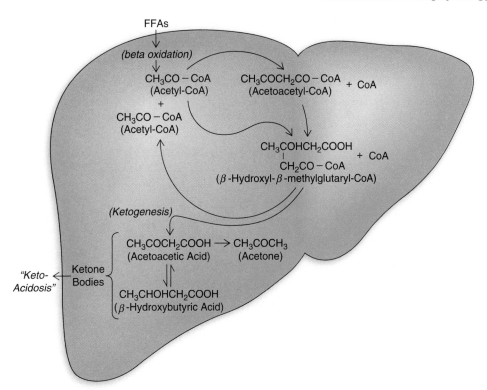

Figure 11.16 Scheme of ketone biosynthesis: The hydroxymethylglutaryl-CoA cycle.

bodies in the urine (ketonuria). This diabetic ketosis may result in a fatal metabolic acidosis [17, 26]. The urinary ketone bodies are excreted as Na^+ salts and large volumes of water are osmotically removed from the plasma, thus intensifying the dehydration already present due to the hyperglycemic diuresis. The loss of Na^+ disturbs the bicarbonate buffering system of the plasma, thus intensifying the blood acidosis. Ketones are also removed through the lungs, producing the characteristic fruity smell of the diabetic in a state of ketosis.

In the absence of insulin, amino acids and glucose cannot enter muscle cells, which results in protein catabolism. The amino acids released through proteolysis from muscle in the diabetic are now available through deamination and transamination for glucose formation within the liver. Use of amino acids in hepatic gluconeogenesis results in a *negative nitrogen balance*. The protein catabolism results in protein depletion and tissue wasting; failure to grow is a symptom of diabetes in animals and children (Fig. 11.17). The protein depletion and accompanying hyperglycemia of the diabetic are also associated with poor resistance to infections.

Obesity can Cause Insulin Resistance and Dysregulation of Insulin Secretion, Leading to NIDDM

Body fat distribution is recognized as an important predictor of the metabolic complications of obesity [4, 38]. Although obesity results in metabolic abnormalities, upper-body obesity is most strongly associated with hyperlipidemia, hypertension, and NIDDM, whereas lower-body obesity is usually not. It has been discovered that fat cells from women with lower-body obesity were of normal size but their numbers were greatly increased. Excessive numbers of adipose cells may be produced by overeating during certain critical periods of childhood. In contrast, upper-body obese women were found to have normal numbers of fat cells, but of greatly increased size. This pattern of cell size may be produced by overeating during adulthood. It has been shown that enlargement of fat cells reduces the number of insulin receptors on their surface. The body then produces more insulin to compensate for the lower numbers of receptors; the hyperinsulinemia may then result in down-regulation of insulin receptors in other tissues. This may account for the elevated blood glucose levels (hyperglycemia) that are the cardinal symptom of diabetes mellitus.

Men tend to have only one pattern of fat distribution: They gain more weight around and above the waist. NIDDM is generally more common in obese men than in obese women but less than that of upper-body obese women. Since upper-body obese women have higher levels of male hormones, this suggests that androgens may stimulate the deposition of fat in a pattern

Figure 11.17
Photograph of a 48-hour-old mouse lacking insulin receptors (right) and a normal litter mate (left). Mice born without insulin receptors are indistinguishable from their wild-type litter mates at birth. With the onset of diabetic ketoacidosis and the ensuing catabolic condition, insulin receptor-deficient mice fail to gain weight. Thus, 48 hours after birth, a sizable difference between the two types of animals is discernable. (From D. Accili, "Insulin receptor knock-out mice." *Trends in Endocrinology and Metabolism* 8:101–4, 1997, with permission.)

similar to that of men. Testosterone has indeed been found to increase the incidence of diabetes, and that may be a contributing factor to NIDDM in these women.

Malignancies of Pancreatic Islet Cells can Cause Profound Metabolic Disturbances

Because of the profound effects of pancreatic hormones on nutrient homeostasis, one should expect that malignancies or neoplasms of pancreatic islet cells would have profound effects on carbohydrate, protein, and fat metabolism. Three neoplasms of the islets are insulinoma, glucagonoma, and somatostatinoma. Other tumors (e.g., gastrinomas, VIPomas) of unknown cellular origin within the pancreas may secrete other peptide hormones that cause dire GI tract disturbances.

Benign and malignant insulin-secreting tumors exhibit complete autonomy of insulin release. If mild, the resulting hypoglycemia can be controlled by an increase in food intake; if severe and intractable, it can lead to convulsions and death if the tumor is not surgically removed [44]. The excessive release of glucagon from an α-cell tumor leads to hyperglucagonemia, and the metabolic disturbances that prevail vary with the capability of the individual to secrete insulin. Development of a somatostatinoma results, not unexpectedly, in hypersomatostatinemia. Patients with such tumors may exhibit hypoinsulinemia and hypoglucagonemia. Because SST may perform a number of functions within the GI tract, it is not surprising that digestive tract functioning may also be impaired. Excessive amounts of VIP are released by all VIPomas and most multiple endocrine adenomas. *Multiple endocrine neoplasia* is characterized by tumors that often occur synchronously in a number of endocrine glands. One type predominantly involves the parathyroid and pituitary glands, and the pancreatic islets.

Improved Insulin Replacement Therapies are Being Explored

In the past, porcine or other mammalian sources of insulin have provided the replacement therapy required by the diabetic. These nonhuman sources of insulin often prove to be immunogenic in some individuals and other sources must be provided. There is hope that DNA recombinant technology will provide a plentiful supply of human insulin (Chap. 4). Two general approaches have been used. Sequences of DNA encoding for the A and B peptide chains of insulin have been ligated separately into the *Escherichia coli* β-galactosidase gene. The individual polypeptide chains produced by the bacterium are then released by enzymatic cleavage from the translation product and purified and recombined to form the biologically active insulin (see Fig. 4.11). An alternate approach has used human preproinsulin DNA inserted into a plasmid that was then used to transform a strain of *E. coli*. The preproinsulin polypeptide sequence was synthesized and correctly cleaved by the bacterium. The polypeptide then could be successfully converted to an insulin-like component by tryptic digestion. This method has proven feasible for the production of adequate amounts of human insulin for therapeutic purposes.

There is also hope that islet transplantation may prove effective in treating insulin-dependent diabetes. Immunoisolation is a potentially important approach to transplanting islets without the need for immunosuppressive drugs. Systems have been designed in which the transplanted tissue is separated from the host's immune system by an artificial barrier (Fig. 11.18). Immunoisolation systems may provide a solution to the problem of human islet procurement by permitting use of the islets isolated from animal pancreases. These devices are referred to as biohybrid artificial organs because they combine synthetic, selectively permeable membranes that block immune rejection with living transplants [30].

Figure 11.18 Canine islets retrieved from a vascular device after >1 year in a diabetic dog. After device removal, the exogenous insulin requirement of the animal increased >20 units/day (hematoxylin/eosin, × 400). (From Lanza et al. [30], used with permission from *Diabetes* 41:1503–10, 1992.)

REVIEW EXERCISES

Match the substrate with its metabolite:

1. Glucose
2. Glucose-1-phosphate
3. Phosphoenolpyruvate
4. Glucose-6-phosphate
5. Fructose-6-phosphate
6. Free fatty acids

A. Glycogen
B. Pyruvate
C. Fructose-1,6-phosphate
D. Glucose-6-phosphate
E. Ketones
F. Glucose-1-phosphate

Think, analyze and discuss:

1. Removal of the pancreas results in a variety of metabolic disturbances that ultimately lead to death. Among the following biochemical processes and physiological parameters, which are increased, decreased, or unchanged following pancreatomy? For each, can you think of a reason why any change would take place?

blood glucose	blood pH	ketogenesis
glycogenolysis	glycogen synthesis	lipolysis
lipogenesis	serum insulin	serum glucagon
hepatic glucose production	polyurea	glucosurea
cellular uptake of amino acids	protein synthesis	proteolysis

2. The loss of insulin-producing pancreatic β cells is thought to be the major cause of the foregoing metabolic disturbances, since insulin replacement therapy can reverse most, if not all of these consequences of pancreatomy. Removal of the pancreas, however, also eliminates glucagon-producing α cells. Are there also profound consequences of the loss of glucagon production, as there are for the loss of insulin production? Why or why not?

3. In IDDM, insulin injections are used to maintain blood glucose levels within a physiological range. What would be the consequence of the accidental injection of excess insulin in these patients? Why would this be dangerous, and possibly lead to death?

4. Glucagon-like peptide has opposite effects on insulin secretion when compared to glucagon. Why would a duplicated gene take on an antagonistic function to its homologue?

5. Glibenclamide and tolbutamide are among a group of drugs called sulfonylureas that bind to one of the subunits of ATP-sensitive potassium channels, and thereby close the channels. What effect would the administration of these drugs have on insulin secretion from pancreatic β cells? Explain how the pharmacological blockade of these channels would be expected to have any such effect.

6. Describe three different mechanisms that can underlie the state of insulin resistance. How does insulin resistance induce compensatory hyperinsulinemia? Why do NIDDM patients exhibit hyperinsulinemia during the development of the disease state, but at later stages they may exhibit insulin deficiency?

7. Most overweight or obese individuals exhibit high serum leptin levels, generally present in proportion to the body fat content. Why is it that elevated leptin in these individuals does not appear to exert its normal anti-appetitive effects? Would administration of exogenous leptin to these hyperleptinemic patients be effective in reducing weight? Why or why not?

8. Compare and contrast "satiety factors" with "adiposity signals." Where do they originate? How are they transmitted to the brain? For each, compare and contrast their receptors and signal transduction mechanisms.

9. Concentrations of glucose required to stimulate insulin secretion from pancreatic tissue in vitro are greater than those needed in plasma to stimulate insulin secretion in vivo. Give three reasons why this would be the case.

10. In hepatocytes treated with a PI-3 kinase inhibitor, would the ability of insulin to stimulate glucose uptake be reduced? Would treatment with the drug actinomycin, an inhibitor of transcription, have any effect on glucose uptake in these cells? Justify your predictions.

11. In what way does glucagon secretion respond differently to a carbohydrate meal versus a protein meal?

12. Pioneering biotechnology is allowing the growth of new organs (i.e., the urinary bladder) from stem (undifferentiated) cells. Explain why the growth and transplantation of new pancreatic islets from a diabetic's own undifferentiated cells would be preferred over transplants from another species or another human.

References

[1] Accili, D., et al. 1992. Insulin resistance due to mutations of the insulin receptor gene: an overview. *J. Endocrinol. Invest.* 15:857–64.

[2] Adler, G., et al. 1995. Neurohormonal control of human pancreatic exocrine secretion. *Pancreas* 10:1–13.

[3] Alzaid, A. A. 1996. Insulin resistance in non-insulin-dependent diabetes mellitus. A review. *Acta Diabetol.* 33:87–99.

[4] Arslanian, S., C. Suprasongsin, and J. E. Janosky. 1997. Insulin secretion and sensitivity in black versus white prepubertal healthy children. *J. Clin. Endocrinol. Metab.* 82:1923–7.

[5] Banting, F. and C. Best. 1922. The internal secretion of the pancreas. *J. Lab. Clin. Med.* 7:465–80.

[6] Bell, G. I., et al. 1996. Glucokinase mutations, insulin secretion, and diabetes mellitus. *Annu. Rev. Physiol.* 58:171–86.

[7] Benoit, S. C., et al. 2004. Insulin and leptin as adiposity signals. *Recent Prog. Horm. Res.* 59:267–85.

[8] Bliss, M. 1989. J. J. R. Macleod and the discovery of insulin. *Q. J. Exp. Physiol.* 74:87–96.

[9] Bogardus, C. and S. Lillioja. 1992. Pima Indians as a model to study the genetics of NIDDM. *J Cell Biochem.* 48:337–43.

[10] Burge, M. R. and D. S. Schade. 1997. Insulins. *Endocrinol. Metab. Clin. North Am.* 26:575–98.

[11] Chang, L., S. H. Chiang, and A. R. Saltiel. 2004. Insulin signaling and the regulation of glucose transport. *Mol. Med.* 10:65–71.

[12] Collins, W., and J. Murlin. 1929. Hyperglycemia following portal injection of insulin. *Proc. Am. J. Physiol.* 264:485–90.

[13] Cryer, P. E. 1993. Glucose counterregulation: prevention and correction of hypoglycemia in humans. *Am. J. Physiol.* 264:E149–55.

[14] Dagogo-Jack, S., and J. V. Santiago. 1997. Pathophysiology of type 2 diabetes and modes of action of therapeutic interventions. *Arch. Intern. Med.* 157:1802–17.

[15] Dorman, J. S. 1997. Molecular epidemiology of insulin-dependent diabetes mellitus. *Epidemiol. Rev.* 19:91–8.

[16] Fehmann, H. C., R. Goke, and B. Goke. 1995. Cell and molecular biology of the incretin hormones glucagon-like peptide-I and glucose-dependent insulin releasing polypeptide. *Endocr. Rev.* 16:390–410.

[17] Fleckman, A. M. 1993. Diabetic ketoacidosis. *Endocrinol. Metab. Clin. North Am.* 22:181–207.

[18] Foa, P., G. Galansino, and G. Pozza. 1957. Glucagon, a second pancreatic hormone. *Recent Prog. Horm. Res.* 13:473–510.

[19] Gohdes, D., S. Kaufman, and S. Valway. 1993. Diabetes in American Indians. An overview. *Diabetes Care* 16:239–43.

[20] Goldstein, B. J. 1993. Regulation of insulin receptor signaling by protein-tyrosine dephosphorylation. *Receptor* 3:1–15.

[21] Hazelwood, R. 1990. *The endocrine pancreas*. Englewood Cliffs, NJ: Prentice Hall.

[22] Hazelwood, R. 1993. The pancreatic polypeptide (PP-fold) family: Gastrointestinal, vascular, and feeding behavioral implications. *Proc. Soc. Exp. Biol. Med.* 202:44–63.

[23] Holz, G. G., and J. F. Habener. 1992. Signal transduction crosstalk in the endocrine system: pancreatic beta-cells and the glucose competence concept. *Trends Biochem. Sci.* 17:388–93.

[24] Inman, L. R., et al. 1993. Autoantibodies to the GLUT-2 glucose transporter of beta cells in insulin-dependent diabetes mellitus of recent onset. *Proc. Natl. Acad. Sci. USA* 90:1281–4.

[25] Iynedjian, P. B. 1993. Mammalian glucokinase and its gene. *Biochem. J.* 293:1–13.

[26] Kecskes, S. A. 1993. Diabetic ketoacidosis. *Pediatr. Clin. North Am.* 40:355–63.

[27] Kimball, C., and J. Murlin. 1923. Aqueous extracts of pancreas III. Some precipitation reaction of insulin. *J. Biol. Chem.* 58:337–46.

[28] Klein, J., et al. 2006. Adipose tissue as source and target for novel therapies. *Trends Endocrinol. Metab.* 17:26–32. Epub 2005 Nov 23.

[29] Korc, M., et al. 1981. Pancreatic islet-acinar cell interaction: amylase messenger RNA levels are determined by insulin. *Science* 213:351–3.

[30] Lanza, R. P., S. J. Sullivan, and W. L. Chick. 1992. Perspectives in diabetes. Islet transplantation with immunoisolation. *Diabetes* 41:1503–10.

[31] Le Douarin, N. M. 1988. On the origin of pancreatic endocrine cells. *Cell* 53:169–71.

[32] Marie, S., et al. 1993. The pyruvate kinase gene as a model for studies of glucose-dependent regulation of gene expression in the endocrine pancreatic beta-cell type. *J. Biol. Chem.* 268:23881–90.

[33] McGarry, J. D. 1992. What if Minkowski had been ageusic? An alternative angle on diabetes. *Science* 258:766–70.

[34] McTernan, P. G., C. M. Kusminski, and S. Kumar. 2006. Resistin. *Curr. Opin. Lipidol.* 17:170–5.

[35] Minkowski, O. 1989. Historical development of the theory of pancreatic diabetes by Oscar Minkowski, 1929: introduction and translation by Rachmiel Levine. *Diabetes* 38:1–6.

[36] Motta, P. M., et al. 1997. Histology of the exocrine pancreas. *Microsc. Res. Tech.* 37:384–98.

[37] Muller-Wieland, D., et al. 1993. Molecular biology of insulin resistance. *Exp. Clin. Endocrinol.* 101:17–29.

[38] O'Dea, K. 1992. Obesity and diabetes in "the land of milk and honey." *Diabetes Metab. Rev.* 8:373–88.

[39] Proud, C. G., and R. M. Denton. 1997. Molecular mechanisms for the control of translation by insulin. *Biochem. J.* 328:329–41.

[40] Romero, G., and J. Larner. 1993. Insulin mediators and the mechanism of insulin action. *Adv. Pharmacol.* 24:21–50.

[41] Rondinone, C. M. 2006. Adipocyte-derived hormones, cytokines, and mediators. *Endocrine* 29:81–90.

[42] Rorsman, P. 1997. The pancreatic beta-cell as a fuel sensor: an electrophysiologist's viewpoint. *Diabetologia* 40:487–95.

[43] Sanger, F. 1959. Chemistry of insulin; determination of the structure of insulin opens the way to greater understanding of life processes. *Science* 129:1340–4.

[44] Service, F. J. 1997. Hypoglycemia. *Endocrinol. Metab. Clin. North Am.* 26:937–55.

[45] Skandalakis, L. J., et al. 1993. Surgical embryology and anatomy of the pancreas. *Surg. Clin. North Am.* 73:661–97.

[46] Steiner, D. F., and A. H. Rubenstein. 1997. Proinsulin C-peptide—biological activity? *Science* 277:531–2.

[47] Taira, M., et al. 1989. Human diabetes associated with a deletion of the tyrosine kinase domain of the insulin receptor. *Science* 245:63–6.

[48] Takata, K. 1996. Glucose transporters in the transepithelial transport of glucose. *J. Electron Microsc. (Tokyo)* 45:275–84.

[49] Thorens, B., and G. Waeber. 1993. Glucagon-like peptide-I and the control of insulin secretion in the normal state and in NIDDM. *Diabetes* 42:1219–25.

[50] Unger, R. 1977. Glucagon and the A cells. *Recent Prog. Horm. Res.* 33:477–517.

[51] Unger, R. 1992. GLUT-2 and the pathogenesis of type II diabetes. *Diabetes Nutr. Metab.* 5:69–9.

[52] Unger, R. H. 1991. Diabetic hyperglycemia: link to impaired glucose transport in pancreatic beta cells. *Science* 251:1200–5.

[53] Woods, S. C. 2005. Signals that influence food intake and body weight. *Physiol. Behav.* 86:709–16. Epub 2005 Nov 2.

[54] Young, T. 1993. Diabetes mellitus among Native Americans in Canada and the United States: An epidemiological review. *Am. J. Human Biol.* 5:399–413.

[55] Zhang, Y., et al. 1994. Positional cloning of the mouse obese gene and its human homologue. *Nature* 372:425–32.

Growth Hormones

*A number of hormones are essential to normal body growth through their actions on bone and other organs such as the gonads and the mammary glands. Although pituitary **growth hormone** (GH) is clearly associated with growth (Chap. 5), most of its actions are mediated indirectly through peptide hormones, the **somatomedins**. Besides the important actions of **insulin** on carbohydrate and fat metabolism, this hormone also plays an important role in growth regulation. **Prolactin** is necessary for mammary gland growth and development during the latter stage of pregnancy. **Placental lactogen** may prove to be significant in maternal and fetal growth during pregnancy. Other putative growth factors affect the growth, proliferation, and differentiation of specific cell types: nerve growth factor, erythropoietin, epidermal growth factor and platelet-derived growth factor, and a number of thymic factors.*

Certain steroid hormones, particularly androgens, play crucial roles in normal growth processes. Other hormones, such as the glucocorticoids and the thyroid hormones, are essential (permissive) for the growth-promoting activities of the peptide growth hormones. The individual roles of growth hormones and their integrated actions of the hormones in growth and development will be discussed. Growth-inhibiting factors, chalones, have also been described [45].

Growth and Cellular Proliferation

All cells in the body are derived from a single cell, the fertilized egg. Although each cell possesses the same genetic information, there are many different kinds of cells. After repeated divisions of the egg to produce cells of a smaller, more uniform size, the cells migrate and continue to divide to produce the embryo. During this process of cell division and subsequent tissue and organ formation, certain genes (proto-oncogenes) are turned on or off, a process that provides the regulatory cues for individual cell differentiation and function. Certain cells are specialized to provide specific functions: Some make hemoglobin, some synthesize keratin, some produce antibodies, and others, such as the hepatocyte, participate in a wide spectrum of cellular activities.

Cells pass through specific stages in their life cycle. The fully mature cell (e.g., skeletal muscle or nerve) is said to be in G_0 (G stands for gap) and is not committed to division (Fig. 12.1). These cells have varying life spans depending on their specific activities. Erythrocytes survive about 120 days in humans; some epithelial cells of the gut live only a few days, and certain neurons in the brain may be as old as the individual. G_1 is a growth phase preparatory to S, the synthetic phase where the DNA is duplicated. The G_2 phase is not clearly defined functionally, but it is a short period (3 to 4 hours) where some protein synthesis occurs. During this time, preparations are made for entry into the complex events of the next phase, mitosis (M). Following mitosis, the daughter cells may re-enter the proliferation cycle or may become resting G_0 cells.

The control point of cell division is believed to be at the transition from G_0 to G_1. Because chemical messengers affect cell division as well as differentiation, it is important to determine whether hormone effects are specific to certain phases of the cell cycle. Hormone receptors

(DNA Synthesis)

$$G_0 \rightleftharpoons G_1 \quad \begin{array}{c} \nearrow S \searrow \\ \\ \searrow M \nearrow \end{array} \quad G_2$$

(Mitosis)

Figure 12.1   The mammalian cell cycle.

may vary in number and/or function throughout the cell cycle and thus affect the responsiveness of the cells to the actions of hormones.

Growth, often defined as simply an increase in size, may occur as a result of three processes: cells may enlarge (become hypertrophic), cells may increase in number (become hyperplastic), and intercellular substances (extracellular matrix) may be produced. These are orderly processes that require exogenous substrates from fuel and from structural components of muscle, bone, adipose tissue, and other organs. Hormones are critical in making these materials available to cells and in stimulating cell division and the secretion of materials (e.g., collagen) for the extracellular framework of the body.

With few exceptions, most hormones stimulate tissue and organ growth, and in their absence target tissues atrophy. For example, in response to melanocyte-stimulating hormone (MSH) integumental melanocytes (in the frog *Xenopus laevis*) increase in number from as few as $10/mm^2$ of epidermis to as many as 1,000 to 2,000 mm^2 (see Fig. 8.11). In the absence of MSH, the melanocytes soon atrophy and disappear from the skin. The size of the human adrenal cortex (Chap. 15) is drastically affected by the levels of ACTH secreted by the pituitary gland.

Growth Hormone and the Somatomedins

The pivotal role of pituitary growth hormone (GH) in the control of growth has been firmly established [1, 3]. Congenital failure to synthesize and secrete GH leads to short stature; hypersecretion of GH, on the other hand, leads to gigantism if overproduction of the hormone is initiated early in life, or to acromegaly if oversecretion occurs in the adult.

Growth hormone causes growth of the epiphyseal regions of the long bones. Growth of bone can be monitored by measuring the incorporation of sulfur (^{35}S) into the epiphyseal cartilage. When bones from young animals are incubated in a medium containing normal serum and the radioactive isotope of sulfur, the sulfur is incorporated into the sulfated polysaccharides of the cartilage. However, when bones are incubated in serum from hypophysectomized animals, no incorporation of ^{35}S takes place. This was initially considered to be due to the lack of GH in the serum. When GH was added to serum from hypophysectomized animals, incorporation of the radioactive sulfur into cartilage still failed to occur. If, however, hypophysectomized animals were injected with GH some hours before blood collection, the serum supported the incorporation of the radioactive sulfur into bone. The conclusion was drawn that GH acts indirectly on bones by way of the production of a *sulfation factor*.

The sulfation factor is now known to consist of several peptides referred to as *somatomedins*. Injected radiolabeled GH rapidly localizes to the liver rather than to the epiphyses of the long bones. Somatomedin is generally used to refer to those growth factors found in the plasma that are under the control of GH, have insulin-like properties, and promote the incorporation of sulfate into cartilage (the "somatomedin hypothesis"). Two substances isolated from the plasma in pure or rather pure form fulfill these criteria: insulin-like growth factors I and II (IGF-I and IGF-II). The peptides bear some structural relationship to proinsulin and, therefore, exhibit some affinity for insulin receptors [26]. Conversely, insulin at high concentration will bind to IGF receptors. IGFs are secreted by the liver and by some other tissues in response to GH stimulation. The somatomedins are not, however, stored in appreciable amounts within the liver; hence, the liver is not a source of extractable growth factors. The growth activity present in the blood cannot be neutralized by antibodies against insulin. The amino acid sequences of these insulin-like growth factors, IGF-I and IGF-II, nevertheless reveal a high degree of similarity to insulin. These polypeptides in the human consist of 70 and 67 amino acid residues, respectively [22], and have a proinsulin-like structure with a shorter connecting peptide of 12 amino acids and an extension of 8 residues at the A-chain terminus (Fig. 12.2). IGF-II is three times more abundant in the adult circulation than IGF-I, yet its origin and function are less well defined.

Insulin is more potent in stimulating metabolic effects in insulin target tissues than are IGF-I and IGF-II. On the other hand, insulin is a less potent stimulator of cell proliferation than these growth factors. From an evolutionary point of view, one precursor hormone of insulin and of IGF-I must have existed that, millions of years ago, was responsible for both the acute regulation of metabolism and the stimulation of the slow processes of growth. Later, a gene duplication must have taken place leading to the diversion of these two functions,

Figure 12.2 Primary
structure of human
IGF-I. The amino acids
in black circles denote
those in identical
position in the A and B
chain of human insulin.
(From Humbel and
Rinderknecht [22],
by permission.)

leaving the second-to-second metabolic regulation to insulin and the regulation of growth to
IGF-I. Although the classic actions of IGFs are thought to be endocrine, physiologically
important IGF concentrations may be generated at the tissue level. The functions of IGFs
are mediated by two main classes of IGF receptors. The IGF-I receptor exhibits ligand-
dependent tyrosine kinase activity and autophosphorylation, causing phosphorylation of the
cytoplasmic proteins, insulin-responsive substrates (IRS), which then activate protein kinase B
and the mitogen-activated protein kinase (MAPK) pathways. The IGF-I receptor has considerable structural and functional similarity to the insulin receptor, but higher affinity for
IGF-I and IGF-II than for insulin (Fig. 12.3). The IGF-II receptor, in contrast, has a different
structure and is homologous with the human mannose-6-phosphate receptor. It has a higher
affinity for IGF-II than IGF-I and does not bind insulin. Both IGF-I and IGF-II can bind,
although at low potency, to the insulin receptor.

According to the somatomedin hypothesis, GH does not have a direct effect on cartilage but
rather stimulates chondrogenesis and subsequent growth indirectly by way of somatomedins.
Nevertheless, local injection of GH into the epiphyseal growth plate of the proximal tibia of
hypophysectomized rats stimulates unilateral longitudinal bone growth. The number of IGF-I
immunoreactive cells in the proliferative zone is increased. It was concluded that IGF-I is produced in proliferative chondrocytes in the growth plate in response to GH and that the number
of IGF-I-containing cells is directly regulated by expansion of differentiated chondrocytes as
stimulated locally through autocrine or paracrine mechanisms or both [32, 35].

GH can induce local IGF-I production in the epiphyseal plate at the level of both mRNA
and protein. In vitro studies of epiphyseal chondrocytes indicate that GH and IGF-I have

Figure 12.3 The insulin and IGF-I
receptors are structurally related
heterotetrameric glycoproteins
consisting of two α and two β subunits.
The α subunits lie entirely
extracellularly, contain cysteine-rich
regions, and bind the ligands. The
transmembrane β subunits are joined
to the α subunits by disulfide bonds and
contain a tyrosine kinase domain in their
cytoplasmic portion. The level of amino
acid similarity between these two
receptors is particularly high (85%)
in the tyrosine kinase domains [26].

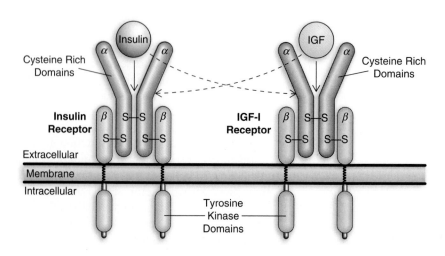

different target cells; they bind to different cell populations and give rise to different clonal types in soft agar suspension cultures. GH, but not IGF-I, stimulates the multiplication of the slowly cycling (label-retaining) cells in the germinal layer of the epiphyseal plate. IGF-I acts only on the proliferation of the resulting chondrocytes. The fact that locally infused IGF-I is able to increase epiphyseal width as well as longitudinal bone growth, together with the finding that IGF-I was unable to increase the number of label-retaining cells in the germinal layer, indicates that the target cells for IGF-I are located in the proliferative cell layer. The cells of the germinal layer may be regarded as the stem cells of the growth plate and the proliferative chondrocytes as "transient amplifying" cells. The growth demonstrated by local or by systemic IGF-I administration could probably be explained by a stimulation of the proliferative cell layer, where extra cell divisions within the transient amplifying cells could result in significant growth. Data support the theory that GH simulates a low differentiated stem cell-like population to start dividing, which gives rise to a clonal expansion, and that IGF-I, on the other hand, enhances the clonal expansion of an already GH-primed cell population [34].

Both triiodothyronine (T_3) and IGF-I interact with epiphyseal chondrocytes and both substances affect cell proliferation and maturation and therefore longitudinal bone growth [27]. IGF-I is important for proliferation of the cells, whereas T_3 may initiate the terminal differentiation of epiphyseal chondrocytes [34].

It is likely that the actions of GH on some other tissues are also mediated by the local production of IGF-I or possibly other somatomedins. In the *dual-effector theory* of somatotropin action, GH directly stimulates the differentiated state of certain cell types. For example, GH, but not IGF-I, directly promotes the differentiation of cultured preadipocytes to adipocytes. The newly differentiated adipocytes were shown to be much more sensitive to the mitogenic actions of IGF-I than were the precursor cells. The result of IGF-I action is, therefore, a selective multiplication of young differentiated cells (a so-called clonal expansion). In this dual-effector system, the target cells of IGF-I action are created by the initial direct action of GH [23]. A model for the direct and indirect actions of GH is provided (Fig. 12.4).

Pituitary GH is essential for normal growth in humans and probably most vertebrates. GH secretion is regulated by stimulating (GH-releasing hormone; GHRH) and inhibiting (somatostatin; SST) factors from the hypothalamus. The extent to which the endogenous GH-secretogogue, ghrelin, may additionally contribute to the physiological regulation of GH secretion remains unclear. Diverse stimuli mediate pituitary GH secretion by their initial actions within the hypothalamus (Chap. 6). In the adult, excess GH secretion results in acromegaly. There is controversy concerning the role of the central nervous system (CNS) in the pathogenesis of acromegaly. The central issue is whether pituitary tumor formation occurs as a consequence of neoplastic transformation in a somatotroph cell(s) or secondary to excessive stimulation by GHRH. Recent molecular biologic studies of two different tumor types support the "pituitary hypothesis." Analysis of these adenomas suggests that

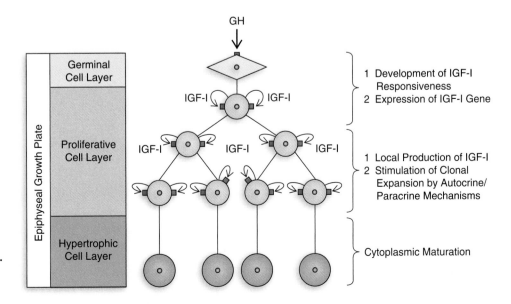

Figure 12.4 Model of the dual-effector hypothesis of GH action. (From Isaksson et al. [23], with permission.)

these tumors are monoclonal, implying that a mutation preceded the tumor's clonal expansion. In other studies, the sequence of the α subunit of the guanine nucleotide binding (regulatory) protein (Gs) in 35–40% of somatotroph adenomas has been shown to contain a common point mutation at one of two sites that is crucial for its intrinsic GTPase activity [43]. The mutations produce a single amino acid substitution that leads to constitutive activation of adenylate cyclase, resulting in enhanced cAMP production (see Figs 21.13 and 21.14). Cyclic AMP has been implicated as a mitogen, as well as a stimulus, to both the synthesis and release of GH. Results from several studies argue in favor of a pituitary defect in the etiology of acromegaly, but they do not exclude a contribution from the CNS, and it is possible that somatotrophs subjected to stimulation by excessive GHRH secretion might be more likely to undergo neoplastic transformation.

IGF-I stimulates hypothalamic SST release and inhibits stimulated pituitary GH release. In addition, intracerebroventricularly injected preparations of IGFs cause a marked decrease in GH secretion. A model for the control of GH secretion and somatomedin production is shown in Figure 12.5.

Replacement therapy in GH-deficient adults alters body composition and energy metabolism through its lipolytic, protein anabolic, and antinatriuretic actions. This results in decreased fat mass, increased fat-free mass, sodium retention, and increased energy expenditure. These observations suggest that after cessation of somatic growth, GH exerts significant diverse metabolic actions in adult life and suggest that the lack of GH may be accompanied by abnormalities in body composition and energy metabolism [21].

Growth hormone regulates growth indirectly through hepatic IGF-I production. IGF-I then affects growth through its action on skeletal tissues and many other connective tissues and organs. Several hormones (e.g., prolactin, placental lactogen, insulin) may also exert part of their growth-promoting activity through effects on hepatic IGF production. The structures of human placental lactogen (hPL) and prolactin (PRL) are similar to that of GH. IGF levels remain normal in hypophysectomized pregnant rats even in the absence of PRL and GH; these levels decline promptly postpartum. Thus, other GH-related factors may be important in IGF production during particular physiological states, such as pregnancy.

Growth hormone has a direct action on a number of target cells in addition to its action on hepatic IGF production. These GH actions have been described as diabetogenic in nature. For example, GH stimulates lipolysis, which provides substrates for glucose formation, and

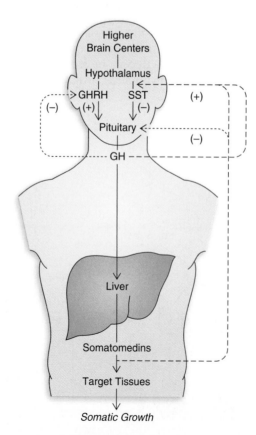

Figure 12.5 Model for the control of GH secretion by somatostatin (SST) and somatocrinin (GHRH).

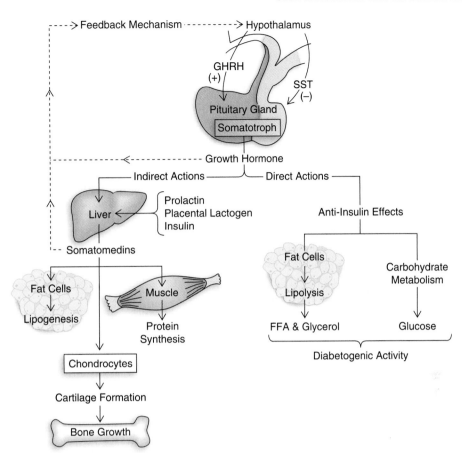

Figure 12.6 Summary scheme of the direct and indirect actions of growth hormone on growth and metabolism.

thus has a sparing effect on direct glucose utilization (Chap. 11). The direct and indirect actions of GH are depicted in Figure 12.6.

Figure 12.7 depicts the relationship between GH and plasma levels of IGFs. Individuals with hypopituitary short stature [1], as might be expected, have very minimal plasma levels of IGF-I and IGF-II. Although levels of IGF-I are greatly increased in acromegalics, levels of IGF-II did not differ from controls. Like IGF-I, IGF-II production is GH-dependent; but this relationship becomes apparent only when GH levels fall below normal. These results indicate

Figure 12.7 Serum immunoreactive (IR) IGF-I and -II levels in normal adults, acromegalic patients, and patients with isolated GH deficiency. (Reproduced from J. Zapf et al. and used by permission from *The Journal of Clinical Investigation,* 1981, vol. 68: 1321–30. © The American Society for Clinical Investigation.)

that production of the two IGFs is regulated differently. Some short children with low sponta-neous GH secretion and high percent increase in serum IGF values in response to provocative GH stimulation benefit from GH or IGF-I treatment by an increased growth rate [16].

Dwarfism in German shepherd dogs may be genetically transmitted by a simple recessive mode of inheritance. Dwarfism in these dogs is caused by GH deficiency resulting in low circu-lating levels of IGF-I. In the dwarf mouse strain, "*little*," decreased growth is associated with a partial deficiency of GH production. The pituitaries of these mice are completely insensitive to GHRH. GH secretion, however, can be stimulated by Db-cAMP or agents that increase cAMP levels. These observations suggested a defect in the early stage of GHRH-stimulated GH release related to receptor binding, a hypothesis confirmed by the finding that the GHRH receptor of *little* mice contains a missense mutation of the extracellular domain that disrupts receptor function [19]. Short stature in the African Pygmy has been an enigma for centuries. Pygmies have decreased circulating levels of IGF-I (Fig. 12.8) and the high-affinity GH-binding protein (GH-BP; see below) [11]. Plasma levels of IGF-II are, in contrast to hypopituitary short stature, within the range found in normal adults [3, 29, 30]. Thus, normal serum levels of IGF-II are inadequate for promotion of normal growth in the absence of IGF-I, at least in Pygmies. The role of IGF-II in growth remains to be clarified. These findings in the African Pygmy may be consistent with undernutrition.

The GH receptor is activated on binding of GH to stimulate the growth and metabolism of muscle, bone, and cartilage cells. This receptor is a member of a group of receptors that are found on various cell types and are generally involved in cell growth and differentiation [2]. All these receptors are grouped together in the cytokine receptor superfamily [17]. Like the receptor tyrosine kinases, members of the cytokine receptor superfamily have a three-domain organization comprising an extracellular ligand binding domain, a single transmembrane segment, and an intracellular domain, which is homologous within the family only within the proximal (near the membrane) sequence. Unlike the receptor tyrosine kinases, the cytokine receptors do not possess intrinsic kinase activity. Binding of GH to the GH receptor induces receptor dimerization, which increases the affinity of the proximal intracellular domain of the receptor for certain cytoplasmic tyrosine kinases called the Janus kinases (JAKs). The binding of JAKs rapidly induces phosphorylation of the JAKs, the receptor, and other cellular proteins that bind to the receptor–JAK complex. The best known targets for JAKs are tran-scription factors known as signal transducers and activators of transcription (STATs). Binding of STATs to phosphorylated sites on the receptor occurs via specialized phospho-tyrosine docking sites referred to as src-homology 2 (SH2) domains. Upon binding to the complex, the STATs undergo phosphorylation, dimerization, and translocation to the nucleus, where they

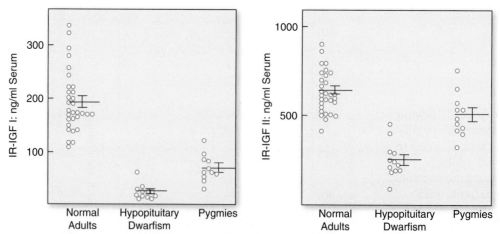

Figure 12.8 Serum concentrations of IGF-I and IGF-II in controls, hypopituitary dwarfism, and Pygmies. IGF-I and IGF-II were measured in the same adult controls. Lines and bars denote means ± SEM. Note that only one Pygmy has an IGF-I value within the lower normal range, whereas all but one have IGF-II values within the normal range. All values are corrected for cross-reactivity. (From Merimee, Zapf, and Froesch, reprinted by permission of *The New England Journal of Medicine*, vol. 305, pp. 965–68, 1981.)

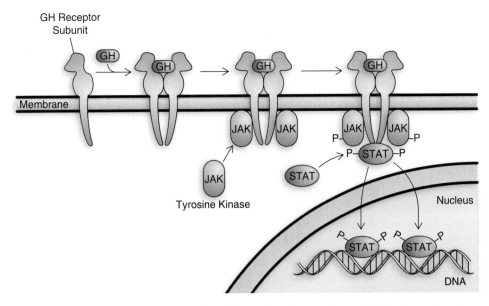

Figure 12.9 Growth hormone signal transduction pathway. GH brings about receptor dimerization by binding first to the extracellular domain (ECD) of one receptor molecule and then to that of another receptor molecule. The signal of GH-binding is probably transmitted via the transmembrane domain (TMD) to bring about conformational changes in the intracellular domain (ICD). This results in the recruitment and binding of the cytoplasmic tyrosine kinase, JAK2, to the receptor. JAK2 undergoes autophosphorylation and activation, which in turn phosphorylates the receptor. Phosphorylated tyrosines on the receptor then function as docking sites for STAT transcription factors, which bind through the SH2 domain and are phosphory-lated. The activated STATs dimerize, translocate to the nucleus, and bind enhancer regions in GH target genes to regulate their transcription.

bind to specific enhancer elements in GH inducible genes, such as those encoding IGF-I or GH-BP [48]. A model for GH action is depicted (Fig. 12.9).

Laron syndrome is due to an autosomal recessive disorder occurring in consanguineous families, and affected individuals are resistant to the effects of endogenous and exogenous GH [4, 8]. Growth hormone from these individuals is, by chemical and biochemical criteria, similar to GH from normal individuals. Unlike short stature due to isolated GH deficiency, individuals with the Laron syndrome have elevated levels of circulating GH. The affected individuals have markedly reduced circulating levels of IGF-I. Laron syndrome is caused by hepatic unresponsiveness to circulating GH due to a defect in the GH receptor [42]. An inbred population with a high incidence of GH receptor deficiency, which is a type of the Laron syndrome, has been described, with the predominance of the affected individuals being females, "the little women of Loja" (Fig. 12.10), and may be the result of the genetic defect being linked to a trait resulting in early fetal death of most affected males [39, 40].

The defect in the GH receptor is an extreme example of the Laron syndrome; several different abnormalities of the GH receptor gene have been demonstrated in this condition: a point mutation in one family, a deletion of a large portion of the extracellular domain of the receptor gene in two other cases [25]. The defect also affects the high-affinity GH-BP; complete absence of GH-binding activity has been demonstrated in the plasma of patients with the Laron syndrome. A high-affinity binding protein has been characterized as a frag-ment of the GH receptor. The assay of the GH-BP can be used as a tool for diagnosis; Laron syndrome is the only situation in which a complete absence of GH-binding activity is observed [15]. This hypothesis, however, has been reevaluated because of the recent description of patients displaying the classic features of the Laron syndrome except for the presence of GH-BP activity similar to that of normal subjects. In this variant form of the Laron syndrome there appears to be a normal GH receptor and GH-BP but a defect in the post-receptor mechanism for the generation of IGF-I [25].

Figure 12.10 The family of patients (#8, #9, #10) with GH receptor deficiency. This photograph shows, from left to right, a sister, 25 years old (height, 158.8 cm); a brother, 18 years old (164.7 cm); Patient 9 (16 years old, 107.1 cm); the father, 52 years old (165 cm); Patient 8 (21 years old, 106.2 cm); a brother, 12 years old (135.9 cm); a sister, 8.5 years old (115.4 cm); and the mother, 46 years old (156.7 cm), holding Patient 10 (6.5 years old, 72 cm). (From A. L. Rosenbloom, J. Guevara Aguirre, R. G. Rosenfeld, and P. J. Fiedler, "The little women of Loja—Growth hormone-receptor deficiency in an inbred population of southern Ecuador." Reprinted by permission of *The New England Journal of Medicine,* 323:1367–74, 1990.)

About 40–50% of circulating GH is complexed to the GH-BP in normal human plasma. The GH-BP complex represents a hormone reservoir, and the presence of the BP modifies the amount of hormone that can have access to the receptors. GH-BP generation in the human probably results from the proteolytic cleavage of the liver membrane receptor. On the other hand, in the rat, alternate splicing of a single primary DNA transcript may give rise to distinct mRNAs; one encodes the full-length membrane receptor, the other a truncated receptor (the extracellular binding domain) [15].

Binding proteins are important modulators of the ligand–receptor interaction on target cells [4, 37]. IGFs circulate in the serum as high-molecular-weight complexes. The majority of the IGFs are complexed as a 150 kDa GH-dependent binding protein complex. Lower-molecular-weight binding proteins occur in fetal plasma and other extracellular fluids. Only low levels of free IGFs are detected in plasma, raising the question as to whether physiologically active IGF is the free or complexed form. The "free hormone hypothesis" as postulated for steroid and thyroid hormones would allow IGF-binding proteins a merely passive role, that of physically transporting the IGFs and of inactivating the IGFs by their being bound. Studies now indicate a more dynamic role for the IGF-binding proteins, that of interacting with target cells and thus facilitating the delivery of hormones to their receptors. IGF-binding proteins themselves bind to some cell surfaces and thus deliver IGF to adjacent IGF receptors [36]. Figure 12.11 illustrates the anatomical and physiological factors related to GH disorders.

Ethical Issues. Growth hormone is already accepted as the conventional treatment for short stature in children with GH deficiency [16], but it is now being given to increasing numbers of children who do not fulfill the classic criteria of growth deficiency. GH will augment the growth of many of these children; however, the effect on final adult heights is as yet unknown. Before trials of GH deficiency are extended beyond children with the classic growth deficiency, ethical and other issues should be considered. There are dangers, for example, that GH might be used to alter people to fit a social norm rather than to treat a disease. Also, it has been questioned whether society should spend resources on "something that really isn't a problem" [44]. Since there has been an increased incidence of neoplasia in females with acromegaly (where there is increased GH secretion), concerns have been raised relative to a possible increase in malignancy in patients receiving GH replacement therapy [9].

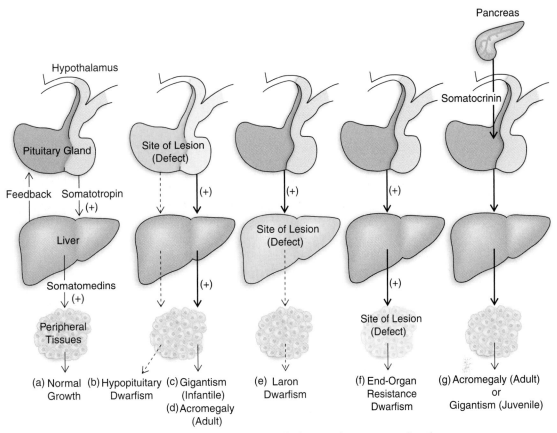

Figure 12.11 Various endocrine disorders relating to the overproduction or underproduction of pituitary GH or to inadequate hepatic or peripheral tissue response to GH or somatomedins.

Safety of Growth Hormone for Animal Use. An independent committee appointed by the National Institutes of Health has examined the available data and concluded that the overall composition and nutritional quality of milk and meat from cows treated with bovine growth hormone (bGH) is equal to that from untreated cows. Similarly, the FDA has concluded that the use of bGH presents no increased health risk to consumers. In addition, there is compelling evidence to indicate that GH poses no increased health risk to the target animal. Thus, GH treatment of farm animals is not only an effective technology for increasing productive efficiency, but one that poses no health risk for either the consumer or the target animal [14].

Insulin

Although insulin plays the dominant role in the control of carbohydrate metabolism in humans and other vertebrates, it also profoundly affects growth processes in animals. Children with diabetes, for example, fail to grow even though GH levels are normal, whereas infants of diabetic mothers with islet hyperplasia and hyper-insulinism are of increased stature. This might not be too surprising considering the structural similarities among insulin, the IGFs, and their receptors. The growth-promoting actions of insulin are amply documented, and protein catabolism is accelerated in the absence of insulin. Insulin is required for the full anabolic effect of GH, an action that may be because insulin, through its action on glucose uptake by muscle, provides the energy substrates necessary for protein synthesis. However, insulin also increases the incorporation of amino acids into muscle by an action that is independent of its effects on glucose metabolism. This may result from the direct action of insulin on the transport of amino acids into cells, as well as activation of ribosomal translational capacity, as protein synthesis per se is not dependent on glucose availability or RNA synthesis. Insulin stimulates the growth of immature hypophysectomized rats, but this action is manifested only when the protein-sparing action of insulin is enhanced by the concomitant feeding of a high carbohydrate diet.

Insulin at a high concentration, as in familial insulin resistance, stimulates general body growth through low-affinity binding to IGF receptors. Although there is insulin-receptor deficiency in this endocrinopathy, the number of IGF receptors appears to be normal. The high circulating levels of insulin thus cause acral (affecting the extremities) overgrowth as well as enlargement of the kidney and adrenal glands; these actions of insulin may result from cross-reactivity with IGF receptors (Fig. 12.3) [37].

Prolactin

In humans, prolactin (PRL) plays an important role in milk synthesis, a function that of necessity requires development and growth of the mammary glands. Because of the close structural similarity between PRL and GH, it is not surprising that many effects of PRL are growth-related; most are usually involved in reproductive processes of the individual (see Chaps 5 and 19).

Prolactin, along with estrogens and adrenal steroids, is essential for ductile branching during the prepubertal and postpubertal period to form the fully developed system of the mammary glands of the mature female (see Fig. 19.6). Large amounts of PRL, even in the absence of adequate amounts of estrogens (as occurs in PRL-secreting tumors in men or postmenopausal women), are usually associated with clinically evident enlargement of the breasts. PRL also stimulates production of somatomedins by the rat liver and could conceivably affect general body growth by a GH-like action.

PRL also has important stimulatory effects on the immune system; it serves as a growth factor for lymphocytes and accelerates T-cell-dependent immune responses [41]. Hyperprolactinemia has been reported in association with autoimmune thyroiditis and systemic lupus erythematosus in humans [47]. PRL is also synthesized and secreted by human blood mononuclear cells and may be an autocrine growth factor for lymphoproliferation [41].

Prolactin also directly affects the growth and function of the ovaries and testes, in some cases by modulating the action of gonadotropins on the gonads. In nonmammalian vertebrates, PRL has growth-related actions such as stimulation of tail and gill growth in amphibians. PRL is required for limb regeneration in the salamander and tail regeneration in lizards. Many structural changes in the skin of the salamander related to "water drive" involve the actions of PRL. Hypertrophy of the pigeon crop-sac mucosa, as well as epidermal hyperplasia related to brood patch formation in the dove, are regulated by PRL. Other physiological actions of this hormone are discussed in Chapters 5 and 19.

The amino acid sequences of human GH and PRL receptors have been deduced from their respective cDNA sequences. There is strong localized sequence identity between the two receptors in both the extracellular and cytoplasmic domains, suggesting that the two receptors originated from a common ancestor. Like the GH receptor, the PRL receptor does not possess tyrosine kinase activity, and signal transduction is mediated by the JAK-STAT signal transduction pathway.

Probably no other hormone has as many effects and possible functions as PRL. This functional versatility may relate to its molecular heterogeneity. Although PRL is encoded by a single gene, molecular variants may arise by alternate splicing of the mRNA along with post-translational modifications of the protein (about 200 amino acids). Diversity of PRL action may result in both molecular heterogeneity of the hormone coupled with structural heterogeneity of the PRL receptor. A differential distribution of these receptors would determine the particular cellular/physiological response [10].

Placental Lactogen

During pregnancy, the placenta secretes hormones that augment maternal pituitary and gonadal functions. In addition to chorionic gonadotropin and a number of steroids, the placenta also synthesizes and secretes chorionic somatomammotropin. Although similar to GH in structure, this hormone lacks significant growth-promoting activity but displays considerable lactogenic activity; it is therefore referred to as placental lactogen (PL). In the human, PL is found in the maternal plasma as early as the sixth week of pregnancy and reaches a concentration three orders of magnitude greater than that of GH during the second trimester. Placental lactogen is synthesized within the *syncytiotrophoblastic* epithelial cells of the chorionic villi of the placenta (Chap. 19).

Placental lactogen increases sulfate uptake into cartilage in hypophysectomized rats, both in vivo and in vitro, and also stimulates growth and induction of milk protein synthesis in mouse mammary explants. Development and maturation of the testes of immature and genetically dwarf mice is also stimulated by PL. All these biological actions are similar to the actions of human PRL. Placental lactogen mimics the action of GH on most of its target tissues but is much less potent than GH. There is no evidence that PL can increase linear growth in hypopituitary short stature. It might be expected, however, that this hormone evolved to play some specific role(s) related to pregnancy and reproductive processes. PL secretion during the second trimester of human pregnancy may supplement the action of choriogonadotropin on the corpus luteum, which is diminishing. The primary role of PL may be to stimulate the development of the mammary glands during pregnancy without actually causing milk secretion. Pituitary PRL then initiates milk secretion soon after parturition. PL may also alter the maternal metabolism so that adequate supplies of glucose, amino acids, and minerals are available to the fetus during the latter part of pregnancy, a time when fetal growth requirements are rapidly increasing. During the second half of pregnancy, PL is one of several factors that counter the effect of insulin in the maternal circulation, thereby facilitating glucose and amino acid availability to the fetus. In this manner, the placental secretion of this hormone indirectly stimulates intrauterine growth. PL may also directly stimulate fetal growth. Ovine PL stimulates glycogenesis in hepatocytes of the fetal rat and sheep and aminoisobutyric acid uptake in diaphragm muscle of the fetal rat. It also stimulates ornithine decarboxylase activity in fetal rat liver and somatomedin secretion in fetal and adult tissue. These observations indicate a role for PL in fetal growth and development (Fig. 12.6).

Human PL and GH are both single-chain polypeptides containing 191 amino acid residues. Both hormones are internally cross-linked through two disulfide bridges and are identical throughout 85% of their primary structures; 162 residues in each polypeptide are identical and occupy similar positions in the hormones. The high degree of structural similarity between hPL and human and ovine GH suggests that the polypeptide arose from a relatively recent duplication of a GH gene (Fig. 12.12), rather than from the more distantly related lactogenic hormones. A placental lactogen immunologically similar to hPL is present in the plasma of the rhesus monkey, baboon, chinchilla, hamster, goat, cow, sheep, and a number of other mammalian species. In general the level of the placental lactogen begins to rise at or before midpregnancy and usually remains elevated until term.

Figure 12.12
Hypothetical scheme for the evolution of growth hormone, prolactin, and placental lactogen.

Neurotropic Growth Factors

Several peptide growth factors regulate the differentiation and growth of both the central and peripheral nervous systems. The etiological basis of one or more disorders (e.g., Alzheimer's disease) may relate to these neurotropic factors.

NGF Promotes Survival of Peripheral Sympathetic and Spinal Neurons During Development

Growth and differentiation of sensory and motor components of the peripheral nervous system are enhanced by factors released from peripheral target tissues [7]. On the other hand, an intact innervation and release of supporting substances from nerve endings are essential for normal development of the innervated target tissues. There is accumulating evidence that specific chemical messengers are important in these reciprocal actions between nerves and target tissues.

Certain mouse sarcomas induce a pathologic hypertrophy of chick embryonic sensory and sympathetic ganglia. This neuronal hypertrophy depends on a humoral protein factor released by the transplanted tumors. This substance was named nerve growth factor (NGF), and its chemistry and biological roles have been well characterized [7]. NGF is also present in snake venom and in the submandibular (submaxillary) salivary glands of adult male mice. NGF is synthesized within tubular cells of the submandibular gland and its production is androgen-dependent. Salivary gland NGF levels in female mice rise during pregnancy and lactation when androgen levels are elevated. Testosterone given to female mice causes tubular cell hypertrophy and the content of salivary gland NGF rises markedly. In contrast, castration of male mice causes tubular atrophy and the salivary gland content of NGF falls dramatically.

The early discovery that mouse submandibular glands synthesize and release into the saliva large quantities of NGF, that the synthesis of the protein molecule is under the control of testosterone and of thyroxine, and that the NGF protein content is about tenfold higher in male than in female mice long remained a puzzling and unexplained finding. The conflicting but negative attempts to reveal the presence of this molecule in the circulating blood, and the lack of any adverse effects on sympathetic and sensory cells by removal of these glands, which deprived these rodents of such a large NGF source, did not support the hypothesis that salivary NGF gains access to target cells. An alternative biological function for salivary NGF has now been hypothesized. Intraspecific fighting experimentally induced in adult male mice by 6 to 9 weeks of social isolation results in massive NGF release into the bloodstream, an event prevented by previous salivary gland removal. Since injections of NGF induce weight and size increase of the adrenal glands and stimulate the synthesis of tyrosine hydroxylase, the key enzyme in catecholamine synthesis (Chap. 14), it was suggested that the release of salivary NGF may be instrumental in defense and/or offense mechanisms of vital significance for male mice that engage in intraspecific fighting among individuals of the same sex.

Peripheral sympathetic postganglionic neurons of the autonomic nervous system (Chap. 14) are the primary target cells for NGF and respond to the protein throughout life. Injections of NGF antiserum in newborn mice or chick embryos cause almost complete destruction of the sympathetic nervous system (immunosympathectomy). Exposure in utero to maternal antibodies to NGF, in addition to producing immunosympathectomy, destroys peripheral nervous system sensory neurons in the dorsal root ganglia. These neurons may depend on NGF for survival during prenatal development. Other dorsal root cells may manifest a temporal difference in their dependence on NGF. NGF antiserum administration to adult animals causes deleterious effects on sympathetic neurons that are reversible after antiserum treatment is stopped. Thus, it appears that an endogenous NGF is critical for sympathetic nervous system development, and NGF may function in the maintenance of sympathetic neurons throughout life.

Mouse salivary gland NGF is a molecular complex consisting of three types of polypeptide chains, designated α, β, and γ. Each of these subunits consists of a pair of identical molecules. The β subunit is held together by noncovalent bonds. Only the β subunit possesses nerve growth-promoting activity. The biological activity of NGF is dependent on the dimeric structure of the molecule. NGF is synthesized as a precursor peptide, a proNGF. The individual β chains of NGF are then cleaved by the γ subunit, which is an endopeptidase. The α subunits may play a role in maintaining the functional integrity of the molecular complex of NGF in the secretory granule.

There is homology between NGF and proinsulin and there are also striking similarities between the biological activities of the two molecules. Both hormones bind initially to cell membranes, which results in an enhancement of a number of ensuing anabolic processes, such as RNA synthesis, polysome formation, and protein and lipid synthesis, characteristic of cellular growth. NGF may be viewed as a hormone whose structural gene may have evolved from an ancestral proinsulin gene and whose mode of action on neurons might, therefore, be somewhat similar to that of insulin on its target tissues. To a limited extent, insulin and proinsulin can compete for the binding of NGF to its receptor, further emphasizing the relationship of NGF to proinsulin.

After an initial interaction with the cell plasma membrane, NGF is internalized and, by retrograde axonal transport, apparently carried to the soma of the cell [37]. Retrograde transport of NGF is specific as other proteins of similar size and charge are transported to a much lesser extent. It is interesting that insulin may be similarly internalized in its target cells to invoke some of its cellular effects. Binding of NGF is specific to target tissue surface receptors because motor neurons that can internalize and transport tetanus toxin fail to do so with NGF. Similarly, cholinergic parasympathetic nerves, which like motor neurons are refractory to the biological actions of NGF, do not transport NGF.

NGF exerts a pleiotropic effect on nerve cells, which includes the synthesis of specific enzymes, tyrosine hydroxylase and dopamine β-hydroxylase, involved in adrenergic nervous transmission [5, 46]. The stimulation by NGF of nerve fiber outgrowth is reflected in the accumulation of large masses of neurofilaments that are found in developing axons. Neurite outgrowth in response to NGF is an RNA-independent event, which suggests that NGF may stimulate fiber outgrowth by acting in a selective fashion on protein synthesis at a stage after transcription. Ornithine decarboxylase is a key enzyme in the biosynthesis of polyamines and may serve an important regulatory role in cell division and growth. In the brain, the intraventricular injection of NGF leads to a marked increase in the activity of this enzyme. Adrenal glucocorticoids appear to be required for NGF to enhance the activity of ornithine decarboxylase.

Clearly, NGF functions in the survival of peripheral sympathetic and spinal sensory neurons during defined periods of their ontogenesis. In addition, NGF directs growing sympathetic nerve fibers toward their corresponding target tissues. The role of NGF as a retrograde messenger between peripheral target tissues and innervating sympathetic and neural crest-derived sensory neurons is supported by the observation that the interruption of the retrograde axonal transport has the same effects as the neutralization of endogenous NGF by anti-NGF antibodies, and by the close correlation between the density of innervation by fibers of NGF-responsive neurons and the levels of NGF and mRNA in their target organs. In situ hybridization experiments have demonstrated that a great variety of cells in the projection field of NGF-responsive neurons synthesize NGF, among them epithelial cells, smooth muscle cells, fibroblasts, and Schwann cells. The continued availability of NGF to sympathetic neurons is essential for neuron survival. A common misconception is that NGF stimulates neuronal cell division. Despite its name, NGF is not mitogenic for neurons. NGF directs neurite outgrowth and guidance to targets; it promotes cell survival in only a few cell populations, which include sympathetic and neural crest-derived sensory neurons.

NGF may also have a physiological role in the mammalian central nervous system as a neurotropic factor. There is evidence that the brain contains NGF, NGF messenger RNA, NGF receptors, and NGF-responsive neurons. One function of NGF in the CNS appears to be the regulation of the differentiation of the cholinergic projection neurons found within various nuclei of the basal forebrain. NGF also prevents the retrograde degeneration of cholinergic neurons within the medial septum of the rat brain that normally occurs following axotomy of these neurons. Lesioned animals suffer from deficits in learning and memory. NGF infusion into the brain of these rats counteracts their learning deficiencies, presumably by prevention of neuronal losses. There is hope that the deterioration of the cholinergic neurons in the brains of Alzheimer's patients might be prevented or retarded by treatment with NGF, related growth factors, or drugs that mimic growth factor activity in the brain [24, 46].

NGF is one Member of a Family of Neurotropins

Considering the diversity of neuronal cell types, it is not unexpected that a number of other neurotropic factors have been identified (see cover photographs and caption).

The NGF Family and Its Receptors.   The gene family of neurotropins includes nerve growth factor (NGF), brain-derived neurotropic factor (BDNF), neurotropin-3 (NT-3), and neurotropin-4 (NT-4). Recently, neurotropin-5 (NT-5), a possible mammalian homologue to NT-4 described in the frog, *Xenopus*, has been cloned in humans and rats. These factors are produced in limited amounts in target tissues and mediate the cell interaction regulating neuron survival during the period of naturally occurring neuronal death in development. The release of these proteins is believed to regulate not only the survival of neurons, but also the extent of innervation of the target tissues. As well as being important in neuronal development, neurotrophic factors also have a function in the adult nervous system [46].

These trophic factors are synthesized as precursor polypeptides that are subsequently cleaved to yield the mature neurotrophins. These molecules are homodimers of 115 to 130 amino acid residues that share at least 50% sequence identity, including six conserved cysteine residues. The structure of NGF has recently been determined from crystallographic data. The similarities between the different neurotropins are substantial within the variable regions, giving specificity to each of the family members. A 140-K tyrosine protein kinase encoded by the proto-oncogene *trk* has been found to bind NGF with high affinity and to evoke the cellular neurotropic responses. In addition, a protein encoded by the *trk*-related gene *trk*B has been shown to bind BDNF. Recently, a third member of the *trk* family, *trk*C, has been cloned and demonstrated to function as a high-affinity receptor for NT-3 [4]. Since NGF acts directly through *trk* tyrosine phosphorylation, many other crucial activities, such as neurite outgrowth, cell survival, chemotaxis, neurotransmitter synthesis and regulation, may be influenced by protein phosphorylation.

There is experimental evidence that NT-4 is a physiological factor influencing "activity-dependent" changes in neuromuscular junctions. The production of NT-4 in rat skeletal muscle, for example, was found to depend on muscle activity. Muscle NT-4 mRNA was decreased after blockade of neuromuscular transmission and was increased during postnatal development and after electrical stimulation. Intramuscular administration of NT-4 induced sprouting of intact motor neurons. Muscle-derived NT-4 may therefore act as an activity-dependent neurotrophic signal for growth and remodeling of adult motor neuron innervation. NT-4 thus may contribute to the effects of exercise and electrical stimulation on neuromuscular performance [18].

Although NGF and NGF receptors have so far not been well described in invertebrates, NGF seems to have effects on neurons from the snail *Lymnaea stagnalis*. Thus, evolution of neurotrophic factors and receptor systems mediating neurotrophic interactions in developmental and neuroplasticity processes may well have begun in ancestors common to several major metazoan phyla. No doubt the flexible system of several neurotropins with partially overlapping activities combined with several receptors has been adopted to fulfill various functions during vertebrate evolution.

Target-Derived Neurotropic Factors.   Treatment of chick embryos in vivo with crude and partially purified extracts from embryonic hindlimbs (days 8 to 9) during the normal cell death period (days 5 to 10) rescues a significant number of motoneurons from degeneration. The survival activity of partially purified extract is dose-dependent and developmentally regulated. The survival of sensory, sympathetic, parasympathetic, and a population of cholinergic sympathetic preganglionic neurons was unaffected by treatment with hindlimb extract. The massive motoneuron death that occurs after early target (hindlimb) removal is partially ameliorated by daily treatment with the hindlimb extract. These results indicate that target-derived neurotropic factors are involved in the regulation of motoneuron survival in vivo.

Insulin and IGFs.   Insulin and insulin-like growth factors I and II (IGF-I and IGF-II) are required for optimal growth and proliferation of a number of cell types. These factors also stimulate proliferation of cultured sympathetic neuroblasts, implicating a regulatory role in the mitogenic cycle of neuroblasts during fetal development. As neurons differentiate terminally, they cease to divide, but they still express receptors for insulin, IGF-I and IGF-II. In mature brain, all three factors can be detected immunochemically, but expression in the brain appears to be restricted to IGF-II and, much less abundantly, to IGF-I. These observations suggest that insulin and IGFs play a role also in the mature nervous system, which seems to include functional maintenance and survival of neurons [38].

Apoptosis can be Triggered by Some Growth Factors and Hormones

Apoptosis is a mode of cell death in which cells are deleted from tissues by a programmed sequence of biochemical events [6]. Apoptosis can be viewed as an equal and opposite force to mitosis and, as such, plays an essential role in the maintenance of renewable tissues. Apoptosis accounts for most or all of the programmed cell death responsible for tissue remodeling in vertebrate development, for the cell loss that accompanies atrophy of adult tissues following diminished endocrine and other stimuli, and for the physiological death of cells in normal tissue turnover. The homeostatic balance of cell number is brought about through the presence or absence of specific hormones or growth factors, such as NGF. The extensive deletion of lymphocytes of the B- and T-cell lineages during negative selection in the immune response is effected by apoptosis, as is a proportion of the target cell death of cell-mediated immune killing [51]. Lymphocytolysis evoked by glucocorticoids is a good example of hormone-mediated cell death. This physiologically mediated cell death is to be contrasted with necrotic death resulting from accidental trauma. Drugs that block protein synthesis prevent apoptosis, demonstrating that this programmed cell death requires specific proteins ("suicide proteins"). Many of the biochemical pathways leading to apoptosis have been delineated [20], and thus the mechanisms by which hormones may trigger or inhibit this process are now being studied.

Hematopoietic Growth Factors

Hematopoiesis is the process of renewal and replacement of the cells and formed elements of blood. Erythropoiesis is a subset of this larger scheme and includes only those events that lead from the appearance of the committed erythroid progenitor cell through the formation of mature red blood cells. Red and white blood cell differentiation and production are regulated by a number of hormones, as will be discussed in what follows.

Erythropoietin Enhances the Formation of New Red Blood Cells

The circulating red cell mass in adult humans is remarkably constant. It has been estimated that a 70 kg individual has about 2.3×10^{13} red blood cells, and that, under normal conditions, they are synthesized at a rate of about 2.3×10^6 per second. Exposing individuals to high altitudes (low oxygen tension, or hypoxia), however, results in increased *erythropoiesis* (from the Greek, *poietin*, to make), whereas hypertransfusion (hyperoxia) results in reduced erythropoiesis. The presence of an erythropoietic factor was implicated in a parabiotic experiment where subjection of one rat to hypoxia resulted in increased erythropoiesis in its parabiotic partner. Transfusion of plasma from anemic animals into normal animals causes erythropoiesis, thus suggesting the existence of a humoral erythropoietic factor (*erythropoietin*, EP [16]). Erythropoietin is elevated by conditions that create tissue hypoxia and decreased by conditions that create tissue hyperoxia (Fig. 12.13). Agents that increase the metabolic rate and oxygen consumption, such as thyroid hormones, or pharmaceutical agents, such as dinitrophenol (an uncoupler of oxidative phosphorylation), produce a state of increased need for oxygen. Under these conditions EP is produced, which leads to increased erythropoiesis. Thus, the ratio of oxygen supply to oxygen need appears to determine the level of EP formation and, therefore, the stimulus to erythropoiesis (Fig. 12.14).

Bilaterally nephrectomized rats, unlike intact animals, do not respond to phlebotomy (blood withdrawal) or red blood cell destruction by increased EP production. In humans, EP levels are low in the serum of anephric patients, but, after successful renal transplantation, EP increases in the blood. Erythropoietic activity is detected in perfusates from isolated kidneys and is also produced by renal cell cultures in vitro. These data establish the kidney as a source of the erythropoietic factor. EP levels are diminished after hypophysectomy and, like the somatomedins, is increased in response to growth hormone. EP is also produced in response to androgen stimulation (Chap. 17). Administration of EP antiserum to normal mice decreases erythropoiesis, providing support for the control of normal erythropoiesis by EP.

EP affects erythroid progenitors in the bone marrow by binding to the EP receptor (EPR). Early- and late-stage erythroid progenitor cells differ in their responsiveness to EP. This is because they express either a truncated (T) or full-length (F) EPR, EPR-T, and EPR-F, respectively. A majority of the early-stage erythroid progenitors expressing EPR-T may die

Erythropoietin (U/l)

Haemoglobin (g/l)

Figure 12.13 Semilogarithomic presentation of the exponential increase in serum erythropoietin with the degree of anemia in 63 subjects with intact kidneys (normal persons and patients with primary hemapoietic disorders; black triangles) and lack of this increase in 22 patients with chronic renal failure (open squares). (From W. Jelkmann and E. Metzen, "Erythropoietin in the control of red cell production." *Annals of Anatomy* 178:391–403, 1996, with permission.)

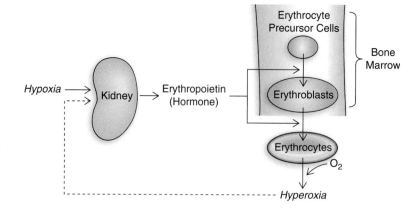

Figure 12.14 Scheme for the biogenesis and actions of erythropoietin.

of apoptosis, but the late-stage erythroid progenitors expressing EPR-F may survive and differentiate into mature erythrocytes in the presence of the same physiological concentration of EP. Thus, a mechanism exists that, under normal conditions, seemingly wastes many early-stage erythroid progenitors, but helps to form a large reservoir of late-stage erythroid precursors, which can be mobilized quickly to restore erythrocyte numbers in response to sudden bleeding or hypoxia [31].

An intrarenal O_2 sensor is thought to monitor the availability of O_2 and to translate this parameter into an altered rate of EP production [16]. Changes in oxygen flux may be detected by the tubular epithelial cells and transmitted to the adjacent peritubular endothelial cells, resulting in an induction of the gene for EP. An alternate hypothesis is that the proximal tubule cells release prostaglandin E_2, which then acts as the chemical messenger to activate EP-producing cells. The severity of hypoxia has no influence on the kinetics of the EP response, which would seem to indicate that the trigger mechanism that activates EP production in the kidney operates in an all-or-none fashion. Several signaling molecules, such as the transcription factor hypoxia-inducible factor-1 (HIF-1), have been shown to be involved in the EP transcriptional response to cellular hypoxia. Factors other than EP may have a stimulatory effect on erythropoiesis and may be necessary for the expression of the EP gene under hypoxic conditions. IGF-I, for example, stimulates erythropoiesis directly, as well as indirectly by increasing EP formation.

EP mRNA should be localized to those cells that produce EP. Using a radioactive probe for the EP mRNA, in situ hybridization and autoradiography demonstrated that a peritubular interstitial cell, outside the tubular basement membrane, was the renal cell that synthesized EP mRNA either under baseline conditions or after hypoxia (Fig. 12.15). These cells were found in

Figure 12.15 Identification of EP-synthesizing cells in murine kidney after in situ hybridization using a ³⁵S-labeled single-stranded RNA probe complementary to EP mRNA. Cells positive for EP mRNA are overlaid with silver grains and clearly lie in the interstitium between tubules. Examples of interstitial cells negative for EP mRNA are indicated by the arrows. (Photomicrograph courtesy of Dr. Stephen T. Koury. From Sanford B. Krantz "Erythropoietin." *Journal of the American Society of Hematology* 77:419–34, 1991, with permission.)

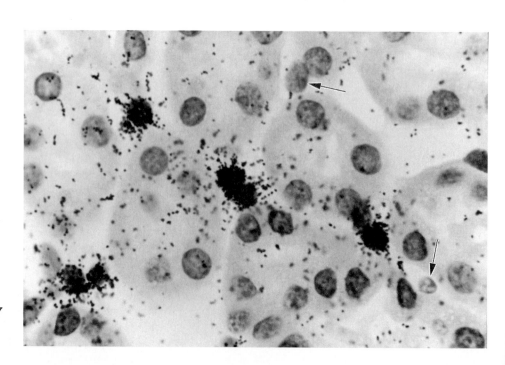

the cortex or outer medulla. When the number of interstitial cells with EP mRNA was measured in relation to increasing anemia, these cells increased in an exponential manner in parallel with the exponential increase in total EP mRNA and serum EP. Thus, increased EP production was related to increased numbers of cells producing the EP mRNA rather than to increased production of the mRNA by the individual EP-producing cells. It was estimated that 20–30% of the total interstitial cell population of the inner cortex, but less than 10% of the interstitial cells in the subcapsular cortex, produced EP. Thus EP-producing cells may represent a specialized cell type within the cortical interstitium rather than a generalized cell type, such as a peritubular capillary endothelial cell.

The kidney is the primary source of EP, but EP also originates in other tissues. A low basal rate of erythropoiesis is maintained by both anephric patients and those with chronic renal failure. This extrarenal source of EP may be the liver; because the liver is the primary producer of fetal EP, it may maintain some degree of that function until adulthood. In the presence of intact kidneys the liver would play an insignificant role in EP production, but if the kidneys were nonfunctional or removed, the liver's role would be of greater importance. Two striking and controversial observations regarding extrarenal EP synthesis have been made. EP may be secreted by bone marrow macrophages. Indeed, this work suggests that EP production by these macrophages may be a principal source of the hormone in the bone marrow microenvironment under normal (nonanemic) conditions.

Plasma EP is a sialoprotein consisting of 165 amino acids. This glycoprotein contains over 40% carbohydrate, consisting of sialic acid and a number of sugars. The sialic acid residues are necessary for biological activity in vivo as in the asialo form it is cleared too rapidly by the liver. Erythropoietin is found in the plasma and urine of many mammalian species, as well as in birds and fishes.

The effects of EP are not noted until 2 to 3 days after stimulation, due to the time it takes for reticulocytes to mature. The half-life of EP is only about 5 hours; this implies that a continuous supply of erythropoietin is not necessary for developing erythroblasts; all that may be needed is a priming stimulus. The role of EP is to enhance proliferation of erythrocyte precursor cells in bone marrow (or fetal liver) into erythroblasts (cells determined to become erythrocytes) and to stimulate proliferation of newly formed erythroblasts. Stimulation of RNA synthesis is the primary event in the mechanism of EP action. EP has its primary effect on the plasma membrane of marrow cells to produce an active cytoplasmic protein intermediate that interacts with the nucleus to stimulate synthesis of a variety of RNAs. DNA synthesis, cell division, and maturation (hemoglobin synthesis) in the responsive cells follow.

The possible role of EP in human diseases has been studied in a variety of clinical conditions. Anemia results from any of a number of events that lead to hemorrhage, hemolysis, or decreased red blood cell production by bone marrow. Some patients with rheumatoid arthritis, chronic infection, and other malignancies may become anemic because of lowered EP levels. Neuraminidase (a sialase enzyme) inactivates EP and may play a role in producing anemia. Chronic renal disease with progressive loss of renal mass also results in decreased production of EP.

Polycythemia (above-normal red cell number) is due to several etiologic factors; in some cases, an inappropriate increase in EP production is the causative factor. A structurally abnormal EPR gene has been identified in a human erythroleukemia cell line. In polycythemia vera, red cell progenitors exhibit exaggerated sensitivity to EP and express only low-affinity EP receptors. Some cases of hereditary polycythemia may be due to a mutant EPR conferring enhanced EP sensitivity. Other pathologic conditions may also be associated with abnormalities of the EPR or its associated molecules. Soluble, immunoreactive EPR is detectable in human serum, but its physiological significance is unknown [50].

Because EP induces marked reticulocytosis and pronounced increases in the circulating red cell mass, EP has potential therapeutic value in the management of certain anemias in which responsive stem cells and erythroid precursors are available but EP plasma levels are low. Commercially produced recombinant human EP is used routinely in the care of patients with renal failure. Patients with renal failure are usually very anemic, and a major factor contributing to their anemia is insufficient production of endogenous EP. Almost all patients respond to the administration of recombinant EP, and frequent transfusions of blood that had been required previously in their care are no longer needed. EP therapy is being tested in patients with anemias due to a wide variety of causes other than renal failure, and its role in clinical medicine will almost certainly increase in the future [16].

Thymic Hormones Stimulate Maturation of T Lymphocytes

The thymus gland is a lobular organ that lies in the upper thorax above the heart and in front of the aorta (Fig. 12.16). In humans and other mammals, the thymus begins to atrophy shortly after puberty [44]. Removal of the gland in the adult animal usually causes no harmful effects. On this basis, the thymus was considered to be an organ without a function. It is now realized that the thymus is an endocrine organ that plays a pivotal role in the development of immunological competence [28].

Thymectomy of mice immediately after birth results in a wasting disease characterized by severe depletion of white blood cells, specifically lymphocytes. Certain lymphocytes synthesize antibodies and, without such molecules, an animal cannot mount an immunological defense. In addition, in the absence of antibody production, an immune imbalance may contribute to the etiology of several diseases. Reimplantation of the thymus into young mice prevents the animals from developing the wasting disease; lymphocytes are produced and the animals are capable of developing an immunological response. A rather puzzling observation was that the lymphocytes in animals receiving a thymus graft were of host origin. It had been thought that the thymus was the source of all the animal's lymphocytes. The results suggested that the thymus was responsible for stimulating proliferation of host lymphocytes. Was the thymus gland the source of a lymphocyte-stimulating hormone? The definitive answer came from an experiment in which a thymus gland was placed in a small plastic capsule with pores so small that no thymus or other cells could escape or enter. Molecules, however, could pass freely in and out through the pores of the capsule. Young mice receiving only a plastic capsule implant developed the wasting disease. Mice receiving a capsule containing a thymus gland, on the other hand, grew and survived like normal animals and were capable of developing an immunological response. The results clearly indicated that the thymus might produce a hormone whose role was to activate lymphocytes for antibody production. An attempt to isolate such a factor from the thymus would be the next step to determine if indeed it were capable of stimulating lymphocyte antibody production.

It was eventually demonstrated that a partially purified thymus gland preparation, called *thymosin fraction five*, could correct some of the immunological deficiencies resulting from a lack of thymic function in a number of animal models, as well as humans with primary and secondary immunodeficiency diseases. This thymosin fraction induced lymphocyte differentiation and enhanced immunologic function in genetically athymic mice, adult thymectomized mice, and strains of mice with autoimmune reactions. Several thymosin fractions are active in various immunological assays, but only a few have been chemically characterized.

Generalized Roles.   White blood cells (leukocytes) are produced in the bone marrow. Stem cells in this hemopoietic tissue give rise to the following white blood cell types: granulocytes (neutrophils, eosinophils, basophils), monocytes (which give rise to some macrophages), and lymphocytes. Lymphocytes may reside within the thymus gland or pass on through to compose

Figure 12.16 Thymus glands from a 9-year-old girl (left) and an 80-year-old man (right). Although size and shape were similar, the gland from the older person was yellow in color and fatty. (From Kendall, Johnson, and Singh, "The weight of the human thymus gland at necropsy." *J. Anat.* 131:485–99, 1980.)

```
                                    5                      10
CH3CONH–Ser–Asp–Ala–Ala–Val–Asp–Thr–Ser–Ser–Glu–Ile–Thr–Thr–Lys ┐
                                                                  │
            ┌─────────────────────────────────────────────────────┘
            └─Asp–Leu–Lys–Glu–Lys–Lys–Glu–Val–Val–Glu–Glu–Ala–Glu–Asn
              15              20              25
```

Figure 12.17 Primary structure of bovine thymosin α_1.

a body of circulating T (thymus-derived) lymphocytes. Other lymphocytes of bone cell origin (B lymphocytes) establish themselves in other lymphoid tissues where they can become transformed into plasma cells that secrete antibodies.

The T lymphocytes become competent to participate in the immune response either by actual passage through the thymus, where they come into contact with one or more thymic hormones, or, alternatively, by being stimulated to become immunologically competent in response to humoral factors (hormones) released by the thymus. Both processes may be components of the maturation process of T lymphocytes. The fully differentiated T cells play a variety of roles in the immune response: They function as killer cells to combat tumor cell development; they release substances (lymphokines) that affect macrophage function; and they may function as helper cells with B cells in antibody production. The lymphocytes are considered to represent a complex group of cells derived from a common origin that are related by a linear or a branching differentiation. The processes that determine the commitment to any one of the pathways of differentiation may be under hormonal control. Clearly, the thymus may be a key element in the complex program, culminating in the fully developed immune system. Abnormalities of thymic function, on the other hand, may be responsible for some pathologies related to the immune system. Excess activity of certain lymphocytes may lead to hyperimmune conditions, whereas impaired function may lead to immunological deficiencies such as agammaglobulinemia (total inability to produce antibodies). Failure of the thymus to develop is manifested in DiGeorge's syndrome, which is characterized by a seriously deficient immune system, usually revealed by an abnormal reaction to vaccination.

The Thymosins. Thymosin is generally used to designate a biologically active class of substances found within extracts of the thymus gland. Subfractionation and purification of these extracts have yielded specific thymosin polypeptides whose primary structures have been determined.

A thymosin polypeptide (thymosin α_1) was isolated from calf thymus that consists of 28 amino acid residues and is highly active in several bioassay systems (Fig. 12.17). This polypeptide is probably derived from a larger precursor molecule and appears to be identical to a similar polypeptide derived from other species (human, pig, sheep, chinchilla, and mouse). The structure of thymosin β_4 has also been reported (Fig. 12.18). This polypeptide appears to act on stem cells to form prothymocytes, whereas thymosin α_1 may act on prothymocytes to induce their differentiation to more mature T cells. Thymosin β_4 is also found in high concentrations in tissues other than the thymus.

Thymosins are being used in clinical tests with children who have primary immunodeficiency diseases. No undesirable side effects have been noted, and significant clinical improvement has been indicated. Immune modulation using thymosins is being considered in the field of immunotherapy for the treatment of cancer. Thymosins appear to trigger maturational progression of several early stages of T-cell development and to augment the capacity of certain mature T cells to respond to antigens. One action of the thymosins may be to act through cGMP to induce the expression of alloantigens (antigen occurring in some, but not all, members of the same species) on the surface of T cells as they develop their functional capacity for immunological competence.

```
        O  1                5                  10                    15
CH3–C //
       \    N–Ser–Asp–Lys–Pro–Asp–Met–Ala–Glu–Ile–Glu–Lys–Phe–Asp–Lys–Ser–Lys–Leu–
     H/

   18      20       23  24  25              30
 –Lys–Lys–Thr–Glu–Thr–Gln–Glu–Lys–Asn–Pro–Leu–Pro–Ser–

   31      33          36  37  38              43       O
 –Lys–Glu–Thr–Ile–Glu–Gln–Glu–Lys–Gln–Ala–Gly–Glu–Ser–C //
                                                          \ OH
```

Figure 12.18 Primary structure of bovine thymosin β_4. Residues 31–43 are aligned with residues 18–30 to indicate regions of internal duplication.

Platelet-Derived Growth Factor (PDGF) Acts Locally on Injured Blood Vessels

Whole blood serum is a requirement for the growth of certain cells (smooth muscle, fibroblasts, 3T3, and glial) in culture. Although there are many factors present in serum that are necessary for viability and growth of cells in culture, serum prepared from cell-free plasma has little or no mitogenic activity. This activity, however, can be restored by adding material released from blood platelets to sera. Thus, the mitogen principle in whole blood serum may be derived from platelets. This *platelet-derived growth factor* (PDGF) is released from platelets during platelet aggregation in the process of blood clot formation. At sites of wounding, the platelets adhere to the endothelial lining of the vessel in such a way as to plug the defect. Platelets also release one or more chemical messengers that stimulate contraction of the injured vessels to prevent further loss of blood. At sites of injury, platelets release PDGF in response to thrombin. The role of PDGF at these sites may be to induce proliferation of smooth muscle cells within the arterial wall—the intima—as a component of a wound-healing process. Animals made thrombocytopenic with an antiplatelet serum fail to produce smooth muscle proliferative lesions in response to vessel injury. These lesions also fail to form in animals whose platelet function is inhibited by drugs (e.g., dipyridamole) that prevent platelet adhesion and granule release at sites of endothelial injury. PDGF is localized within α granules of the platelet; interaction of platelets with localized surfaces of damaged blood vessels provides for a site-specific release mechanism of PDGF to act as a local hormone. The wide distribution of smooth muscle cells throughout the body would, indeed, necessitate such a specialized mode of hormone delivery.

Atherosclerosis is recognized as a principal cause of death in the western hemisphere. Atherosclerotic lesions are localized to the innermost layers of the artery wall, the tunica intima and tunica media. This disease process, which results from endothelial disruption due to a number of possible causes, involves smooth muscle proliferation, formation of large amounts of a collagen matrix by the proliferated smooth muscle cells, and the deposition of lipids within these cells and the surrounding connective tissue. These atherosclerotic plaques impede blood flow in affected vessels, which may lead to brain stroke, heart attack, or other complications, depending on the particular vascular bed concerned. Although PDGF serves an important role in the healing process of the vascular system, it may play a dominant part in the development of atherosclerosis. It has been demonstrated that PDGF is also a potent vasoconstrictor, and it is possible that this peptide may be responsible, in part, for the increased vasoreactivity that occurs primarily at the site of atherosclerotic lesions.

PDGF consists of a family of molecules wherein each peptide is a heterodimer composed of an A and B chain. The two chains share 60% sequence identity and can dimerize to form PDGF-AA, PDGF-BB, and PDGF-AB. The dimer composition of PDGF isolated from human platelets has shown that PDGF-AB is the predominant form obtained, but PDGF-AA and PDGF-BB are also present. There are two PDGF receptor subtypes: one that recognizes all three PDGF varieties and a second that binds only the BB variety. It is believed that the existence of two receptor forms is biologically important and that they have different functions. The existence of genes encoding two PDGF receptors that interact in a distinct manner with three different PDGF isoforms likely confers considerable regulatory flexibility in the functional responses to PDGF.

Other Peptide Growth Factors

Other peptide growth factors have been discovered, and it is likely still others will be found in the future. Although their physiological roles have not been fully determined, these factors are important peptides for the study of the growth requirements of cells maintained in tissue culture. These peptides also provide important insights into evolution of hormone structure and common mechanisms of hormone action. These growth factors may eventually prove to be of immense medical importance.

Epidermal Growth Factor Stimulates Proliferation and Keratinization of Epidermal Tissue

Administration of partially purified nerve growth factor (NGF) from mouse submaxillary glands to newborn mice results in an early opening of the eyelids and precocious eruption of the teeth. A heat-stable protein, distinct from NGF, was isolated from these extracts that

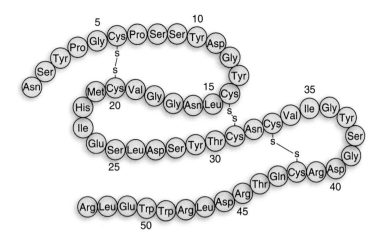

Figure 12.19 Primary structure of mouse epidermal growth factor (EGF).

possessed the ability to accelerate tooth eruption and eyelid opening in neonatal mice and rats. The biological activity was subsequently found to be due to a direct stimulation of the proliferation and keratinization of epidermal tissue. Autoradiography using [³H]thymidine revealed that this epidermal growth factor (EGF) enhanced cell proliferation in the basal layer of the skin.

Mouse EGF consists of 53 amino acids and is conformationally restricted by three intrachain disulfide bonds (Fig. 12.19). EGF is found within the salivary gland combined with an EGF-binding protein that is an arginine esterase. This observation is interesting because NGF is also found within the submaxillary glands. NGF is associated with other proteins, and one of the subunits of this complex is also an arginine esterase, which may be similar but not identical to the EGF-binding esterase as the latter does not complex with NGF. EGF and NGF appear to be derived from inactive precursors, and the biosynthesis and activation of both may be similar, perhaps under the control of the same genetic locus. This is further substantiated by the discovery that the synthesis of both peptides is androgen-dependent.

Release of the peptide from the salivary glands (in mice) may be under nervous system control because α-adrenergic agonists (Chap. 14) increase serum levels of EGF, as does electrical stimulation of the superior cervical ganglia. Although mouse EGF is found in duct cells of the submaxillary glands, these glands are not the sole source of the peptide, as removal of the glands does not eliminate immunoreactive EGF-like material from the blood.

In addition to effects on tooth eruption, eyelid opening, and skin proliferation in the neonate and embryo, EGF stimulates growth in a number of cultured normal epithelial cells. In epithelia, EGF rapidly stimulates the transport of small molecules into cells, followed by an increase in the rate of RNA synthesis and a conversion of pre-existing ribosomes into polysomes. One consequence of the binding of EGF to membrane receptors is a rapid activation of a cAMP-independent phosphorylating system.

Some known biological effects of EGF in the mammal include the following:

- enhanced proliferation and differentiation (keratinization) of the epidermis
- increased growth and maturation of the fetal pulmonary epithelium
- stimulation of ornithine decarboxylase activity and DNA synthesis in the mucosa of the digestive tract
- acceleration of the healing of wounds of the corneal epithelium, and phosphorylation of membrane and nuclear proteins.

Human milk is mitogenic to a number of cultured cell lines, an activity that is neutralized by antibodies to human EGF. These observations and other experimental results identify EGF as a major growth-promoting agent in breast milk. Because EGF is not entirely destroyed in the digestive tract, it might act directly on tissues of the digestive tract.

Most interesting is the discovery that EGF promotes plant-shoot growth and possibly growth of roots. It has been hypothesized, therefore, that EGF or EGF-like substances may control plant community productivity [13]; that is, the presence of a growth factor, such as EGF, in the saliva of an herbivorous animal might provide the stimulus for plant regrowth after grazing.

Many animals lick their wounds. Is it possible that the EGF present in the saliva of some animals may be a stimulus to the wound-healing process? Several lines of evidence suggest that salivary EGF plays a role in wound healing of the skin and gastric mucosa. It has been shown that wound healing of the skin is enhanced by licking, that is, transfer of saliva to the wound. In addition, topical application of EGF to the skin promotes wound healing. Healing of gastric ulcer is retarded in rats by sialoadenectomy (removal of the submandibular glands) and can be restored by intragastric administration of EGF but not EGF-free saliva. EGF produced in the submandibular glands also promotes wound healing of the tongue. It is suggested that EGF-rich excreta such as saliva, duodenal juice, and tears may play important roles in the promotion of wound healing [33].

A surprising finding is that peptic ulcer in humans undergoes remission during pregnancy, and urine contains a potent inhibitor of gastric acid secretion. This substance, *urogastrone*, consists of a single polypeptide chain of 53 residues with three disulfide bonds. It was then discovered that mouse EGF is of the same length and differs from urogastrone in only 16 of the 53 residues (see Fig. 10.11). Urogastrone is a gastrointestinal peptide that is inhibitory to gastric acid (HCl) secretion directly at the level of the gastric mucosa. Urogastrone, like EGF, induces premature opening of eyes in young mice. Both peptides stimulate DNA synthesis within human fibroblasts, and at submaximal concentrations their effects are additive. Binding data also reveal that they share the same receptor site on fibroblasts. Immunocytochemical studies indicate that cells of the human submandibular gland contain urogastrone-like activity. In the GI tract, urogastrone appears to be localized to cells of Brunner's glands. Urogastrone in the human and EGF in the mouse are known to be elevated during pregnancy. Because androgen levels are also elevated during pregnancy, it is possible that elevated levels of these peptides in the blood reflect the changing hormonal status of the female. Present evidence suggests, therefore, that urogastrone is the human hormonal equivalent of mouse EGF.

Activation of the EGF receptor initiates a cascade of cellular events. On binding ligand, the intrinsic tyrosine kinase activity is triggered, and this is immediately followed by a rise in cytosolic Ca^{2+} concentration and receptor internalization, which results in receptor degradation. Specific gene transcription is stimulated within minutes. Hours later, DNA synthesis and cell division occur. It has been shown that the tyrosine kinase activity of the receptor is necessary for all subsequent receptor actions, including internalization [49].

Tumor-Derived Growth Factors also Play Important Roles in Normal Development

Angiogenesis is the formation of blood vessels in situ and involves the orderly migration, proliferation, and differentiation of vascular cells. For tumors to grow, they must become vascularized to provide the nutrients and oxygen necessary for cellular proliferation. It was shown experimentally that tumor cells isolated within a Millipore filter could induce the growth of new capillary vessels despite separation of the cells from the vascular bed of the host. This provided evidence for the release of a diffusible tumor-derived *angiogenic factor*, although an alternative explanation might be that the tumor enhanced the degradation of an inhibitor of tumor growth. The *angiogenins* fall into two groups: those that act directly on vascular endothelial cells to stimulate locomotion or motility, and those that act indirectly through mobilizing host cells (cellular elements of the blood) to release endothelial growth factors. The angiogenic peptides are not restricted to tumors but are also present in normal tissues. Their release must therefore be tightly regulated. Besides fibroblast growth factor, these polypeptides include *angiogenin* and *transforming growth factors* (TGFs).

In addition to the angiogenesis induced by tumors, it now appears that a number of non-neoplastic diseases may be considered angiogenic diseases because they are characterized by the pathologic growth of capillary blood vessels. It will be important to now determine whether angiogenic factors administered in vivo, either locally or systemically, can be used to accelerate the healing of wounds and fractures, or to increase neovascularization of the ischemic or infarcted heart.

Fibroblast Growth Factors.   The fibroblast growth factor (FGF) family consists of polypeptide growth factors characterized by amino acid sequence homology, heparin-binding avidity, the ability to promote angiogenesis, and mitogenic activity towards cells of epithelial, mesenchymal, and neural origin. Members of the FGF family appear to have roles in development, tissue repair, maintenance of neurons, and the pathogenesis of disease. Aberrant expression of FGFs may cause cell transformation by an autocrine mechanism. Moreover, FGFs may enhance tumor growth and invasiveness by stimulating blood vessel growth into the tumor or by inducing production of proteases such as plasminogen activator.

The FGF family includes acidic and basic FGFs (bFGFs), the keratinocyte growth factor, and several other peptides. The actions of acidic and basic FGF are mediated through binding to high-affinity cell-surface receptors. It is not known whether each FGF interacts with a different receptor or whether the different forms of FGF share the same receptor. Of all the growth factors that have been identified to date, none has such a wide range of effects on so many cell types.

bFGF is a single-chain peptide composed of 146 amino acids that can also exist in an NH_2-terminally truncated form missing the first 15 amino acids. The truncated form of βFGF is as potent as the native form, thus indicating that this NH_2 terminus region of βFGF is not involved either in biological activity or in binding to FGF cell-surface receptors. Acidic FGF is a 140-amino-acid peptide that can also exist in an NH_2-terminally truncated form missing the first six amino acids. βFGF has been well conserved through evolution. In the case of bovine and human βFGF, only 2 of the 146 amino acids are different, giving an overall amino acid sequence homology of 98.7%. Avian βFGF has the same amino acid composition and cross-reacts on an equimolar basis with bovine βFGF in radioimmunoassay. This suggests that homologous epitopes are well conserved across species. αFGF seems to be less well conserved, and the bovine form differs from the human by 11 of the 140 residues. The high degree of homology between αFGF and βFGF suggests that they are derived from a single ancestral gene. The recent cloning of the genes and analysis of the complementary DNA (cDNA) sequences of both βFGF and αFGF suggest that through processes of gene duplication and evolutionary divergence, they have become separate gene products.

βFGF has been purified from many mesoderm- and neuroectoderm-derived tissues that have been shown to be FGF-sensitive either in vitro or in vivo. These include the brain, pituitary, retina, corpus luteum, adrenal gland, kidney, placenta, prostate, thymus, bone, immune system (macrophages-monocytes), and various tumors such as melanoma, chondrosarcoma, and hepatoma. Depending on the organ from which it is purified, either the complete (146aa) or truncated (des 1–15aa) forms of βFGF may be present. In the pituitary, brain, and retina, the complete form predominates, whereas in the kidney and corpus luteum, only the truncated form can be detected. In the adrenal gland and placenta, both forms coexist. It is not known whether these various forms coexist in the tissues, or whether they are artifactually created by specific proteases during FGF extraction and subsequent isolation. So far, αFGF has been found only in the brain and retina. The complete (140aa) and truncated form (des 1–6aa) seem to be present in stoichiometric amounts. Most of the organs from which bFGF has been purified share in common a strong angiogenic potential as well as being heavily vascularized. This suggests that cells of the vascular system might be responsible for bFGF production.

Probably one of the most important questions to be resolved is the in vivo role of FGF. The high degree of structural conservation of bFGF through species as diverse as mammals, birds, and amphibians, as well as its presence in all vertebrates studied to date, including fish, indicates that in vivo FGF could have a primordial role. It has been shown that bFGF can act as a morphogen at one of the earliest embryonic stages, including the transformation of cells designed to be ectodermal into mesenchymal cells. This is consistent with the in vitro properties of bFGF, which have been shown to act as mitogen as well as morphogen for all mesenchymal cells studied to date. It is also in agreement with the ability of bFGF to support the regeneration process in lower vertebrates.

Transforming Growth Factors. Two structurally distinct TGFs, TGFα and TGFβ, have been purified and their primary sequences determined [8]. TGFα is composed of 50 amino acids and bears sequence homology to EGF and binds to the EGF receptor. TGFα exhibits some homology with the amino acid sequences of human and mouse EGFs. If TGFα plays some role in normal development, one might wonder why there is an apparent duplicity of growth factors such as the TGFα and EGF. Maybe TGFα plays a local role under normal conditions requiring autocrine or paracrine stimulation of growth, as in embryogenesis and tissue regeneration. EGF, on the other hand, which is secreted by glands, may fulfill an endocrine type of role. Topical application of TGFα in an antibiotic cream to partial thickness second-degree burns increased the rate of epidermal regeneration. This finding suggests that topical application of selected growth factors may be useful in accelerating the healing of wounds.

The *TGFβ superfamily* of signaling molecules contains structurally related proteins that play numerous regulatory roles in development. TGFβ is a homodimer consisting of 112 amino acids per chain. TGFβ occurs in three related forms (TGFβ$_1$, TGFβ$_2$, and TGFβ$_3$). TGFβ has structural homology to other members of the superfamily, which includes the inhibins and activins (Chap. 16), bone morphogenetic proteins, and Müllerian inhibiting substance (MIS) (Chap. 18). It is of interest that both inhibin and MIS, like TGFβ, can exhibit strong growth-inhibitory activities. Depending on the experimental condition, TGFβ can stimulate or inhibit growth of certain nonendothelial cells depending on whether the cells are anchored or not and whether EGF is present or absent.

It has been suggested that TGFβ acts as a bifunctional regulator of cell growth in vitro. In fact, "transforming growth factor" may be a misnomer, since TGFβ more often than not has an inhibitory effect on the proliferation of most cell types, with the exception of fibroblasts. It is possible that the loss of responsiveness of cells to TGFβ may contribute to the uncontrolled division of cancer cells. Human breast cancer cells produce several growth-promoting factors, including TGFβ. Breast cancer patients who have estrogen-dependent tumors may be treated with an antiestrogen (Chap. 19). Antiestrogens, for example, increase TGFβ production, an effect that may contribute to their ablity to inhibit growth. Estrogens themselves decrease TGFβ production. TGFβ might be considered to be a chalone, as discussed later. Although TGFβ inhibits the proliferative actions of some hormones on cells, it does not inhibit protein synthesis induced by these hormones; thus, the action of TGFβ is to stabilize the differentiated state induced by other hormones and to allow cellular hypertrophy and phenotypic expression.

Normal skeletal growth results from a balance between the processes of bone matrix synthesis and resorption. These activities are regulated by both systemic and local factors. Bone turnover is dynamic, and skeletal growth must be maintained throughout life. Although many growth promoters are associated with bone matrix, it is enriched particularly with TGFβ activity. Experimental evidence indicates that TGFβ regulates replication and differentiation of mesenchymal precursor cells, chondrocytes, osteoblasts, and osteoclasts. TGFβ activity in skeletal tissue may be controlled at multiple levels by other local and systemic agents. Consequently, the intricate mechanisms by which TGFβ regulates bone formation are likely to be fundamental to understanding the processes of skeletal growth during development, maintenance of bone mass in adult life, and healing subsequent to bone fracture [8].

Cytoplasmic determinants influence the development of embryonic cells. A critical early stage in this development is formation of the three germ layers, known as the endoderm, the ectoderm, and the mesoderm, from which the specific tissues of the organism later differentiate. The TGFβ family of peptides has now been linked to early embryonic development of the frog egg, specifically to mesoderm formation. Both TGFβ and bFGF are produced by the amphibian egg and induce mesoderm formation. TGFβ is made at the appropriate site, the cells of the vegetal pole of the egg, and at the right time in development for mesoderm induction. Transforming growth factor β$_2$ but not TGFβ$_1$, was active in α-actin induction, whereas addition of fibroblast growth factor had a small synergistic effect. Medium conditioned by *Xenopus* XTC cells (XTC-CM), known to have powerful mesoderm-inducing activity, was shown to contain TGFβ-like activity as measured by a radioreceptor-binding assay, colony formation in NRK cells, and growth inhibition in CCL64 cells. The activity of XTC-CM in mesoderm induction and growth inhibition of CCL64 cells was inhibited partially by antibodies to TGFβ$_2$ but not by antibodies to TGFβ$_1$. Thus, a TGFβ$_2$-like molecule may be involved in mesoderm induction.

The cellular effects of TGFβ and other members of the TGFβ superfamily are varied and complex, yet the signal transduction pathways that mediate their actions are relatively stereotyped. All members of the family bind to plasma membrane receptors that directly phosphorylate and activate transcription factors, collectively known as *Smads*. The receptors for each are dimeric transmembrane proteins with serine/threonine kinase activity in their cytosolic domains. TGFβ binds directly with a constitutively active serine-threonine kinase receptor, the TGFβ type II receptor (TβRII). This causes recruitment and activation of a type I receptor (TβRI). Activated TβRI transphosphorylates Smad proteins (Smad2 or Smad3), which then bind a co-Smad (Smad 4) and translocate to the nucleus of the cell. Transcriptional co-regulators present in the nucleus associate with the Smad complex, bind response elements in the regulatory regions of target genes, and regulate their transcription.

Cytokines can have Both Immunological and Physiological Functions

A cytokine may be defined as a soluble protein, synthesized by immune or nonimmune cells, that mediates intercellular communication. Cytokines transmit information to target cells through receptor–ligand interactions and thereby regulate immunologic and physiologic events. This class of mediators is represented by growth and differentiation, cytolytic, chemotactic, and immunoenhancing factors. Many of these factors appear to have multifunctional immunologic and physiologic activities. Interleukins may be the best known but least understood group; the eight or more known interleukins have diverse biologic activities. The term *interleukin* originally described a leukocyte-derived protein with activity for other leukocytes. It is now understood that both immune and nonimmune cells synthesize interleukins and other cytokines that are important in inflammation. Indeed, many cytokines have physiologic and immunologic activities far beyond those originally discovered.

Chalones are Mitotic Inhibitors

Many hormones stimulate synthetic processes within cells of their target tissues. An increase in cell function and cell size (hypertrophy) is often followed by cell proliferation (hyperplasia). As noted, growth factors are potent mitogens. Mitotic activity of the many tissues of the body is variable. Brain cells, for example, seldom divide, whereas epithelial cells, especially those of the epidermis or the intestinal lining, divide at a much higher rate to replace those cells lost from the surface. When epidermal cells are destroyed by tissue damage, the rate of cell production in the basal layer of the skin increases to restore the lost cells. A balance of cellular mitotic activity could probably not be maintained unless controlled by some type of feedback mechanism. The critical moment in the life of an epidermal cell may be when it emerges from mitosis: it must prepare for division again or for keratin synthesis and death.

When the epidermis is damaged, the mitotic rate of nearby cells is enhanced. It was thought that mitosis was in response to a "wound hormone." The opposite view is now favored: The epidermis normally contains a mitotic inhibitor whose loss from the damaged area permits the increase in mitotic activity of the adjacent cells. It has been proposed that these substances be referred to as *chalones* (from the Greek *chalan*, to slacken, slow down), which suggests that they act as mitotic inhibitors. A number of classic experiments have provided strong support for the chalone hypothesis.

Growth Factors, Receptors, and Cancer

Neoplastic transformation in some cases may relate to cellular growth factors and their receptors [12]. It has become evident that cells stimulated by growth factors and cells transformed by viruses are quite similar, suggesting common stimulation pathways of cellular proliferation in viral-transformed and growth-factor-stimulated cells. Oncogenes are genes whose coding sequence contains the information necessary to initiate and maintain neoplastic proliferation. Oncogenes were first discovered in transforming viruses, but it is now appreciated that these genes were actually acquired from normal host genes (proto-oncogenes) of infected cells by genetic transduction. Proto-oncogenes can be expressed in many different tissues and provide a potential for malignant transformation. These proto-oncogenes are probably the same genes that were once activated through inductive processes during embryonic development. The inadvertent activation of these genes in the differentiated state by mutational mechanisms may lead to their irreversible activation, and through ensuing cellular proliferation may lead to cancer growth and metastases. Proto-oncogenes can release growth-factor-like peptides that are released extracellularly and then stimulate proliferation of cells through autocrine and paracrine mechanisms.

Proto-oncogene activation within virally infected cells is another way for cancerous cellular proliferation to become manifested. A relationship between growth-factor receptors and transforming proteins of oncogenes has also been noted. There is a marked homology between certain growth-factor receptors (e.g., for EGF) and proteins coded for by certain viruses. Viral-induced transformation might relate to the overproduction and expression of GH receptor proteins by infected cells, thus leading to their uncontrolled proliferation.

The role of protein kinase C (PKC) in signal transduction was reviewed in Chapter 3. Activation of PKC is a stimulus to cellular proliferation. Phorbol esters—like diacylglycerol, which is the natural second messenger of PKC activation—also activate the enzyme. Phorbol esters share a structural similarity to diacylglycerol, and this probably explains their mitogenic actions. These observations point out how exogenous ligands (carcinogens) can be responsible for cellular activation, possibly leading to tumor growth and spread.

Rapidly growing transformed cells, which frequently secrete growth-promoting polypeptides, also produce high amounts of proteolytic activity. Since high proteolytic activity is usually associated with malignant or proliferating cells, a possible explanation is that malignant cells produce autocrine growth factors or other factors that regulate their proteolytic activity. A few growth factors have been previously found that affect the proteolytic balance of cultured cells. Recent work has indicated that, in fact, several growth factors have an ability to modulate the expression of proteolytic enzymes. However, disturbances in proteolytic balance and overexpression of proteolytic enzymes by malignant cells may result from inappropriate regulation of these activities and can be related to excessive production of certain growth factors or inadequate production of other ones.

REVIEW EXERCISES

Match the growth factor with receptor and/or signaling molecules:

	Receptor type *(tyrosine kinase, serine/threonine kinase, cytokine receptor)*	Intracellular signaling pathway *(JAK-STAT, IRS/PI-3 kinase, Smads)*
1. Prolactin	_____	_____
2. TGFβ	_____	_____
3. **GH**	_____	_____
4. insulin	_____	_____
5. EGF	_____	_____
6. IGF-1	_____	_____

Match the stages of the cell cycle:

1. Apoptosis
2. G_0 stage
3. G_2 stage
4. G_1 stage
5. S stage
6. M stage

A. A growth stage in preparation for DNA synthesis
B. A cell division stage
C. A resting stage
D. A short growth stage
E. The DNA synthesis stage
F. A stage of programmed-cell-death

Think, analyze and discuss:

1. Laron syndrome is characterized by short stature and can be caused by an inactivating mutation of the GH receptor. Short stature is also the major feature of isolated GH deficiency.
   a. In Laron syndrome and isolated GH deficiency, would you expect to find increased, decreased, or unchanged concentrations of IGF-I in serum? Why?
   b. What is the reason that GH levels in Laron syndrome are typically elevated?
   c. If the concentrations of somatostatin and GHRH could be measured in the hypophysial portal blood of an individual with Laron syndrome, would you expect them to be increased, decreased, or unchanged? Why?

   d. Some individuals with Laron syndrome do not have genetic mutations that alter GH receptor structure. Can you think of a likely alternative explanation for the pathophysiological basis of the syndrome? What tests could you perform to test your hypothesis?

2. Insulin and IGF-I can both stimulate proliferative and metabolic effects on target cells. However, IGF-I is a more potent stimulator of cell proliferation than insulin, while insulin is more potent in stimulating metabolic effects than IGF-I. Can you provide a plausible explanation for these observations, based on the receptors and signal transduction pathways that may be stimulated by these two proteins?

3. Prolactin functions as the major lactogen that stimulates mammary growth and milk production after parturition. Which lactogen stimulates mammary growth during pregnancy? In which tissue is this hormone produced? Describe the putative evolutionary relationship between this hormone, prolactin, and GH. Does it share more structural homology with GH or prolactin?

4. Nerve growth factor is produced by certain target tissues during development and exerts its effects on certain parts of the the developing nervous system. Describe these effects, and the cellular mechanisms that may mediate them. Gene targeting methods have been used to generate mice that lack the NGF gene and hence, do not express the NGF protein. Can you predict some of the abnormalities observed in the adult nervous systems of these mice?

5. Is it more likely that the growth and invasiveness of a tumor be enhanced or suppressed by increased production of FGFs? Why? Is it more likely that cancer cell proliferation would be enhanced or suppressed by increased production of TGFβ? What may be the effect of the loss of responsiveness to TGFβ by cells? Why?

6. Would you expect EP concentrations in serum to be elevated, decreased, or unchanged in an individual who has suffered a hemorrage and resultant loss of blood? In an individual suffering from kidney failure? In an individual who takes a trip to a high-altitude location? What is the rationale for athletes to conduct their aerobic exercise training at higher altitudes?

7. Foot ulcers are relatively common in diabetic patients, and it has been proposed that certain growth factors might be useful in promoting the healing of these tissues. PDGF is one growth factor that has been approved for local use in this clinical condition. Considering that damage to the microvasculature is involved in the development of diabetic foot ulcers, can you think of how PDGF might be particularly effective in promoting healing in this situation?

References

[1] Aarskog, D., et al. 1997. Pituitary dwarfism in the R271W Pit-1 gene mutation. *Eur. J. Pediatr.* 156:829–34.

[2] Argetsinger, L. S., and C. Carter-Su. 1996. Mechanism of signaling by growth hormone receptor. *Physiol. Rev.* 76:1089–107.

[3] Baumann, G., M. A. Shaw, and T. J. Merimee. 1989. Low levels of high-affinity growth hormone-binding protein in African pygmies. *N. Engl. J. Med.* 320:1705–9.

[4] Baxter, R. 1993. Circulating binding proteins for insulin-like growth factors. *TEM* 4.

[5] Bonni, A., and M. E. Greenberg. 1997. Neurotrophin regulation of gene expression. *Can. J. Neurol. Sci.* 24:272–83.

[6] Bowen, I. D. 1993. Apoptosis or programmed cell death? *Cell Biol. Int.* 17:365–80.

[7] Bradshaw, R. A., et al. 1993. Nerve growth factor revisited. *Trends Biochem. Sci.* 18:48–52.

[8] Centrella, M., et al. 1994. Transforming growth factor-beta gene family members and bone. *Endocr. Rev.* 15:27–39.

[9] Cheung, N. W., and S. C. Boyages. 1997. Increased incidence of neoplasia in females with acromegaly. *Clin. Endocrinol. (Oxf.)* 47:323–7.

[10] Clapp, C., and G. M. d. l. Escalera. 1977. Prolactins: novel regulators of angiogenesis. *News Physiol. Sci.* 12:231–37.

[11] Davila, N., et al. 2002. Growth hormone binding protein, insulin-like growth factor-I and short stature in two pygmy populations from the Philippines. *J. Pediatr. Endocrinol. Metab.* 15:269–76.

[12] Dhanasekaran, N., L. E. Heasley, and G. L. Johnson. 1995. G protein-coupled receptor systems involved in cell growth and oncogenesis. *Endocr. Rev.* 16:259–70.

[13] Dyer, M. 1980. Mammalian epidermal growth factor promotes plant growth. *Proc. Natl. Acad. Sci. USA* 77:4836–37.

[14] Etherton, T. D. 1991. Clinical review 21: The efficacy and safety of growth hormone for animal agriculture. *J. Clin. Endocrinol. Metab.* 72:957A–957C.

[15] Fontoura, M., et al. 1991. Regulation of the growth hormone binding proteins in human plasma. *Acta Endocrinol. (Copenh.)* 124:10–3.

[16] Fried, W. 1995. Erythropoietin. *Annu. Rev. Nutr.* 15:353–77.

[17] Fuh, G., et al. 1992. Rational design of potent antagonists to the human growth hormone receptor. *Science* 256:1677–80.

[18] Funakoshi, H., et al. 1995. Muscle-derived neurotrophin-4 as an activity-dependent trophic signal for adult motor neurons. *Science* 268:1495–9.

[19] Godfrey, P., et al. 1993. GHRH receptor of little mice contains a missense mutation in the extracellular domain that disrupts receptor function. *Nat. Genet.* 4:227–32.

[20] Hail, N., Jr., et al. 2006. Apoptosis effector mechanisms: A requiem performed in different keys. *Apoptosis* 13:13.

[21] Ho, K. K., and D. M. Hoffman. 1995. Defining growth hormone deficiency in adults. *Metabolism* 44:91–6.

[22] Humbel, R., and E. Rinderknecht. 1979. From NSILA to IGF (1963–1977). In: G. Giordano, J. J. Van Wyk, and F. Minuto, eds. *Somatomedins and growth.* London: Academic Press, pp. 61–64G.

[23] Isaksson, O. G., et al. 1988. Action of growth hormone: current views. *Acta Paediatr. Scand. Suppl.* 343:12–18.

[24] Kromer, L. F. 1987. Nerve growth factor treatment after brain injury prevents neuronal death. *Science* 235:214–16.

[25] Laron, Z. 1995. Prismatic cases: Laron syndrome (primary growth hormone resistance) from patient to laboratory to patient. *J. Clin. Endocrinol. Metab.* 80:1526–31.

[26] LeRoith, D., P. C. Sampson, and C. T. Roberts, Jr. 1994. How does the mitogenic insulin-like growth factor I receptor differ from the metabolic insulin receptor? *Horm. Res.* 41:74–8; discussion 79.

[27] LeRoith, D., et al. 1995. Molecular and cellular aspects of the insulin-like growth factor I receptor. *Endocr. Rev.* 16:143–63.

[28] Levy, R. 1964. The thymus hormone. *Sci. Am.* 211:66–77.

[29] Merimee, T. J., J. Zapf, and E. R. Froesch. 1981. Dwarfism in the pygmy. An isolated deficiency of insulin-like growth factor I. *N. Engl. J. Med.* 305:965–8.

[30] Merimee, T. J., et al. 1987. Insulin-like growth factors in pygmies. The role of puberty in determining final stature. *N. Engl. J. Med.* 316:906–11.

[31] Nakamura, Y., N. Komatsu, and H. Nakauchi. 1992. A truncated erythropoietin receptor that fails to prevent programmed cell death of erythroid cells. *Science* 257:1138–41.

[32] Nilsson, A., et al. 1986. Regulation by growth hormone of number of chondrocytes containing IGF-I in rat growth plate. *Science* 233:571–4.

[33] Noguchi, S., Y. Ohba, and T. Oka. 1991. Effect of salivary epidermal growth factor on wound healing of tongue in mice. *Am. J. Physiol.* 260:E620–5.

[34] Ohlsson, C., et al. 1992. Effects of tri-iodothyronine and insulin-like growth factor-I (IGF-I) on alkaline phosphatase activity, [3H]thymidine incorporation and IGF-I receptor mRNA in cultured rat epiphyseal chondrocytes. *J. Endocrinol.* 135:115–23.

[35] Ohlsson, C., et al. 1992. Growth hormone induces multiplication of the slowly cycling germinal cells of the rat tibial growth plate. *Proc. Natl. Acad. Sci. USA* 89:9826–30.

[36] Ooi, G. T. 1990. Insulin-like growth factor-binding proteins (IGFBPs): more than just 1, 2, 3. *Mol. Cell. Endocrinol.* 71:C39–43.

[37] Oppenheim, R. W. 1996. The concept of uptake and retrograde transport of neurotrophic molecules during development: history and present status. *Neurochem. Res.* 21:769–77.

[38] Plum, L., M. Schubert, and J. C. Bruning. 2005. The role of insulin receptor signaling in the brain. *Trends Endocrinol. Metab.* 16:59–65.

[39] Rosenbloom, A., and J. Guevara-Aguirre. 1994. Prismatic cases: Bienvenidosa mi terra de soledad: from poetry to molecular biology in southern Ecuador. *J. Clin. Endocrinol. Metab.* 79:690–702.

[40] Rosenbloom, A. L. 1999. Growth hormone insensitivity: physiologic and genetic basis, phenotype, and treatment. *J. Pediatr.* 135:280–9.

[41] Sabharwal, P., et al. 1992. Prolactin synthesized and secreted by human peripheral blood mononuclear cells: an autocrine growth factor for lymphoproliferation. *Proc. Natl. Acad. Sci. USA* 89:7713–16.

[42] Shiverick, K. T., and A. R. Rosenbloom (eds.). 1995. *Human growth hormone pharmacology, basic and clinical aspects.* Boca Raton, FL: CRC Press.

[43] Spada, A., et al. 1990. Clinical, biochemical, and morphological correlates in patients bearing growth hormone-secreting pituitary tumors with or without constitutively active adenylyl cyclase. *J. Clin. Endocrinol. Metab.* 71:1421–6.

[44] Stone, R. 1992. NIH to size up growth hormone trials. *Science* 257:739.

[45] Tattersall, R. 1996. A history of growth hormone. *Horm. Res.* 46:236–47.

[46] Thoenen, H. 1995. Neurotrophins and neuronal plasticity. *Science* 270:593–8.

[47] Walker, S., S. Allen, and R. McMurray. 1993. Prolactin and autoimmune disease. *TEM* 4.

[48] Waters, M. J., et al. 2006. New insights into growth hormone action. *J. Mol. Endocrinol.* 36:1–7.

[49] Wells, A., et al. 1990. Ligand-induced transformation by a noninternalizing epidermal growth factor receptor. *Science* 247:962–4.

[50] Winkelmann, J. C. 1992. The human erythropoietin receptor. *Int. J. Cell Cloning* 10:254–61.

[51] Wyllie, A. H. 1993. Apoptosis (the 1992 Frank Rose Memorial Lecture). *Br. J. Cancer* 67:205–8.

CHAPTER 13

Thyroid Hormones

Anatomists of the fifteenth and sixteenth centuries described the thyroid gland in detail, and an enlargement of the thyroid as the anatomical basis for goiter was subsequently noted [16]. The etiological basis for goiter, however, was only discerned centuries later after a number of important discoveries in chemistry. Courtois, a French pharmacist, discovered iodine (Greek: violet) in 1811 and Davy, an English chemist, discovered its elemental nature in 1813. Gay-Lussac, a French chemist, named the element iodine in 1814. Iodine was discovered to be abundant in seaweed and other marine products; if eaten, these marine substances had a beneficial effect on goiter. Burnt sponge was recommended as a treatment for goiter in the mid-thirteenth century. It was subsequently surmised and proven correct that iodine might aid in the cure of goiter. Evidence for a connection between iodine deficiency and endemic goiter was obtained from studies of several European locales; the suggestion was put forward in 1849 that the disease was due to a deficiency of iodine in drinking water [12, 16].

In 1895, Magnus-Levey demonstrated that the feeding of dried animal thyroids to normal men increased their metabolic rate. This suggested that the thyroid gland might contain a substance that affected the cellular activity of other organs. It was hypothesized that thyroid tissue might contain iodine, which was known to be beneficial to hypothyroid individuals. In 1895, Kocher of Bern demonstrated the high amount of iodine in a thyroid concentrate. He named this substance iodothyrin. Iodothyrin was active in hypothyroid patients, whereas an iodine-free fraction of the thyroid was not. In 1918, an American scientist, Kendall, isolated the active component of the thyroid that he named thyroxin (**thyroxine**), and proposed its structural formula. Harrington in England revised the constitution of thyroxine and synthesized the definitive structure of L-thyroxine (Fig. 13.1). Thyroxine was later isolated from the thyroid gland in pure form.

It was soon discovered that the physiological activity of thyroid material could not be accounted for entirely by its thyroxine content. Kendall suggested that the "active" hormone might contain less iodine than thyroxine. Gross and Pitt-Rivers, British scientists, were then able to isolate a triiodinated thyronine from animal thyroid glands. In 1952, **triiodothyronine** (Fig. 13.1) was synthesized and found to be more active than thyroxine. It was then suggested that triiodothyronine (T_3) was the peripheral physiological hormone and thyroxine (T_4) its precursor [28].

The Thyroid Gland

The thyroid gland is derived from endoderm of the cephalic portion of the embryo's alimentary canal [17]. A saclike diverticulum first appears in the midline of the ventral surface of the pharynx. This glandular organ becomes bilobed but remains connected to the pharynx by

Thyroxine (3,5,3′,5′-Tetraiodothyronine, T₄)   Triiodothyronine (3,5,3′-Triiodothyronine, T₃)

Figure 13.1   Structures of thyroxine (T$_4$) and triiodothyronine (T$_3$).

Figure 13.2   The human thyroid gland.

a thyroglossal duct. The thyroglossal duct becomes a solid stalk that usually atrophies. The two lateral lobes of the human thyroid become solid masses of tissue and remain connected to each other by a narrow isthmus of tissue. The thyroid tissue in mammals lies over the trachea at a position just below the cricoid cartilage (see Fig. 9.1). A pyramidal lobe near the isthmus of the thyroid may persist as a remnant of the thyroglossal stalk (Fig. 13.2). The thyroid gland of humans weighs about 15 to 20 g. In nonmammalian species, the thyroid gland consists of a pair of glands separated from each other at varying distances lateral to the esophagus. The functional components of the thyroid gland are the individual thyroid follicles, which consist of a cuboidal epithelium arranged as a single layer surrounding a lumen that contains a colloid material (Fig. 13.3). In humans, an individual thyroid follicle may reach a diameter of almost 1 cm [37].

In the mammal, so-called clear (C) cells are present within the follicular wall and the extracellular space between the follicles. These cells are the source of *calcitonin*, an important hormone involved in Ca^{2+} homeostasis in some animals (Chap. 9). The follicular cells synthesize a protein, *thyroglobulin*, which is released into the colloid space by vesicular exocytosis. Thyroglobulin is the substrate for tyrosine iodination and the subsequent synthesis of thyroid hormones. In response to endocrine stimulation, follicular cells engulf the colloid by phagocytosis. The colloid within the endocytotic vesicles is enzymatically degraded to yield thyroid hormones that are released from the follicular cells into the extracellular space where they enter the abundant capillaries.

The thyroid is richly supplied with sympathetic postganglionic neurons that not only serve a vasomotor function, but in some species may innervate the individual follicular cells. In mice, unilateral sympathetic stimulation induces secretion of thyroid hormones from those areas supplied by the stimulated nerve. Sympathetic innervation of the thyroid may provide a means for effecting prompt, short-term alterations in the rate of thyroid hormone secretion [21]. Amine-containing mast cells are present between the thyroid follicles of mammals; they respond to TSH by releasing histamine and serotonin (5-hydroxytryptamine, 5-HT), as well as other substances. The released biogenic amines may act directly on the follicle cells to initiate thyroid hormone secretion or to increase blood flow throughout the gland.

Figure 13.3
Diagrammatic histological representation of the human thyroid gland.

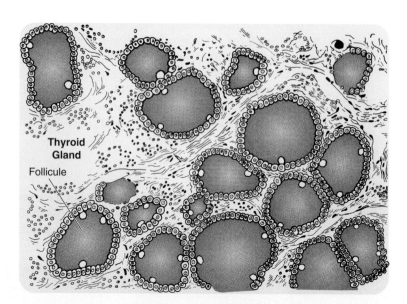

Synthesis and Chemistry

Thyroid hormones are unique in that they are complexed through covalent bonds to iodine. The availability of iodine to the terrestrial vertebrate is limited and, therefore, some interesting cellular mechanisms have evolved for the ultimate utilization and conservation of the element. The thyroid follicular cells are able to trap iodide at the base of the cell and transport it against an electrical gradient across the cell. Accumulation of iodide by the thyroid is an energy-requiring mechanism. Its Na^+ dependence was recognized and an Na^+-I^- cotransport system was demonstrated. Iodide uptake into the thyroid cell (thyrocyte) is an example of a secondary active transport mechanism, sometimes improperly referred to as the "iodide pump." The Na^+-I^- symporter (NIS) is inserted into the basolateral membrane of the thyrocyte. Its activity is dependent on the Na^+ gradient across the membrane and therefore on Na^+/K^+-ATPase. A second porter protein, termed *pendrin*, is located on the apical membrane of the thyrocyte, where it transports iodide across the membrane into the follicular lumen. The protein is the product of the PDS gene, which is mutated in Pendred syndrome, a rare genetic disorder characterized by a lack of thyroid hormone synthesis. Pendrin is a large porter protein with 11 transmembrane-spanning domains, and it is required for iodide transport from the follicular cell cytoplasm into the follicular lumen, where it is used in the synthesis of the thyroid hormones.

After transport into the follicular lumen, iodide is then converted by a *peroxidase* at the luminal surface of the cell, to an oxidized species of iodine that is incorporated into tyrosyl groups of thyroglobulin (TG) as monoiodotyrosine (MIT) and diiodotyrosine (DIT) residues [32]. Within the TG, iodinated tyrosines undergo an *oxidative coupling* that results mainly in the formation of T_4 and smaller amounts of T_3. This oxidative coupling may be catalyzed by the same peroxidase responsible for conversion of iodide to iodine. Iodination of TG tyrosyl residues and subsequent oxidative coupling to form *iodothyronines* may be facilitated by intraluminal ciliary action and the subsequent movement of TG to reactive sites of the apical surface of the follicular cells.

Through the processes of micropinocytosis and macropinocytosis, the colloid is engulfed by follicular cell pseudopods and transported into the cells as *colloid droplets*. These colloid-containing vesicles then fuse with lysosomes and are referred to as *secondary lysosomes*. Much of the TG within these vesicles is degraded by lysosomal proteolytic enzymes. The thyroid hormones are then released (presumably by diffusion) into the cytoplasm and enter the extracellular space by diffusion, apparently through the basal or lateral follicular membranes [40]. Exocytosis of vesicular products, including T_3 and T_4, is not excluded as TG is also secreted into the circulation. The iodinated tyrosines that are released into the cytosol through lysosomal proteolysis are then deiodinated by a *deiodinase* and recycled for use within the cell. A scheme of the events involved in thyroid hormone synthesis and secretion is depicted (Fig. 13.4).

Thyrotropin Induces Expression and Activation of Proteins Controlling Thyroid Hormone Synthesis

Follicular thyroid hormone synthesis is regulated through the action of thyrotropin (thyroid-stimulating hormone; TSH) (Chap. 5). Continued stimulation of the thyroid by TSH results in a great increase in the quantity and activity of the synthetic machinery (rough endoplasmic reticulum and Golgi) of the follicular cells. The cells become columnar in shape and the luminal content of the colloid is greatly decreased. In the absence of TSH, synthesis of thyroid hormones is minimal or nonexistent. Subsequently, there is a loss of most protein-synthesizing elements of the cell; the individual follicular cells become flattened and the lumen remains enlarged and full of colloid.

In response to TSH there is an immediate activation of follicular cell thyroid hormone-synthesizing activity (Fig. 13.4). TSH interacts with follicular cell membrane receptors with resulting activation of adenylate cyclase and cAMP production. The thyrotropin receptor (TSRH) has been cloned and its primary structure determined [15]. The TSHR and the receptor for luteinizing hormone/choriogonadotropin constitute a subfamily of G-protein-coupled receptors with distinct sequence characteristics (see Fig. 19.2). All the subsequent follicular activities may be mediated through cAMP-induced gene expression and activation of NIS, TG, peroxidase, and other proteins involved in iodine uptake and

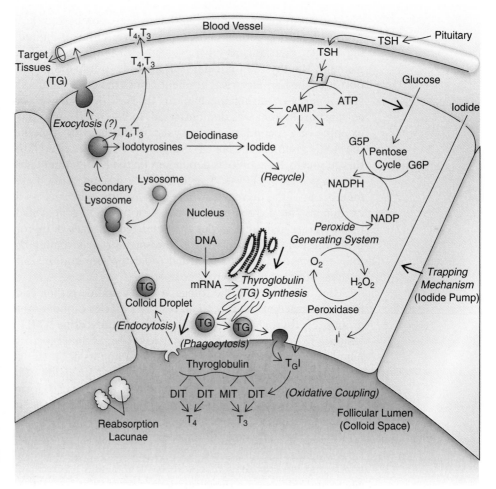

Figure 13.4 Summary scheme of thyroid hormone biosynthesis and secretion. The actual oxidative coupling of iodinated tyrosine residues probably takes place at the apical surface of the follicular cell, rather than in the lumen. From Van Herle, A. J., G. Vassart, and E. Dumont. 1995. "Control of thyroglobulin synthesis and secretion." The New England Journal of Medicine. 301:239–49, 307–314.

thyroid hormone formation. Thus, theophylline and cAMP analogs added to thyroid tissue mimic most actions of TSH, such as the stimulation of TG gene expression and incorporation of iodide into thyroglobulin. In response to TSH, oxygen consumption is increased in incubated thyroid tissue and glucose is taken up from the medium and metabolized via the *pentose monophosphate shunt*. In this pathway, NADPH is generated from NADP; this reduced adenine nucleotide is required for the reduction of molecular oxygen to hydrogen peroxide. The H_2O_2 is then used in the oxidation of iodide to an active form. The reaction is catalyzed by a thyroidal peroxidase that may be present within the Golgi-derived vesicles containing newly synthesized TG. Conversion of iodide to active iodide and organification of iodide into tyrosine residues of TG may occur as TG is secreted into the follicular lumen.

Immediately on stimulation of the thyroid by TSH, there is enhanced pinocytotic activity at the apical follicular membrane. Thus, colloid is actively engulfed and carried into the cell by this endocytotic process. Active removal of colloid from the lumen can be visualized microscopically as so-called *reabsorption lacunae* (Figs 13.3 and 13.4).

Thyroglobulin is composed of two identical subunits, each containing a 330 kDa polypeptide. The primary structure of the subunit has been determined. Although tyrosyl residues are essential for iodine incorporation, the actual amount of tyrosine within TG is low (about 2%). The main intrathyroidal storage form of thyroid hormones is TG, and the individual iodinated thyronines are liberated from TG as T_4 and T_3 within the colloid droplets by the action of proteolytic enzymes. Iodination of TG initially requires the conversion of inorganic iodide to some molecular species of "active iodide." This active iodide then reacts with tyrosine moieties of the TG. Incorporation of a single iodide into the

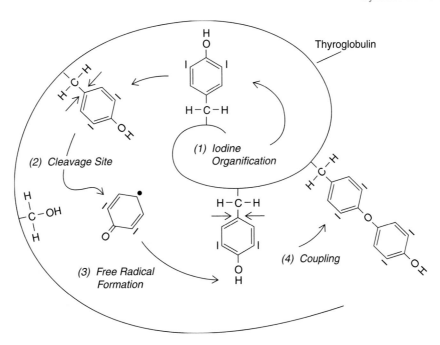

Figure 13.5
Hypothetical coupling scheme for iodothyronine formation.

phenolic ring of tyrosine yields a 3-monoiodotyrosine (MIT). A second iodide may be incorporated into the 5 position to yield a 3,5-diiodotyrosine (DIT). Iodination specifically involves initial iodination of the 3 position, which is usually followed by iodination of the 5 position as 5-monoiodotyrosine is never formed.

Coupling of iodinated tyrosyl residues within TG is undoubtedly assisted by the three-dimensional structure of TG, but the exact mechanism remains undetermined. For example, the extent to which intramolecular or intermolecular coupling by tyrosyl moieties predominates is unknown. Coupling is enzymatically controlled and apparently involves the cleavage of a phenolic ring from tyrosine, and its incorporation through an ether (—O—) linkage, to another iodinated tyrosine. Coupling usually involves the joining of two DIT moieties to form 3,5,3',5'-tetraiodothyronine, T_4, whereas the addition of MIT to a DIT residue yields 3,5,3'-triiodothyronine, T_3. All iodinated tyrosines do not become coupled, and much extractable organic iodide remains in the form of MIT or DIT.

One suggested coupling scheme involves free-radical formation. In this model, free DIT radicals are generated within the TG matrix through the action of thyroperoxidase. In this particular pathway, a serine residue would remain in the position formerly occupied by the phenolic residue cleaved from the tyrosine (Fig. 13.5). The formation of T_3 may occur by a similar scheme, except the coupling would be between MIT (contributing a phenolic group) and DIT.

Antithyroid Drugs can Suppress Thyroid Hormone Synthesis

Certain drugs inhibit thyroid function by antagonizing formation of thyroid hormones. These drugs are generally classified into those compounds that inhibit iodide transport (iodide trapping) into the thyroid gland and those that inhibit iodine incorporation into tyrosine. Univalent inhibitors of iodide transport include thiocyanate and other mono-valent anions (perchlorate, chlorate, periodate, etc.). Even iodide in large doses is transiently inhibitory to thyroid function (Wolff–Chaikoff effect), but the mechanism of this inhibition remains unexplained. Iodide uptake inhibitors probably antagonize iodide transport through *competitive inhibition*. Other antithyroid compounds include the thionamides, the sulfonamides (e.g., para-aminobenzoic acid), and the sulfonylureas (carbutamide, tolbutamide). Maintenance of an effective serum concentration of these antithyroid drugs for a sufficient time will usually cause thyroid hypertrophy and goiter. These agents are therefore often referred to as *goitrogens*. A number of these drugs are of clinical importance in the treatment of excess thyroid hormone production (thyrotoxicosis) (Fig. 13.6).

Thiourea

Thiouracil

Propylthiouracil (PTU)

Methimazole

Figure 13.6 **Structures of some thionamide type antithyroid drugs.**

Figure 13.7 Synthesis and structure of goitrin.

Dietary goitrogens are responsible for *endemic goiter* in certain parts of the world. *Cyanogenic glucosides* (found in cassava, sorghum, sweet potatoes, maize, apricots, cherries, almonds) are hydrolyzed by glucosidases in the gut and release free cyanide that is converted to thiocyanate. Thioglucosides found in certain plants (e.g., genus *Brassica*: cabbage, Brussels sprouts, cauliflower, turnips, and rutabagas (swedes)) are metabolized within the body to thiocyanates and isothiocyanates (Fig. 13.7). These plant products are usually not consumed in large enough quantities to produce goiter, although they may augment endemic goiter in areas deficient in iodine. Involvement of dietary goitrogens in the pathogenesis of human goiter has been discovered in a population of natives in Zaire, Africa [8, 22]. Cassava forms an important part of the natives' diet, and it has been shown that ingestion of cassava from this area depresses radioiodide uptake by the normal human thyroid. The nature of the putative goitrogen remains unclear. Congenital goiter in lambs of ewes fed various mustard greens has also been reported.

Thyroid Hormones or Thyroid Hormone?

Normally, thyroxine (T_4) is produced in greater quantity than triiodothyronine (T_3). In human serum, the concentration of T_4 is about 50 times greater than the T_3 level. Because T_4 is converted to T_3 in athyreotic human subjects, extrathyroidal monodeiodination of T_4 appears to be the major source of T_3 in the body. If T_3 is the physiologically relevant hormone, is T_4 therefore the prohormone of T_3? Is it possible that both T_4 and T_3 are hormones, each with its own specific target tissues? There is strong evidence that T_3 is the major physiologically active thyroid hormone regulating cellular activity in many species, but T_4 is thought to exert a negative feedback action on the hypothalamus. In newborn infants, serum T_3 levels are very low in cord blood, whereas T_4 concentrations are high, suggesting that T_4 may serve a direct functional role during certain developmental stages of animals. In this text, the term *thyroid hormones* will refer to the putative activities of both T_3 and T_4, but it must be understood that T_3 is the most effective thyroid hormone under normal serum levels of iodothyronines, at least in mammals [38].

Other Iodothyronines in Biological Fluids

Although T_4 and T_3 are the major thyroid hormones in the human circulation, other iodothyronines are also present [38] (Fig. 13.8). The relative concentrations of these iodinated thyronines vary in healthy and diseased states, but the significance of these differences is presently unknown. T_3, T_4, triac (3,5,3'-triiodothyroacetic acid), and tetrac (3,5,3',5'-tetraiodothyroacetic acid) have calorigenic activity; the relative potency of these compounds is approximately 300 : 100 : 21 : 11, respectively. Although reverse triiodothyronine (3,3',5'-triiodothyronine, rT_3) has little thermogenic activity, it is more potent than T_3 in a number of systems. Nevertheless, it is argued that the concentrations of these iodothyronines required to cause physiological responses in vitro exceed by several orders of magnitude those concentrations present in vivo. Thus, the physiological significance, if any, of the actions of these iodothyronines is questionable.

The T_3 and rT_3 present in body fluids are derived from monodeiodination of T_4 within peripheral tissues. Subsequent metabolism of these iodothyronines provides the major sources of the T_2's and $3'$-T_1. Ultimately, these iodinated thyronines are made soluble through sulfation or glucuronide formation within the liver and are excreted in the urine or with bile salts. High concentrations of T_0 (completely deiodinated thyronine) are present in the plasma and urine and may represent a major end product of thyronine deiodination in humans.

Figure 13.8 appears here with the structural formulas of the iodothyronines:

3'-Monoiodothyronine (3'-T_1)

3,3',5'-Triiodothyronine (Reverse-T_3)

3,3'-Diiodothyronine (3,3'-T_2)

3',5'-Diiodothyronine (3',5'-T_2)

3,5,3'-Triiodothyronine (T_3)

3,5,3',5'-Tetraiodothyroacetic Acid (Tetrac)

3,5,3',5'-Tetraiodothyronine (Thyroxine, T_4)

3,5,3'-Triiodothyroacetic Acid (Triac)

Figure 13.8 Structural formulas of iodothyronines found in human plasma.

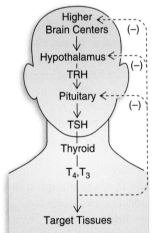

Figure 13.9 Central nervous system pituitary-thyroid axis.

Control of Thyroid Hormone Secretion

Thyroid hormone secretion is regulated by TSH from the pituitary gland that, in turn, is controlled by thyrotropin-releasing hormone (TRH) of hypothalamic origin (Chap. 6). Thyroid hormones feed back at the pituitary and hypothalamic levels to inhibit TRH and TSH secretion (Fig. 13.9). TSH secretion is inhibited by stress in a number of species, including humans [24]. The action of TRH follows its specific high-affinity binding to the thyrotroph plasma membrane receptor. Hydrolysis of phosphatidylinositol followed by altered intracellular Ca^{2+} are the proximal events in the secretion of TSH, whereas cAMP appears not to be involved.

In many mammals, activation of the pituitary-thyroid axis occurs during exposure to a lowered ambient temperature. Acute cold exposure of the rat, for example, leads to a rapid release of TSH, probably involving a neuroendocrine reflex mechanism. TSH release in response to a cold stimulus occurs in infants but is minimal or absent in adult humans. Present evidence suggests that an acute neuroendocrine reflex exists for TSH release in some mammals, including human infants, which is mediated initially by peripheral sensory receptors, then relayed to the hypothalamus where stimulation of TRH release occurs. This is substantiated by the observation that prior administration of T_4 inhibits pituitary TSH release in response to a cold stimulus. In addition, peripheral plasma levels of TRH increase in hypophysectomized cold-exposed rats. Finally, TRH synthesis is increased in vitro in hypothalamic tissue taken from cold-exposed rats.

In addition to the well-established negative feedback action of T_4 on pituitary TSH production, T_4 controls TRH synthesis by regulating gene expression of the TRH prohormone in the "thyrotrophic area" of the hypothalamus. The negative feedback effect of T_4 on the synthesis of the TRH prohormone is specific for TRH-producing neurons located in the medial division of the paraventricular nucleus (PVN), whereas TRH neurons elsewhere in the hypothalamus or in extrahypothalamic locations are not affected by changes of thyroid status. For example, TRH in the hypothalamus, but not olfactory lobe, is regulated by thyroid hormone. In the hypothalamus, hypothyroidism enhances not only proTRH synthesis, but also release of TRH and another proTRH-derived peptide [6].

Circulation and Metabolism

The thyroid hormones are water-insoluble molecules that require specific binding proteins in the plasma and the cell cytosol to gain access to nuclear receptors. This protein-bound iodine (PBI) consists of two major thyroxine-binding proteins present in human plasma: *transthyretin* and *thyroxine-binding globulin* (TBG). Transthyretin has a molecular weight of 55,000 and is composed of four identical subunits, each consisting of 127 amino acid residues arranged in a tetrahedral symmetry and possessing a pair of T_4-binding sites. These binding sites are located deep inside a cylindrical channel that runs completely through the molecule and are almost completely isolated from the surrounding medium. TBG consists of a single polypeptide chain; although it is similar in molecular weight to transthyretin, much less is known about its chemical constitution. About 70–75% of T_4 is bound to TBG, about 20% to transthyretin, and 5–10% may be bound to albumin. These binding proteins are synthesized within the liver.

During pregnancy in humans there is a doubling of TBG concentration, which may result from estrogen stimulation of binding protein synthesis within the liver. Increased TBG production is followed by increased thyroid T_4 synthesis and secretion, but the plasma concentrations of unbound iodothyronines remain unchanged. In normal individuals, less than 0.5% of the total serum T_4 and about 0.3% of the serum T_3 are present in the free or unbound state. Any factor that alters the serum-binding proteins, particularly TBG, may affect the total T_4 concentration in the absence of thyroid dysfunction [34]. Mutations in the transthyretin gene can lead to inappropriate levels of circulating T_4 [29]. Pregnancy and estrogen-containing medications increase TBG concentrations; testosterone, corticosteroids, severe illness, cirrhosis, and nephrotic disorders can lower TBG concentrations. Teleost fishes lack high-affinity T_4-binding plasma proteins. If one function of the binding proteins is to provide a large extrathyroidal pool of iodide, these proteins may not be required in a marine environment where iodide is always abundant.

Physiological Roles

The first scientific experiment to determine the role of the thyroid gland was reported in 1858 and involved the removal of the gland from dogs. The animals died soon after surgery. Transplantation of thyroid tissue from a thyroidectomized animal into the body cavity resulted in survival of the animals for a long duration, thus demonstrating that death was due to an absence of the thyroid rather than to the operation itself. Many experiments led to the erroneous belief that the thyroid gland is essential to life. Only later was it realized that death from thyroidectomy was due to removal of the parathyroid glands present within the thyroid tissue. The essential role of the thyroid glands in the control of numerous physiological processes is now well documented.

Thyroid hormones influence most bodily functions [4, 44]. They directly affect a number of physiological processes and, although without observable actions, they are often required (permissive) for the actions of other hormones on these functions. For example, they are obligatory, along with growth hormone (GH), for early growth and development. Thyroid hormone deficiencies in humans produce major abnormalities in growth, development, reproduction, behavior, and metabolism. Thyroid hormones are unique in that they exert effects within almost every tissue of the body throughout the life of an individual.

Thyroid Hormones are Required for Normal Growth and Development

The absence of thyroid hormones results in severe growth retardation, which is associated with arrest of bone elongation as well as retarded bone maturation [44]. Growth hormone secretion is diminished in the absence of thyroid hormones and is renewed when thyroid hormones are administered. Thus one cause of growth retardation is the absence of circulating levels of GH. Nevertheless, administration of GH to hypothyroid individuals is without effect if thyroid hormones are not also given. Thus, the role of thyroid hormones in normal growth is twofold; they are required both for the production of GH and for its systemic actions.

Levels of hyaluronic acid are high in proliferating tissue and decrease as division ceases and the cells become more differentiated. The enzyme *hyaluronidase* (an endoglycosidase), which splits hyaluronic acid into smaller oligosaccharides, is apparently induced at a time when tissues mature and therefore, may serve as a signal for differentiation. Thyroid hormones stimulate tadpole tissue differentiation, which is paralleled by a decrease in hyaluronic acid levels and an increase in hyaluronidase concentrations. In myxedematous tissue from subjects with hypothyroidism there is an increase in hyaluronic acid. These observations suggest that thyroid hormones stimulate differentiation tissue through stimulation of hyaluronidase production.

Thyroid hormones in concert with prolactin (PRL) regulate mouse mammary gland development. Decreased serum levels of thyroid hormones result in retarded growth of the ductal system and little or no alveolar development. Thyroid hormones may also be required for the synthesis of normal levels of PRL by the pituitary gland. Thyroid hormones are required for the normal development of the brain; without these hormones there is decreased protein synthesis, decreased myelinogenesis, and retarded axonal ramifications. These developmental processes, unlike general body growth, are irreversibly compromised and lead to mental deficiency, as is particularly evident in cretins. Nerve growth factor (NGF) induces dendritogenesis and regeneration of sympathetic neurons (Chap. 12). It may be significant, therefore, that thyroid hormone administration increases the concentration of NGF in the brain. These observations suggest that thyroid hormones may control CNS development through stimulation of NGF biosynthesis. Thyroid hormones also accelerate axonal regeneration in the cerebrum of lesioned adult rats, and the hormones appear to be selectively concentrated within adrenergic nerve terminals.

Thyroid Hormones Stimulate Thermogenesis and Oxygen Consumption

The evolution from poikilothermy to homeothermy required the acquisition of some mechanism for heat production. Active sodium transport uses a high proportion (possibly as much as 20–40%) of the total cellular energy supply. In the process of ATP hydrolysis by the Na^+ pump, heat is liberated, which contributes greatly to the maintenance of an elevated body temperature in homeotherms (sodium pump theory of thermogenesis). The activity of the sodium pump requires a source of ATP, which is produced mainly within the mitochondria. Thyroid hormones stimulate mitochondrial oxygen consumption and production of ATP. The T_3-induced increase in Na^+/K^+-ATPase activity results from an increase in the amount of the enzyme rather than a change in the affinity of the enzyme for substrates or in the catalytic properties of the enzyme. Na^+/K^+-ATPase expression is controlled at multiple levels, including transcriptional, translational, and post-translational activities. T_3 regulation of this important enzyme is highly tissue specific and may be mediated by one or more of these regulatory mechanisms operating simultaneously. Inhibition of Na^+/K^+-ATPase activity by ouabain and other sodium pump antagonists markedly reduces the action of thyroid hormones on heat production and oxygen consumption.

Diet can Alter Thyroid Hormone Production and Function

An increase of caloric intake (mixed diet or carbohydrates) in individuals results in an increased diet-induced thermogenesis. The production of T_3 is increased during short-term overfeeding; the increased serum levels of T_3 apparently derive from altered (increased) peripheral conversion of T_4 to T_3 and a decreased conversion of T_3 to rT_3. Individuals fed isocaloric diets low in carbohydrates or containing no carbohydrates develop changes in T_3 and rT_3 opposite to those resulting from feeding excess carbohydrates. Here may be an adaptation in which the resting metabolic rate is increased in the presence of excess poor-quality food (carbohydrates) to provide enough of a scarce nutrient, such as protein or even minerals, without the burden of weight gain.

Plasma levels of T_3 decrease during prolonged fasting, which is correlated with a decrease (down-regulation) in hepatic nuclear T_3 receptors. A decrease in serum T_3 concentration per se does not diminish hepatic nuclear T_3 receptor content as brain T_3 receptor number is not concomitantly changed. A particular cell type may be able to modify its nuclear T_3 receptor content in response to its own metabolic status, which "infers the possibility of individual target cell acceptance or rejection of the hormonal directive" [33]. This may represent a homeostatic protective mechanism to prolong survival of the organism under conditions of food deprivation.

Thyroid Hormones and Aging.   Food restriction alters the aging process. In rats, long-term reduction in food consumption increases longevity, decreases the frequency of occurrence and severity of age-related diseases, and retards much of the physiological decline seen with aging. The mechanism by which food restriction exerts its antiaging action is not known, but may be mediated by altering endocrine and/or neural regulatory systems.

TABLE 13.1 Some physiological roles and actions of thyroid hormones in mammals

Feedback inhibition of hypothalamic TRH and pituitary TSH secretion
Permissive to the action of many other hormones:
    Enhances lipolytic response of adipose tissue to hormones
    Required for the growth-promoting activity of GH
Increases activity of the sympathoadrenal system
Regulates basal metabolic rate:
    Increases mitochondrial oxidative phosphorylation
Required for hepatic conversion of carotenes to vitamin A
Required for bone growth and maturation
Required for nervous system differentiation in early development
Required for pituitary prolactin and growth hormone synthesis
Increases the rate of intestinal glucose absorption
Increases human red blood cell Ca^{2+}-ATPase activity
Induces enzyme synthesis:
    Na^+/K^+-ATPase (or a protein component or activator of the sodium pump)
    Carbamoyl phosphate synthetase (a phosphotransferase)
    α-Lactalbumin (lactose synthetase system proteins)
    Hepatic pyruvate carboxylase (converts pyruvate to oxaloacetate)
    Chromatin protein kinase
    Mitochondrial α-glycerophosphate dehydrogenase
    Malic dehydrogenase (converts malic acid to oxaloacetate)
    Hyaluronidase (dissolves intercellular ground substance)
Induction of cellular proteins (other than enzymes):
    Prolactin, growth hormone, lung surfactants, brain nerve factor (NGF)

The thyroid hormone system represents one potential coupler of food restriction with aging. Since this endocrine system is sensitive to changes in food consumption, several studies have suggested that the thyroid is involved in the aging process per se.

Many Actions of Thyroid Hormones are "Permissive"

Thyroid hormones are required for the actions of other hormones on target tissues. This permissive action is also a characteristic of gonadal and adrenal steroids on some of their target tissues. Because thyroid and steroid hormones mediate most of their actions at the level of the genome to induce protein synthesis, it is likely that these proteins function as substrates in the action pathway of other hormones (see Fig. 3.16).

Thyroid hormones induce GH production in cultured rat pituitary tumor (GH1) cells. Glucocorticoids also stimulate GH synthesis, but only in the presence of thyroid hormones. There is a dramatic synergistic activation of GH production when both hormones are present together in the medium, suggesting that the ability of glucocorticoids to stimulate GH synthesis is controlled by thyroid hormones. This is another example of the permissive action of thyroid hormones.

The enzyme ornithine decarboxylase (ODC) is essential for polyamine biosynthesis and is intimately related to the regulation of nucleic acid and protein biosynthesis. Growth hormone stimulates ODC activity in brain tissue, but only in the presence of thyroid hormones. Thyroid hormones, however, do not stimulate brain ODC activity. This demonstrates dramatically the permissive action of a hormone. In the liver, in contrast, GH and thyroid hormones stimulate ODC activity independently of each other. These results demonstrate the tissue specificity to the actions of these hormones within an individual animal. Some of the more prominent actions of thyroid hormones are summarized in Table 13.1.

Mechanisms of Action

The action of T_3 is analogous to the model for steroid hormone action (Chaps 4, 9, and 17) [43, 45]. There are two known thyroid hormone receptor (TR) genes: thyroid hormone receptor β (TRβ) on chromosome 3 and thyroid hormone receptor α (TRα) on chromosome 17. Both genes encode isoform products by alternative mRNA splicing. The TRβ gene produces TRβ1 and TRβ2 proteins, and the TRα gene produces TRα1 and an α2 isoform.

The TRβ1, TRβ2, and TRα1 proteins appear to be physiologic thyroid hormone receptors that avidly bind T_3 and regulate subsequent thyroid hormone-responsive gene transcription. The α2 isoform does not bind T_3 and is thus not a receptor, but is believed to inhibit the transcriptional effects of TRβ1, TRβ2, and TRα1. TRβ1 and TRα1 receptors are present in many tissues, but TRβ2 appears to be restricted to the pituitary gland and some areas of the central nervous system. The TRs are intranuclear proteins (ligand-activated transcription factors) that have distinct domains for binding to T_3 and DNA and for forming homodimers with nearby TRs or heterodimers with other nuclear receptors (retinoic acid receptors, retinoid X receptors), or thyroid hormone receptor auxiliary proteins (TRAPs) [18]. Under normal circumstances, circulating T_4 and T_3 traverse the cell membrane by an energy-dependent process. T_4 is then converted to T_3, which enters the nucleus where it binds to the TR. The T_3–TR complexes bind as monomers, homodimers, or heterodimers to specific thyroid-response elements present in thyroid hormone-regulated genes. This initiates the activity of RNA polymerase, which controls transcription of the structural gene regions into mRNA. Subsequently, mRNA is translated into protein products that ultimately mediate thyroid hormone tissue effects (Fig. 13.10).

The actions of T_3 may not be restricted to a genomic locus; rather, they may induce effects on the plasma membrane and mitochondria. Thyroid hormones stimulate human red cell

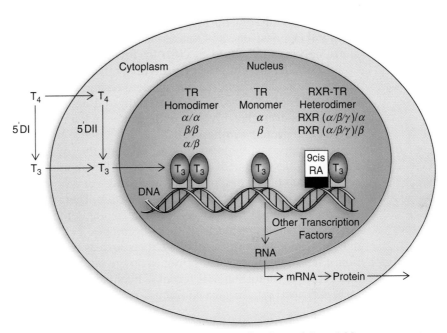

Figure 13.10 Model for the action mechanism of thyroid hormone on target tissues. The active form of thyroid hormone, triiodothyronine (T_3), is produced by deiodination of thyroxine (T_4) by the enzymes $T_4$5'-deiodinase (5'-D) types I and II. Type I $T_4$5'-deiodinase is found predominantly in the liver and kidneys; its action is responsible for the production of two-thirds of the total T_3 in the body. Type II $T_4$5'-deiodinase is responsible for most of the T_3 found in the pituitary, the brain, and brown fat. T_3 enters the cell or is produced locally and then transported into the nucleus. Transcriptionally active forms of thyroid hormone receptors (TR) include monomers, homodimers, and heterodimers with nuclear protein partners, such as the retinoid X receptor (RXR). The T_3–receptor complex interacts with specific sequences in DNA regulatory regions and modifies gene expression. T_3 causes both increases and decreases in gene expression and may also influence the stability of messenger RNA (mRNA). 9-cis RA denotes 9-cis-retinoic acid, the ligand for RXR. (From Brent, with permission. Reprinted by permission of *The New England Journal of Medicine.* "The molecular basis for thyroid hormone action," 331:847–53. © 1994 Massachusetts Medical Society.)

Ca^{2+}-ATPase activity, which clearly documents the extranuclear actions of these hormones. Thyroid hormones stimulate the rapid uptake of amino acids into cells, an action not blocked by actinomycin D or puromycin. These results again suggest a direct action of thyroid hormones at the level of the plasma membrane. In addition, 2-deoxyglucose (a nonmetabolizable glucose substrate) uptake into cells is rapidly stimulated by T_3 at physiological concentrations. These effects are also not blocked by inhibitors of transcriptional and translational processes. Thyroid hormones also stimulate plasmalemmal Na^+/K^+-ATPase (the sodium pump). This enhanced activity may be an indirect action of the hormones and result from an increased number of pump units rather than any direct increase in the activity of the ATPase. Newly synthesized ATPase derives from actions of the thyroid hormones at the level of the genome.

For many years, there was argument whether thyroid hormones mediated their effects through direct actions on mitochondria. The following data provide convincing evidence that, indeed, mitochondria are another site of thyroid hormone action. In the hypothyroid state, mitochondria are altered both morphologically and functionally, and the uptake of ADP by mitochondria is increased after administration of T_3 or T_4 to thyroidectomized rats. A specific receptor for T_3 and T_4 is a component of the inner mitochondrial membrane, which is known to be the site of oxidative phosphorylation. These receptors are present in mitochondria from thyroid hormone-responsive tissues, but not in spleen and testes, tissues known to be refractory to thyroid hormones. Most interesting is the observation that mitochondria from neonatal rat brain, but not from brain tissues of older animals, possess thyroid hormone receptors. These data are compatible with the known temporal responsiveness of this tissue to thyroid hormones. Finally, mitochondrial oxygen consumption is increased in vitro by thyroid hormones. This effect is not inhibited by cycloheximide, an inhibitor of protein synthesis, suggesting an acute action of the hormones on the mitochondria. The marked changes in mitochondrial nucleic acid synthesis in vivo that are associated with altered thyroid states suggest that thyroid hormone action in mitochondria may involve both acute and long-term actions, the latter involving mRNA and protein synthesis.

In summary, thyroid hormones act on a number of cellular receptor sites. The actions of most hormones that mediate their effects at the plasmalemma involve changes in the intracellular levels of one or more cyclic nucleotides or other second messengers, whose activities appear restricted to substrate phosphorylation. There appears to be no single intracellular effector mechanism for thyroid hormone action; rather, several pathways contribute to an integrated cellular response of these hormones. The nuclear actions of thyroid hormones may be related to slower anabolic effects such as those involved in growth and differentiation. The actions of thyroid hormones on the plasmalemma (sodium pump hypothesis) and mitochondria (mitochondrial receptor hypothesis) are rapidly initiated events that control increased heart rate, oxygen consumption, and ATP production.

Pathophysiology

Because thyroid hormones affect many physiological processes and are necessary for the optimal activity of numerous hormones, it is not surprising that abnormalities of thyroid function lead to gross alterations in the normal physiology of an individual [30]. Thyroid hormone underproduction or overproduction, referred to as hypothyroidism or hyperthyroidism, respectively, can occur at birth (congenital) or later in life. A defect at the level of the pituitary or hypothalamus (see case studies provided) would result in decreased or increased production and secretion of TSH with resulting secondary or tertiary hypothyroidism or hyperthyroidism, respectively [46, 47]. Abnormalities of thyroid function may be familial (genetic) in nature and involve failure in growth or normal function of the thyroid gland. Other genetic defects may result in biosynthetic defects related to thyroid hormonogenesis, iodine trapping or organification, defective thyroglobulin synthesis and secretion, and other abnormalities [7, 30].

TSH is a member of a group of closely related glycoprotein hormones, all of which are heterodimeric molecules consisting of common α and specific β subunits [10]. Several clinical cases show congenital, isolated TSH deficiencies associated with cretinism, displaying severe mental and growth retardation with the failure to go through puberty. One family with two patient siblings has been analyzed intensively. These patients showed no TSH in the blood even in the hypothyroid state, but showed normal levels of other glycoprotein hormones, such as luteinizing hormone (LH) and follicle-stimulating hormone (FSH), which share the same α subunit with TSH. On administration of TRH, a dramatic increase of the α subunit was observed in the bloodstream, but not of the heterodimeric TSH or the free β subunit, suggesting that the patients do not produce active β subunits. The absence of the β subunit could either be due to a failure to produce the polypeptide or to the production of an inactive subunit. It was shown that the patients' β subunit genes carry a mutation in the 29th amino acid codon, and that the mutant gene may produce a conformationally abnormal β subunit that cannot associate with the α subunit [11, 20, 27].

Thyrotropin (TSH) controls thyroid function by binding to its receptor at the basolateral membrane of the thyroid follicular cells. Mutations in the gene encoding the TSH receptor can lead to hypothyroidism (see case study provided) or to hyperthyroidism. Activating mutations of TSH receptors result in clonal expansion of the thyrotrophs into a hyperfunctional adenoma (toxic nodule) [31]. In rare instances, hyperthyroidism may result from the ectopic production of TSH [10] or even from a trophoblastic (placental) tumor secreting either excessive amounts of choriogonadotropin (structurally somewhat related to TSH) or of a TSH-like molecule. Primary hyperthyroidism may derive from development of a thyroidal adenoma or carcinoma and involve gross overproduction of thyroid hormones [31, 36, 41, 46].

Overstimulation of the thyroid may result from an autoimmune response involving antibodies to the TSH receptor [3]. *Thyroid-stimulating antibody* (TSAb) is the name given to the antibody once believed responsible for TSH receptor stimulation. This type of hyperthyroidism has been referred to as Graves' disease (exophthalmic or toxic goiter) [3]. Graves' thyrotoxicosis is uniquely associated with an exophthalmos (protruding of the eyes). *Cretins* are individuals who suffer from a deficiency or total absence of thyroid hormones. The major symptoms of cretinism are failure of skeletal growth and maturation and a marked retardation in development of intellect. *Athyreotic cretinism* may result from an in utero (congenital) thyroiditis or from a failure in thyroid development. Thyroid dysgenesis is responsible for decreased thyroid function in most infants with hypothyroidism and is most prevalent in females. Although sporadic, it may be familial in origin and may also occur in association with maternal autoimmune thyroiditis. Congenital goiter may also be associated with thyroid dyshormonogenesis due to hereditary defects in hormone synthesis or metabolism. Hypothyroidism in the adult is referred to as *myxedema* (from the Greek *myxa*, mucus and *oidema*, swelling) because of the characteristic mucinous protein deposit in the subcutaneous tissues.

A genetic failure in development of thyroid hormone receptors results in a familial peripheral (end organ, target tissue) resistance with resulting hypothyroidism [2, 23, 29, 47]. Generalized resistance to thyroid hormone (GRTH), in which most or all of the tissues of the body are variably resistant to thyroid hormone, has been described in more than 200 cases (see case study provided). Selective pituitary resistance to thyroid hormone (PRTH), in which predominantly the pituitary gland is resistant, has been reported in at least 32 cases, and selective peripheral resistance to thyroid hormone (PerRTH), in which only peripheral tissues are resistant, has been described. In the *low T_3 syndrome*, hypothyroidism results from a failure in the peripheral conversion of T_4 to T_3, which is probably the physiologically relevant thyroid hormone [19].

The clinical manifestations of tissue resistance to the action of thyroid hormones differ dramatically depending on the tissues involved. Individuals with the general resistance syndrome are clinically euthyroid; they may have goiter, and plasma levels of thyroid hormones may even be elevated. The variable biochemical defects responsible for end organ thyroid hormone resistance may be caused by the following: (1) decreased binding affinity; (2) decreased binding capacity (decrease in receptor number); and (3) an abnormal post-receptor mechanism. For example, a genetic defect in development of thyroid hormone receptors results in a familial peripheral resistance with resulting clinical hypothyroidism that is not, however, characterized by goiter. On the other hand, individuals with a pituitary (thyrotroph) resistance to thyroid hormone feedback are hyperthyroid

Figure 13.11 Diffuse thyromegaly (goiter) in a 12-year-old girl with euthyroid autoimmune thyroiditis. (From Foley, with permission. *Endocrinology and Metabolism Clinics of North America* 22:593–606, 1993.)

and, as might be expected, plasma TSH and thyroid hormone levels are elevated. This example of TSH-dependent hyperthyroidism represents one of the *syndromes of inappropriate TSH secretion.*

Failure of the thyroid to produce T_4 and T_3 may lead to the development of a goiter (Fig. 13.11) since, in the absence of any negative feedback to the hypothalamus and pituitary gland, there is excessive secretion of TSH. In the absence of thyroid hormone production, TSH stimulation continues to lead to hypertrophy of the thyroid follicular cells. Thyroid glands from such hypothyroid individuals are hyperplastic and exhibit grossly columnar follicular cells with a decreased amount of colloid (due to enhanced engulfment and degradation). Goiters may also develop under conditions of thyroiditis due to autoantibodies against thyroid TSH receptors. In the past, a lack of iodine in the diet resulted in hypothyroidism; with the general availability of iodized salt this problem has been eradicated throughout much of the world. Clinically, endemic (simple, nontoxic) goiter is treated with iodized salt, but prolonged hypothyroidism in early childhood may lead to irreversible stunting and cretinism.

About one billion people worldwide are potentially at risk from iodine deficiency disorders. Endemic goiter is the most common manifestation, and its prevalence rises directly with the degree of iodine lack, reaching 100% in communities with severe iodine deficiency. The greatest morbidity of severe iodide deficiency arises not by its primary consequences on thyroid gland enlargement, but by its secondary effects on thyroid hormone homeostasis resulting in deficits in neonatal brain development. This is expressed clinically in its extreme as endemic cretinism, a disorder of profound mental and physical disability [5, 22].

The integrity of the thyroglobulin structure as a protein is essential for adequate synthesis of thyroid hormone. Mutations in TG gene or hyposialylated TG, due to defective sialyltransferase activity, cause a structurally defective protein and severely impair the function of TG. Defective TG synthesis and secretion can cause goiter and hypothyroidism [42]. Inactivating mutations in the sodium/iodide symporter gene, producing iodide transport defects and congenital hypothyroidism, have also been described (see Molecular Medicine Case Studies, this chapter).

Thyroxine has been used as replacement therapy in hypothyroidism. For the treatment of thyrotoxicosis, such antithyroid drugs as propylthiourea, methimazole, or carbimazole are used most commonly (Fig. 13.6). These thionamide-type drugs inhibit the coupling of iodotyrosyl residues in thyroglobulin to form T_4 and T_3. Propylthiourea (PTU) is the preferred drug as, in addition to the effects in the thyroid common to all these drugs, it blocks the peripheral conversion of T_4 to T_3 in the liver. Radioactive (cytotoxic) iodide, administered

TABLE 13.2 Major physiological manifestations of hyperthyroidism and hypothyroidism

Hyperthyroidism	Hypothyroidism
Elevated T_4-T_3 levels	Decreased (or absent) T_4-T_3 levels
Elevated basal metabolic rate (BMR) (hypermetabolism)	Low basal metabolic rate (BMR) (hypometabolism)
Increased perspiration	Decreased perspiration
Rapid pulse (increased cardiac output, hypertension)	Slow pulse (decreased cardiac output, hypotension)
Increased body temperature (sensation of warmness)	Lowered body temperature (sensation of coldness)
Heat intolerance	Cold intolerance
Warm, moist palms	Coarse, dry skin, subdermal thickening
Nervousness, anxiety, excitability, restlessness, insomnia	Lethargy, decreased mentation, depression, paranoia, sleepiness, tiredness
Weight loss	Weight gain
Muscle wasting	Loss of hair, dry and brittle texture
Increased appetite	Edema of face and eyelids
Menstrual irregularities	Menstrual irregularities
Exophthalmos (in some individuals)	Carotenemia (increased plasma levels of carotenes)
Goiter (primary or secondary origin)	Goiter (may or may not be present)

one time only, is a preferred treatment of hyperthyroidism in patients who have difficulty adhering to the medical regimen of taking antithyroid drugs three times a day for a year or more.

The general symptoms of hypothyroxinemia and thyrotoxicosis are summarized in Table 13.2. Many general manifestations of underproduction or overproduction of thyroid hormones relate to decreased or increased activity of the sympathoadrenal system (Chap. 14). A summary of the general etiology of hypothyroidism and hyperthyroidism is provided in Table 13.3 and Figure 13.12.

TABLE 13.3 Pathophysiology of the human thyroid gland

Hypothyroidism (hypothyroxinemia)
  Primary hypothyroidism
    Familial or congenital thyroid dysgenesis
    Failure of thyroid hormonogenesis (usually of genetic origin)
  Secondary hypothyroidism
    Hypothalamic hypothyroidism (tertiary hypothyroidism)
  Cretinism (childhood hypothyroidism)
    Goitrous cretinism (endemic; lack of dietary iodide)
    Athyreotic cretinism (congenital absence of thyroid; thyroid dysgenesis)
  Myxedema (adult hypothyroidism)
    Simple goiter (endemic; lack of dietary iodide)
    Primary myxedema
      Idiopathic (atrophic thyroiditis of unknown origin)
      Iatrogenic (surgical removal or chemical inactivation)
      Spontaneous (autoimmune destruction: Hashimoto's thyroiditis)
  Familial peripheral (end-organ) resistance to thyroid hormones (e.g., lack of or defective T_3, T_4 receptors)
  Familial thyroid hormone-binding protein defects or levels
  Low T_3 syndrome (failure of peripheral conversion of T_4 to T_3)
  Thyroid gland resistance to TSH
Hyperthyroidism (thyrotoxicosis)
  Primary hyperthyroidism
    Neoplasia (adenoma, carcinoma producing excessive TSH)
  Secondary hyperthyroidism
    Hypothalamic hyperthyroidism (tertiary hyperthyroidism)
    TSH-dependent hyperthyroidism (pituitary thyrotroph unresponsiveness to T_3 feedback inhibition)
    Ectopic TSH secretion (rare)
  Thyroid-stimulating antibody (TSAb) (autoimmune agonistic antibodies of thyroid TSH receptors) (Graves' disease) [9, 38]

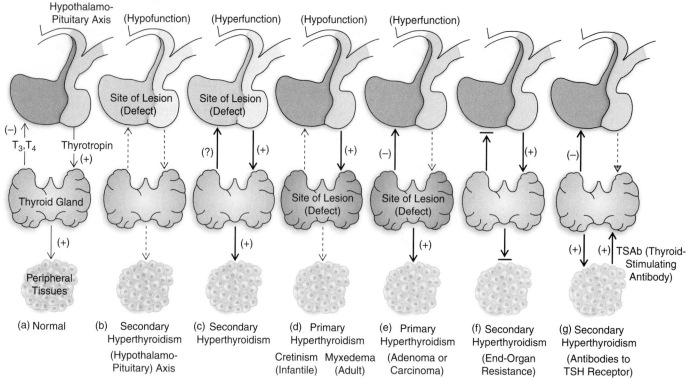

Figure 13.12 Various endocrine disorders relating to the overproduction or underproduction of TSH or to inadequate thyroid- or peripheral-tissue responses to TSH or thyroid hormones.

MOLECULAR MEDICINE CASE STUDIES

Four case studies of hypothyroidism involving mutations in different receptors (T3, TSH, TRH) and the sodium/iodide symporter are provided.

The thyroid hormone receptor-beta gene mutation R383H is associated with isolated central resistance to thyroid hormone (J. D. Safer, M. G. O'Connor, S. D. Colan, S. Srinivasan, S. R. Tollin, F. E. Wondisford. *J. Clin. Endocrinol. Metab.* 84(9):3099–109, 1999). "Resistance to thyroid hormone (RTH) action is due to mutations in the beta-isoform of the thyroid hormone receptor (TR-beta). RTH patients display inappropriate central secretion of TRH from the hypothalamus and of TSH from the anterior pituitary despite elevated levels of thyroid hormone (T_4 and T_3). RTH mutations cluster in three hot spots in the C-terminal portion of the TR-beta. Most individuals with TR-beta mutations have generalized resistance to thyroid hormone, where most tissues in the body are hyporesponsive to thyroid hormone. The affected individuals are clinically euthyroid or even hypothyroid depending on the severity of the mutation. Whether TR-beta mutations cause a selective form of RTH that only leads to central thyroid hormone resistance is debated. Here, we describe an individual with striking peripheral sensitivity to graded T_3 administration. The subject was enrolled in a protocol in which she received three escalating T_3 doses over a 13-day period. Indexes of

central and peripheral thyroid hormone action were measured at baseline and at each T_3 dose. Although the patient's resting pulse rose only 11% in response to T_3, her serum ferritin, alanine aminotransferase, aspartate transaminase, and lactate dehydrogenase rose 320%, 117%, 121%, and 30%, respectively. In addition, her serum cholesterol, creatinine phosphokinase, and deep tendon reflex relaxation time fell (25%, 36%, and 36%, respectively). Centrally, the patient was sufficiently resistant to T_3 that her serum TSH was not suppressed with 200 μg T_3, orally, daily for 4 days. The patient's C-terminal TR exons were sequenced revealing the mutation R383H in a region not otherwise known to harbor TR-beta mutations. Our clinical evaluation presented here represents the most thorough documentation to date of the central thyroid hormone resistance phenotype in an individual with an identified TR-beta mutation" (Fig. 13.13).

Two novel mutations in the thyrotropin (TSH) receptor gene in a child with resistance to TSH (R. J. Clifton-Bligh et al., *J. Clin. Endocrinol. Metab.* 82:1094–1100, 1997). "The TSH receptor is a G protein-coupled receptor that mediates the effects of TSH in thyroid development, growth, and synthetic function. We report here that a child with features of TSH resistance, including markedly increased serum TSH concentrations and low normal

Figure 13.13 Location of the R383H TRβ point mutation in a patient with central resistance to thyroid hormone (CRTH). The wild-type (WT) sequence of the TRβ amino acid 383 (CGC; *bold*) and adjacent amino acids is shown on the *left*. On the *right* is the sequence of an affected subject's mutant allele across the same area (R383H, CGC to CAC). (From Safer, J. D., M. G. O'Connor, S. D. Colan, S. Srinivasan, S. R. Tollin, F. E. Wondisford, The thyroid hormone receptor-beta gene mutation R383H is associated with isolated central resistance to thyroid hormone. *J. Clin. Endocrinol. Metab.* 1999, with permission.)

thyroid hormone levels, is a compound heterozygote for two novel mutations in the TSH receptor gene. One allele has a G to A transition corresponding to an arginine to glutamine change at codon 109 (R109Q) in the extracellular domain of the receptor. The other allele has a G to A transition corresponding to a premature termination codon at tryptophan 546 (W546X) in the fourth transmembrane segment. Each parent is heterozygous for one mutation, and both parents have normal thyroid function. Cells transiently transfected with R109Q mutant exhibit reduced membrane binding of [^{125}I]TSH and impaired signal transduction in response to TSH. In contrast, the W546X mutant was nonfunctional, with negligible membrane radioligand binding. Our findings indicate that a single normal TSH receptor allele is sufficient for normal thyroid function, but that the compound abnormality in the proband leads to TSH resistance."

A novel mechanism for isolated central hypothyroidism: inactivating mutations on the thyrotropin-releasing hormone receptor gene (R. Collu et al., *J. Clin. Endocrinol. Metab.* 82:1561–65, 1997). "Isolated central hypothyroidism, characterized by insufficient TSH secretion resulting in low levels of thyroid hormones, is a rare disorder. We report a boy in whom isolated central hypothyroidism was diagnosed at 9 yr of age. Complete absence of TSH and PRL responses to TRH led us to speculate that he had an inactivating mutation of the TRH receptor gene. The patient's genomic DNA was isolated,

and the entire coding region of the TRH receptor was amplified by the PCR method and sequenced directly. Confirmation of the mutations and haplotyping of the family was performed using restriction enzymes. The biological activity of the wild-type and mutated TRH receptors was verified by evaluating the binding of labeled TRH and stimulation by TRH of total inositol phosphate accumulation in transfected HEK-293 and COS-1 cells. The patient was found to be a compound heterozygote, having inherited a different mutated allele from each of the parents; both mutations were in the 5'-part of the gene. Mutated receptors were unable to bind TRH and to activate total inositol phosphate accumulation. Our report is the first description of naturally occurring inactivating mutations of a G protein-coupled receptor linked to the phospholipase C second-messenger pathway. The prevalence and phenotypic spectrum of TRH receptor mutations in isolated central hypothyroidism remain to be established."

A novel peculiar mutation in the sodium/iodide symporter gene in Spanish siblings with iodide transport defect (S. Kosugi S, H. Okamoto, A. Tamada, F. Sanchez-Franco, *J. Clin. Endocrinol. Metab.* 87(8):3830–6, 2002). "Previously, we reported two Spanish siblings with congenital hypothyroidism due to total failure of iodide transport. These were the only cases reported to date who received long-term iodide treatment over 10 yr. We examined the sodium/iodide symporter (NIS) gene of these patients. A large deletion was observed by long

(Continued)

(Continued)

and accurate PCR using primers derived from introns 2 and 7 of the NIS gene. PCR-direct sequencing revealed a deletion of 6,192 bases spanning from exon 3 to intron 7 and an inverted insertion of a 431-base fragment spanning from exon 5 to intron 5 of the NIS gene. The patients were homozygous for the mutation, and their mother was heterozygous. In the mutant, deletion of exons 3–7 was suggested by analysis using programs to predict exon/intron organization, resulting in an in-frame 182-amino acid deletion from Met(142) in the fourth transmembrane domain to Gln(323) in the fourth exoplasmic loop. The mutant showed no iodide uptake activity when transfected into COS-7 cells, confirming that the mutation was the direct cause of the iodide transport defect in these patients. Further, the mutant NIS protein was synthesized, but not properly expressed, on the cell surface, but was mostly accumulated in the cytoplasm, suggesting impaired targeting to the plasma membrane."

Comparative Endocrinology

Some classical experiments in endocrinology were performed early last century on amphibian larvae, most often the anuran (frog, toad) tadpole. These experiments established a role for the thyroid in the control of metamorphosis in the amphibian [1, 14, 35, 39]. The following experimental observations were made:

1. Preparations (desiccated tissue) of the thyroid gland fed to frog tadpoles induced metamorphosis.
2. Removal of the thyroid glands prevented metamorphosis of tadpoles.
3. Implantation of thyroid glands into tadpoles caused accelerated development.
4. Hypophysectomy of tadpoles resulted in thyroid gland atrophy and prevented metamorphosis.
5. Injections of pars distalis extracts induced metamorphosis of hypophysectomized tadpoles.
6. Implantation of the pars distalis, but not the neurointermediate lobe, accelerated development in normal and hypophysectomized larvae, but not in thyroidless tadpoles.

The conclusion that emerged was that "metamorphosis is due to the combined action of both the anterior lobe of the hypophysis and the thyroid gland" [1]. Evidence has now shown that a thyroid-stimulating hormone (TSH) is specifically produced by thyrotrophs of the pars distalis and that thyrotropin of any source will stimulate metamorphosis of larval amphibians. Both thyroxine and triiodothyronine induce metamorphosis of amphibian larvae, and they are the likely thyroid hormones controlling metamorphosis in these animals.

Metamorphosis involves radical changes in body structure and function to allow successful transition of the amphibian from an aquatic to a terrestrial habitat (Fig. 13.14). The following metamorphic changes occur in amphibians:

1. Loss of the tail as a locomotory organ and acquisition of the characteristic tetrapod appendages.
2. Change in the integument from a smooth, moist skin (for respiration and increased locomotion) to a thicker, keratinized skin that is more resistant to water loss.
3. Loss of the major respiratory structure, the gills, and acquisition of lungs.
4. Radical changes in structural components of the GI tract: loss of the horny, rasping beak-like mouth and development of a new mouth with distensible tongue; shortening of the long intestine (needed for an essentially vegetarian diet) to a much shorter one for a generally carnivorous diet.
5. Development of corneal reflex, eyelids, and ocular muscles to control eye movements (eye movements in larvae are essentially nonexistent).
6. Biochemical changes in numerous organs:
   a. From predominantly amylase to protease production within the GI tract.
   b. From larval hemoglobins to adult hemoglobins. Larval hemoglobins bind more avidly to O_2 than do adult hemoglobins because O_2 is usually more limiting in the aquatic environment than in the terrestrial habitat.

Figure 13.14
Metamorphic change of the salamander, *Ambystoma tigrinum*, as induced by thyroxine (T_4) added to the aquarium water.

    c. From larval visual pigments to those of the adult, a change from predominantly rhodopsin to mostly porphyropsin.

    d. From ammonia excretion (ammonotelism) to urea excretion (ureotelism).

Amphibian larvae are voracious omnivores and spend most of their time eating and converting the ingested metabolic substrates into body structures, essentially proteins. After reaching a particular body size, or in response to environmental cues, larvae undergo irreversible metamorphic changes that ultimately lead to their adult forms. Clearly, thyroid hormones control metamorphic change, but what are the particular endocrine events involved? Are circulating levels of thyroid hormones increased? If so, what physiological events are responsible for such changes? What causes the destruction of one tissue (e.g., the tail) and the development of another (e.g., tongue)? The activity of the thyroid gland (amount of rough ER, follicular height) is clearly increased at metamorphic climax. A popular hypothesis is that the low circulating levels of thyroid hormones in the premetamorphic tadpole cause a slow maturation of hypothalamic neurosecretory centers, in time resulting in greater thyroid hormone secretion. The increase in these hormones, in turn, provides a positive feedback to the hypothalamus, which causes an accelerated maturation of the hypothalamus and its neurosecretory neurons. The resulting activation of TRH secretion and subsequent stimulation of pituitary TSH secretion would provide the final stimulus to thyroid gland maturation and maximal T_4-T_3 secretion [9]. Injection of a minute amount of T_4 directly into the hypothalamus is capable of activating the hypothalamo-hypophysial-thyroid axis in larval salamanders [25].

A body of evidence suggests that prolactin is a larval growth hormone with antimetamorphic actions in amphibians. Normal metamorphic processes may depend on an interplay between PRL and thyroid hormones. For example, thyroxine-induced metamorphosis in the frog is accelerated by injections of antiserum to PRL. Hypophysectomized larval amphibians administered PRL continue to grow with time, even beyond their normal size range; although they never metamorphose, they may be made to do so by injections of high concentrations of thyroid hormones. Both in vivo and in vitro experiments have provided data that PRL antagonizes the action of thyroid hormones on metamorphic processes. For example, thyroxine added to tadpole tails incubated in vitro causes their resorption, a process that normally takes place in the intact animal during metamorphosis. In contrast, PRL added to the incubation medium inhibits the actions of thyroid hormones on tail resorption. It was proposed that the actions of the PRL are also exerted at the level of the thyroid to inhibit thyroid hormone synthesis and secretion (a goitrogenic action). In the *hypothalamic maturation model of metamorphosis* the action of thyroid hormones at the level of the hypothalamus would also involve the establishment of an inhibitory influence on the release of pituitary PRL secretion. This might be effected by the developmental acquisition of functional PRL-inhibiting factor neurons, resulting in establishment of a tonic inhibitory control over pituitary PRL secretion, as in mammals [9].

Acceleration of the metamorphic process may involve more than an increase in circulating levels of thyroid hormones. There appears to be an increased sensitivity of target tissues, such as the tail, during the progress of metamorphosis. Experimental evidence suggests that the number of binding sites for T_3 in nuclei from tail tissue increases during spontaneous metamorphosis; nuclear receptors for T_3 increase after exposure of intact cells to thyroid hormones. It has been proposed, therefore, that the elevated levels of endogenous thyroid hormones at the onset of metamorphic climax in the tadpole regulate the number of their own nuclear receptors, thus increasing tissue sensitivity to the hormones.

Further evidence for thyroid hormone–prolactin interactions during amphibian metamorphosis is available and provides interesting insights into the developmental roles of these two hormones. Certain urodeles, such as the red-spotted newt (*Notophthalmus viridescens*), undergo a second metamorphosis. After an initial metamorphosis from an aquatic larva to a terrestrial tetrapod, the young salamander migrates back to water (so-called "water drive"). Young newts can be induced to undergo precocious water drive by injections of PRL. Thyroid hormones, on the other hand, antagonize the actions of PRL. Not all actions of PRL and thyroid hormones are exerted in opposition to each other; their actions are indeed often synergistic. For example, binding of PRL to the kidney of the bullfrog tadpole increases during metamorphic climax and in response to treatment with thyroxine. It was suggested that, during metamorphosis, the role of PRL as a growth-promoting agent is lost, along with its ion regulation of the gill. The osmoregulatory function of PRL may nevertheless persist beyond the larval period and be directed through the actions of the thyroid hormones from the gills (which are lost) to the kidneys.

Thyroid Hormones Play Additional Roles in Other Vertebrates

Evidence is lacking for a clearly defined role of the thyroid gland in cyclostomes and elasmobranchs. In teleost fishes, the thyroid gland is required for normal gonadal maturation. Thyroxine increases the sensitivity of the teleost olfactory epithelium to detection of salinity [26]. Thyroid hormones also increase O_2 consumption in fishes and amphibians, but the increase in metabolic activity is easily obscured by other factors. In reptiles, a calorigenic action of thyroid hormones has been documented under certain environmental conditions. Thyroid hormones in birds appear to assume roles similar to those in mammals. In amphibians, reptiles, and birds, thyroid hormones have prominent effects on the growth and differentiation of the integument and are required for molting of feathers and shedding of skin. Thyroxine is involved in the normal molting of the pelage in mammals; in addition, it stimulates the rate of hair growth in rodents and increases the rate of wool growth in sheep.

It has been hypothesized that in the evolution of endothermy, thermoregulatory responses to cold, thyroxine, and the sodium pump are related functionally and phylogenetically. In this evolutionary scheme, thyroxine was selected as the hormonal regulator because its major role in fishes is ion regulation. Thyroxine increases spontaneous motor activity in all classes of vertebrates; thus, thyroxine enhances behavioral thermoregulation through heat generation from muscular activity. Any increase in oxygen demand results in a concomitant stimulation of the Na^+ pump, and it is speculated that the evolution of nonshivering (metabolic) thermogenesis involved a bypassing of behavioral thermogenesis to a direct stimulation of the Na^+ pump by thyroid hormones to produce heat [13, 14].

REVIEW EXERCISES

Match the symptom to its cause:

1. Low basal metabolic rate
2. Cold intolerance
3. Rapid pulse
4. Decreased T_3-T_4 levels
5. Elevated basal metabolic rate
6. Weight gain

A. Hyperthyroidism
B. Hypothyroidism

Think, analyze and discuss:

1. Graves' disease is characterized by hyperthyroidism resulting from autoimmune antibodies that activate the TSH receptor. There are various tests that have been devised to detect the presence of these autoimmune TSAbs in the serum of patients with the disease. Devise a simple in vitro bioassay for the detection of TSAbs in human serum. You can assume that you have cultured rat thyroid follicular cells, as well as a biochemical assay, to measure cAMP levels in the cultures. How would you perform the bioassay? Describe the results that you might expect to obtain in tests of sera from a normal (euthyroid) individual, a Graves' disease patient, and a patient with some other form of hyperthyroidism.

2. It has been demonstrated in healthy volunteers that the administration of recombinant TSH stimulates radioactive iodine uptake (RAIU) in the thyroid gland. If the RAIU test is performed within a few hours after TSH administration, relatively little uptake occurs; by 24 hours after TSH administration, however, RAIU is maximally stimulated; at time intervals greater than 24 hours, RAIU is again diminished. Consider the cellular actions of TSH, as described in this chapter, and then propose a logical reason that RAIU is maximal at a 24-hour delay following TSH administration. How might you test your hypothesis in experimental animals? What measurements might you make and how would you interpret them?

3. Immunohistofluorescence can be performed to examine the expression of proteins in thyroid follicular cells. Assuming sufficient microscopic resolution of proteins at the subcellular level, where in thyroid follicular cells would you expect to observe high levels of the following proteins: NIS, pendrin, TG, peroxidase? For each of these proteins, explain why their localization is critically important for their specific cellular functions.

4. Dietary iodine deficiency can lead to hypothyroidism.
   a. In this condition, would serum TSH, serum thyroid hormones, and RAIU be high, low, or normal? If any of these measures would be abnormal, explain why.
   b. What are the metabolic symptom manifestations of hypothyroidism?
   c. Why is this condition often associated with the development of a goiter?
   d. Why is this condition of particular concern in children?

5. Which of the following conditions would produce a stimulation of proTRH synthesis? Which would lead to an inhibition of proTRH synthesis? Explain your answers.
    a. Thyroidectomy
    b. Thyroid hormone administration
    c. Cold stress
    d. Targeted deletion of thyroid hormone receptor genes
    e. Iodine deficiency
    f. TRH administration
6. What might be the pathophysiological consequences of an inactivating mutation in the gene encoding thyroxine-binding globulin, transthyretin?
7. Describe at least two possible cellular mechanisms by which thyroid hormones can stimulate thermogenesis. Why does the drug ouabain reduce the action of thyroid hormones on heat production?
8. Thyroid hormones are said to be permissive for the actions of other hormones. Name one such hormone and describe how thyroid hormones permit its effects.
9. A doctor examines a patient who reports that he has experienced excessive sweating, irritability, and feverish episodes. Assay of hormones in blood reveal that thyroid hormone levels are abnormally high, and TSH levels are low. An RAIU scan reveals a "hot spot" on the thyroid, indicating a localized region of intense iodine uptake. What do you predict that this patient's diagnosis will be? How would you attempt to treat such a condition?

References

[1] Allen, B. M. 1927. Influence of the hypophysis upon the thyroid gland in amphibian larvae. *Univ. Calif. Publ. Zool.* 31:53–78.

[2] Abramowicz, M. J., et al. 1997. Familial congenital hypothyroidism due to inactivating mutation of the thyrotropin receptor causes profound hyperplasia of the thyroid gland. *J. Clin. Invest.* 99:3018–24.

[3] Akamizu, T., T. Mori, and K. Nakao. 1997. Pathogenesis of Graves' disease: Molecular analysis of anti-thyrotropin receptor antibodies. *Endocrinol. J.* 44:633–46.

[4] Bernal, J. 2005. Thyroid hormones and brain development. *Vitam. Horm.* 71:95–122.

[5] Boyages, S. C., and J.-P. Halpern. 1993. Endemic cretinism: Toward a unifying hypothesis. *Thyroid* 3:59–69.

[6] Bruhn, T. O., J. H. Taplin, and I. M. D. Jackson. 1991. Hypothyroidism reduces content and increases in vitro release of prothyrotropin-releasing hormone peptides from the median eminence. *Neuroendocrinology* 53:511–15.

[7] Cooper, D. S., and B. M. Wenig. 1996. Hyperthyroidism caused by an ectopic TSH-secreting pituitary tumor. *Thyroid* 6:337–43.

[8] Ermans, A. M., et al. 1972. Possible role of cyanide and thiocyanate in the etiology of endemic cretinism. In: J. G. Stanbury and R. L. Kroc, eds. *Human development and the thyroid gland.* New York: Plenum.

[9] Etkin, W. 1978. The thyroid: A gland in search of a function. *Perspec. Biol. Med.* 22:19–30.

[10] Grossmann, M., B. D. Weintraub, and M. W. Szkudlinstri. 1997. Novel insights into the molecular mechanisms of human thyrotropin action: Structural, physiological, and therapeutic implications for the glycoprotein hormone family. *Endocr. Rev.* 18:476–501.

[11] Hayashizaki, Y., et al. 1990. Deoxyribonucleic acid analyses of five families with familial inherited thyroid stimulating hormone deficiency. *J. Clin. Endocr. Metab.* 71:792–96.

[12] Hoskins, R. G. 1946. *The tides of life.* New York: W. W. Norton.

[13] Ismail-Beigi, F. 1993. Thyroid hormone regulation of Na,K-ATPase expression. *TEM* 4:152–55.

[14] Johnson, L. G. 1997. Thyroxine's evolutionary roots. *Perspec. Biol. Med.* 40:529–35.

[15] Kosugi, S., H. Sugawa, and T. Mori. 1996. TSH receptor and LH receptor, 1996. *Endocrinol. J.* 43:595–604.

[16] Lason, A. H. 1946. *The thyroid gland in medical history.* New York: Frogen Press.

[17] Mansberger, A. R., and J. P. Wei. 1993. Surgical embryology and anatomy of the thyroid and parathyroid glands. *Surg. Clin. North Am.* 73:727–46.

[18] Marill, J., et al. 2003. Retinoic acid metabolism and mechanism of action: a review. *Curr. Drug. Metab.* 4:1–10.

[19] Masiukiewicz, U. S., and G. N. Burrow. 1999. Hyperthyroidism in pregnancy: diagnosis and treatment. *Thyroid* 9(7):647–52.

[20] Mediros-Neto, G., L. de Lacerda, and F. E. Wondisford. 1997. Familial congenital hypothyroidism caused by abnormal and bioinactive TSH due to mutations in the β-subunit gene. *TEM* 8:15–20.

[21] Melander, A., et al. 1974. Sympathetic innervation of the mouse thyroid and its significance in thyroid hormone secretion. *Endocrinology* 94:959–66.

[22] Moreno-Reyes, R., et al. 1993. Endemic juvenile hypothyroidism in a severe endemic goiter area of Sudan. *Clin. Endocrinol.* 38:19–24.

[23] Munoz, A., and J. Bernal. 1997. Biological activities of thyroid hormone receptors. *Eur. J. Endocrinol.* 137:433–45.

[24] Nillni, E. A., and K. A. Sevarino. 1999. The biology of pro-thyrotropin-releasing hormone-derived peptides. *Endocr. Rev.* 20(5):599–648.

[25] Norris, D. O., and W. A. Gern. 1976. Thyroxine-induced activation of hypothalamo-hypophysial axis in neotenic salamander larvae. *Science* 194:525–7.

[26] Oshima, K., and A. Gorbman. 1966. Olfactory responses in the forebrain of goldfish and their modification by thyroxine treatment. *Gen. Comp. Endocrinol.* 7:398–409.

[27] Paschke, R., et al. 1996. The TSH receptor and thyroid diseases. *Baillière's Clin. Endocrinol. Metab.* 10:9–27.

[28] Pitt-Rivers, R. 1978. The thyroid hormones: Historical aspects. In: C. H. Li, ed. *Hormonal proteins and peptides* (vol. 6). New York: Academic Press, pp. 391–422.

[29] Refetoff, S., et al. 1996. A new family with hyperthyroxinemia caused by transthyretin Val[109] misdiagnosed as thyrotoxicosis and resistance to thyroid hormone—A clinical research center study. *J. Clin. Endocrinol. Metab.* 81:3335–40.

[30] Refetoff, S., J. E. Dumont, G. Vassart. 2001. Thyroid disorders. In: C. R. Scriver, ed. *The metabolic and molecular bases of inherited diseases* (vol. 3). New York: McGraw-Hill, pp. 4029–76.

[31] Russo, D., et al. 1997. Molecular insights into TSH receptor abnormality and thyroid disease. *J. Endocrinol. Invest.* 20:36–47.

[32] Sawin, C. T., and D. V. Becker. 1997. Radioiodide and the treatment of hyperthyroidism: The early history. *Thyroid* 7:163–76.

[33] Schussler, G. C., and J. Orlando. 1978. Fasting decreases triiodothyronine receptor capacity. *Science* 199:686–7.

[34] Schussler, G. C. 2000. The thyroxine-binding proteins. *Thyroid* 10(2):141–9.

[35] Shi, Y.-B. 1994. Molecular biology of amphibian metamorphosis: A new approach to an old problem. *TEM* 5:14–20.

[36] Studer, H., and M. Derwahl. 1995. Mechanisms of non-neoplastic endocrine hyperplasia—A changing concept: a review focused on the thyroid gland. *Endocr. Rev.* 16:411–26.

[37] Studer, H., H. J. Peter, and H. Gerber. 1989. Natural heterogeneity of thyroid cells: The basis for understanding thyroid function and nodular goiter growth. *Endocr. Rev.* 10:125–35.

[38] Sypniewski, E. 1993. Comparative pharmacology of the thyroid hormones. *Ann. Thorac. Surg.* 56:S2–8.

[39] Tata, J. R. 1996. Amphibian metamorphosis: An exquisite model for hormonal regulation of post-embryonic development in vertebrates. *Develop. Growth Differ.* 38:223–31.

[40] Van Herle, A. J., G. Vassart, and J. E. Dumont. 1979. Control of thyroglobulin synthesis and secretion. *N. Engl. J. Med.* 301:239–49, 307–14.

[41] Vassart, G., et al. 1996. Activating mutations of the TSH receptor gene cause thyroid diseases. *Ann. Endocrinol. (Paris)* 57:50–4.

[42] Vono-Toniolo, J,. et al. 2005. Naturally occurring mutations in the thyroglobulin gene. *Thyroid* 15(9):1021–33.

[43] Weiss, R. E., and H. E. Ramos. 2004. Thyroid hormone receptor subtypes and their interaction with steroid receptor coactivators. *Vitam. Horm.* 68:185–207.

[44] Weiss, R. E., and S. Refetoff. 1996. Effect of thyroid hormone on growth. *Endocrinol. Metab. Clin. North Am.* 25:719–30.

[45] Wondisford, F. E. 2003. Thyroid hormone action: Insight from transgenic mouse models. *J. Invest. Med.* 51(4):215–20.

[46] Wonerow, P., et al. 2001. Thyrotropin receptor mutations as a tool to understand thyrotropin receptor action. *J. Mol. Med.* 79(12):707–21.

[47] Yen, P. M. 2003. Molecular basis of resistance to thyroid hormone. *Trends Endocrinol. Metab.* 14(7):327–33.

Catecholamines and the Sympathoadrenal System

T*he physiologically relevant catecholamines are* **epinephrine** *(E),* **norepinephrine** *(NE), and* **dopamine** *(DA). The chemical structure of E was the first determined; the structure of NE (also referred to as noradrenaline) was elucidated much later. Although E (also referred to as adrenaline) has generally been considered a classic example of a hormone (a humoral messenger) and NE a truly representative neurotransmitter, it is now realized that both catecholamines function reciprocally as humoral effectors or as neurotransmitters. Dopamine's major physiological roles are relegated to the central nervous system (CNS) and certain autonomic nervous system ganglia. A chronological history of research related to the catecholamines provides a fascinating example of the growth and development of endocrine physiology [8].*

Historical Perspective

1895 Oliver and Schafer discovered that extracts of the suprarenal (adrenal) glands (specifically, the chromaffin component) of a number of mammalian species produced a pressor response when injected into animals [37].

1899 The pressor principle of the adrenal gland was isolated and named epinephrine by Abel.

1901 The true structural identity of epinephrine was determined by Aldrich (Fig. 14.1).

1898–1901 Lewandowsky and Langley noted that injections of adrenal extracts produced effects similar to stimulation of sympathetic neurons.

1904 Elliot postulated that sympathetic nerve impulses release an epinephrine-like substance onto adjacent effector cells. This was the first suggestion of a neurohumor and the concept of neurotransmission.

1904–1905 Stolz (1904) and subsequently Dakin (1905) synthesized epinephrine.

1905 Administration of epinephrine was found to exhibit both excitatory (vasopressor) and inhibitory (vasodepressor) effects on the cardiovascular system. Langley therefore proposed that autonomic effector cells may possess excitatory and inhibitory receptive substances and that the particular response elicited depended on which substance was present.

1906 Dale discovered that a drug, an ergot alkaloid, specifically antagonized the pressor activities of sympathetic nervous stimulation or epinephrine administration [9, 13, 14]. Indeed, the drug actually reversed the actions of such stimuli, producing instead a vasodepressor response. These observations again revealed that epinephrine could elicit two opposing actions, even in the same tissue.

1910 Barger and Dale studied the action of a large number of synthetic amines related to epinephrine in structure and termed the actions of these drugs as sympathomimetic.

Figure 14.1 **Structures of norepinephrine and epinephrine.**

1921   Loewi provided evidence that, indeed, an excitatory substance similar to epinephrine is released from the vagus nerve on electrical stimulation. In this same year, Cannon and Uradil noted that although stimulation of certain sympathetic neurons released an epinephrine-like substance that increased blood pressure and heart rate, other smooth-muscle responses differed qualitatively from the effects produced by epinephrine. Cannon and Bacq referred to the substance released as sympathin. Barger and Dale had noted earlier (1910) that the effects of sympathetic nerve stimulation were more similar to those of a primary amine than epinephrine or other secondary amines.

1931   Bacq advanced the thesis that sympathin might be norepinephrine (noradrenaline).

1933   Cannon and Rosenblueth formulated the concept that two sympathins might exist, a sympathin E (excitatory) and a sympathin I (inhibitory) [10].

1935   Although Bacq realized that sympathin was not identical to epinephrine, he objected to the view that both a sympathin E and I existed. Rather, a catecholamine could have opposite effects on the same cell.

1946   Von Euler established that the neurotransmitter released from the postganglionic neurons of the sympathetic system was norepinephrine (Fig. 14.1). Although the chemical nature of sympathin was elucidated, this putative neurotransmitter, norepinephrine, could elicit either smooth muscle contraction or relaxation depending on the particular muscle preparation studied. The hypothesis of two sympathins was still in vogue.

1948   Ahlquist studied a large number of sympathomimetic amines and determined that for each tissue a certain potency ranking could be established for the biological actions of these agents. He formulated the concept of dual adrenoceptors where different receptors controlled smooth muscle contraction and relaxation. These receptive substances were referred to as α- and β-adrenoceptors, respectively. Although the *adrenoceptor hypothesis* was not accepted immediately, the discovery of drugs that specifically inhibit either α- or β-adrenoceptors firmly established the validity of the concept.

1962   Sutherland and his colleagues discovered cAMP and proposed that this cyclic nucleotide be considered an intracellular second messenger of hormone action. It was subsequently revealed that β-adrenoceptor stimulation always leads to cAMP production, whereas in some tissues α-adrenoceptor stimulation lowers cellular cAMP levels.

In retrospect the confusion relating to the roles and actions of the catecholamines is understandable. Both E and NE are similar in structure and are released from the adrenal or from neurons in response to a variety of stimuli. Also, both catecholamines can produce similar or opposing physiological responses within the same tissue; their actions at a particular concentration may even be different. The formulation of the adrenoceptor hypothesis by Ahlquist [1] substantiated the early suggestion of Langley that cells might possess different "receptive substances" (in this context, adrenoceptors) and that the particular response of a cell depended on which substance (receptor) was activated. A more thorough historical discussion of catecholamines and adrenoceptors is available [8].

The Sympathoadrenal System

Epinephrine and norepinephrine are hormones of the adrenal chromaffin tissue and sympathetic neurons, respectively. Because these two catecholamines have similar structures and biological actions, it is customary to discuss their endocrine roles together, as components of the *sympathoadrenal system*. It is first necessary to review the general anatomical components of the autonomic nervous system (ANS), because both sympathetic neurons and chromaffin tissue are integral structural and functional components of the ANS.

The Autonomic Nervous System Includes Sympathetic and Parasympathetic Divisions

The *peripheral nervous system* consists of those nerves that arise from the brainstem and spinal cord—the cranial and spinal nerves, respectively. Cranial and spinal nerves that innervate skeletal (voluntary) muscle make up the somatic component (*somatic nervous system*) of the peripheral nervous system. The cell bodies of the somatic neurons lie within the spinal column, and the long axons of these nerves directly innervate skeletal muscle. The other nerves of the peripheral nervous system make up the ANS. These nerves supply the skin and all visceral organs (heart, blood vessels, gastrointestinal (GI) tract, pancreas, adrenals, kidneys, etc.). These nerves are mainly *vasomotor* and *secretomotor* in function; that is, the neurons innervate smooth muscles of blood vessels, and they innervate exocrine (salivary, pancreas) and endocrine (adrenals, pancreas) glands. Other smooth muscles of the GI tract, gallbladder, urinary bladder, spleen capsule, hair follicles, as well as the cardiac muscle of the heart, are also innervated by neurons of the ANS.

The ANS can be subdivided into nerves that comprise the *parasympathetic nervous system* and the *sympathetic nervous system*. The nerves of both systems are composed of *preganglionic* and *postganglionic* neurons. The cell bodies of the preganglionic fibers of both divisions, which reside within the spinal cord, synapse with a second neuron within various ganglia. The postganglionic neurons then directly innervate the various *autonomic effector organs*. Neurotransmission between preganglionic and postganglionic neurons is effected by *acetylcholine* release from the presynaptic neurons. The neurotransmitter of the postganglionic neurons of the parasympathetic system is also acetylcholine, but the neurotransmitter released by the postganglionic neuron of the sympathetic system is norepinephrine.

Parasympathetic nerves arise in the cranial-sacral segments of the spinal column, whereas sympathetic neurons arise in the thoracolumbar region of the spinal cord. The very long parasympathetic preganglionic fibers usually synapse with postganglionic neurons within ganglia located in the autonomic effector organs that they regulate. The sympathetic preganglionic fibers, on the other hand, usually synapse with postganglionic neurons within ganglia located some distance from the target tissues they innervate. The general anatomy of the autonomic nervous system and its effector organs is shown (Fig. 14.2).

The parasympathetic system is concerned mainly with the so-called vegetative (resting) states of the body. Most of its actions are related to those processes concerned with the movement and digestion of food within the GI tract, the transit of metabolic substrates into the body proper, and the conservation (storage) of these substrates within organs such as the liver, adipose tissue, and muscle. The sympathetic nervous system, in contrast, is concerned with those processes related to the more active states of the body and plays a particularly important role under conditions of stress. The sympathetic system generally prepares the body for "fight or flight" [9]. Here for example, the muscular and secretory activities of the GI tract are depressed, whereas the force and rate of the heartbeat are increased, and consequently blood flow is increased, particularly to those areas, such as muscle, that are most active. Blood flow to the brain and coronary arteries is enhanced, whereas circulation to the skin, digestive tract, and kidneys is diminished.

Although the individual actions of acetylcholine and NE are often viewed as opposite, they are actually complementary to each other. For example, NE contracts the heart and forces blood out into the circulatory system. Acetylcholine, on the other hand, relaxes the heart so that it can again fill up with blood. The movement of food through the GI tract results from peristalsis, a process that involves the alternate contraction and relaxation of individual segments of the gut in temporal unison. Contractions of the gut are regulated by acetylcholine, whereas NE relaxes smooth muscles of the gut. Although their actions are opposite in direction, both neurotransmitters participate in the rhythmic (peristaltic) movement of food through the gut.

The Adrenal Medulla is Comprised of Chromaffin Tissue

The adrenal gland of many vertebrates is composed of two distinct cellular types of different embryological origin that secrete structurally very different hormones [11]. Chromaffin cells (pheochromoblasts) are derived from the neural crest, whereas the steroidogenic component of the adrenal is of mesodermal origin (Chap. 15). In most mammals, the chromaffin tissue is surrounded by an outer adrenal cortex composed of steroid-producing cells. Therefore, the chromaffin tissue is often referred to as the *adrenal medulla*. In most nonmammalian species, however, the chromaffin tissue is not associated with any surrounding mass of cortical tissue; hence, the term adrenal medulla is without anatomical justification unless used in reference to

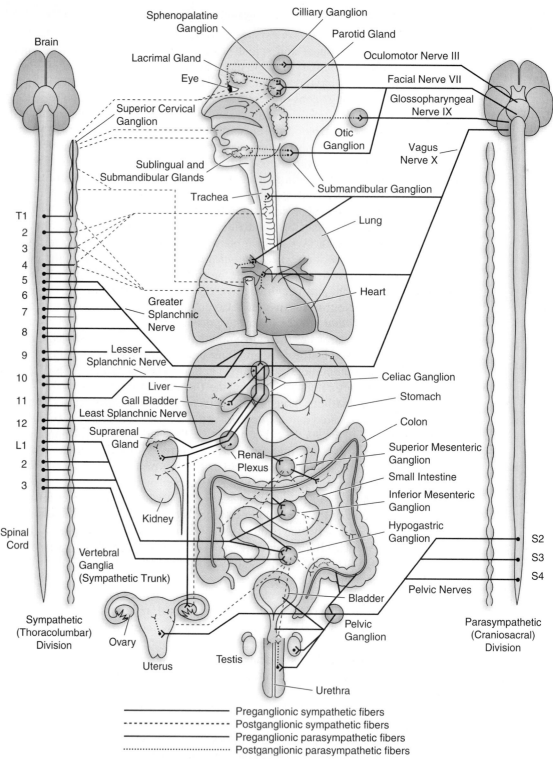

Figure 14.2 The autonomic nervous system. (From William F. Evans, *Anatomy and Physiology*, 2nd edn, p. 187. © 1976. Reproduced by permission of Prentice Hall, Inc., Englewood Cliffs, NJ.)

a restricted number of mammalian species. The term chromaffin (from the Greek *chroma*, or color, and the Latin *affinis*, or affinity) tissue derives from the observation that the pheochromocytes become brown when placed in contact with oxidizing agents such as chromate.

The human adrenal medulla consists of two cell types: adrenaline(A)-storing cells and noradrenaline(N)-storing cells. (The terms adrenaline and noradrenaline are interchangeable with epinephrine and norepinephrine, respectively). Chromaffin cells contain granules composed of catecholamines, adenine nucleotides (mainly ATP), proteins, and lipids. The protein of these granules is referred to as *chromogranin* [44]. Histochemical studies demonstrate that the cells are not biochemically identical: The A cells apparently contain more glycoproteins. The ratio of these two cell types differs between species; the chromaffin tissue of the human and the guinea pig, for example, consists mainly of A cells. Less information is available relative to nonmammalian species, but the same two cell types have been recognized in species of elasmobranchs, amphibians, birds, and reptiles.

Extra-adrenal chromaffin tissue occurs as encapsulated and nonencapsulated masses scattered throughout the abdominal prevertebral sympathetic plexuses of the human fetus. The encapsulated masses predominate and are richly vascularized from adjacent blood vessels. These numerous chromaffin masses are of varying size and are referred to as para-aortic bodies or *paraganglia*. The larger para-aortic bodies lie on the aorta near the origin of the inferior mesenteric artery and are known as the *organs of Zuckerkandl*. These groups of isolated chromaffin cells probably represent neural crest cells that "fail" to migrate into the adrenal during embryonic development. The extra-adrenal chromaffin tissue involutes after birth, but tumors may appear later from this tissue. The para-aortic chromaffin tissue may also proliferate (compensatory hypertrophy) and achieve a functional role if the adrenals are surgically removed or destroyed by disease.

Large amounts of extra-adrenal chromaffin tissue are present in the fetus. Although this tissue only contains NE, it is not known if it is secreted into the fetal circulation. The tissue, however, does have an endocrine appearance. Because the sympathetic nervous system is still incompletely developed at the time of birth, the vascular tone of the fetus may be under humoral control by NE produced by the para-aortic bodies; during postnatal life this function may be replaced by NE of sympathetic origin [12].

Comparative anatomical studies reveal that the distribution of chromaffin tissue and adrenal steroidogenic tissue differs considerably among the vertebrates. In elasmobranchs and teleost fishes, the two tissues are well separated, whereas in mammals and birds, they are always intermingled. The association of the two tissues in amphibians and reptiles is variable. The functional significance of what appears to have been an evolution of the two tissues to come together as a single anatomical entity—the adrenal gland—is nebulous. There is clearly a biochemical correlation between the degree of anatomical association of the two tissues and the relative amounts of NE and E produced by the chromaffin tissue [36].

In the dogfish shark, where the chromaffin tissue is entirely separated from steroidogenic tissue, NE is the only catecholamine produced. In the frog, where chromaffin tissue is intermingled with steroidogenic tissue, NE accounts for about 55 to 70% of the catecholamines. In primates and other mammals, where the two tissues are closely intermingled, very little NE is produced and E may be the exclusive product of the chromaffin tissue. Apparently the proximity of the adrenal steroidogenic tissue determines the degree to which NE is methylated to E in the chromaffin tissue.

Adrenal Chromaffin Cell Development Depends on Both Genetic Programming and Environmental Cues

Elegant experimental techniques have provided fascinating observations related to the embryology of the ANS and continue to provide new insights into factors that may influence the autonomic neurons and chromaffin cells during development [2, 4, 5, 30]. There are preferential pathways located at precise levels of the embryo that direct neural crest cells to their definitive anatomical destinations. Nevertheless, differentiation of the autonomic neuroblasts is controlled by the environment in which the crest cells become localized at the end of their migration. Neural crest cells destined to populate the ANS express an overt noradrenergic phenotype only on reaching the primordium of the sympathetic chain. The initial metabolic commitment, however, appears to be mutable (plastic), and further differentiation may be influenced by the environment within which the cells reside. For example, those cells that populate sympathetic ganglia remain noradrenergic, whereas those that invade the adrenal gland begin to synthesize E [4, 5].

The expression of the adrenergic phenotype of chromaffin tissue precursor cells in the embryonic adrenal gland has been studied in some detail. In the 13.5-day-old mouse, the medullary precursors lying in the sympathetic ganglia primordia—those migrating toward the adrenal as well as those within the adrenal—express noradrenergic characteristics (tyrosine hydroxylase and dopamine-β-hydroxylase activities). Phenylethanolamine-*N*-methyltransferase (PNMT), the enzyme required for conversion of NE to E, is not present but is detectable 3.5 days later at 17 days gestation. This initial expression of PNMT is not dependent on normal glucocorticoid levels and cannot be induced prematurely by glucocorticoids; it is also independent of the pituitary adrenal axis [5]. The normal ontogenetic increase in the activity of this enzyme after the initial expression has occurred does require the presence of an intact pituitary-adrenal axis [8]. The synthesis of PNMT within the CNS indicates that development within the adrenal environment is not an absolute requirement for PNMT biosynthesis. Extra-adrenal chromaffin tissue is also capable of expressing PNMT activity in response to glucocorticoid stimulation.

Sympathetic neurons and adrenal chromaffin tissue derive from a common neuroectodermal origin; the morphology and enzymatic profiles of the two cell types, however, differ considerably. Neural crest cell differentiation into sympathetic neurons is controlled by nerve growth factor (NGF). Prenatal and postnatal injections of NGF into rats can divert partially differentiated chromaffin cells into nerve cells that are morphologically and ultrastructurally indistinguishable from sympathetic neurons. NGF can channel chromaffin cell precursors toward nerve cell differentiation, an action that apparently must override the effects of glucocorticoids that normally induce enzymes required for E synthesis. Sympathetic neurons disconnected from their autonomic effector organs die unless supplied with exogenous NGF. Apparently, the effector organs normally provide a continuous supply of NGF to the sympathetic neurons, which is a requirement for their structural and functional integrity. In the absence of NGF administration, the transformed sympathetic cells undergo destruction (apoptosis); injections of antisera to NGF into the rat fetus produce massive destruction of chromaffin cell precursors. Isolated adrenal medullary cells treated with NGF occasionally develop neurites, sometimes even in the absence of exogenous NGF. Addition of a glucocorticoid to the incubation can inhibit neurite development. These results demonstrate that normal growth and development of adrenal chromaffin tissue may depend on the temporal interactions of NGF and glucocorticoids (Chap. 12).

Synthesis, Chemistry, and Metabolism of Catecholamines

The pathways of catecholamine biosynthesis within the CNS, sympathetic postganglionic neurons, and adrenal chromaffin tissue appear to be identical. The number of steps in each pathway, however, depends on the definitive product—DA, NE, or E—to be secreted [8] (Fig. 14.3).

Figure 14.3 Pathway of catecholamine biosynthesis.

Synthesis.   The conversion of tyrosine to E involves four steps: (1) hydroxylation at the three position of the phenolic ring; (2) side-chain decarboxylation; (3) side-chain hydroxylation; and (4) N-methylation. Hydroxylation of phenylalanine, although essential for tyrosine production, may not make an important contribution to tyrosine availability within sympathetic neurons and chromaffin cells. Tyrosine is transported into the cell where it is converted to dihydroxyphenylalanine (DOPA) by the enzyme *tyrosine hydroxylase*. This is the rate-limiting enzyme in catecholamine biosynthesis. The activity of this enzyme is regulated by feedback (end-product) inhibition by cytoplasmic catecholamines. Chronic stimulation of catecholamine synthesis and secretion leads to elevation of cellular tyrosine hydroxylase levels. In the subsequent step DOPA is decarboxylated to dopamine (DA) by DOPA *decarboxylase*, a nonspecific decarboxylase (L-aromatic amino acid decarboxylase) found in many tissues. Dopamine is then hydroxylated by *dopamine β-hydroxylase* (DBH) by addition of an —OH group to the side-chain carbon (β-carbon adjacent to the phenolic ring). Dopamine is an important neurotransmitter within the CNS [16]. In dopaminergic neurons, DA is the final step in catecholamine biosynthesis. In noradrenergic cells or neurons DA is then converted to NE within the chromaffin granule. The NE produced is converted to E by PNMT outside the granule; this enzyme is found only in cells that synthesize E (adrenal chromaffin tissue of many vertebrates, and within specific neuronal tracts in the brain). It should be noted that NE is a primary amine, whereas E is a N-methylated secondary amine; these differences provide an important structural basis for the differing potency of these two catecholamines on adrenoceptors.

In species where the chromaffin tissue is separated from the adrenal steroidogenic tissue, NE is usually the main synthetic product. In those species (e.g., human, rat) where the chromaffin cells are contiguous with steroidogenic tissue, however, E is the predominant catecholamine synthesized. Levels of PNMT decline in hypophysectomized rats, and normal levels are restored by administration of ACTH or glucocorticoids. These results suggest a role for pituitary corticotropin in adrenal medullary catecholamine biosynthesis (see above).

Storage and Release.   Catecholamines are stored within granules wherein they are complexed with ATP and a specific protein, *chromogranin*, and DBH [3, 44]. The secretory vesicles are released through a stimulus-secretion coupling requiring calcium (Ca^{2+}). All the contents of the storage granules are released during vesicular exocytosis.

Metabolism.   Catecholamines are catabolized by two enzymes, catechol-amine-*O*-methyltransferase (COMT) and monoamine oxidase (MAO). Norepinephrine and E are metabolized extracellularly by COMT to normetanephrine and metanephrine, respectively (Fig. 14.4). COMT is localized within the cytosol of sympathetic effector cells and is also

Figure 14.4   **Pathways of catecholamine metabolism.**

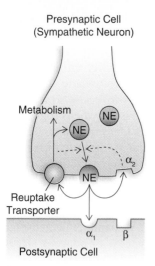

Presynaptic Cell
(Sympathetic Neuron)

Metabolism

NE

NE

α_2

NE

Reuptake
Transporter

α_1 β

Postsynaptic Cell

Figure 14.5
Sympathetic negative feedback mechanisms for inhibition of sympathetic neuron secretion.

found extracellularly in close proximity to adrenoceptors of autonomic effectors. Increased activity of COMT in response to catecholamines provides a homeostatic mechanism for the rapid removal of catecholamines from the circulation and the synaptic cleft. MAO is found in the surface of the outer membrane of mitochondria where it limits the accumulation of catecholamines within the cytoplasm. Because of the sequential action of these two enzymes, the main metabolite of catecholamines excreted in the urine is 3-methoxy-4-hydroxymandelic acid (also known as vanillylmandelic acid, VMA) (Fig. 14.4). After release into the synaptic junction, catecholamines can be removed by active transport into the presynaptic terminal via specific norepinephrine reuptake transporters [23]. Upon reuptake into the axon terminal, most NE is either transported into the secretory vesicles or destroyed by MAO. It is clear that a feedback mechanism operates in the synaptic junction, where the NE accumulated within the synaptic cleft either feeds back to stimulate α_2-adrenergic receptors within the presynaptic membrane, or undergoes reuptake, and these processes function in part to inhibit further synthesis of NE (Fig. 14.5).

Sympathoadrenal System Receptors

The terms *adrenergic* and *cholinergic* were introduced by Dale to designate those nerves that release the sympathetic transmitter (unknown at that time) and acetylcholine, respectively. These terms are now used to designate the receptors through which these neurotransmitters of the postganglionic neurons of the sympathetic (norepinephrine) and parasympathetic (acetylcholine) nervous system mediate their effects. These receptors are localized to the postsynaptic membranes of the innervated effector cells (e.g., smooth muscle, salivary gland cells).

Nicotinic and Muscarinic Cholinergic Receptors are Pharmacologically and Structurally Distinct

Cholinergic receptors respond to acetylcholine and several related analogs of acetylcholine [46]. Two plant substances, *nicotine* and *muscarine*, also stimulate cholinergic receptors and are appropriately referred to as *cholinomimetic* agents. The effects of these two cholinergic agonists are tissue-specific. Nicotine, for example, stimulates skeletal muscle and autonomic postganglionic neurons. Muscarine, on the other hand, stimulates autonomic effector cells such as smooth muscle. These observations demonstrate that these nicotinic and muscarinic cholinoceptive receptor sites are not identical. This is further substantiated by the observation that the drug curare (and also tubocurare) specifically blocks *nicotinic* receptors, whereas the drug atropine is inhibitory to acetylcholine stimulation of *muscarinic* cholinergic receptors. For example, the muscles lining the gut of a teleost fish, the tench, are composed of both striated and smooth muscle. Electrical stimulation of the vagus nerve innervating these muscles results in contraction of both types of muscle, producing a recorded response that contains both a quick and a slow component of contraction. After curarization, however, only the slow component can be elicited. After blockade by atropine, on the other hand, only the fast component of contraction is evident. The slow and fast components of muscle contraction are both abolished, however, after administration of both curare and atropine [8]. Autoantibodies against skeletal cholinergic receptors block their normal response to acetylcholine, resulting in a pathological condition known as myasthenia gravis [34].

Until recently, all muscarinic receptors were thought to be alike. However, at least three different pharmacologically identifiable types and at least five different molecular forms have now been delineated. These glycosylated proteins have single chains of 460 to 590 amino acids and span the plasma membrane seven times, creating four extracellular domains, seven helical hydrophobic transmembrane domains, and four intracellular domains. In structure and evolution, muscarinic receptors are quite distinct from nicotinic receptors and belong to the large family of seven-helix G-protein-coupled receptors, GPCRs (see Fig. 3.2). This family includes the adrenoceptors, at least three subtypes of serotonin receptors, substance K receptors, rhodopsin, and opsin. The GPCRs bind the ligand and transduce their intracellular signals through one or more species of guanosine triphosphate-binding proteins (G proteins) (Chap. 3) [42].

Adrenergic Receptors (Adrenoceptors) Mediate the Actions of Norepinephrine and Epinephrine

After studying the actions of a number of sympathetic amines on smooth muscle contraction and relaxation, Ahlquist concluded that two types of adrenergic receptors (ARs) might exist: α- and β-ARs or, as they are also designated, α- and β-adrenoceptors [1]. These putative receptors differed in their relative responsiveness (sensitivity) to certain sympathetic amines. The response of α-ARs provided the following potency ranking: epinephrine (E) > norepinephrine (NE) > (ISO). The potency ranking for β-ARs was (ISO) > (E) > (NE). The α-ARs subserve smooth muscle contraction, the β-ARs relaxation. A number of drugs were then discovered that could stimulate specifically the putative ARs or antagonize the response of these receptors to catecholamines. It was noted, for example, that phenylephrine was a very specific agonist of α-ARs, whereas isoproterenol was a very specific β-AR agonist. Used at high (unphysiological) concentrations, sympathoamines usually can stimulate either AR, as these agents are structurally related.

After α-AR blockade certain smooth muscle preparations relaxed rather than contracted as they normally did in response to E [35]. This "epinephrine reversal" was reminiscent of that noted by Dale [13] using an ergot alkaloid preparation. The subsequent discovery of a compound that specifically blocked β-AR-stimulated smooth muscle relaxation provided an explanation for the phenomenon of E reversal [17, 26]. E stimulates both α- and β-ARs simultaneously, but the actions of the hormone on α-ARs dominate (Fig. 14.6). However, in the presence of α-AR blockage, the response of the "silent" β-AR is revealed. Simultaneous incubation of smooth muscle in the presence of both α- and β-AR antagonists (blocking agents) totally inhibits smooth muscle responses to the agonists. The *dual-receptor hypothesis* provided a rational explanation for the contrasting effects of catecholamines on autonomic effectors. It was no longer necessary to think of a sympathin E and a sympathin I to account for the excitatory and inhibitory activities of a catecholamine; rather, a single sympathetic neurotransmitter exists whose actions are determined by the nature of the particular ARs stimulated.

The adrenoceptor family consists of at least nine distinct GPCRs that mediate the varied effects of only two physiological agonists, E and NE. At least five subtypes of these catecholamine receptors, the α_1-, α_2-, β_1-, β_2, and β_3-adrenoceptors (α_1-, α_2-, β_1-, β_2-, and β_3-ARs), have been identified on the basis of their pharmacological properties and physiological effects. Chemical agents that selectively block or stimulate these receptors are used extensively in clinical medicine [21, 40]. The genes encoding each of the α_1-, α_2-, β_1-, β_2-, and β_3-ARs have been isolated [24, 41, 42]. Like other members of the GPCR superfamily they are products of homologous genes that encode integral membrane receptors with seven membrane-spanning domains, N-terminal extracellular and C-terminal intracellular tails, three intracellular loops, and two extracellular loops (see Figs. 3.2 and 14.9).

Dopamine (Dopaminergic) Receptors.   Dopaminergic receptors are mainly restricted to the brain wherein they subserve a multitude of functions. As for other adrenoceptors, DA receptors can be further subdivided into two or more subclasses based on their relative affinities for DA and their relative antagonism by pharmaceutical agents (e.g., DA_1 and DA_2 receptors) [16]. It is now well accepted that in the periphery, specific DA receptors are present in many tissues, including those of the cardiovascular and autonomic nervous system.

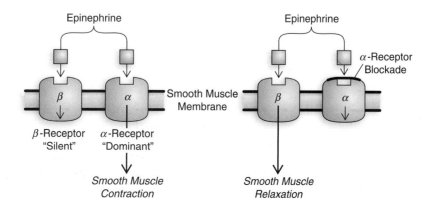

Figure 14.6 Experimental demonstration of epinephrine (catecholamine) reversal.

Epinephrine

Epinephrine

α-Receptor / Blockade

Smooth Muscle Membrane

β-Receptor "Silent"   α-Receptor "Dominant"

β   α

Smooth Muscle Contraction

Smooth Muscle Relaxation

Phenylephrine
(α_1-Agonist)

Phentolamine
(Mixed α-Adrenoceptor
Antagonist)

Clonidine
(α_2-Agonist)

Figure 14.7   Examples of α-AR agonist and antagonist structures.

They seem to be involved in vasodilation of certain vascular beds, inhibition of neurotransmitter release during electrical nerve stimulation, diuresis and natriuresis, renin release and aldosterone release. Dopaminergic receptors regulate pituitary prolactin (Chap. 19) and α-melanotropin (Chap. 8) secretion, whereby DA of hypothalamic origin is inhibitory to the secretion of these two hormones.

α-Adrenoceptors.   Arterial vasoconstriction in a wide array of vascular beds is mediated by a mixed population of postjunctional vascular α_1- and α_2-adrenoceptors [36, 38]. The physiologic function and/or distribution of these receptors has been extensively studied. By using a variety of α_1-selective, α_2-selective, and nonselective α-adrenoceptor antagonists, it was observed that pressor responses to exogenously administered catecholamines were selectively antagonized by α_2-adrenoceptor blockers. Conversely, the pressor response evoked by sympathetic nerve stimulation was selectively antagonized by α_1-adrenoceptor blockers. It was postulated that postsynaptic vascular α-adrenoceptors located at the neuroeffector junction (i.e., junctional receptors) were of the α_1-subtype, whereas those located away from the neuroeffector junction (i.e., extrajunctional receptors) were of the α_2-subtype. Presynaptic α_2-ARs occur at all noradrenergic synapses where they subserve an autoinhibition (negative feedback) in which released NE inhibits its own further release (Fig. 14.5) [43]. The structures of phenylephrine and clonidine, α_1- and α_2-AR agonists, respectively, are shown, as is the structure of a mixed α-AR antagonist, phentolamine (Fig. 14.7).

It is clear that α-adrenoceptors are not pharmacologically homogeneous [18, 19]. Evidence from radioligand-binding studies, functional studies of smooth muscle contractile responses, and studies of receptor-mediated second-messenger accumulation shows substantial differences in the affinities and efficacies of agonists, and the affinities of antagonists for α_1-ARs in different tissues. Based on these differences, the existence of at least three discrete subtypes of α_1-ARs (α_{1A}, α_{1B}, α_{1D}) and three subtypes of α_2-ARs (α_{2A}, α_{2B}, α_{2C}) seems clear [18, 21, 28, 38, 42].

β-Adrenoceptors.   There is evidence that β-ARs represent at least two pharmacologically different subgroups. The lipolytic response of adipose tissue and the contraction of cardiac muscle typify β_1-ARs, where the potency ranking for certain agonists is ISO » E $\cong$ NE. Bronchodilation and vasodepression, on the other hand, are regulated by β_2-ARs, where the agonist potency profile is ISO > E » NE. The major difference between β_1- and β_2-ARs is their sensitivity to norepinephrine. The β_1-receptors respond readily to circulating E or to neurally released NE. On the other hand, the natural agonist of the β_2-ARs is probably E. From these observations, it has been suggested that the β_2-receptor is a hormonal AR, whereas the β_1-AR is a neuronal AR.

β-AR blocking agents do not block responses associated with α-ARs, and they do not inhibit the actions of other hormones or drugs. For example, E and glucagon both stimulate hepatic glycogenolysis, but only the actions of E are antagonized by the blocker (see Fig. 11.11). On the adipocyte, β-AR antagonists block the lipolytic action of E but not ACTH. The structures of β-AR agonists and antagonists bear resemblance to isoproterenol (Fig. 14.8).

Since the classification of β-adrenergic receptors into β_1 and β_2 subtypes, additional β-ARs have been implicated in the control of various metabolic processes by catecholamines. A human gene has been isolated that encodes a third β-AR, the "β_3-AR." Exposure of eukaryotic cells transfected with this gene to E or NE promotes the accumulation of cAMP; only two of eleven classical β-AR blockers efficiently inhibited this effect, whereas two others behaved as β_3-AR agonists. The potency order of β-AR agonists for the β_3-AR correlates with their rank order for stimulating various metabolic processes in tissues where atypical adrenergic sites are thought to exist. The β_3-AR has been shown to play an important role in the regulation of lipid metabolism in both brown and white adipose tissue [33], and thus it is considered a possible target for anti-obesity drug therapies.

The Silent β-AR.   The adrenoceptor hypothesis of Ahlquist adequately explains the vasopressor and vasodepressor responses of smooth muscle to catecholamines. The presence of dominant α-ARs also explains the vasodepressor response to E or NE after α-AR blockade. Nevertheless, catecholamine reversal is a pharmacological phenomenon. The physiological significance of the β-AR in the presence of the dominant α-AR is unclear. Although there are examples of smooth muscles that lack α-ARs and only possess β-ARs, there apparently are no examples of smooth muscles that possess α-ARs in the absence

Figure 14.8 Examples of β-AR agonist and antagonist structures.

Practolol
(β1-Antagonist)

Butoxamine
(β2-Antagonist)

Prenalterol
(β1-Agonist)

Salbutamol
(β2-Agonist)

Isoproterenol

of β-ARs. It is reasonable to hypothesize, therefore, that the β-ARs provide a mechanism for *autoinhibition*. For example, although there is an initial smooth muscle contraction in response to dominant α-ARs, there follows a reversal of the vasopressor response due to a slowly developing β-AR response. Autoinhibition can be prevented by β-AR blockade. The silent β-AR may provide a mechanism for protection against continuous vascular vasoconstriction that would lead to oxygen deprivation and gangrene in the peripheral extremities. Indeed, certain drugs, ergot alkaloids, which establish an irreversible vasoconstriction, have been known to cause gangrene of the legs.

Adrenoceptor Structure

Understanding ligand binding and the coupling of ARs to specific biochemical pathways depends on determining the structures of the family members of these related receptors. The molecular cloning of the gene and complementary DNA (cDNA) for the hamster and human β_2-AR and the cDNA for the human β_1-AR, all of which stimulate adenylate cyclase, was reported [21, 25, 42, 45]. An avian β-AR, which also stimulates adenylate cyclase, and two subtypes of muscarinic cholinergic receptors, which are coupled to stimulation of polyphosphoinositide turnover and the inhibition of adenylate cyclase, have also been cloned. The deduced structures of these receptors reveal that they are homologous to each other and to the visual light pigment, rhodopsin [40].

Analysis of the amino acid sequence of the β-AR has revealed that the protein contains seven regions of hydrophobic amino acids (20–30 residues in length) that form membrane-spanning helices that are typical for the G-protein-coupled receptor superfamily (Fig. 14.9). These hydrophobic domains are connected by short hydrophilic segments, which form extramembranous loops. The tertiary structure predicted for the receptor is similar to that proposed for the visual pigment rhodopsin, which acts through G proteins to stimulate cGMP phosphodiesterase. The receptor shares significant amino acid similarity with rhodopsin. This primary sequence conservation is highest in the putative transmembrane regions that in opsin comprise the binding site for the ligand retinal. In contrast, there is little or no similarity in sequence within the hydrophilic loop regions. It has been hypothesized that the ligand-binding site lies in the transmembrane domain of the receptor [25] (Fig. 14.9).

The function of specific structural domains of these receptors was determined after construction and expression of a series of chimeric α_2-, β_2-AR genes. Studies with chimeric ARs and muscarinic cholinergic receptors implicate the putative 3rd intracellular loop as the major, but not the sole, determinant of selective coupling to their respective G proteins [20]. Chimeric receptors are proving useful for elucidating the structural basis of receptor function [25].

Figure 14.9 Topological model of the ligand-binding pocket of the β_2-adrenergic receptor, which is inserted in the membrane. The ligand-binding region formed by the seven transmembrane domains is buried in the lipidic bilayer. (From A. D. Strosberg, with permission, from *Molecular Neurobiology* 4:211–50, 1990. ©1992 by Humana Press, Inc.)

Adrenoceptor Signal Transduction

NE or E of neural or humoral origin, respectively, interacts with ARs of the plasma membrane of target cells. Depending on the nature of the AR, ligand binding is followed by signal transduction and second-messenger production as described in what follows.

A number of neurotransmitter and hormone receptors elicit their responses via biochemical pathways that involve transduction elements known as guanine nucleotide regulatory (G) proteins (Chap. 3). Among these are several types of receptors for E; these adrenergic receptor subtypes are of particular interest because they are coupled to each of the major second-messenger pathways that are known to be linked through G proteins. Thus the β_1- β_2- and β_3-ARs stimulate adenylate cyclase; the α_1-AR stimulates breakdown of polyphosphoinositides, and the α_2-AR inhibits adenylate cyclase (Fig. 14.10). Studies of chimeric AR receptor proteins have revealed that the third intracellular loop of ARs is the region of these receptor proteins that determines the specificity of the G-protein coupling.

α-Adrenoceptors. It is now well established that activation of α_1-adrenergic receptors by NE or other agonists increases hydrolysis of phosphoinositol (PIP_2), through an intermediary $G_{\alpha q}$ protein. The resulting release of $Ins(1,4,5)P_3$ and diacylglycerol into the intracellular milieu mobilizes Ca^{2+} stored in intracellular pools, such as the endoplasmic and sarcoplasmic reticulum, and activates protein kinase C (see Fig. 3.12). These primary events appear to be responsible for many of the effects of α_1-adrenergic receptor activation in many tissues [39].

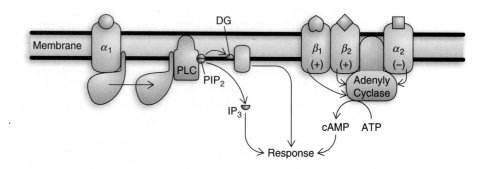

Figure 14.10
Multiple mechanisms
of adrenoceptor signal
transduction.

α_1-Adrenergic receptor responses in some tissues may be mediated through a signal transduction mechanism unrelated to breakdown of PIP_2. Increases in Ca^{2+} influx, arachidonic acid release, and cyclic GMP accumulation have all been reported in response to α_1-AR activation, and some of these effects have been clearly differentiated from activation of inositol phospholipid breakdown. The possibility that different α_1-AR subtypes use different signal transduction mechanisms is increasingly attractive [18]. A hypothesis consistent with most available data is that the α_{1A}-AR primarily promotes influx of extracellular Ca^{2+} through dihydropyridine-sensitive channels, while the α_{1B}-AR initiates signals through the well-characterized inositol phospholipid pathway. Overall, the existence of pharmacologically distinct subtypes of α_1-ARs linked to different signal transduction mechanisms raises interesting questions concerning the basic mechanisms by which receptor activation controls the intracellular, free Ca^{2+} concentration (Fig. 14.10). The α_2-ARs are usually coupled via $G_{\alpha i}$ to the inhibition of adenylate cyclase and the generation of cAMP. However, they are also known to activate certain potassium channels in some cells, and to signal as well through the mitogen-activated protein kinase transduction pathway. Further characterization of these adrenoceptor subtypes may also lead to the development of more selective and useful therapeutic agents for treating a variety of physiological disorders.

β-Adrenoceptors.   In Sutherland's initial studies it was established that cAMP is the intracellular second messenger in the hepatic glycogenolytic response to β-AR stimulation by E. All subsequent studies have established that cellular responses to β-AR stimulation, with only rare exceptions [49], are linked to adenylate cyclase activation and cAMP formation [32]. Although both glucagon and E stimulate hepatic glycogenolysis, they do so through separate receptors that are, nevertheless, linked through a common adenylate cyclase (see Fig. 11.11). Similarly, E and ACTH stimulate fat cell lipolysis and do so through separate receptors again linked to a common adenylate cyclase (Fig. 14.11). The transduction mechanisms linking ACTH receptors to cyclase activation requires Ca^{2+}, whereas activation of the enzyme through β-AR stimulation is without such a divalent metal ion requirement. This lack of Ca^{2+} requirement for β-AR signal transduction appears to be a common feature of this receptor in many, but possibly not all, tissues.

Adrenoceptor Autoinhibition.   The myometrium of the uterus provides a good model for understanding the role of the cyclic nucleotides in autoinhibition of uterine muscle contractility in response to E. In vitro, the isolated uterus always contracts in response to E, a response that can be blocked by α-AR antagonists. However, the contractile response to subsequent doses of E is usually completely inhibited. This autoinhibition can be prevented by the β-AR antagonist propranolol; each subsequent addition of E to the uterus

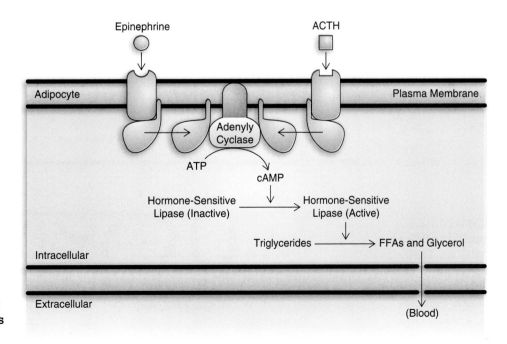

Figure 14.11 Lipolytic action of catecholamines on adipocytes.

will produce a contraction as long as a β-antagonist is present. E stimulates adenylate cyclase activity of uterine muscle, an action antagonized by β-AR antagonists. (Bu)$_2$ cAMP added to the incubation medium mimics the inhibitory action of E. Thus, the initial contractile response to the myometrium to E is mediated through α-ARs, but simultaneous stimulation of silent β-ARs elevates the intracellular levels of cAMP, which are then inhibitory to myometrial contractility (autoinhibition).

Adrenoceptor Desensitization. Stimulation of plasma membrane β-ARs with catecholamines results in increases in the intracellular levels of cAMP. Detectable increases in the concentration of this second messenger occur within a few seconds of exposure to agonists. Following removal of agonist stimulation of the β-AR, the intrinsic GTPase activity of Gα$_s$ hydrolyzes the bound nucleotide, GTP, to GDP (Chap. 3). An interesting feature of the cAMP response is that even when the agonist is continuously present, intracellular cAMP levels generally plateau or even return to near basal levels within a few minutes. This waning of the stimulated response in the face of continuous agonist exposure has been called desensitization. Desensitization has been demonstrated in many other hormone- and neurotransmitter-receptor systems, including those that activate different G proteins and effector systems. In addition, many pharmacological agents targeted at hormone receptors show diminished effectiveness (tachyphylaxis) with time. Desensitization of signal transduction may occur through a variety of processes, including receptor internalization or receptor uncoupling mediated by receptor phosphorylation [15, 27].

Agonist-induced β-AR desensitization appears to be due to a rapid attenuation of the stimulated rate of cAMP generation. Plasma membrane preparations derived from desensitized cells exhibit markedly diminished adenylate cyclase activities upon restimulation by the desensitizing agonists. The molecular mechanisms underlying rapid β-AR desensitization do not appear to require internalization of the receptors, but rather an alteration in the functioning of β-AR themselves that uncouples the receptors from Gα$_s$. This uncoupling phenomenon involves phosphorylation of the β-AR by at least two kinases, PKA and the β-AR kinase (β-ARK), which are activated under different desensitizing conditions (Fig. 14.12). Receptor phosphorylation by the two kinases leads to desensitization of the receptor response via distinct biochemical mechanisms, and additional cytosolic factors appear to be involved in the case of β-ARK [27, 45].

Hormonal Modulation of Adrenoceptors

The tissue density of ARs varies and depends on the presence or absence of stimulation; ARs increase (up-regulation) in the absence of stimulation and decrease (down-regulation) under continuous stimulation. The density of β$_1$- and β$_2$-ARs can be independently regulated, providing strong evidence that the receptors are separate. An increase in the

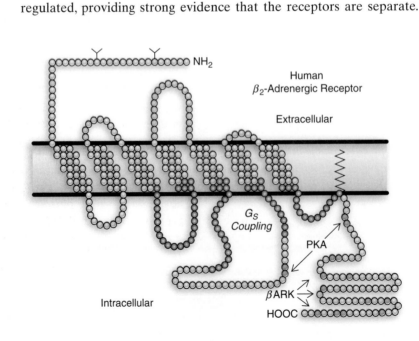

Figure 14.12
Mechanisms of β-AR desensitization. (From Hausdorff et al., 1990. "Turning off the signal: Desensitization of β-adrenergic receptor function." *FASEB J.* 4:2881–9.)

sensitivity of adrenergic effector organs to catecholamines has been noted after denervation. The denervated heart of the dog and the denervated rat pineal, for example, respond to catecholamines by an enhanced production of cAMP over that of intact control tissues. This *denervation supersensitivity* is due to an increase in tissue β-ARs. On the other hand, the density of these receptors decreases in tissues subjected to continued elevated levels of the β-AR agonist isoproterenol.

Gonadal Steroid Hormones.   AR responses to catecholamines are affected by gonadal steroids. Steroid hormones affect sympathetic function by modulating AR responses to catecholamines. Estrogen and progesterone may modulate sympathoadrenal activity by altering catecholamine metabolism and, in addition, produce qualitative changes in the contractile response of smooth muscle to stimulation by catecholamines. The response of the oviduct and uterus from humans and several other species changes from contraction to relaxation, depending on the concentrations of gonadal steroids present. Contraction is mediated through α-ARs in the estrogen-dominated uterus, whereas β-AR-induced relaxation predominates during pregnancy or when the uterus is incubated in vitro in the presence of progesterone (Chap. 19).

Adrenal Steroid Hormones.   Glucocorticoids play a permissive role in regulating cAMP-mediated effects of hormones on the liver and other organs. In adrenalectomized rats, the stimulation of liver gluconeogenesis and glycogenolysis in response to catecholamines is greatly reduced. The lipolytic response of adipose tissue to epinephrine in vitro is blunted in tissues removed from adrenalectomized animals. Glucocorticoid treatment restores the lipolytic response of fat tissue removed from adrenalectomized animals. Catecholamine-induced pressor effects on the cardiovascular system are dependent on permissive actions of glucocorticoids. One mechanism of glucocorticoid enhancement of cardiovascular responses to catecholamines may involve inactivation of COMT. Glucocorticoids therefore play vital roles in the regulation of tissue responses to catecholamines during stress.

Thyroid Hormones.   Thyroid hormones profoundly affect the activity of the sympathoadrenal system. Sympathoadrenal activity is enhanced under conditions of hyperthyroidism and depressed under conditions of low levels of thyroid hormones, as in myxedema. Therefore, the major symptoms of patients with a thyroid dysfunction relate to functional alterations of those organs regulated by the sympathetic nervous system (see Table 13.2).

Sympathoadrenal Functions

The role of the sympathoadrenal system is to maintain the constancy of the internal environment of the body [9, 10]. Any decrease in blood pressure, blood glucose level, or oxygen availability leads to an acute enhancement of sympathoadrenal activity with resulting elevation in plasma catecholamines. In addition, the sympathoadrenal system is activated in anticipation of events that may adversely affect an individual. Stress is a term generally used to designate the state resulting from events (stressors) of external or internal origin, real or imagined, that tend to affect the homeostatic state. Although an acceptable definition of stress may not be available, in the present context stress refers to any condition tending to elevate plasma catecholamine levels in response to exogenous or endogenous stimuli. For example, the early experiments of Cannon [9, 10] revealed that the barking of a dog was a stimulus to E secretion from the adrenal gland of a cat. In humans, plasma levels of NE and E are immediately elevated on standing, during exercise, during and after surgery, and whenever plasma glucose levels fall below normal [48]. The neural signals for adrenal E release are transmitted via preganglionic fibers carried in the splanchnic nerve. Thus, a physical or psychological stress, or decrease in blood pressure, blood glucose level, or oxygen availability, activates the sympathetic outflow to target tissues and stimulates adrenal E release.

Norepinephrine is released by sympathetic neurons to provide localized autonomic effector control, whereas E is released from the adrenal as a humoral messenger that may also provide an additional stimulus to autonomic effectors. Since catecholamines communicate with their effector cells through ARs, the distribution and nature of these receptors will determine the response generated. These tissues therefore must possess the "correct" type of AR to provide the response that will be most appropriate (adaptive) under conditions of stress. By inference, therefore, it should be possible to predict the nature of both the response and the type of AR that characterize a particular tissue. The following guidelines should assist in the formulation of such predictions:

1. Autonomic effector cells may possess α- and β-ARs or only β-ARs in addition to cholinergic receptors.

2. Smooth muscle contraction, with few exceptions (intestinal smooth muscle), is regulated through α-ARs, whereas relaxation, with one exception (cardiac muscle), is controlled through β-AR stimulation.

3. Where α-ARs are present, they dominate (mask) β-ARs.

4. The β-ARs are generally stimulatory to cellular secretion, whereas α-ARs (with few exceptions) are inhibitory to cellular secretion.

5. When β-ARs of smooth muscle control relaxation, cholinergic receptors will regulate contraction.

6. When α-ARs regulate smooth muscle contraction, acetylcholine will normally regulate relaxation.

Catecholamines Regulate Intermediary Metabolism

Carbohydrate Metabolism. One would expect that under conditions of stress, blood glucose levels would need to be elevated to provide this metabolic substrate for energy production within critical tissues (brain, heart, skeletal muscle). Glycogen is available as a storage form of glucose within the liver. E is stimulatory to hepatic glycogenolysis and glucose release through its action on β-ARs. Skeletal muscle may provide an even greater total source of glycogen and, in response β-AR stimulation, glycogen is converted through the glycolytic pathway to lactic acid. This lactic acid is cycled to the liver and through E-stimulated gluconeogenesis converted to glucose.

Most interesting is the demonstration that catecholamines are inhibitory (through α-ARs) to pancreatic B cell insulin secretion. On the other hand, catecholamines are stimulatory to glucagon secretion through an action on β-ARs of pancreatic A cells. Therefore, under conditions of stress, elevated circulating levels of E would be stimulatory to numerous physiological processes that would elevate blood glucose levels. The inhibition of insulin secretion, in contrast, would prevent removal of glucose from the general circulation.

If the blood glucose concentration is reduced by fasting or administration of insulin, an immediate release of E follows [22]. The denervated adrenal is, however, insensitive to a hypoglycemic stimulus. Adrenal catecholamine secretion in response to hypoglycemia can be blocked by local anesthetic application to the hypothalamus and adjacent brain areas. In addition intracerebroventricular injection of a nonmetabolizable analog, 5-thioglucose, increases sympathoadrenal-mediated hyperglycemia. These observations suggest that some glucoreceptors that regulate sympathoadrenal discharge reside within the brain. The cellular receptors that mediate the hyperglycemic response to glucoprivation are apparently localized caudal to the forebrain [22].

Fat Metabolism. Adipose tissue cells possess β-ARs and, in response to catecholamines of either sympathetic or adrenal origin, lipolysis is stimulated. Epinephrine-induced cAMP production activates a hormone-sensitive lipase, triglyceride lipase, which metabolizes fats into free fatty acids (FFAs) and glycerol (Fig. 14.11). The FFAs released into the blood are then used directly by certain tissues (brain, cardiac muscle) as sources of energy (a glucose-sparing action), or they may be used within the liver in the formation of glucose.

The demonstration that not all lean individuals gain weight when overfed, coupled with a number of studies pointing to a metabolic defect in the obese, has led to the notion that there are two necessary conditions for the development of obesity: (1) an ample supply of food, and (2) a genetic predisposition for a high efficiency in the conversion of food to body fat. It is toward the latter condition that current pharmaceutical work on obesity is directed; that is to say, there is an active search for drugs that will raise metabolic rate (i.e., thermogenic drugs). The use of thermogenic drugs in the treatment of obesity is now directed toward a search for stimulants of the sympathetic nervous system (SNS). This approach follows several lines of evidence that suggest an important role for the SNS in the control of diet-induced thermogenesis, and that an impairment in its functional state could lead to obesity. A reduced release of norepinephrine (NE), rather than insensitivity to the neuro-transmitter, has been implicated in the thermogenic defect of the obese. Drugs that mimic the activity of the SNS and increase metabolic rate therefore offer considerable therapeutic potential and provide a rational approach for the treatment of obesity.

Protein Metabolism.   Epinephrine acting through β-ARs and cAMP decreases the release of amino acids from skeletal muscle. A reduced rate of muscle proteolysis appears to be the mechanism responsible for adrenergic inhibition of amino acid release. This adrener-gic modulation of protein degradation may be of physiological importance to the short-term fight or flight response associated with increased adrenal E secretion. Under these condi-tions, lactate, glycerol, and glucose levels would be increased and additional gluconeogenic substrates might not be needed.

The Sympathetic Nervous System Regulates Thermogenesis

The sympathetic nervous system plays a critical role in the regulation of mammalian ther-mogenic responses to cold exposure and dietary intake [7, 29]. Both fasting and feeding induce changes in sympathoadrenal activity. In rats, fasting suppresses and overfeeding stimulates the sympathetic nervous system. It was hypothesized that during fasting sup-pression of sympathetic activity would conserve calories by decreasing metabolism and heat production, whereas during feeding the increased sympathetic activity would expend the excess calories. Increased sympathetic activity might account for some of the increased incidence of cardiac arrhythmias, angina, and hypertension in populations known for overeating.

Shivering Thermogenesis.   Thermogenesis associated with muscular activity is a by-product, rather than a goal, of the activity. The heat produced by shivering, however, has heat production as the major objective. Piloerection (goose pimples) is controlled by the SNS.

Nonshivering (Chemical) Thermogenesis.   Catecholamine-stimulated thermogenesis is mediated by β-ARs [28, 29]. In the rat, brown adipose tissue (BAT) is the major site of metabolic heat production in response to both cold (nonshivering thermogenesis) and diet-induced thermogenesis. Measurements of NE turnover rate in interscapular BAT of the rat demonstrate increased sympathetic activity in response to both cold exposure and overfeed-ing. Injections of NE trigger a coordinated proliferation of brown adipocytes and endothe-lial cells in vitro that is similar to those observed after cold exposure. It has also been suggested that cold exposure stimulates BAT growth by increasing the release of NE from sympathetic nerves and that the neurohormone activates mitoses in BAT precursor cells via β-AR pathways. In adult humans, a physiologically significant role for BAT has not been established, but cannot be excluded.

Adrenergic Receptors Mediate Cardiovascular Responses to Stress

Epinephrine increases both the force and rate of the heartbeat through stimulation of car-diac muscle β-ARs [19]. There are no other examples known where β-ARs induce muscle contraction. From an adaptive standpoint, it is obvious that enhanced pumping of blood through the heart would be desirable. The particular distribution of vascular smooth muscle ARs provides a mechanism for the shunting of blood to various body compartments during stress. For example, blood is shunted from the skin, mucosa, connective tissue, and kidneys; as expected, vascular smooth muscles of these organs possess α-ARs. In contrast, smooth muscle of coronary arteries, as well as skeletal muscle, possess β-ARs. If dominant α-ARs were present, blood flow to these vital organs would be diminished when these organs were maximally active. The decreased blood flow to the kidneys reduces glucose clearance from the circulation, and this reduced clearance may be primarily responsible for the prolonged hyperglycemia induced by catecholamines.

The spleen capsule is contracted through catecholamine stimulation of α-ARs, which increases the circulating levels of erythrocytes. These erythrocytes provide the blood with an increased capacity for oxygen uptake from the lungs. Epinephrine enhances blood platelet adhesiveness and reduces clotting time by its actions on platelet α-ARs.

In those smooth muscles where α-ARs subserve contraction, the parasympathetic nervous system, through the release of its neurotransmitter, acetylcholine, controls relaxation. This holds true for cardiac muscle as well. Since β-ARs also regulate relaxation of smooth muscle, acetylcholine regulates the contractile component of the muscle.

β-Adrenergic Receptors Mediate Dilation of Bronchial Passageways

Bronchial smooth muscle is relaxed in response to catecholamines and only β-ARs are present. Relaxation of these muscles dilate the bronchial passageways so that increased amounts of air containing oxygen are made available to the blood under conditions of increased exertion.

Sympathoadrenal, Hypothalamic-Pituitary-Adrenal, and Parasympathetic Stress Responses are Integrated

Both postganglionic sympathetic neurons and adrenal chromaffin cells are directly innervated by cholinergic neurons. Under stress, adrenal chromaffin cell enzymes are regulated by both neuronal and endocrine pathways. Tyrosine hydroxylase and DBH are regulated mainly by neuronal transynaptic stimulation, whereas PNMT is primarily under endocrine control. For example, denervation of an adrenal gland by cutting the splanchnic nerve prevents elevations in tyrosine hydroxylase and DBH in response to stress, whereas PNMT is still enhanced. PNMT and DBH activities in the adrenal decrease following hypophysectomy and can be restored by administration of ACTH or glucocorticoids. Levels of tyrosine hydroxylase, on the other hand, are increased by ACTH, but not by glucocorticoids.

Discrepancies between perceptions of internal or external circumstances and innate or acquired expectations lead to patterned stress responses involving several homeostatic systems, of which the sympathoadrenomedullary system (SAMS) is one. Severe, generalized threats such as hypoglycemia, hypoxia, hemorrhage, circulatory collapse, and fight/flight situations elicit generalized SAMS activation, including cardiac stimulation; splanchnic, cutaneous, and renal vasoconstriction, and usually preserved skeletal muscle blood flow. Patterned sympathetic neural responses, resulting in redistribution of blood volume or changes in glandular activity, occur during orthostasis, exercise, altered environmental temperature, the postprandial state, and performance of attention-requiring tasks. In all these situations, SAMS activity is coordinated with that of the parasympathetic nervous system, the pituitary-adrenocortical system, and probably several neuropeptide systems.

Norepinephrine may Function as Both Neurotransmitter and Hormone in Humans

Epinephrine, in humans at least, is generally considered the only humoral catecholamine normally serving an endocrine function. Nevertheless, NE does escape into the circulation during sympathetic activity. Is this extrasynaptic NE destined only for metabolic degradation, or might it also subserve some role as a hormone? NE was infused into normal men and a variety of physiological parameters were monitored concomitantly. Only NE levels in excess of 1,800 pg/ml caused hemodynamic and metabolic effects. Thus, under usual conditions, NE's biological actions may relate only to its sympathetic neurotransmitter function. Because NE levels can exceed 1,800 pg/ml during stress, it is conceivable that NE might subserve some role in stress along with epinephrine of adrenal origin [48]. Also, posturally-associated NE concentrations occur in normal, and even adrenalectomized individuals, suggesting that the adrenals are not the only source of plasma NE.

Sympathoadrenal Pathophysiology

β-Adrenoceptor antagonists ("β-blockers") play an important role in the pharmacological therapy of such cardiovascular disorders as hypertension, ischemic heart disease, and arrhythmias [17]. Rapid relief of symptoms is often achieved using β-AR antagonists and with few side effects. The demonstration that ARs can be classed into subgroups based on their selective response to pharmaceutical agonists and antagonists raises hopes that other drugs might be developed that would be selective for these AR subtypes; such selectivity might also decrease the severity of any side effects. β$_1$- and β$_2$-ARs are components of many tissues and this may therefore limit their effectiveness until further specificities of the receptors are discovered [40].

Adrenal Chromaffin Tumors. Neuroblastoma is a highly malignant neoplasm of early life that arises from primitive sympathetic cells and neuroblasts. Tumors may arise within the sympathoadrenal system. Adrenal chromaffin tumors (pheochromocytomas), although generally benign, are nevertheless life-threatening. Although pheochromocytomas are found wherever sympathetic nervous tissue is located, it most often arises from the adrenal medulla or along the sympathetic chain [31]. Pheochromocytomas that contain only E are comprised entirely of A cells, whereas those containing only NE consist entirely of N cells. Both cells are present in mixed pheochromocytomas containing both NE and E. The excessive secretion of catecholamines, characteristic of pheochromocytoma and neuroblastoma, results in severe hypertension, as well as increased basal metabolic rate, increased oxygen consumption, weight loss, psychosis, tremulousness, and increased respiratory rate. Medical treatment with antihypertensive drugs, including α_1-receptor antagonists and calcium channel antagonists, are commonly prescribed until successful surgical removal of adrenal pheochromocytomas [6].

Adrenoceptor Hypothesis of Asthma. It has been suggested that the symptoms and pathophysiology of asthma may be explained in terms of reduced pulmonary β-AR function [8]. The status of β-AR function in asthmatics has been extensively investigated for many years, but it remains controversial. Studies both in vitro and in vivo have shown that asthmatics do not necessarily have diminished bronchial β-AR function. Furthermore, it is well established that blockade of β-ARs of nonasthmatics does not induce asthma or bronchial hyperresponsiveness. These findings indicate that β-AR dysfunction is not a fundamental cause of asthma. Since β_2-agonists are widely used and are an effective treatment for asthma, it is also clear that significant β-AR function is maintained in most asthmatics. Nevertheless, a definite decrease in β-AR function has been detected in bronchial smooth muscle removed from severe asthmatics. Evidence suggests that the reduction in β-AR function involves both receptor uncoupling and a decrease in receptor number. The marked worsening of asthma produced by β-blockers illustrates the role of effective β-AR function in maintaining adequate airway caliber in asthmatics. Thus significant β-AR hypofunction, secondary to asthma, may contribute to the further deterioration of this disease by rendering the subject more vulnerable to spasmogens and less responsive to β-agonist therapy.

Adrenoceptors, Fat Cells, and Heart Disease. ARs play important roles in fat cell metabolism, lipogenesis, and lipolysis. α-AR stimulation results in fat storage, whereas β-AR activation results in catabolic metabolism within the cells. The relative distribution of ARs may determine gender differences in fat distribution in humans. Gender differences in distribution of α-ARs may partly explain the tendency of the male to look like an apple rather than like a pear as in some females. Female shape may have to do with differences in fat cell number and size in the hips, thighs, and buttocks, whereas the male potbelly may be due to a greater number of α-ARs in abdominal adipose tissue [40].

Recent epidemiological studies have confirmed an earlier observation of a relationship between anatomical distribution of fat and the risk of diabetes, hypertension, stroke, ischemic heart disease, and early death. Among individuals with the same degree of relative adiposity, those whose adipose tissue is located predominantly in the upper body (android distribution) have higher rates of diabetes, hypertension, stroke, ischemic heart disease, and early death than those whose fat is located primarily in the hips, buttocks, and thighs (gynecoid distribution). The biological reasons for these epidemiologic associations are not known.

Comparative Endocrinology

The comparative physiology and pharmacology of ARs in vertebrates has not been studied systematically. Because NE, E, and possibly DA are the only catecholamines produced by the sympathoadrenal system, it might be expected that the ARs of all vertebrates are similar, although the particular response elicited might show some species specificity. (The turkey erythrocyte, for example, has been used for detailed studies on the β-AR.) Melanosome aggregation and dispersion within dermal melanophores of elasmobranchs, teleosts, amphibians, and reptiles are stimulated by catecholamines interacting through α- and β-AR, respectively. These responses can be blocked by the classical α- and β-AR antagonists (Chap. 8).

Evidence to date supports the hypothesis that adrenergic and cholinergic receptors existed for hundreds of millions of years and that the same receptor molecules have been put to a variety of uses in different species and tissues. The extent of structural homology among these proteins became apparent with the cloning and sequence analysis of genes encoding adrenergic and muscarinic cholinergic receptors from a variety of species. Gene cloning and sequencing have provided data that have proven that a high degree of structural homology exists between a number of neurotransmitter receptors and the opsins. It has been proposed that an evolutionary relationship exists between adrenergic and muscarinic cholinergic receptors and that they evolved from one common ancestor via gene duplication [47].

REVIEW EXERCISES

Match the substrate with its enzyme:

1. Phenylalanine
2. Dopa
3. Tyrosine
4. Norepinephrine
5. Dopamine
6. Epinephrine

A. Tyrosine hydroxylase
B. Dopamine β-hydroxylase
C. Phenylalanine hydroxylase
D. Phenylethanolamine-*N*-methyltransferase
E. L-aromatic amino acid decarboxylase
F. Monoamine oxidase

Fill in the blanks to complete the comparisons between the parasympathetic and sympathetic nervous systems:

Attributes	Parasympathetic nervous system	Sympathetic nervous system
Relative length of preganglionic fibers		
Relative length of postganglionic fibers		
Spinal cord regions giving rise to fibers		
Preganglionic neurotransmitter		
Postganglionic neurotransmitter		
Active in resting state or stress		
Discrete or mass response		

Think, analyze and discuss:

1. Chromaffin tissues in some species are anatomically distinct from adrenal steroidogenic tissue, while in others the two tissues are either loosely intermingled, or closely intermingled to make a single anatomical entity. To what degree would these two tissues be separate, loosely intermingled, or closely intermingled in teleost fishes? In frogs? In birds and mammals? Rank these different animals in increasing order of epinephrine production, as opposed to norepinephrine production, in their chromaffin tissues.

2. The normal growth and development of adrenal chromaffin tissue appears to depend upon the appropriate temporal interactions between NGF and glucocorticoids. What would be the likely result of blockade of NGF actions in the fetus? What would happen as a result of glucocorticoid receptor antagonism at 17 days of gestation or later?

3. Norepinephrine is the precursor for epinephrine in the catecholamine biosynthetic pathway. It is thus difficult to unambiguously identify A cells versus N cells using immunohistochemistry in sympathoadrenal tissues.
   a. Devise a strategy for immunohistofluorescence analysis of chromaffin tissues, with which you could be reasonably sure that you have made this distinction. Which molecule(s) would you attempt to immunochemically analyze? Predict the results that you would obtain using tissues from a teleost fish versus a primate.
   b. Dopamine is the precursor for norepinephrine in the catecholamine biosynthetic pathway. Devise a second immunohistochemical strategy for identifying dopaminergic, as opposed to noradrenergic or adrenergic neurons in brain tissues. You may utilize double-labeling immunohistofluorescence methods in your study. Which molecule(s) would you attempt to immunochemically analyze?

4. Consider an experiment in which a smooth muscle tissue culture preparation is used to assess contractile/relaxation responses to drugs. Which response would you likely observe when the following test substances were applied alone, or coadministered with E:

	Contraction	Relaxation	No response
E			
phenylephrine			
isoproterenol			
phentolamine + E			
propranolol + E			
phentolamine + propranolol + E			

5. Using recombinant DNA technology, genes can be constructed that encode the β-AR with the "wild-type" (normal) amino acid sequence, or receptors with one or more portions of the molecule replaced with a segment normally found in another receptor. If a β$_1$-AR

molecule containing the normal amino acid sequence is expressed in host cells that do not make the protein normally, which second messenger system would likely be activated? If the sequence comprising the third intracellular loop (i3) is replaced by the corresponding sequence from an α_1-AR, which signaling pathway would be activated by E? If the i3 is replaced by one from a α_2-AR, which signaling pathway would be activated by E? If the α_1-AR molecule containing the i3 of the β_1-AR were expressed, which signaling pathway would be activated by E?

6. A significant drop in blood glucose invariably evokes the release of epinephrine from the adrenal medulla. The reduction in blood glucose is most likely registered by glucose responsive neurons in the brain, which then initiate neural signals that descend through the spinal cord, ultimately reaching the adrenal medulla and prompting release of E. Draw a line graph of the serum E and glucose levels that you would expect to see before, and at several time points after, the injection of a bolus of insulin in an experimental rat. Draw a second line to indicate the changes in these variables over time in an insulin-injected rat in which the splanchnic nerve is sectioned.

References

[1] Ahlquist, R. P. 1948. A study of the adrenotropin receptors. *Am. J. Physiol.* 153:586–600.

[2] Anderson, D. J. 1992. Cell fate determination in the peripheral nervous system: the sympathoadrenal progenitor. *J. Neurobiol.* 24:185–98.

[3] Aunis, D., and K. Langley. 1999. Physiological aspects of exocytosis in chromaffin cells of the adrenal medulla. *Acta Physiol. Scand.* 167(2):89–97.

[4] Black, I. B. 1982. Stages in development of autonomic neurons. *Science* 214:1198–204.

[5] Bohn, M. C., M. Goldstein, and I. B. Black. 1981. Role of glucocorticoids in expression of the adrenergic phenotype in rat embryonic adrenal gland. *Dev. Biol.* 82:1–10.

[6] Bravo, E. L., and R. Tagle. 2003. Pheochromocytoma: state-of-the-art and future prospects. *Endocr. Rev.* 24(4):539–53.

[7] Bray, G. A. 1993. The nutrient balance hypothesis: peptides, sympathetic activity, and food intake. *Ann. N.Y. Acad. Sci.* 676:223–41.

[8] Brunton, L., J. Lazo, and K. Parker. 2006. *Goodman and Gilman's The pharmacological basis of therapeutics.* 11th ed. New York: McGraw-Hill.

[9] Cannon, W. B. 1932. *The wisdom of the body.* New York: W. W. Norton.

[10] Cannon, W. B., and A. Rosenblueth. 1937. *Autonomic neuroeffector systems.* New York: Macmillan.

[11] Carmichael, S. W., and S. L. Stoddard. 1993. *The adrenal medulla, 1989–1991.* Boca Raton, FL: CRC Press.

[12] Coupland, R. E. 1953. On the morphology and adrenaline-noradrenaline content of chromaffin tissue. *J. Endocrinol.* 9:194–203.

[13] Dale, H. H. 1906. On some physiological actions of ergot. *J. Physiol.* 3:163–206.

[14] Dale, H. H. 1934. Chemical transmission of the effects of nerve impulses. *Br. Med. J.* 1:835–41.

[15] Dawson, T. M., et al. 1993. β-Adrenergic receptor kinase-2 and β-arrestin-2 as mediators of odorant-induced desensitization. *Science* 259:825–8.

[16] Glickstein, S. B., and C. Schmauss. 2001. Dopamine receptor functions: lessons from knockout mice. *Pharmacol. Ther.* 91(1):63–83.

[17] Goldstein, S. 1996. β-Blockers in hypertensive and coronary heart disease. *Arch. Intern. Med.* 156:1267–76.

[18] Graham, R. M., et al. 1996. α_1-Adrenergic receptors subtypes: Molecular structure, function, and signaling. *Circ. Res.* 78:737–49.

[19] Guarino, R. D., D. M. Perez, and M. T. Piascik. 1996. Recent advances in the molecular pharmacology of the α_1-adrenergic receptors. *Cell. Signal.* 8:323–33.

[20] Gudermann, T., F. Kalkbrenner, and G. Schultz. 1996. Diversity and selectivity of receptor-G protein interaction. *Annu. Rev. Pharmacol. Toxicol.* 36:429–59.

[21] Hieble, J. P., W. E. Bondinell, and R. R. Ruffolo, Jr. 1995. α- and β-adrenoceptors: From the gene to the clinic. 1. Molecular biology and adrenoceptor subclassification. *J. Med. Chem.* 38:3415–44.

[22] Himsworth, R. L. 1970. Hypothalamic control of adrenaline secretion in response to insufficient glucose. *J. Physiol.* 206:411–17.

[23] Keller, N. R., et al. 2004. Norepinephrine transporter-deficient mice exhibit excessive tachycardia and elevated blood pressure with wakefulness and activity. *Circulation* 110:1191–6.

[24] Kobilka, B. K., et al. 1987. Cloning, sequencing, and expression of the gene coding for the human platelet α_2-adrenergic receptor. *Science* 238:650–6.

[25] Kobilka, B. K., et al. 1988. Chimeric α_2-, β_2-adrenergic receptors: delineation of domains involved in effector coupling and ligand binding specificity. *Science* 240:1310–16.

[26] Kotlikoff, M. I., and K. E. Kamm. 1996. Molecular mechanisms of β-adrenergic relaxation of airway smooth muscle. *Annu. Rev. Physiol.* 58:115–41.

[27] Kozasa, T. 2004. The structure of GRK2-G beta gamma complex: intimate association of G-protein signaling modules. *Trends Pharmacol. Sci.* 25(2):61–3.

[28] Lafontan, M., and M. Berlan. 1995. Fat cell α_2-adrenoceptors: the regulation of fat cell function and lipolysis. *Endocr. Rev.* 16:716–38.

[29] Landsberg, L., M. E. Saville, and J. B. Young. 1984. Sympathoadrenal system and regulation of thermogenesis. *Am. J. Physiol.* 247:E181–9.

[30] Le Douarin, N. M. 1986. Cell line segregation during peripheral nervous system ontogeny. *Science* 231:1515–22.

[31] Lenders, J. W., et al. 2005. Phaeochromocytoma. *Lancet* 26;366(9486):665–75.

[32] Levitzki, A. 1988. From epinephrine to cyclic AMP. *Science* 241:800–6.

[33] Lowell, B. B., and J. S. Flier. 1997 Brown adipose tissue, β-adrenergic receptors, and obesity. *Annu. Rev. Med.* 48:307–16.

[34] Marx, A., et al. 1997. Pathogenesis of myasthenia gravis. *Virchows Arch.* 430:355–64.

[35] Nickerson, M., and L. S. Goodman. 1947. Pharmacological properties of a new adrenergic blocking agent: N,N-dibenzyl-β-chloroethylamine (Dibenamine). *J. Pharmacol. Exper. Ther.* 89:167–85.

[36] Nussdorfer, G. G. 1996. Paracrine control of adrenal cortical function by medullary chromaffin cells. *Pharmacol. Rev.* 48:495–530.

[37] Oliver, G., and E. A. Schafer. 1895. The physiological effects of extracts from the suprarenal capsules. *J. Physiol. Lond.* 18:230–76.

[38] Piascik, M. T., et al. 1996. α-Adrenoreceptors and vascular regulation: molecular, pharmacologic and clinical correlates. *Pharmacol. Ther.* 72:215–41.

[39] Piascik, M. T., and D. M. Perez. 2001. Alpha1-adrenergic receptors: new insights and directions. *J. Pharmacol. Exp. Ther.* 298(2):403–10.

[40] Ruffolo, R. R. Jr., W. Bondinell, and J. P. Hieble. 1995. α- and β-adrenoceptors: From the gene to the clinic. 2. Structure-activity relationships and therapeutic applications. *J. Med. Chem.* 38:3681–716.

[41] Strosberg, A. D. 1997. Structure and function of the β3-adrenergic receptor. *Annu. Rev. Pharmacol. Toxicol.* 37:421–50.

[42] Strosberg, A. D. 1993. Structure, function, and regulation of adrenergic receptors. *Protein Sci.* 2:1198–209.

[43] Szabadi, E., and C. M. Bradshaw. 1996. Autonomic pharmacology of α2-adrenoreceptors. *J. Psychopharmacol.* 10(Suppl. 3):6–18.

[44] Taupenot, L., K. L. Harper, and D. T. O'Connor. 2003. The chromogranin-secretogranin family. *N. Engl. J. Med.* 348(12):1134–49.

[45] Tesmer, V. M., et al. 2005. Snapshot of activated G proteins at the membrane: The Galphaq-GRK2-Gbetagamma complex. *Science* 310(5754):1686–90.

[46] van Koppen, C. J., and B. Kaiser. 2003. Regulation of muscarinic acetylcholine receptor signaling. *Pharmacol. Ther.* 98(2):197–220.

[47] Venter, J. C., et al. 1988. Evolution of neurotransmitter receptor systems. *Prog. Neurobiol.* 30:105–69.

[48] Wortsman, J. 2002. Role of epinephrine in acute stress. *Endocrinol. Metab. Clin. North Am.* 31(1):79–106.

[49] Zhen, M., et al. 2005. Emerging concepts and therapeutic implications of β-adrenergic receptor subtype signaling. *Pharmacol. Ther.* 108:257–68.

Adrenal Steroid Hormones

T*he adrenal gland of most vertebrates is composed of two tissues of different origin that produce two classes of hormones unrelated in structure. Nevertheless, the hormones of both the adrenal* **steroidogenic** *tissue and the adrenal* **chromaffin** *tissue play important roles in response to stress. The discoveries that led to present knowledge of the adrenal steroidogenic tissue hormones and their role in endocrine physiology are presented in the following chronological summary. A number of treatises on adrenal structure and function are available [23, 24, 49].*

Historical Perspective

1815   Meckel described the gross comparative anatomy of the adrenals.

1846   Ecker provided a detailed description of the histology of the adrenal medulla and cortex.

1854   Kölliker recognized the cortex and medulla as functionally different structures in humans.

1855   Addison described a disease (Addison's disease) that involved a degeneration of the adrenals.

1856   Brown-Séquard studied the effects of adrenalectomy in animals and concluded that the glands are indispensable for life.

1866   Arnold described the cellular zonation of the cortex.

1927   Baumann showed that longevity in animals after adrenalectomy was prolonged by injections of sodium salts. Other investigators noted that there was excessive excretion of sodium and chloride by the kidneys in the absence of normal adrenal function.

1927–1930   Smith established that although the adrenals of the rat atrophied after hypophysectomy, they could be restored to normal size by administration of pituitary extracts.

1928–1931   Baumann and colleagues were among the first to employ adrenal cortical extracts as replacement therapy in adrenalectomized animals and in patients with Addison's disease. In 1931, Swingle and Pfiffer, and in 1930, Hartman and Brownell, described the beneficial actions of adrenal extracts on survival of adrenalectomized animals.

1936   Kendall and co-workers obtained crystalline extracts of the adrenal cortex and demonstrated the effectiveness of compound E (cortisone) in ameliorating the symptoms of adrenalectomy in rats.

1936   Selye described the general adaptation syndrome, which provided a major impetus to stress research and the subsequent recognition of the essential role of the adrenal in the stress response.

1940   Long and associates established the importance of the adrenal cortex relative to carbohydrate metabolism.

1945	By 1945, 6 active and more than 20 inactive steroids were extracted from the adrenal cortex. The four compounds with greatest biological activity were 11-dehydrocorticosterone, corticosterone, cortisone, and hydrocortisone (cortisol).
1950	Hench and associates described the effectiveness of cortisone in relieving the symptoms of rheumatoid arthritis. It was noted, however, that patients treated with ACTH excreted cortisol rather than cortisone. Cortisol was found to be the principal glucogenic steroid secreted by patients with Cushing's disease.
1951	It was established that cortisol is the major steroid released from the human adrenal gland following stimulation by ACTH.
1952	Tait and Simpson and colleagues demonstrated the presence of an adrenal steroid that is extremely active in retaining sodium.
1954	The structure of the salt-retaining hormone, aldosterone, was determined by Simpson and Tait and colleagues.
1955	Conn described primary hyperaldosteronism (Conn's disease) [10].
1955	Li and co-workers isolated the pituitary factor ACTH (corticotropin), which regulates adrenal cortisol secretion. As early as 1940, Swann proposed that there were separate controls for adrenal glucocorticoid and mineralocorticoid secretion.
1960	Laragh described the renin–angiotensin system that controls adrenal aldosterone secretion.

*These studies established that **cortisol**, a glucocorticoid, and **aldosterone**, a mineralocorticoid, play important roles in carbohydrate and Na^+ balance, respectively, in humans and many other vertebrates. Abnormal secretion of either of these hormones has profound pathophysiological consequences in humans.*

The Adrenal Glands

The adrenal gland is composed of steroidogenic as well as chromaffin tissue. In many mammals, the steroidogenic tissue forms a cortical mass surrounding an inner medullary component of chromaffin tissue. In humans and many other mammals, these tissue components may appropriately be referred to as the adrenal cortex and adrenal medulla. In many vertebrates, including some mammals, these two tissues are intermingled; in some poikilotherms, the two endocrine components are totally separate masses of tissues, therefore, the comparative endocrinologist prefers the functional designations adrenal steroidal and adrenal chromaffin tissue [5, 21].

Adrenomedullary and Adrenocortical Tissues have Separate Embryological Origins

Steroidogenic and chromaffin tissues originate from separate primordia. Chromaffin cells are derived from the neural crest (Chap. 14), whereas the steroidogenic tissue arises from the coelomic mesoderm (corticogonadal anlagen) in the genital ridge of the embryo. During migration to definitive anatomical sites, some steroidogenic tissue becomes located in extra-adrenal sites. These aberrant adrenal *rests* may hypertrophy and become more active after adrenalectomy. In humans, adrenal rests are usually distributed in the celiac plexus and the adjacent fatty tissue, or along the path of the spermatic cord.

In the primate, the adrenals are located adjacent to the upper surface of each kidney (Fig. 15.1). Each human adrenal gland weighs approximately 3.5 to 4.5 g and is well vascularized by arterial branches from the aorta. Smaller arterial branches spread over the adrenal capsule, pierce it, and pass as sinusoids between adjacent rows of cortical cells to a subcapsular plexus at the corticomedullary junction. A few venules flow through the medullary chromaffin tissue to a central vein that connects directly or indirectly (via the renal vein) to the inferior vena cava.

The Adrenal Functional Unit.   In humans and many other mammals, the chromaffin tissue is surrounded by steroidogenic tissue and the vascular relationships are such that the secretory products of the cortex perfuse the medulla through a portal network. In addition, sphincter-like muscles in the central adrenal vein may alter the rate of flow of

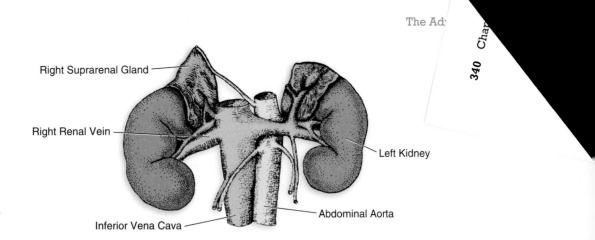

Figure 15.1 Gross anatomy of the human adrenal glands.

Right Suprarenal Gland

Right Renal Vein

Left Kidney

Inferior Vena Cava

Abdominal Aorta

adrenal cortical effluent. Adrenal chromaffin epinephrine synthesis is dependent on steroid hormonal support (Chap. 14). There is evidence that chromaffin tissue has the capacity to carry out many enzymatic reactions characteristic of the cortex and is therefore capable of converting incomplete steroid intermediates passing through the medulla into active glucocorticoids. The close anatomical coupling and the functional interrelationship between the cortex and medulla suggest that these two tissues, although of diverse origin, may constitute an integrated functional unit, at least in higher vertebrates. This relationship may be of particular adaptive importance under conditions of stress when both epinephrine and glucocorticoids are in particular demand.

Histology

In most mammals, the adrenal cortical tissue can be divided into three morphologically and functionally different layers: a thin outer *zona glomerulosa*; a thicker middle *zona fasciculata*; and an innermost, moderately thick *zona reticularis* (Fig. 15.2). Steroidogenic cells are filled with lipid droplets (liposomes) containing cholesterol, the substrate for steroid biosynthesis. These droplets are stainable with lipid-soluble dyes such as Sudan red or Sudan black. In the typical alcohol dehydration preparation, the cells appear full of vacuoles due to extraction of the lipids from their contained vesicles; these cells are often referred to as *spongiocytes*. Ultrastructurally, the steroidogenic cells (like those of the gonads) contain abundant mitochondria and an especially conspicuous smooth endoplasmic reticulum. Although the cortical tissue may be grossly divided into three separate regions,

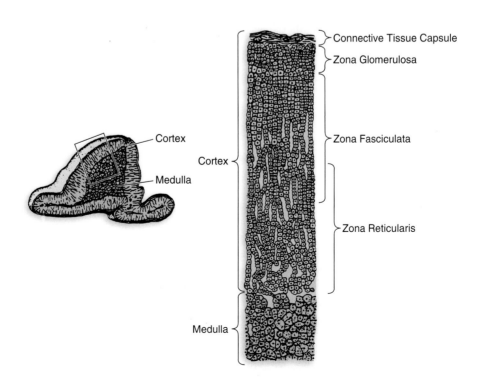

Figure 15.2 Diagrammatic representation of the microanatomy of the human adrenal cortex.

Cortex

Medulla

Cortex

Medulla

Connective Tissue Capsule

Zona Glomerulosa

Zona Fasciculata

Zona Reticularis

the histological picture reveals that the three cell types are parts of the same cords of cells that extend from the capsule to the medulla. These cell cords are surrounded by a capillary network, thus providing steroids ready access into the blood.

The Fetal Adrenal Cortex Regresses Towards the End of Gestation

In the fetus, a specialized region of the human adrenal cortex has been described between the maturing (permanent) cortex and the medulla. This primate *fetal adrenal cortex* may exceed the size of the kidney; the fetal cortex regresses during the last month of gestation and is then only one-tenth or less the size of an individual kidney. A transient fetal adrenal cortex is also present in the monkey, armadillo, sloth, members of the cat family, elephant seal, and pig [21, 22].

In the mouse, the cortex possesses a juxtamedullary zone where morphological expression varies according to sex and age. This zone, generally referred to as the *X zone*, degenerates in the male at maturity and in the female early during the first pregnancy. Castration of the male mouse before puberty allows the X zone to survive, apparently in response to increased secretion of pituitary luteinizing hormone (LH). Injections of LH into the postpubertal castrated mouse reestablish the X zone. The X zone does not disappear in the unmated female. Androgens of gonadal origin appear to be responsible for degeneration of the X zone in some strains of mice, but possibly not in other strains. The adrenal X zone degenerates in Tfm mutant mice whose cells are insensitive to androgens, suggesting that in this strain, the X zone atrophy is not directly dependent on androgens [42]. The product(s) that the X zone might secrete is unknown as is the significance of this specialized area of the adrenal gland.

Chemistry and Synthesis

Cholesterol, a sterol consisting of 27 carbon atoms, is the precursor for both gonadal and adrenal steroid hormone biosynthesis [34, 40, 45]. The first step in the biosynthetic pathway of steroidogenesis involves cleavage of the terminal six carbons of the side chain of cholesterol, resulting in the formation of pregnenolone. Key enzymes, collectively known as the *desmolase system (cytochrome p450scc)*, are requisite for side-chain cleavage. From pregnenolone a number of pathways lead to the formation of metabolic intermediates that give rise ultimately to the definitive steroid hormones characteristic of the species (Fig. 15.3). The steroid hormones of the adrenal glands may be categorized into three groups according to their principal effects: glucocorticoids, mineralocorticoids, and androgens. Cortisol and aldosterone are the major glucocorticoid and mineralocorticoid hormones, respectively, of humans. Note that all the steroids of the adrenal contain the *cyclopentanoperhydrophenanthrene* nucleus (Fig. 15.4).

Several different systems of nomenclature are used to refer to individual steroid structures (Tables 15.1 and 15.2). The Greek capital letter Δ (delta) is often used to indicate a double bond, and it is important to note that a Δ^4 bond is common to nearly all the adrenal steroids. The orientation of hydroxyl groups at either the 11 or 17 position of the steroid nucleus is indicated by a β sign and a solid line (—OH), or an α sign and a dashed line (—OH). The latter designation indicates that the group projects below the plane of the steroid nucleus, and the former indicates that it is above. Cortisol, for example, has a Δ^4-3-keto configuration in the A ring and β- and α-hydroxyl groups at positions 11 and 17, respectively, of the molecule. Aldosterone is unique in having an aldehyde group at the 18 position of the molecule. The systemic names of some steroids are provided in Table 15.2.

The double bond between positions 4 and 5 and the presence of the keto group at position 3 of the A ring are essential for the biological activities of adrenal steroids. Introduction of a Δ^2 double bond in cortisone (prednisone, Δ^1-cortisone) or cortisol (prednisolone, Δ^1-cortisol) enhances the ratio of glucocorticoid to mineralocorticoid activity by increasing the former. Incorporation of fluoride into the 9α position enhances both the glucocorticoid and mineralocorticoid activity of cortisol (9α-fluoro-cortisol). Dexamethasone (9α-fluoro-16α-methylprednisolone) is a very potent glucocorticoid with minimal salt-retaining activity.

Conversion of cholesterol to pregnenolone occurs within the mitochondria. Pregnenolone is then released from the mitochondria and, in the smooth endoplasmic reticulum, the double bond is shifted from the 5 to the 4 position and the hydroxyl group at position C-3 is oxidized to

Figure 15.3 Pathways of adrenal steroid hormone biosynthesis.

a keto group by an enzyme, Δ^5,3-β-hydroxysteroid dehydrogenase-dehydrogenase-isomerase. All the remaining steps in corticosteroidogenesis consist of additional hydroxylations, at either positions 11, 17, or 21, by various NADPH-dependent hydroxylases. The pathway leading to aldosterone synthesis involves an initial hydroxylation at position 18 followed by dehydrogenase activity, resulting in formation of an aldehyde group at that position.

The bulk of adrenal cholesterol is derived by uptake from plasma cholesterol rather than by intracellular synthesis as previously believed [26]. Low-density lipoproteins (LDLs) are the major cholesterol transport complexes in human plasma. Cholesterol esters, with triglycerides, are packaged into lipoprotein particles where they form a hydrophobic core surrounded by a monolayer of polar phospholipids and small amounts

Cyclopentanoperhydro-
phenathrene Nucleus

"C 21" Steroid
(Progesterone)

"C 19" Steroid
(Dehydroepiandrosterone)

**Figure 15.4 Steroid
hormone structure and
nomenclature.**

TABLE 15.1   Terms used in steroid nomenclature

Term	Description
Hydroxy-	Indicates an —OH (hydroxyl) group
-ol	Indicates an —OH (hydroxyl) group
Oxy-	Indicates an =O (keto) group
Keto-	Indicates an =O group
-one	Indicates an =O (keto) group
-al	Indicates an aldehyde (—CHO) group
Δ	Signifies location of a double bond in the steroid nucleus (e.g., Δ^4 = double bond between C-4 and C-5 positions)
-ene[a]	Indicates one double bond in the steroid nucleus
-diene	Indicates two double bonds in the steroid nucleus
-triene	Indicates three double bonds in the steroid nucleus
α- and β-	Designates if a substituted group lies below (α) or above (β) the plane of the molecule
Estrane[b](C18)	Indicates basic steroid skeleton with methyl group attached at C-13 in addition to the 17 carbon atoms of the ring structure
Androstane[b](C19)	Indicates steroid skeleton with methyl groups at both the C-13 and C-10 positions
Pregnane[b](21)	Indicates basic steroid skeleton with methyl groups at C-13 and C-10 and a two-carbon atom side chain attached at the C-17 position

[a]The suffix -ene is currently used more often than Δ.
[b]Hypothetical parent compound.

of proteins called *apolipoproteins*. The apolipoproteins bind to LDL receptors of adrenal target cells, which may stimulate endocytosis and the transport of the lipoproteins into the cells, an event enhanced by ACTH. Subsequent to receptor binding, the lipoproteins are internalized by receptor-mediated endocytosis and catabolized in lysosomes [26]. The number of LDL binding sites is highest in membranes of the adrenal cortex and ovarian corpus luteum, two tissues that synthesize steroids and therefore have a high requirement for cholesterol [19].

Receptor-mediated endocytosis of LDL is a regulatory event in cellular cholesterol homeostasis. The complete sequence of metabolic events associated with the binding, uptake, and degradation of these cholesterol-rich lipoprotein particles by mammalian cells has been called the "LDL receptor pathway" [26]. This important process supplies cells with cholesterol, thereby mediating the removal of cholesterol-rich lipoproteins from the circulation. Also, it protects cells from overaccumulation of cholesterol, because the cholesterol derived from lysosomal hydrolysis of LDL cholesterol esters exerts a series of feedback control mechanisms designed to maintain a constant level of cholesterol within the cell.

TABLE 15.2   Systematic names of vertebrate steroids

Class name	Trivial name	Systematic name
Glucocorticoids	Cortisol (hydrocortisone)	11β, 17α, 21-Trihydroxy-pregn-4-ene-3, 20-dione
	Corticosterone	11β, 21-Dihydroxy-pregn-4-ene-3, 20-dione
Mineralocorticoids	Aldosterone	11β, 21-Dihydroxy-pregn-4-ene-3, 20-dione-18-al
	11-Deoxycorticosterone	21-Hydroxy-pregn-4-ene-3, 20-dione
Androgenic steroids	Dehydroepiandrosterone	3β-Hydroxy-androst-5-ene-17-one
	Testosterone	17β-Hydroxy-androst-4-ene-3-one
Estrogenic steroids	Estradiol	1, 3, 5(10)-Estratriene-3, 17β-diol
Progestens	Pregnenolone	3β-Hydroxy-pregn-5-ene-20-one
	Progesterone	Pregn-4-ene-3, 20-dione

Thus, high extracellular concentrations of LDL reduce cellular synthesis of cholesterol by suppression of the activities of 3-hydroxy-3-methyl-glutaryl-CoA synthase and reductase (rate-limiting enzymes in cholesterol synthesis); stimulate its re-esterification; and decrease the number of LDL receptors, preventing further cellular entry of cholesterol.

The uptake of cholesterol-rich lipoprotein particles into cells provides the pool of cholesterol esters that are subsequently metabolized to produce bioactive steroids. The cholesterol esters are hydrolyzed by cholesterol ester hydrolases, and the resultant free cholesterol is transported from the outer mitochondrial membrane to the inner mitochondrial membrane by a steroid acute regulatory protein (StAR) [9, 44]. On the inner mitochondrial membrane, cholesterol is acted upon by a cholesterol side-chain cleavage enzyme, e.g. cytochrome P450 side-chain cleavage enzyme 11A (CYP11A), which converts the cholesterol to pregnenolone. When the pregnenolone moves back into the cytoplasm, it is thereafter subject to modification by a series of enzymatic reactions in the endoplasmic reticulum and mitochondria, ultimately producing the predominant steroid hormone (glucocorticoid, mineralocorticoid, or androgen) in the adrenocortical cell. The type of steroid hormone produced in a particular adrenocortical cell is dictated by the types of cytochrome P450 enzymes that are expressed in that cell. Thus, the enzymes present in cells within the zona glomerulosa, zona fasciculata, and zona reticularis are specifically capable of catalyzing the production of mineralocorticoids, glucocorticoids, and androgens, respectively.

A model for cholesterol homeostasis in the adrenal gland is presented in Figure 15.5. In the basal state, the amount of cholesterol delivered to the cell by LDLs is balanced by cholesterol conversion to steroid hormones that are then secreted. The metabolically active pool of free cholesterol is derived from LDL internalization, limited endogenous synthesis (through acetyl CoA), and hydrolysis of cholesterol esters. In response to ACTH, there is an enhancement of cholesterol ester hydrolase, leading to an increase in the pool of free cytoplasmic cholesterol, and a stimulation of StAR expression, producing an increased rate of cholesterol transfer into the mitochondria. Both actions contribute to an increase in steroid synthesis. Esterified cholesterol reserves are limited, and endogenous cholesterol synthesis is insufficient to supplement the required pool of cholesterol; consequently, extracellular lipoproteins must provide all of the cholesterol for continued steroid hormone biosynthesis. This is apparently accomplished by an increase in the number of LDL receptors (Fig. 15.5).

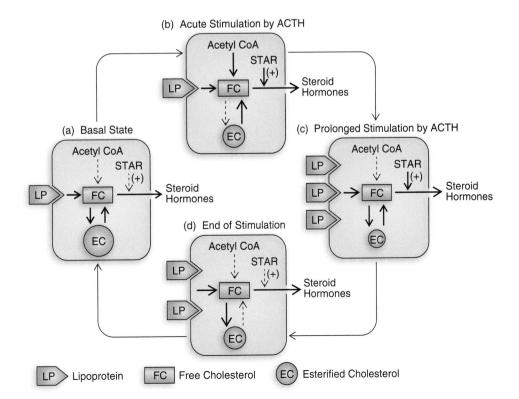

Figure 15.5 Model for cholesterol homeostasis in the adrenal. (Adapted from Brown, M. S., P. T. Kovanen, and J. L. Goldstein. 1979. Receptor-mediated uptake of lipoprotein-cholesterol and its utilization for steroid synthesis in the adrenal cortex. *Rec. Prog. Horm. Res.* 35:215–57, with permission).

The Adrenal Cortex is Composed of Three Separate Functional Zones

In most mammals, mineralocorticoids are produced in the zona glomerulosa, glucocorticoids in the zona fasciculata, and androgens in the zona reticularis. Functional separation of the zones was suggested when Greep and Deane [18] noted that the zona fasciculata may atrophy or become grossly hyperactive without any conspicuous alteration in the zona glomerulosa. These investigators also noted that, on a gross morphological basis, the gland could be separated into two zones, and they were the first to comment on the dual nature of the adrenal cortex control. The mammalian zona glomerulosa lacks a 17α-hydroxylase and therefore synthesizes corticosterone, a glucocorticoid that does not contain a 17α-hydroxyl group. Sequential actions by the enzymes 18-hydroxylase and 18-hydroxysteroid dehydrogenase convert corticosterone to aldosterone. The latter enzyme is found only in the glomerulosa. In humans and cattle, 17-hydroxysteroids are produced by the zona fasciculata and zona reticularis [49].

Control of Synthesis and Secretion

The biological roles of adrenal glucocorticoids and mineralocorticoids differ considerably. It is not unexpected, therefore, that the control of synthesis and secretion of these two classes of steroid hormones is also different. Adrenal glucocorticoid synthesis and secretion are controlled by pituitary adrenocorticotropin (ACTH), whereas aldosterone secretion is controlled primarily by the *renin–angiotensin system* (RAS) [49].

Pituitary ACTH Regulates the Synthesis and Secretion of Glucocorticoids

Glucocorticoid production by cells of the zona fasciculata is regulated by pituitary ACTH. The release of ACTH is in turn regulated by a hypothalamic corticotropin-releasing hormone (CRH) as discussed in Chapters 6 and 7. Unilateral adrenalectomy is followed by contralateral adrenal hypertrophy and hyperplasia. After bilateral adrenalectomy or in primary adrenal insufficiency (Addison's disease), there is a striking increase in plasma ACTH levels. These elevated levels of ACTH can be returned to normal by administration of glucocorticoids, demonstrating a negative feedback regulation of ACTH secretion by the steroids. Glucocorticoid negative feedback is mediated at the level of the pituitary, hypothalamus, and even higher brain centers (Fig. 15.6).

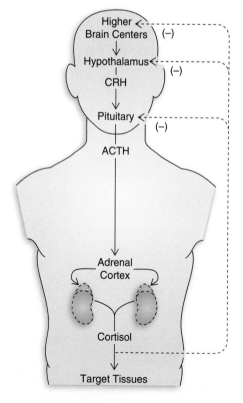

Figure 15.6 Brain-pituitary-adrenal axis.

ACTH interacts with its cognate G-protein-coupled receptor, the melanocortin 2 receptor (MC2-R), in the plasmalemma of zona fasciculata cells to increase intracellular cAMP levels; activation of protein kinase A (PKA) follows. During ACTH stimulation, increased cAMP production and PKA activation precede the steroidogenic event. Calcium is required for ACTH activation of adenylate cyclase, but not for binding of the peptide to adrenal cells. The effects of ACTH on adrenal fasciculata cell steroidogenesis are mimicked by methylxanthines and cAMP analogs, revealing that cAMP is the major second messenger regulating ACTH action. The stimulation of cAMP production and PKA activation, in turn, appears to concurrently evoke several cellular responses, and these collectively mediate ACTH-induced glucocorticoid production and secretion. Among the best characterized of these are ACTH-stimulated cholesterol ester hydrolase activity and StAR expression. While increased cholesterol ester hydrolase activity enlarges the pool of free cholesterol to be utilized as the precursor for steroidogenesis, augmented StAR expression leads to enhanced cholesterol transfer into mitochondria and conversion to pregnenolone by P450scc enzymes. The latter effect is thought to be a most important action of ACTH in adrenocortical cells, as StAR-mediated cholesterol transfer is thought to be the rate-limiting step in steroidogenesis.

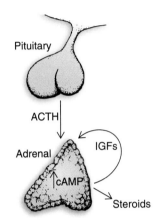

Figure 15.7   Model for the role of IGFs in the control of adrenal steroidogenesis.

Incubation of primary cultures of human fetal adrenal cells with ACTH or cAMP also results in an accumulation of insulin-like growth factor II (IGF-II) mRNA. The time-course and dose–response curves of IGF-II mRNA and P450scc mRNA accumulation rose in parallel. ACTH and other hormones exerted this action on IGF-II production in a strictly tissue-specific fashion: human chorionic gonadotropin (hCG) did not affect adrenal cells, and ACTH, prolactin, and growth hormone did not affect the IGF-II or p450scc mRNAs in granulosa cells (Chap. 18). The stimulation of IGF-II mRNA was not secondary to steroidogenesis, as exogenously added steroid hormones did not affect IGF-II mRNA. These results suggest that the hypertrophy and hyperplasia of the adrenal seen in response to ACTH may be due to IGF-II production, which then acts locally as an autocrine/paracrine growth factor (Fig. 15.7). When IGF-I or IGF-II is added to the culture medium, the responses of P450c17 and P450c21 mRNAs to ACTH were not altered compared to controls. By contrast, exogenously added IGF-I or -II significantly reduced the ACTH-stimulated accumulation of IGF-II mRNA in the same cells. This experiment supports the hypothesis that trophic hormones stimulate adrenal growth via stimulation of IGF-II, which is autoregulated by short-loop feedback.

In humans and other animals, there is a circadian rhythm of ACTH and 17-hydroxycorticoid secretion (e.g., cortisol). The rhythm appears to be directed by a rhythmic signal emanating from cells comprising the biological clock in the suprachiasmatic nucleus of the hypothalamus; this signal appears to drive a circadian rhythm in CRH neurosecretion, which in turn stimulates corresponding rhythms in ACTH and cortisol secretion. The CRH, ACTH and cortisol rhythms are phase-locked with the sleep–wake habits of the individual. In those individuals who sleep regularly at the same hours each day, a rise in ACTH and cortisol secretion occurs during the third to fifth hour of sleep and becomes maximal just before awakening. Minimal levels of these hormones are reached a few hours before and after resumption of sleep. In humans this circadian rhythm of secretion is first established at about 3 months of postnatal life. The circadian rhythm has a cycle length of about 24 hours and cannot be synchronized with environmental lighting regimes. In a free-running environment with an absence of clues to the true local time, the rhythm persists but is slightly and consistently longer or shorter than 24 hours. The cortisol rhythm may serve as an adaptive anticipatory mechanism, mobilizing energy stores in preparation for physiological and behavioral activity during waking hours.

Aldosterone Synthesis and Secretion is Regulated by the Renin-Angiotensin System

Aldosterone secretion from the zona glomerulosa is mainly controlled by *angiotensin II* (AII, Ang II), an octapeptide that is derived from a decapeptide, angiotensin I, through the action of a *converting enzyme*. Angiotensin I (AI) is derived from a precursor protein, appropriately designated as *angiotensinogen* (or renin substrate), which originates in the liver. The conversion of angiotensinogen to AI results from the enzymatic action of an enzyme, *renin*, which is released from specialized granular cells, *juxtaglomerular (JG) cells*, in the afferent arteriole of the vascular pole of the renal glomerulus. The action of AII on adrenal glomerulosa cells

Angiotensinogen (Renin Substrate) Asp–Arg–Val–Tyr–Ile–His–Pro–Phe–His–Leu–Leu–Val–Tyr–Ser–Protein

Renin

Angiotensin I Asp–Arg–Val–Tyr–Ile–His–Pro–Phe–His–Leu + Leu–Val–Tyr–Ser–Protein

Converting Enzyme

Angiotensin II Asp–Arg–Val–Tyr–Ile–His–Pro–Phe + His–Leu

Angiotensinases

Smaller Fragments

Figure 15.8 Angiotensin biosynthesis.

is terminated by *angiotensinases*, which split the octapeptide into smaller inactive fragments (Fig. 15.8). Extrarenal sources of renin, *isorenins*, have been described (brain, uterus, adrenal glands), but their significance is undefined [34, 35]. Angiotensin I converting enzyme has been localized to a variety of vascular beds. The presence of this enzyme in these vessels may be indicative of a functional role of angiotensins in the local control of blood flow. These extrarenal sites of angiotensin production make up so-called tissue angiotensinogenase systems [16, 35, 36].

Renin is secreted in response to hypovolemia or to an increase in the osmolarity of the blood [11]. According to the *baroreceptor hypothesis*, the afferent arteriole responds to a change in mean renal perfusion pressure. These changes result in either a stretching or a decreased transmural (vessel wall) pressure in the afferent arteriole, which results in an observable altered JG cell granularity (the granules being the cellular source of renin). In this theory, the JG cells are modified smooth muscle cells and function as baroreceptors.

Another theory suggests that specialized cells of the distal tubular epithelium play a pivotal role in the control of renin release. These cells are in close apposition to the JG cells; they may function as chemoreceptors and monitor the urinary Na^+ load within the distal tubule. According to the *macula densa theory*, this information is in some manner relayed to the JG cells where appropriate modifications of renin release take place. The renal functional unit of renin secretion, which consists of the macula densa cells and the JG cells, is referred to as the *juxtaglomerular apparatus* (Fig. 15.9).

Renin secretion is also regulated by the autonomic nervous system. Renin release is increased in response to sympathetic nerve stimulation, and catecholamines stimulate renin release from kidney slices incubated in vitro. Norepinephrine released from sympathetic neurons acts on β-adrenoceptors of the JG cells, and the resulting increase in cAMP is the stimulus to vesicular exocytosis of the renin secretory granules.

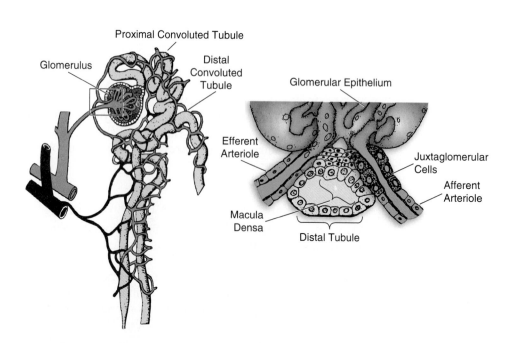

Figure 15.9 Renal juxtaglomerular apparatus.

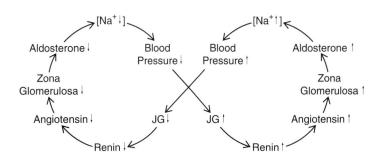

Figure 15.10 Renin–angiotensin system and Na$^+$ homeostasis. Arrows indicate increases (↑) or decreases (↓) in the factors indicated. (From Goss, R. J. 1978. *The physiology of growth*. New York: Academic Press, with permission.)

Vascular smooth muscle contraction and the release of aldosterone from the adrenal gland were the first recognized biological actions of AII [47]. Within the kidney, AII is a vasoconstrictor. Both afferent and efferent arteriolar resistances are modulated by AII, and these actions influence glomerular filtration rate.

Removal of the N-terminal aspartic acid residue from AII gives rise to a heptapeptide referred to as angiotensin III. Although originally considered only a degradative product of AII metabolism, this peptide produces levels of aldosterone secretion in the rat similar to that of AII, but possesses very little pressor activity. It has been suggested, therefore, that AIII may serve as a specific hormone for aldosterone secretion. On the glomerulosa cell, AIII is as potent as AII.

Recent investigations have focused on the possible role of an intra-adrenal renin–angiotensin system as an important regulator of aldosterone biosynthesis. As in many other tissues, renin, angiotensinogen, and AII have all been demonstrated in the adrenal gland, especially in the zona glomerulosa. Dietary modifications of both K$^+$ loading and Na$^+$ restriction increase adrenal renin content. Therefore, the activity of the adrenal renin system may play a role in determining the stimulatory effects of these diets. It has been shown that Na$^+$ restriction increases zona glomerulosa AII content, but reduces the content of AI. This suggests that Na$^+$ restriction not only increases angiotensin generation, but also selectively increases the conversion of AI to AII.

Aldosterone mediates its action at the level of the distal convoluted tubules and the cortical collecting tubules of the kidney. Sodium resorption increases the osmolarity of the blood, which is monitored by the JG cells, and they respond by decreased renin secretion (Fig. 15.10). Increasing the plasma Na$^+$ concentration may be a direct inhibitory stimulus to further aldosterone secretion. In the absence of aldosterone, the ratio of K$^+$ to Na$^+$ increases; high K$^+$ is a direct stimulus to aldosterone secretion. Besides its action on the cells of the zona glomerulosa, AII stimulates vasoconstriction. This adaptive vasopressor response results in elevation of the blood pressure. Afferent sensory neurons respond to the vasoconstriction and, by a reflex mechanism, inhibit sympathetic stimulation of renin secretion.

A Renal Kallikrein–Kinin System Activates Vasoactive Peptides

Kinins are peptide hormones released from plasma protein precursors by plasma and tissue enzymes termed *kallikreins* [28]. The protein precursors are referred to as *kininogens*, and they serve as substrates for the enzymatic actions of the kallikreins, which may themselves become activated after they are enzymatically released from proenzymes referred to as *prekallikreins*. The kinins are subsequently inactivated by enzymes referred to as *kininases* (Fig. 15.11). Glandular kallikreins are a group of kinin-forming enzymes found in many

Figure 15.11 Kallikrein role in renin activation and bradykinin production. (From Inagami, T., and K. Murakami. 1981. Prorenin. *Biomed. Mater. Res.* 1:456–75, with permission.)

glands such as the kidney. Glandular kallikreins from diverse tissues differ in primary structure. Activation of these enzymes (isozymes) and their subsequent activation of kininogens may provide a mechanism for the local production of kinins. Within the kidney, kallikrein activation leads to the production of a decapeptide, *lysylbradykinin* (Lys-Arg-Pro-Pro-Gly-Phe-Ser-Pro-Phe-Arg), which is then converted (apparently by an angiotensinase) to the nonapeptide *bradykinin* by the removal of the terminal lysine.

In the kidney, renin is derived from an inactive zymogen precursor, a prorenin. There is some evidence that renal kallikrein is responsible for the enzymatic activation of renin from prorenin, in addition to its role in the activation of a kininogen to bradykinin, but this remains controversial [41]. Most interesting is the discovery that the AI-converting enzyme is apparently identical to kininase II. Thus, this enzyme is responsible for the conversion of AI to its active form, AII, as well as the conversion of bradykinin to inactive fragments (Fig. 15.11).

It is interesting that renal kallikrein participates in the activation of two peptides that have vasoactive actions. Angiotensin II can be considered a systemic vasoconstrictor whose direct actions on the arterial tree elevate blood pressure. Within the kidney, on the other hand, bradykinin may function as a localized vascular smooth muscle relaxant. It has been suggested that the concurrent release of two enzymes that produce peptides with diametrically opposing actions would seem counterproductive. However, it would be important that maintenance of blood pressure via constriction does not occur at the expense of renal blood flow. The role of bradykinin would be confined to the renal vascular bed so that kidney perfusion is protected. Thus, this dual system would function to maintain a normal renal blood flow and at the same time increase systemic pressure [41].

Within the kidney, kallikrein is localized to the basal membrane of the epithelial cells of the distal tubules. There is evidence that aldosterone increases kallikrein excretion in humans and other animals and also enhances renin activity. A stimulus may be required to release prorenin so that it can be acted on by a kallikrein. There is strong evidence that bradykinin mediates its renal vasodepressor action through activation of one or more E-series prostaglandins. Bradykinin also increases the concentration of PG-like substances in the renal venous blood. PGs released from renal tissues therefore may participate in the regulation of renin release. Prostacyclin I_2 (PGI_2) appears to be the arachidonic acid product that is responsible for renin release. It is possible that the roles of PGE_2 and PGI_2 vary in different compartments of the kidney. A summary scheme of the possible relationships of aldosterone and the renal kallikrein–bradykinin system to renin production is shown (Fig. 15.12).

An Atrial Natriuretic Factor (ANF) Inhibits Renal Tubular Reabsorption

A number of early experimental observations suggested that variations in glomerular filtration rate and aldosterone secretion were insufficient to fully account for renal responses to volume expansion. It was therefore postulated that a humoral substance regulated volume overload by inhibiting reabsorption by the renal tubules, thereby promoting diuresis and natriuresis. There is now evidence that a hormone released by the atria of the heart may mediate some of the physiological responses to volume expansion [6, 7].

This *atrial natriuretic factor* (ANF), also known as atriopeptin, or atrial natriuretic peptide (ANP), was localized (as its name implies) to the atria [6, 7]. Atrial cardiocytes contain granular

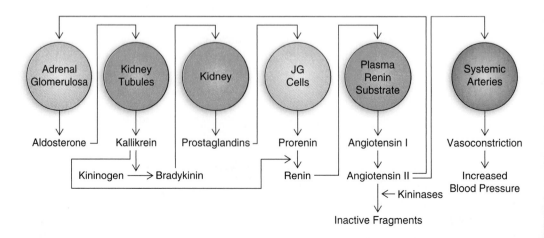

Figure 15.12
Summary scheme of the role of aldosterone in renal renin production.

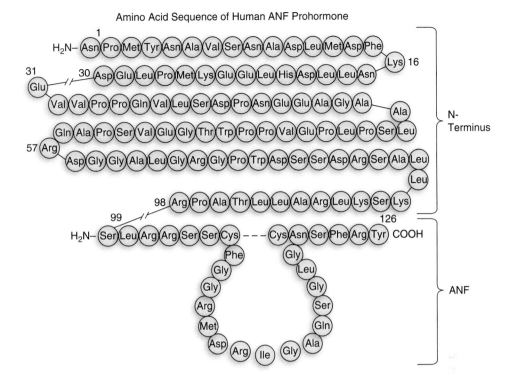

Figure 15.13 Primary structure of atrial natriuretic factor (ANF). (From Vesely, D. L. 1991. *The atrial peptides*, Prentice Hall Endocrinology Series. Englewood Cliffs, NJ: Prentice Hall, with permission).

inclusions that are the source of ANF. Injections of atrial, but not ventricular, extracts induce a rapid diuresis and natriuresis in experimental animals. Immunohistochemical studies using antibodies to the peptide have localized the hormone to the granules of atrial myocytes. The ventricles as well as the atria of nonmammalian vertebrates contain secretory granules, suggesting that a restriction of the hormone to the atria is a more recent evolutionary acquisition.

ANF is a peptide composed of 28 amino acids and is derived from a 126-amino-acid precursor (pro-ANF) (Fig. 15.13). Most interesting is the observation that pro-ANF gives rise to three structurally unrelated fragments that all exhibit ANF activity to varying degrees. ANF affects diuresis and natriuresis by several physiological actions:

1. it inhibits aldosterone production by the adrenal glomerulosa cells
2. it inhibits the release of renin (which indirectly stimulates aldosterone secretion)
3. it inhibits vasopressin secretion from the pituitary, as well as the action of vasopressin at the level of the kidney
4. it causes relaxation of blood vessels (possibly by antagonizing the vasoconstrictor actions of AII).

All these ANF actions effectively reduce the retention of Na^+ and water, and therefore decrease volume expansion (Fig. 15.14).

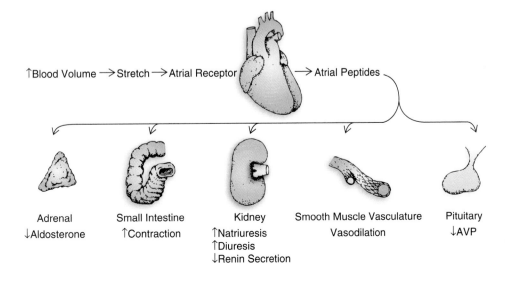

Figure 15.14 Biological roles of ANF. (Revised from Vesely, D. L. 1991. *The atrial peptides*, Prentice Hall Endocrinology Series. Englewood Cliffs, NJ: Prentice Hall, with permission).

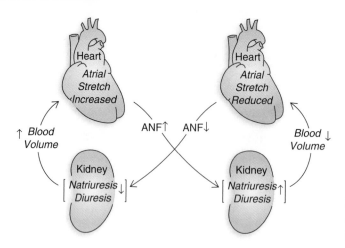

Figure 15.15 The role of atrial natriuretic factor (ANF) in blood volume homeostasis.

In addition, ANF may have a central role in suppression of fluid and salt intake (drinking and salt appetite, respectively) and of vasopressin secretion, actions that again would result in processes leading to reduction in body salt and fluid levels and peripheral blood pressure. Thus, ANF contributes to the reestablishment of intravascular volume homeostasis in states of acute volume overload (Fig. 15.15). Conversely, ANF levels (in dogs) are reduced during hypotension due to hemorrhage, thus protecting the hypovolemic organism from further volume loss. It has been shown that ANF has biological effects in humans at physiological plasma concentrations.

Although some experimental evidence is consistent with the concept that ANF is an important physiological regulator of renal Na^+ excretion, this hypothesis remains unproven [2]. Evidence also suggests that ANF does not contribute to the process that elicits a post-prandial natriuresis, a process that presumably is of primary importance in the physiological regulation of Na^+ balance. A number of common physiological, experimental, and patho-physiological conditions reveal that circulating ANF does not correlate with renal Na^+ excretion. This lack of correlation may suggest that systemic ANF is not an important regulator of Na^+ excretion in these situations. Evidence that the kidneys produce their own natriuretic peptide may partly explain why investigations of the effects of endogenous ANF on renal Na^+ excretion often have yielded inconsistent results. This inconsistency has led to a gradual evolution of opinion concerning the functional role of ANF. Based on current data, it is postulated that ANF is primarily a regulator of the cardiovascular system and that renal natriuretic peptide (urodilatin?) participates locally in the intrarenal regulation of Na^+ and chloride transport.

ANF (ANP) was the first described member of a family of polypeptide hormones that regulates salt and water balance and blood pressure. Subsequent to the isolation and characterization of ANP, two related hormones have been described: brain natriuretic peptide (BNP), isolated from both brain and heart; and C-type natriuretic peptide (CNP), purified from porcine brain. Like ANP, both of these hormones can elicit vasore-laxant, natriuretic, and diuretic responses in bioassay systems. These natriuretic peptides share a common structural motif consisting of a 17-amino-acid loop formed by an intramolecular disulfide linkage. Only 5 of the 17 amino acids in the ring differ among the three peptides isolated from the pig, whereas the NH_2- and COOH-terminals vary in both amino acid composition and length. Among different species, the structures of both ANP and CNP are highly conserved, whereas the amino acid sequence of BNP varies as much as 50%. The physiological significance of these ANF-related peptides remains to be determined.

Circulation and Metabolism

Steroid hormones are only sparingly soluble in water, and most are transported to their target tissues by plasma proteins. Within the plasma, cortisol is reversibly bound to two proteins, *transcortin* or *corticosteroid-binding globulin* (CBG) and, to a lesser extent, an

Figure 15.16 One pathway of cortisol metabolism and glucuronide formation.

α-2 globulin. About 6% of cortisol is unbound, and it is this pool that apparently represents the hormone available for uptake by target tissues ("free hormone hypothesis"). The bound cortisol provides a larger buffer pool of the corticosteroid that can be made immediately available as the free cortisol.

More than 50% of circulating aldosterone is unbound. The biological half-life of cortisol in the human is about 80 minutes, whereas the half-life of aldosterone is about 30 minutes. The short half-life of aldosterone may be because most aldosterone circulates in an unbound form and is therefore readily available for metabolism and excretion [12]. Metabolism of adrenal steroids occurs primarily in the liver, where side-chain and A-ring reductions take place. Structurally altered steroids are then conjugated to glucuronic acid or sulfates to form water-soluble derivatives [20, 46]. One pathway of cortisol metabolism is shown in Figure 15.16.

Physiological Roles

In humans, the biological roles of cortisol and aldosterone, the major glucocorticoid and mineralocorticoid, respectively, are quite different. In pathophysiological states of cortisol hypersecretion (Cushing's disease) or aldosterone hypersecretion (Conn's disease), each hormone, however, may exhibit both glucocorticoid and mineralocorticoid activity because they share structural similarities.

Glucocorticoids Regulate Key Physiological Processes in Response to Prolonged Stress

Intermediary Metabolism. Glucocorticoids affect carbohydrate, lipid, and protein metabolism. They increase synthesis of a number of key enzymes in the gluconeogenic pathway within hepatocytes. Although the actions of glucocorticoids on the liver are anabolic, the actions on skeletal muscle and adipose tissue are catabolic. Catabolic actions may result because glucose uptake by these tissues is inhibited by glucocorticoids. In the absence of a metabolic substrate for ATP production, proteolysis of muscle proteins and lipolysis of fat occur. The free fatty acids (FFAs) and amino acids that are released from these tissues become available as substrates for gluconeogenesis within the liver (Fig. 15.17). The glucose produced is either stored as glycogen or released into the blood. Excessive secretion of glucocorticoids is antagonistic to the actions of insulin and predisposes the individual to diabetes mellitus as the actions of glucocorticoids elevate blood glucose levels. Glucocorticoids also reduce the affinity of certain cells for insulin, which further aggravates the diabetic hyperglycemia.

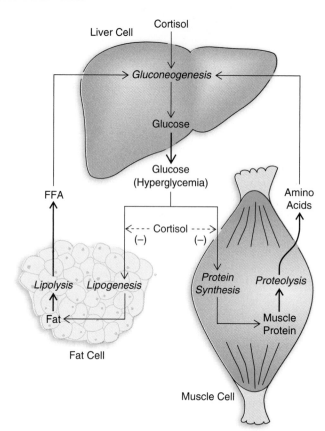

Figure 15.17 Major effects of excess cortisol in intermediary metabolism.

Permissive Actions. Most, if not all, effects of glucocorticoids may be considered permissive to the actions of other hormones. In particular, glucocorticoids are required for functioning of the sympathoadrenal system. Under conditions of stress, and in the absence of glucocorticoids, there is vascular collapse, which usually leads to death. Glucocorticoids are necessary for catecholamine synthesis within sympathetic nerve terminals and for the process of catecholamine reuptake from the synaptic cleft; they may also decrease the rate of catecholamine degradation by catechol-amine-O-methyltransferase (COMT). Evidence for these statements includes a diminished sympathoadrenal activity in the absence of glucocorticoids. Fat mobilization in response to catecholamines is impaired after hypophysectomy but is corrected by treatment with ACTH or glucocorticoids. Glucocorticoids themselves have little, if any, fat-mobilizing activity, but they apparently maintain levels of lipolytic enzymes that are activated through the actions of catecholamines. Hypothermia usually follows adrenalectomy, and adrenalectomized animals soon die under conditions of cold stress. Glucocorticoids maintain body temperature in homeotherms through their permissive actions on liver gluconeogenesis and adipose tissue metabolism.

Role in Reproduction. In sheep and other domestic animals, the pituitary-adrenal axis is clearly involved in the process of parturition. Plasma levels of corticosterone increase in fetal sheep several days before birth, and infusions of ACTH or dexamethasone induce premature parturition. The fetal adrenal is relatively unresponsive to ACTH until 7 to 9 days before term, but no adequate explanation is available as to why adrenal sensitivity to ACTH changes just prior to parturition (Chap. 19). Cortisol and prolactin are the principal hormones required for lactogenesis in the mouse mammary gland. In mammary tissue, the actions of cortisol are expressed through a specific glucocorticoid receptor. There is about an 85% decrease in the level of casein mRNA after adrenalectomy. A single injection of cortisol then can cause an increase in casein mRNA to a level above that of the adrenalectomized animal.

Nervous System Effects. Neonatal administration of corticosterone can reduce both the basal level and amplitude of the diurnal rhythm of plasma corticosterone in the adult rat, depending on the age at which exposure to the steroid occurs. This suggests that, as for gonadal steroids, adrenal steroids of fetal or maternal origin may play an important role in early "imprinting" of the central nervous system (Chap. 16). It is also possible that the presence of maternal steroids in excessive concentrations adversely affects the normal development of the fetal nervous system and thus contributes to birth defects.

Certain hormones influence the survival of neurons in the developing brain and are necessary for maintenance of the structural integrity of the mature brain. The hippocampus, a brain region involved in learning, memory, and a number of neurological disease states, is a target of adrenal steroids and is thought to play a role in the endocrine functions of the adrenal-hypothalamic-pituitary axis. Adrenalectomy of adult male rats results in a nearly complete loss of hippocampal granule cells by 3 to 4 months after surgery. Granule cell loss is selective; that is, there is no apparent loss of hippocampal pyramidal cells or of several types of hippocampal interneurons. The hippocampal CA1 pyramidal cells of adrenalectomized animals exhibit normal electrophysiological responses to afferent stimulation, whereas responses evoked in the dentate gyrus are severely attenuated. Corticosterone replacement prevents both the adrenalectomy-induced granule cell loss and the attenuated physiological response. Thus, the adrenal glands play a role in maintaining the structural and functional integrity of the normal adult brain [43].

Steroids can rapidly alter neuronal function and behavior through poorly characterized, direct actions on neuronal membranes. In the classic model of steroid hormone action, steroids bind to intracellular receptors, which act as ligand-dependent transcription factors that regulate gene expression. Steroids may also alter brain functions through nongenomic mechanisms. For example, in rats, short-term exposure to progesterone is associated with rapid changes in behavior, and this effect occurs in the absence of new protein synthesis. Gonadal and adrenal steroid hormones can alter neuronal firing activity within milliseconds to minutes of administration; these responses can occur in brain regions lacking classic steroid receptors or if steroid access to intracellular receptors is blocked. These events appear to be mediated by direct steroid action on neuronal membranes [27].

Anti-inflammatory and Immunosuppressive Actions of Glucocorticoids. At higher than physiological concentrations, as in Cushing's disease, glucocorticoids inhibit inflammatory and allergic reactions. These actions may result from stabilization of lysosomal membranes that prevents the secretion of enzymes that normally occurs during inflammation. Glucocorticoids inhibit the infiltration of leukocytes into the affected tissue and also exert an immunosuppressive action through their lympholytic actions.

In addition to the catabolic actions of glucocorticoids on muscle tissue and the protein matrix of bone, glucocorticoids cause atrophy of the lymphatic system (lymph nodes, thymus gland, spleen), which results in decreased levels of circulating lymphocytes. Ultimately, this lymphocytopenia results in failure of the body to provide antibodies during an infection. Although glucocorticoids may be useful in combating the undesirable effects of local infections, excessive use of these agents may render the individual susceptible to severe systematic bacterial infection as many protective mechanisms are suppressed, but the underlying cause of the disease remains.

Interleukin-1 (IL-1), a member of a family of polypeptides produced by activated monocytes and other cells, has an important role, not only in stimulating the immune cells, but also in eliciting a variety of physiological reactions observed during infection, inflammation, and injury. Stimulation of ACTH release may be one of these important nonimmune responses that can be induced by the monokine. Stimulation of ACTH release induced by IL-1β may contribute to a homeostatic regulation of the immune function. Increased hypothalamopituitary-adrenal activity results in an increased secretion of glucocorticoids that suppress immune responses, and hence, unfavorable overstimulation of the immune reaction, during infection or other conditions. Increased secretion of glucocorticoids could represent a way for the body's natural defense mechanism to control or remedy undesirable symptoms and conditions, such as arthritis, induced by increased production of IL-1β as observed in various infections, such as Lyme disease. These findings suggest that IL-1 may play an important role as a carrier of messages from the immune system to the neuroendocrine system. Numerous other data indicate that there is bidirectional communication between the immune system and the neuroendocrine system.

Glucocorticoids and the General Adaptation Syndrome. In 1936, Selye published the paper "A Syndrome Produced by Diverse Nocuous Agents." This syndrome was later referred to as the *general adaptation syndrome*, or GAS. In response to stress, a body responds in a stereotypic manner, which, if the stress is prolonged, may proceed through a number of stages: (1) an initial *alarm reaction*; (2) *resistance*; and eventually (3) *exhaustion* [39]. These stages may be characterized more precisely if one understands the underlying physiological processes involved in the adaptation syndrome.

In response to stress, the sympathoadrenal system is activated (Chap. 14). Through the actions of epinephrine released from the adrenal chromaffin tissue and norepinephrine released from sympathetic nerve endings, the general body metabolic and motor activity is increased (alarm reaction). The basal metabolic rate is elevated and blood flow is increased, particularly to those organs that are more physiologically active. A major effect of circulating catecholamines is the utilization of liver glycogen stores for the production of glucose. This depot source of readily available carbohydrate, though limited, may be sufficient for an immediate stress (alarm) response.

The release of adrenal glucocorticoids is also activated in response to stress. Through the permissive actions of these hormones there is an enhancement of sympathoadrenal activity. In fact, in the absence of adrenal steroids, sympathoadrenal actions are generally depressed, which may lead to the individual's demise. Glucocorticoids enhance the lipolytic actions of catecholamines on adipose tissue. The FFAs released from fat cells provide metabolic substrates necessary for survival in the absence of hepatic glycogen stores. Hepatic glycogen depots are also restored through gluconeogenesis resulting from FFA utilization. The actions of glucocorticoids are slower than the initial rapid actions of catecholamines on metabolic processes, but they provide the secondary response (resistance) necessary for continued sympathoadrenal activity and hepatic gluconeogenesis.

Under prolonged conditions of stress, the individual enters the third stage of the adaptation syndrome, exhaustion. In effect, the prolonged hypercortisolism eventually leads to muscle wasting, hyperglycemia (diabetes mellitus), atrophy of the immune system, vascular derangements, gastrointestinal ulceration, and other symptoms of excessive sympathoadrenal activity.

Adrenal Hormones and Self-Regulation of Mammalian Populations. Within natural populations of animals adrenal hormones may play an important role in the control of population density. Some mammalian populations establish social hierarchies where there is a dominant animal, a second-ranking animal, and so on, to the lowest-ranking animal that is subordinate to all others [8]. Adrenocortical morphology and function (corticosterone output) are negatively related to social rank or dominance in these populations. In subordinate animals adrenal hypertrophy is followed by thymic involution, diminished resistance to disease, and many symptoms related to excessive glucocorticoid and sympathoadrenal activity. Increases in population density also enhance the number of encounters between members of a group that can lead to further subordination of the less dominant individuals. Increased mortality follows, as well as diminished reproductive capacity. Therefore, the ultimate effect of increased population density is, through the actions of adrenal hormones, to inhibit recruitment of new individuals into the population and thus to maintain the population at a level below that which might exhaust environmental resources [8].

It is clear that adrenal steroid hormones are essential for survival under stress. Continued stress eventually leads to gross pathophysiological alterations of bodily processes due to prolonged excessive actions of adrenal hormones. A little stress may be of adaptive necessity; too much, however, may be disastrous.

Aldosterone Stimulates Sodium Reabsorption in Renal Tubules

Aldosterone's major role is to regulate Na^+ homeostasis and, indirectly, volume homeostasis by influencing water reabsorption from the nephron. Like parathormone, which also regulates blood electrolyte (Ca^{2+}) composition, aldosterone is essential for life.

Sodium/Potassium Homeostasis. Aldosterone accelerates the reabsorption of Na^+ by the kidney distal and cortical collecting tubules, salivary and sweat glands, and gastrointestinal mucosa. Through its major action on renal tubular Na^+ retention, aldosterone also profoundly affects the plasma concentration of K^+ and hydrogen ions. In the nephron, the uptake of Na^+ in response to aldosterone is usually balanced by a concomitant loss of K^+ (Fig. 15.18). Under conditions of plasma K^+ deficiency (hypokalemia), there is an increase in distal tubular H^+ secretion, whereas during states of K^+ excess, distal tubular secretion of K^+ is enhanced. One of the important elements in acclimatization to heat is the ability of

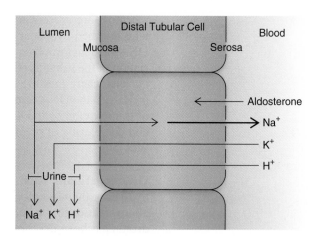

Figure 15.18 Physiological effects of aldosterone on renal distal tubular Na$^+$ resorption and K$^+$ and H$^+$ excretion. In response to aldosterone, sodium is actively transported across the tubular serosal membrane into the peritubular space. Potassium and hydrogen ions are passively shunted across the mucosal membrane in exchange for sodium.

an animal to reduce the amount of Na$^+$ in sweat. Injections of a mineralocorticoid into an individual not exposed to heat produce a drop in the Na$^+$ content of sweat within 2 to 3 days. These observations suggest that the Na$^+$ concentration of sweat is regulated in the human by aldosterone. High-affinity sites for aldosterone have been identified in the rat brain. These receptors may represent extrarenal sites of aldosterone action, and one of these may affect salt intake.

Physiological Roles of Adrenal Androgens have yet to be Clarified

The production of androgens by the adrenal is minimal compared to the production of these hormones by the gonads. In the female, adrenal androgens may contribute to pubertal changes (adrenarche), and postmenopausally these androgens may serve as substrates for extragonadal estrogen production. Abnormal adrenal steroid production, due to a defect in the normal steroidogenic pathway or to a tumorous condition, has profound morphogenetic consequences, particularly in the pregnant female. There is evidence that adrenal steroids may help support growth of mammary and prostatic carcinomas. Regression of steroid-dependent tumors, although accelerated after gonadectomy, is further enhanced by adrenalectomy.

Mechanisms of Action

Adrenal steroid hormones, like other steroid hormones, mediate their actions through genomic mechanisms.

Glucocorticoids Exert Actions Through Intracellular Glucocorticoid Receptors

Glucocorticoids regulate the activity of a variety of tissues. Most actions are mediated by activation of intracellular glucocorticoid receptors (GRs), which are ligand-induced transcription factors that modulate de novo synthesis of cellular proteins, most often enzymes. In addition, glucocorticoids, as well as other steroid hormones, enhance guanylate cyclase activity at physiological concentrations in a variety of tissues. Glucocorticoids also inhibit prostaglandin synthesis possibly by an inhibition of phospholipase A$_2$ activity. One mechanism of glucocorticoid action may be to modulate the number of cell membrane receptors for hormones.

Enzyme Induction. Glucocorticoids increase the activity of a number of enzymes. This action could come about either by controlling the number of mRNA templates for enzyme synthesis or by changing the translational efficiency of a fixed level of mRNA. There is evidence that glucocorticoids stimulate the de novo synthesis of mRNA; thus, glucocorticoids stimulate both transcriptional and translational processes related to protein synthesis. Many of these enzymes, such as hepatic tyrosine amino transferase, play important roles in the anabolic actions of steroid hormones. A majority of the actions of cortisol are, however, catabolic in nature.

Glucocorticoid Receptors. Glucocorticoids exert their effects on target tissues through intracellular receptors that are hormone-dependent transcription factors. In cells, the unliganded receptors are present as heteromeric structures consisting of a pair of steroid-binding proteins attached to a heat shock protein. On hormone binding, they are rapidly activated to a DNA-binding form by a process known as "activation" or "transformation" that involves dissociation of the subunits (Chap. 3). The activated hormone-receptor complexes translocate to the nucleus, where they are thought to associate as dimers with glucocorticoid response elements (GREs) in the DNA through which they activate or repress regulated genes [53]. The regulation of transcription by the ligand-activated glucocorticoid receptors typically involves recruitment and complexing of several transcriptional co-activator and co-repressor proteins at the GRE sites [50].

Glucocorticoid Resistance.   The essential nature of the glucocorticoid receptor in mediating the physiologic effects of glucocorticoid hormones is underscored by the clinical abnormalities that result from receptor deficiency or receptor defects. A rare familial syndrome has been described in which primary cortisol resistance is caused by a glucocorticoid receptor present at normal concentration, but with decreased affinity for cortisol. The syndrome is characterized by hypercortisolism without the features of Cushing's syndrome. In the affected patients, compensatory production of adrenocorticotropic hormone may cause hyperpigmentation, hypertension, hypokalemia, and precocious puberty.

Aldosterone's Actions are Mediated by Intracellular Mineralocorticoid Receptors

Both the kidney and the toad urinary bladder have been used extensively for studies on the mechanism of aldosterone action. Aldosterone increases the rate of Na^+ transport across epithelial cells of these organs. This movement of Na^+ is generally viewed as a two-step process: (1) there is entry of Na^+ from the fluid bathing the mucosal surface of the cell; and (2) there is subsequent extrusion of Na^+ through the serosal membrane into the interstitial space (Fig. 15.18). Numerous experiments have been directed toward determining which step in the transport process is stimulated by aldosterone.

Aldosterone mediates its action through the induction of the synthesis of proteins within target tissues. Three different mechanisms have been postulated by which these hormone-inducible proteins augment transepithelial Na^+ transport (Fig. 15.19). The sodium pump theory postulates that these proteins directly stimulate the activity of a sodium pump that is localized in the serosal side of the cell. The metabolic theory suggests that the aldosterone-inducible proteins increase the supply of ATP to the pump. In the permease theory, these proteins enhance the permeability of the luminal mucosal membrane to Na^+. Experimental evidence strongly supports the view that both the passive apical entry of Na^+ and the active extrusion of Na^+ across the basal-lateral serosal membranes depend on the induction of enzymes that

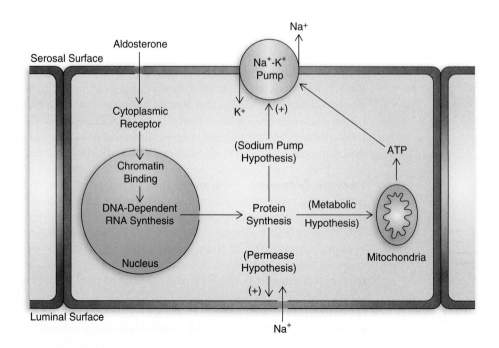

Figure 15.19
Hypothetical mechanisms of aldosterone action on the kidney.

modulate energy metabolism. Aldosterone also stimulates fatty acid synthesis and the turnover of membrane phospholipid fatty acids in the toad bladder. Aldosterone alteration of the lipid composition of membranes may be an important component of its action mechanism.

Vasopressin (AVP) also increases the rate of Na^+ transport and the permeability to water of the urinary bladder of the toad, two responses mediated through cAMP (Chap. 7). Although aldosterone stimulates Na^+ transport in these tissues, it does so without affecting permeability to water. Aldosterone stimulation of Na^+ transport does not involve cAMP production, but it enhances cAMP-induced Na^+ transport and water permeability. The action of the steroid may involve the inhibition of the degradation of cAMP, as suggested by the following observations. In response to AVP or theophylline, cAMP levels are higher in aldosterone-treated tissues, and the activity of cyclic nucleotide phosphodiesterase, the enzyme that catalyzes the degradation of cAMP, is depressed.

Mineralocorticoid Receptors.   Mineralocorticoid receptors, from tissue extracts and when recombinant-derived, have equal affinity for the physiological mineralocorticoid aldosterone and for the glucocorticoids, cortisol and corticosterone, which circulate at much higher concentrations than aldosterone [1]. Such receptors are found in mineralocorticoid target tissues (kidney, parotid, and colon) and in nontarget tissues, such as hippocampus and heart. Given this equal receptor affinity and the much higher circulating levels of cortisol or corticosterone than aldosterone, additional mechanisms must operate to allow selective mineralocorticoid action in mineralocorticoid target tissues. In mineralocorticoid target tissues, the receptors are selective for aldosterone in vivo because of the presence of the enzyme 11β-hydroxysteroid dehydrogenase, which converts cortisol and corticosterone, but not aldosterone, to their 11-keto analogs. These analogs cannot bind to mineralocorticoid receptors [31].

Angiotensin II Actions are Mediated by Cognate G-Protein-Coupled Receptors, AT_1 and AT_2

The recent availability of pure AII antagonists has established that there are at least two types of angiotensin receptors, now referred to as AT_1 and AT_2 subtypes. The cardiovascular effects of AII are mediated by the AT_1, receptor subtype and include the following actions: aldosterone secretion from the adrenal, pressor and tachycardiac (increased heart beat) responses, increased water intake (polydipsia), and contraction of certain vascular smooth muscles. The role(s) of the AT_2 receptor subtype remains to be defined. The rat AII receptor, AT_1, has been cloned. As for many other peptide hormones, seven hydrophobic domains are postulated to transverse the cell membrane [4]. Numerous second messengers have been implicated in the actions of AII, as depicted in Figure 15.20.

Pathophysiology

The clinical manifestations of abnormal levels of adrenal glucocorticoids or mineralocorticoids in humans are predictable from an understanding of the biological actions of these corticosteroids (Table 15.3) [38]. A total loss of adrenal function may derive from a congenital developmental defect or adrenal destruction during a particular disease state (e.g., tuberculosis). The adrenal abnormality may be of primary origin and involve a failure of glucocorticoid or mineralocorticoid biosynthesis due to a genetic defect related to an absence or faulty structure of a particular enzyme. Overproduction of a particular corticoid may be due to an adrenocortical adenoma or carcinoma, resulting in excess cortisol (Cushing's syndrome) or, as in primary aldosteronism, in excess aldosterone secretion (Conn's disease). Hyposecretion or hypersecretion of adrenal steroids may be of secondary origin and involve a defect in mechanisms involved in the control of cortisol or aldosterone secretion (Fig. 15.21).

Disorders of Cortisol Secretion Include Syndromes of Cortisol Deficiency and Excess

Addison's Disease.   In a manuscript published in 1855, "On the Constitutional and Local Effects of Disease of the Supra-Renal Capsules," Addison provided the classical description of the disease that bears his name. The disease may be of primary origin and involve total destruction of the glands ("primary adrenocortical failure"). Most often the

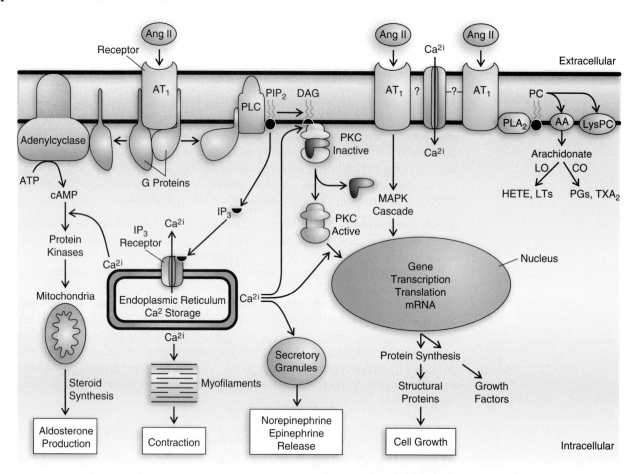

Figure 15.20   AII receptor-cellular response coupling. PLC, phospholipase C; DAG, diacylglycerol; IP$_3$, inositol triphosphate; G protein, guanosine triphosphate-binding protein; PKC, protein kinase C; AA, arachidonic acid; PC, phosphatidylcholine; LysPC, lysophosphatidylcholine; LO, lipoxygenase; CO, cyclooxygenase; HETE, hydroxy-eicostatetraenoic acid; TXA$_2$, thromboxane A$_2$; PGs, prostaglandins (e.g., prostaglandin E$_2$); channel, calcium channel; PIP$_2$, phosphatidylinositol diphosphate; LTs, leukotrienes. (Modified from Timmermans et al., 1993. "Angiotensin II receptors and angiotensin II receptor antagonists." *Pharmacol. Res.* 45:205–51.)

etiology is due to bilateral tubercular destruction of the glands. Atrophy due to tuberculosis involves the medulla as well as the cortex, whereas in idiopathic (unknown cause) atrophy usually only the cortex is affected. The most frequent symptoms of Addison's disease include weakness, increased melanin pigmentation of the skin, weight loss, hypotension, salt craving, and hypoglycemia. These symptoms result from a combination of both glucocorticoid and mineralocorticoid deficiencies. The increased integumental pigmentation, a cardinal symptom of the disease, is because in the absence of cortisol feedback to the hypothalamus, excessive amounts of ACTH are secreted. Because nearly the complete structure of α-MSH is contained within the ACTH molecule (see Fig. 8.1), it is probable that ACTH acts on integumental melanocytes to increase melanin production of the skin. In Addison's disease of secondary or tertiary origin, the defect may reside at the level of the pituitary or hypothalamus, respectively [30]. A failure of the hypothalamus to secrete CRH or the absence of functional pituitary corticotrophs could explain the etiology of some forms of adrenal insufficiency (Fig. 15.21).

Cushing's Syndrome.   This disease, first described by Cushing in 1932, refers to any clinical entity due to excessive and prolonged secretion and action of glucocorticoids, although the cause of the disease may relate to any one of a number of origins. Primary hypercortisolism may be due to an adrenal cortical tumor (adenoma or carcinoma). Cushing's disease of secondary origin may derive from a pituitary tumor secreting an excess of ACTH, or to ectopic ACTH production, or to pituitary corticotroph hyperplasia. The simultaneous measurement of

TABLE 15.3   Endocrine pathophysiology of the adrenal cortex

Adrenocortical hypofunction
  Addison's disease
    Primary adrenocortical insufficiency
    Secondary adrenocortical insufficiency
      Pituitary origin (no ACTH secretion)
      Hypothalamic origin (no CRH secretion?)
  Hypoaldosteronism
    Primary (adrenocortical insufficiency)
    Secondary
      Hyporeninemic hypoaldosteronism
Adrenocortical hyperfunction
  Syndromes of excess cortisol secretion (Cushing's disease)
    Cushing's syndrome (primary origin)
      Adrenal adenoma or adenocarcinoma
    Cushing's syndrome (secondary origin)
      Bilateral adrenal hyperplasia
        Pituitary origin (microadenoma secreting ACTH, Nelson's syndrome)
        Hypothalamic origin
        Ectopic ACTH syndrome
  Syndromes of excess aldosterone secretion
    Primary hyperaldosteronism, Conn's syndrome (adrenal adenoma/aldosteronoma)
    Secondary hyperaldosteronism
      Bartter's syndrome (hyperreninism)
      Malignant hypertension (due to decreased renal perfusion pressure)
      Renin-secreting tumor (hyperreninemic hyperaldosteronism)
      Glucocorticoid-suppressible aldosteronism (GSA)
  Syndromes of excess adrenal androgen secretion (virilizing adrenal tumors)
    Male (precocious pseudopuberty in the preadolescent boy)
    Female (masculinization)
  Syndromes of excess estrogen production (feminizing adrenal tumor)
    Male (gynecomastia)
    Female (precocious puberty in the preadolescent girl)
Adrenal enzyme deficiency syndromes
  Congenital (lipoid) adrenal hyperplasia (fatal)
  Congenital virilizing adrenal hyperplasia
    3β-Dehydrogenase deficiency
    11β-Hydroxylase deficiency (hypertensive form)
    21β-Hydroxylase deficiency (salt-losing form)
  Congenital 17α-hydroxylase deficiency
  Corticosterone methyl oxidase (type II) deficiency (hypoaldosteronism)
  Syndrome of apparent mineralocorticoid excess (due to a defect of 11β-hydroxy oxide-reductase)

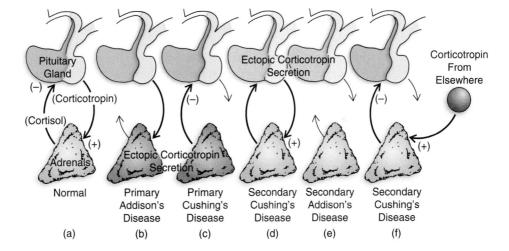

Figure 15.21
Summary scheme of the etiology of hypocortisolism and hypercortisolism.

plasma ACTH and cortisol is useful in differentiating between adrenal hyperplasia (due to excess pituitary ACTH stimulation) and adrenal tumors as the cause of Cushing's syndrome. In patients with adrenal tumors, plasma cortisol levels are high but the concentration of ACTH is low or undetectable. In contrast, both cortisol and ACTH plasma levels are elevated in bilateral adrenal hyperplasia, and both can be lowered by exogenous dexamethasone (a synthetic glucocorticoid) administration. A summary scheme of the etiological basis for Cushing's disease is shown (Fig. 15.21).

Some symptoms of cortisol excess are central (trunkal) obesity, hypertension, glucose intolerance, hirsutism, osteoporosis, polyuria, and polydipsia. The hyperglycemia resulting from excess glucocorticoids leads to a so-called "steroid diabetes," where prolonged elevated levels of glucose in time, may lead to pancreatic β-cell exhaustion (diabetes mellitus). The change in fat distribution is due to the lipolytic action of ACTH and glucocorticoids on the normal fat depots. The redistribution of fat may not be due to the direct actions of glucocorticoids but rather to the insulin that is secreted in response to increased hepatic glucose formation. Although the actions of insulin on the normal fat depots are apparently antagonized by cortisol, insulin appears able to exert a lipogenic effect in other areas of the body, such as the face, upper back, and supraclavicular fat pads. The catabolic actions of glucocorticoids on skeletal muscle cause thinning of the extremities. Loss of the protein matrix of bones causes severe osteoporosis, which may severely affect the spinal column [25]. The excess androgens produced are the cause of hirsutism in the female. Again, the hyperpigmentation that may be present in Cushing's disease of secondary origin may be due to the presence of increased circulating levels of ACTH [37]. Polyuria and polydipsia are due to the loss of large volumes of water as a result of solvent drag during the process of excessive glucose excretion by the kidneys.

Disorders of Aldosterone Secretion Include Syndromes of Aldosterone Excess or Deficiency

Conn's Syndrome. In 1955, Conn published a classical report, "Primary Aldosteronism: A New Clinical Entity" [10]. The cause of aldosterone hypersecretion is almost always an adrenal adenoma, but in some instances it may be due to adrenal carcinoma, hyperplasia, or other unknown causes [17, 52]. The oversecretion of aldosterone increases renal distal tubular excretion of K^+ (K^+ diuresis) and H^+ in exchange for reabsorbed Na^+. This leads to the cardinal findings of plasma *hypernatremia* and *hypokalemia*; because hydrogen ions are also lost, this leads to serum *alkalosis* and nephropathy. The hypernatremia is usually associated with water retention, leading to severe hypertension. Therefore, plasma renin levels are low in primary aldosteronism.

Renin-Secreting Tumors. The rare but fatal occurrence of a renin-secreting tumor is associated with hypertension, due to excessive renin secretion (primary reninism). Renin-secreting tumors show that, in humans, hypertension can be produced and maintained by hypersecretion of renin, as shown by the complete reversal of hypertension after removal of the tumor. The hypertension can be totally reversed, even if the duration of hypertension lasted more than 10 years.

Malignant Hypertension. This disease state develops whenever renovascular damage decreases the flow of blood to the afferent arteriole of the glomerulus. The localized decrease in blood pressure is the stimulus to renin secretion that becomes excessive due to the constancy of the restricted blood flow to the glomerulus. The resulting overproduction of AII, due to increased renin secretion, causes a chronic hypertension [11].

Hyporeninemic Hypoaldosteronism. As the clinical name implies, this disease state is associated with reduced plasma renin levels. It is not known, however, whether the etiology involves a defect in stimulatory cues to renin secretion or resides at the level of the JG cell itself. Clinical evidence suggests that in some cases, the defect involves destructive lesions of the JG cells, most often associated with diabetes mellitus.

Bartter's Syndrome. Hyperaldosteronism due to hyperreninism has been associated with hyperplasia of the JG cells in some individuals. This disease is usually associated with increased urinary excretion of E-series prostaglandins. The increased production of these PGs may contribute to several functional abnormalities usually associated with this syndrome. Prostacyclins are directly stimulatory to JG cell renin secretion and may be implicated in JG cell hyperplasia.

Glucocorticoid-Suppressible Aldosteronism (GSA). This is a rare form of hyperaldosteronism inherited as an autosomal dominant trait. The unique feature of this disorder is that the hypersecretion of aldosterone and the elevation of blood pressure are corrected by chronic glucocorticoid therapy. Aldosterone secretion in these patients is regulated by ACTH. During adrenal cell migration, it is likely that during the transition from one type of cells to another, intermediate cell type(s) are formed. These hybrid cells will have some of the characteristics of glomerulosa and fasciculata cells, and they have been called "transitional cells." In the normal adrenal cortex, a small population of such transition cells coexist between the well-developed glomerulosa and fasciculata cells. Thus, these cells are able to synthesize cortisol and aldosterone, as well as the hybrid steroids (18-hydroxycortisol and 18-oxocortisol), having both 17- and 18-hydroxylation by the action on cortisol of the same enzyme(s) responsible for the final steps of aldosterone synthesis [13–15].

Disorders of Steroid Secretion can be Caused by Genetic Mutations Producing Adrenal Enzyme Defects

Genetic defects can lead to inherited inborn errors of metabolism related to specific enzymatic deficiencies in the biosynthesis of adrenal steroids. The severity of such a defect depends on whether the block occurs early or late in the steroidogenic biosynthetic pathway.

Congenital Adrenal Lipoidal Hyperplasia. This rare and fatal condition results from a defect in the conversion of cholesterol to pregnenolone [32]. In the absence of cortisol production and negative feedback to the hypothalamus or pituitary, there is enhanced secretion of ACTH. Corticotropin stimulates adrenal cortical cells; although cholesterol is taken up, it is not used as substrate for steroid hormone production. This leads to a condition referred to as adrenal lipoidal hyperplasia. This defect in enzyme activity in the initial stage of steroid biosynthesis would also involve a concomitant failure in synthesis of gonadal steroids.

Congenital Virilizing Adrenal Hyperplasia. A defect in 3β-hydroxysteroid dehydrogenase, 11β-hydroxylase, or 21β-hydroxylase leads to virilizing syndromes of differing severity, depending on whether the defect is partial or complete. In the absence of 3β-hydroxysteroid dehydrogenase activity there is impaired formation of both cortisol and aldosterone, thus this defect in steroidogenesis is usually fatal [3]. Because ACTH secretion is elevated and the desmolase system is intact, as is 17α-hydroxylase activity, the major product formed is dehydroepiandrosterone. Although a weak androgen with minimal masculinizing activity, excessive levels of this androgen are indeed masculinizing. Excessive androgen production causes virilization of affected newborns. About two-thirds of the cases have an associated mineralocorticoid defect leading to impaired renal tubular resorption of sodium ("salt losing") that can result in shock and death.

In the absence of 11β-hydroxylase activity, diminished cortisol secretion leads to excessive ACTH secretion, resulting in adrenal cortical hyperplasia. The subsequent excessive production of cortisol precursors leads to an increased availability of substrates for androgen production (mainly androstenedione), causing excessive virilization in both male and female. There is enhanced deoxycorticosterone production (at the expense of cortisol synthesis), and the excessive secretion of this mineralocorticoid leads to hypertension. Glucocorticoid replacement therapy will correct the abnormal steroid synthesis and secretion by suppressing the excessive pituitary ACTH production.

A defect in 21β-hydroxylase may be partial or complete. In the female, the excessive secretion of androgens may lead to complete masculinization of the external genitalia (Chap. 16). In the salt-losing form of the syndrome, there is an almost total lack of 21β-hydroxylase activity essential for mineralocorticoid production. Both mineralocorticoid and glucocorticoid replacement therapies are essential for survival.

Corticosterone Methyl Oxidase (Type II) Deficiency. Hypoaldosteronism, due to an inborn error in the terminal step of aldosterone biosynthesis, has been discovered within related members of a family. These individuals exhibit hyperreninemia and elevated plasma and urinary levels of specific 18-hydroxysteroids. The genetic basis for this disease involves a defect in the function of corticosterone methyl oxidase (type II), the enzyme involved in the oxidation of the hydroxyl group at the C-18 position to the aldehyde [29, 48, 51].

17-Hydroxylase Deficiency. Deficient activity of 17-hydroxylase results in deficient biosynthesis of cortisol and androgens. The enzymic defect is also in ovarian tissue and, as testosterone is the precursor to estradiol synthesis, estrogen deficiency is also present, resulting in primary amenorrhea and defeminization (breast and genital atrophy), depending on whether the defect is congenital or occurs later in life. With diminished 17-hydroxylase activity adrenal metabolism is shunted toward increased production of aldosterone, as well as the production of the precursor mineralocorticoids, 11-deoxycorticosterone, and corticosterone. Absence of glucocorticoid feedback to the brain results in enhanced ACTH secretion and an aggravated production of precursors to mineralocorticoid synthesis (Fig. 15.22). The resulting hypertension can be alleviated by the administration of dexamethasone, which feeds back to the hypothalamus, resulting in decreased ACTH secretion.

Syndrome of Apparent Mineralocorticoid Excess. This disorder has thus far been reported only in children and young adults. Its clinical presentation is like that of primary aldosteronism with hypertension, hypokalemic alkalosis, and suppressed plasma renin activity. The response of these clinical manifestations to spironolactone (mineralocorticoid antagonist) suggests the presence of a circulating mineralocorticoid; however, levels of aldosterone and all known mineralocorticoids are either very low or absent. It is likely that the functioning mineralocorticoid in this disorder is cortisol, circulating in normal amounts, but exerting a mineralocorticoid effect because of incomplete metabolism at target tissues. Normally, cortisol has little mineralocorticoid activity in vivo or in mineralocorticoid receptor preparations. It has been shown that the pure mineralocorticoid receptor, as well as preparations from nonmineralocorticoid target tissues, possesses equal affinity for both mineralocorticoids and glucocorticoids. The abnormality in steroid metabolism in the syndrome appears to be due to a decreased intracellular conversion of cortisol to cortisone. Normally, a reversible 11β-hydroxy oxidoreduction leads to an equilibrium mixture of approximately equal amounts of cortisol and cortisone. Cortisone itself is biologically inactive [31].

Defects in LDL Receptor Function are Linked to Development of Atherosclerosis

The term atherosclerosis encompasses a range of degenerative phenomena that affect the arterial wall. Lipid, though present in variable amounts, plays a key role in the development of atherosclerotic plaques. Numerous clinical studies have shown a close association between lipoprotein abnormalities and coronary heart disease (CHD) susceptibility. The

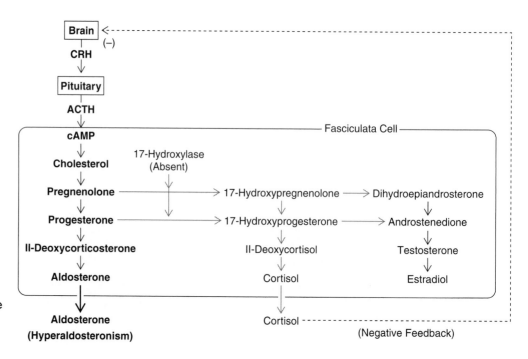

Figure 15.22 Genetic defect in 17α-hydroxylase activity leading to hyperaldosteronism.

primary carrier of cholesterol in the blood is LDL. Epidemiological studies have clearly implicated elevated serum LDL levels in the premature development of CHD. LDL is formed by the action of lipoprotein lipase on its precursor, intermediate-density lipoprotein. Both LDL and intermediate-density lipoprotein are recognized by a specific receptor called the LDL receptor.

There is now compelling evidence linking a defect in the activity of the LDL receptor to the etiology of atherosclerosis. The link between the two comes from an "experiment of nature" called familial hypercholesterolemia (FH). In this genetic disorder, there is a relative or absolute deficiency of LDL receptor function leading to accumulation of cholesterol in the plasma and resulting in occlusive vascular disease. Most afflicted individuals are heterozygous for the disease and possess only about half the normal complement of hepatic LDL receptors. The liver possesses most of the body's LDL receptors. In true receptor-negative homozygous FH, no receptors are present. The LDL receptor is expressed in virtually all cells, but the hepatic expression of LDL receptor is primarily responsible for modulating cholesterol homeostasis in vivo. Transplantation of a liver that expresses normal levels of LDL receptors into patients with homozygous deficiency leads to near normalization of serum cholesterol level, illustrating the importance of hepatic LDL receptor expression. Traditional pharmacologic therapy for hypercholesterolemia in LDL receptor-expressing patients, in fact, is based on up-regulation of residual hepatic LDL receptor function. Drugs such as 3-hydroxy-3-methylglutaryl coenzyme A reductase inhibitors and bile acid binders result in diminished intracellular hepatic-free cholesterol, which leads to derepression of the LDL receptor gene, increased LDL catabolism, and decreased serum cholesterol level [26].

Apolipoprotein E, a protein constituent of several plasma lipoproteins, serves as a high-affinity ligand for the LDL receptor. A major function of apo-E is the transport of lipids (especially cholesterol) among various cells of the body from sites of synthesis or absorption to sites of utilization (peripheral tissues) or excretion (liver). Equally important is its role in the local redistribution of lipid within a tissue during normal cholesterol homeostasis, especially during injury and repair. The elaborate system for storing, releasing, and reusing cholesterol depends on a coordinated regulation of apo-E synthesis and LDL receptor expression. Genetic variability of apo-E, resulting from different alleles coding for proteins with single amino acid substitutions, has been most informative in defining, at a cellular and molecular level, the role of this protein in normal and abnormal lipoprotein metabolism. The genetic disorder type III hyperlipoproteinemia, which is associated with premature atherosclerotic disease, is secondary to the presence of a variant apo-E that does not bind normally to the LDL receptors.

Adrenal Steroid Hormone Pharmacology

A number of drugs have been produced that are useful in the treatment of overproduction or underproduction of adrenal steroids or their actions. One approach to secondary hyperaldosteronism is to prevent the production of AII from its precursors by inhibition of AI converting enzyme activity (ACE inhibitors). Potent and specific renin inhibitors would constitute an interesting alternative to ACE inhibitors for two reasons: (1) the first step in the renin–angiotensin system, the hydrolysis of angiotensinogen by renin, is rate-limiting; and (2) renin has a unique specificity for angiotensinogen, as there is no other known substrate for this enzyme. Inhibitors with an exceptionally high specificity and affinity for renin have been developed in recent years; however, most of the structures are peptidic in nature and have relatively large molecular weights, which might explain their low oral availability and their rapid metabolism. Other enzyme inhibitors have been developed to prevent specific enzyme-related hydroxylations in the aldosterone biosynthetic pathway. Renin secretion may normally be regulated by a renal prostaglandin; indomethacin, an inhibitor of PG synthesis, has been used successfully in some cases to lower renin secretion and aldosterone production in Bartter's syndrome.

Spironolactone, an aldosterone antagonist, is a competitive inhibitor of aldosterone binding to receptors, primarily those of the distal renal tubule. Spironolactone is used clinically to suppress the action of excess aldosterone on renal Na^+ retention. Metyrapone, an inhibitor of cortisols production, is used to test the capacity of the pituitary to respond to decreased circulating levels of plasma cortisol. Metyrapone is particularly useful in the differential diagnosis of Cushing's syndrome, as it will usually enhance ACTH secretion if the disease is of pituitary origin but not if the excess cortisol is due to ectopic production of ACTH.

Match the steroid with its general classification:

1. Cortisol
2. 11-Deoxycorticosterone
3. Aldosterone
4. Progesterone
5. Corticosterone
6. Dehydroepiandrosterone

A. Progesten
B. Glucocorticoid
C. Androgen
D. Mineralocorticoid

Think, analyze and discuss:

1. Adrenomedullary and adrenocortical tissue are anatomically associated despite their different embryological origins. What may be the adaptive significance of this anatomical relationship? Describe at least three ways in which one tissue may regulate the endocrine functions of the other.

2. Describe the three functional divisions of the adrenal cortex. Which zones produce which steroid hormones? Cells in which zone are stimulated by ACTH? By angiotensin II? How might immunohistochemical methods be used to distinguish cells in the three zones? (Hint: which enzymes would be differentially expressed in the three divisions?)

3. The gene that encodes the StAR protein has been subject to targeted deletion in StAR gene knockout (StAR-KO) mice. What effect would this have on the synthesis and secretion of steroid hormones? Why? Without any postnatal treatments, these animals die shortly after birth. Provide a plausible explanation for this finding. To allow these animals to survive into adulthood, which single hormonal treatment could be administered? Why would it likely be effective?

4. Certain tissues are only responsive to mineralocorticoids or glucocorticoids even though their receptors bind both classes of steroid with equal affinity. Provide a plausible explanation for this phenomenon.

5. The adrenal X zone has an unknown function. How would you determine its function?

6. Removal of one adrenal gland results in the hypertrophy of the remaining gland. What is the explanation for this phenomenon? Using line graphs, plot the levels of serum ACTH, as well as local adrenal concentrations of IGF-II, that you would expect to observe before and over time following unilateral adrenalectomy.

7. Atrial natriuretic factor (ANF) has numerous actions that all serve to counteract fluid volume expansion, by promoting diuresis and/or natriuresis. List the major actions of ANF, and the net effect that each of these has on diuresis and natriuresis. Devise an in vitro or in vivo bioassay that might be used to measure ANF activity in extracts of the atrium. Provide a graph containing a hypothetical standard curve that might be generated in the use of this assay. Label both axes of the graph.

8. Renin is secreted in response to hypovolemia or to an increase in the osmolarity of the blood.
   a. Provide three possible mechanisms by which these conditions may stimulate renin secretion.
   b. What are the consequences of increased renin secretion that lead to increased aldosterone secretion? Draw this sequence of events.
   c. Why are angiotensin converting enzyme (ACE) inhibitors used as a common therapy for hypertension? How do they influence blood pressure?
   d. Are plasma levels of renin elevated or depressed in a patient with Conn's disease? Why?

9. Describe three possible cellular mechanisms that may mediate the ability of aldosterone to stimulate Na^+ retention in the renal tubules.

10. The symptoms of Cushing's disease include abdominal obesity, hypertension, glucose intolerance (steroid diabetes), hirsutism, osteoporosis, polyuria, and polydipsia.
    a. Describe the consequences of cortisol excess that would produce each of these symptoms.
    b. Which tests can be performed to determine if a patient has primary or secondary Cushing's disease. What would the results of these tests be for each type of disease?

11. Individuals with Addison's disease commonly exhibit an increased pigmentation of the skin. Propose a mechanism that can account for the development of this symptom.

References

[1] Arai, K., and G. P. Chrousos. 1995. Syndromes of glucocorticoid and mineralocorticoid resistance. *Steroids* 60:173–9.

[2] Awazu, M., and I. Ichikawa. 1993. Biological significance of atrial natriuretic peptide in the kidney. *Nephron* 63:1–14.

[3] Bose, H. S., et al. 1996. The pathophysiology and genetics of congenital lipoid adrenal hyperplasia. *N. Engl. J. Med.* 335:1870–8.

[4] Botarri, S. P., M. De Gasparo, and N. R. Levens. 1993. Angiotensin II receptor subtypes: Characterization, signalling mechanisms, and possible physiological implications. *Front. Neuroendocrinol.* 14:123–71.

[5] Callard, I. P., and G. V. Callard. 1978. The adrenal gland in reptilia. In: I. Chester Jones and I. W. Henderson, eds., *General, comparative and clinical endocrinology of the adrenal cortex*, vol. 2. New York: Academic Press, pp. 419–94.

[6] Christensen, G. 1993a. Cardiovascular and renal effects of atrial natriuretic factor. *Scand. J. Clin. Lab. Invest.* 53:203–9.

[7] Christensen, G. 1993b. Release of atrial natriuretic factor. *Scand. J. Clin. Lab. Invest.* 53:91–100.

[8] Christian, J. J. 1971. Population density and reproductive efficiency. *Biol. Reprod.* 4:248–94.

[9] Clark, B. J., and D. M. Stocco. 1997. Steroidogenic acute regulatory protein: The StAR still shines brightly. *Mol. Cell. Endocrinol.* 134:1–8.

[10] Conn, J. W. 1955. Primary aldosteronism: A new clinical entity. *J. Lab. Clin. Med.* 45:3–17.

[11] Corvol, P., and X. Jeunemaitre. 1997. Molecular genetics of human hypertension: Role of angiotensinogen. *Endocr. Rev.* 18:662–77.

[12] Fardella, C. E., and W. L. Miller. 1996. Molecular biology of mineralocorticoid metabolism. *Am. Rev. Nutr.* 16:443–70.

[13] Funder, J. W. 1995. Apparent mineralocorticoid excess. *Endocrinol. Metab. Clin. North Am.* 24:613–21.

[14] Funder, J. W., et al. 1988. Mineralocorticoid action: Target tissue specificity is enzyme, not receptor, mediated. *Science* 242:583–5.

[15] Ganguly, A. 1991. Glucocorticoid-suppressible hyperaldosteronism: A paradigm of arrested adrenal zonation? *Clin. Sci.* 80:1–7.

[16] Ganong, W. F. 1993. Blood, pituitary, and brain renin-angiotensin systems and regulation of secretion of anterior pituitary gland. *Front. Neuroendocrinol.* 14:233–49.

[17] Gittler, R. D., and S. S. Fajans. 1995. Prismatic case: Primary aldosteronism (Conn's syndrome). *J. Clin. Endocrinol. Metab.* 80:3438–41.

[18] Greep, R. O., and H. W. Deane. 1947. Cytochemical evidence for the cessation of hormone production in the zona glomerulosa of the rat's adrenal cortex after prolonged treatment with desoxycorticosterone acetate. *Endocrinology* 40:417–25.

[19] Grossman, M., and J. M. Wilson. 1992. Frontiers in gene therapy: LDL receptor replacement for hypercholesterolemia. *J. Lab. Clin. Med.* 119:457–60.

[20] Hobkirk, R. 1993. Steroid sulfation. Current concepts. *TEM* 6:69–74.

[21] Holmes, W. N., and J. G. Phillips. 1976. The adrenal cortex of birds. In: I. Chester Jones and I. W. Henderson, eds., *General, comparative and clinical endocrinology of the adrenal cortex*, vol. 1. New York: Academic Press, pp. 293–420.

[22] Idelman, S. 1978. The structure of the mammalian adrenal cortex. In: I. Chester Jones and I. W. Henderson, eds., *General, comparative and clinical endocrinology of the adrenal cortex*, vol. 2. New York: Academic Press, pp. 1–199.

[23] Jones, I. C., and I. W. Henderson (eds.). 1976. *General, comparative and clinical endocrinology of the adrenal cortex*, vol. 1. New York: Academic Press.

[24] Jones, I. C., and I. W. Henderson (eds.). 1978. *General, comparative and clinical endocrinology of the adrenal cortex*, vol. 2. New York: Academic Press.

[25] Kemink, S. A. G., et al. 1997. Nelson's syndrome: A review. *The Endocrinologist* 7:5–9.

[26] Li, Y., J. Cam, and G. Bu. 2001. Low-density lipoprotein receptor family: Endocytosis and signal transduction. *Mol. Neurobiol.* 23(1):53–67.

[27] Makara, G. B., and J. Haller. 2001. Non-genomic effects of glucocorticoids in the neural system. Evidence, mechanisms and implications. *Prog. Neurobiol.* 65(4):367–90.

[28] Margolius, H. S. 1995. Kallikreins and kinins. *Hypertension* 26:221–9.

[29] Müller, J. 1993. Final steps of aldosterone biosynthesis: Molecular solution of a physiological problem. *J. Steroid Biochem. Mol. Biol.* 45:153–9.

[30] Nishihara, E., et al. 1997. A case of adrenal insufficiency due to acquired hypothalamic CRH deficiency. *Endocrinol. J.* 44:121–6.

[31] Palermo, M., M. Quinkler, and P. M. Stewart. 2004. Apparent mineralocorticoid excess syndrome: An overview. *Arq. Bras. Endocrinol. Metabol.* 48(5):687–96.

[32] Pang, S. Y. 1997. Congenital adrenal hyperplasia. *Endocrinol. Metab. Clin. North Am.* 26:853–92.

[33] Parker, K. L., and B. P. Schimmer. 1997. Steroidogenic factor 1: A key determinant of endocrine development and function. *Endocr. Rev.* 18:361–77.

[34] Penning, T. M. 1997. Molecular endocrinology of hydroxysteroid dehydrogenases. *Endocr. Rev.* 18:281–305.

[35] Phillips, M. I., E. A. Speakman, and B. Kumura. 1993. Levels of angiotensin and molecular biology of the tissue renin angiotensin systems. *Regul. Pept.* 43:1–20.

[36] Re, R. N. 2004. Tissue renin angiotensin systems. *Med. Clin. North Am.* 87:441–57.

[37] Reid, I. R. 1997. Glucocorticoid osteoporosis—mechanisms and management. *Eur. J. Endocrinol.* 137:209–17.

[38] Schild, L., et al. 1995. A mutation in the epithelial sodium channel causing Liddle disease increases channel activity in the *Xenopus laevis* oocyte expression system. *Proc. Natl. Acad. Sci. USA* 92:5699–703.

[39] Selye, H. 1976. *The stress of life.* New York: McGraw-Hill.

[40] Sewer, M. B., and M. R. Waterman. 2001. Insights into the transcriptional regulation of steroidogenic enzymes and StAR. *Rev. Endocr. Metab. Disord.* 2(3):269–74. Review.

[41] Shen, B., and S. S. El-Dahr. 2006. Cross-talk of the renin-angiotensin and kallikrein-kinin systems. *Biol. Chem.* 387(2):145–50.

[42] Shire, J. G. M. 1976. Degeneration of the adrenal X-zone in Tfm mice with inherited insensitivity to androgens. *J. Endocrinol.* 71:445–6.

[43] Sloviter, R. S., et al. 1989. Selective loss of hippocampal granule cells in the mature rat brain after adrenalectomy. *Science* 243:535–8.

[44] Stocco, D. M. 2001. Tracking the role of a star in the sky of the new millennium. *Mol. Endocrinol.* 15(8): 1245–54.

[45] Stocco, D. M., et al. 2005. Multiple signaling pathways regulating steroidogenesis and steroidogenic acute regulatory protein expression: More complicated than we thought. *Mol. Endocrinol.* 19(11):2647–59.

[46] Strott, C. A. 2002. Sulfonation and molecular action. *Endocr. Rev.* 23(5):703–32.

[47] Ullian, M. E., and J. J. Fine. 1994. Mechanisms of enhanced angiotensin II-stimulated signal transduction in vascular smooth muscle by aldosterone. *J. Cell. Physiol.* 161:201–8.

[48] Veldhuis, J. D., et al. 1980. Inborn error in the terminal step of aldosterone biosynthesis. *N. Engl. J. Med.* 303:117–21.

[49] Vinson, G., and B. Whitehead. 1992. *Adrenal cortical steroid hormones*, Prentice Hall Endocrinology Series. Englewood Cliffs, NJ: Prentice Hall.

[50] Weigel, N. L. 1996. Steroid hormone receptors and their regulation by phosphorylation. *Biochem. J.* 319:657–67.

[51] White, P. C. 2004. Aldosterone synthase deficiency and related disorders. *Mol. Cell. Endocrinol.* 31:217(1–2): 81–7.

[52] Young, W. F., Jr., 1997. Primary aldosteronism: Update on diagnosis and treatment. *The Endocrinologist* 7:213–21.

[53] Zhou, J., and J. A. Cidlowski. 2005. The human glucocorticoid receptor: One gene, multiple proteins and diverse responses. *Steroids* 70(5–7):407–17.

CHAPTER

16

Endocrinology of Sex Differentiation and Development

N o other component of the vertebrate endocrine system is as complex as the reproductive system. Although the **genetic sex** of an individual is determined by the chromosomal complement of the fertilized egg, the direction in which the gonads differentiate to produce either ovaries or testes depends on hormones secreted by the gonads. The **gonadal sex** then regulates the **phenotypic sex**. Even the development of the brain into a male or female type is dependent on early exposure to gonadal steroid hormones. The brain, in turn, affects the temporal characteristics of pituitary gonadotropin secretions that regulate further development of the gonads into functional organs capable of producing mature gametes. In addition, adult behavior is dependent on both early and late effects of gonadal steroids on the brain (Fig. 16.1).

Compared to the human male, the human adult female might be considered to possess a rather dynamic reproductive system. After puberty, the male reproductive system is rather invariant in its structural and functional characteristics. The female, on the other hand, is cyclic in her hormonal output and gonadal function. She may become pregnant, which entails radical changes in the reproductive organs to provide an environment for fetal growth and development. Unique female hormones are involved in the maintenance of pregnancy and in the induction of parturition, and additional hormones are required for milk synthesis and milk secretion. These sexually dimorphic female functions are regulated by a variety of hormones acting in concert or sequentially.

Sex Determination, Differentiation, and Development

Genetic sex, established at the time of conception, governs the development of the gonadal sex of the individual [20, 32, 50, 56]. Gonadal sex, in turn, regulates the development of phenotypic sex, that is, the differentiation of internal and external sex organs as well as attainment of adult secondary sexual characteristics [24].

Sex Chromosomes Define Genetic Sex

The genetic sex of an individual is realized at the moment the egg is fertilized by a sperm. The genes specifically related to the determination of sex are grouped together on particular chromosomes. Initially, all cells of the human body contain 22 pairs of somatic chromosomes (*autosomes*) plus a pair of *sex chromosomes*. The female possesses a pair of X chromosomes (homogametic sex), whereas the cells of the male contain an X and a Y chromosome (heterogametic sex). During gametogenesis, the diploid number of chromosomes is reduced through meiotic division to the haploid number. The female can normally only contribute an X chromosome, whereas the male may contribute either an X or a Y chromosome. The fertilized egg, the zygote, will normally develop in a female or male direction depending on whether a pair of XX or XY chromosomes are present, respectively. The Y chromosome in

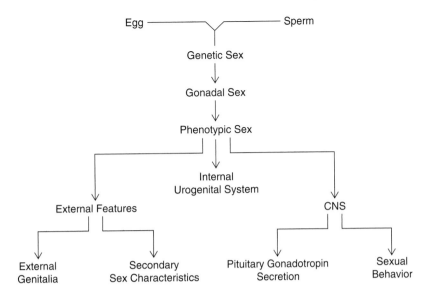

Figure 16.1
Sequential events in the determination of genetic, gonadal, and phenotypic sex.

the mammal appears to be responsible mainly for sex differentiation as any embryo without a Y chromosome develops as a female. Even humans with as many as four X chromosomes and a single Y chromosome develop into males. Random union of the male gamete with the egg ensures that approximately half the progeny will be females and half will be males. Differential survival or other attributes of the X- and Y-bearing sperms may thwart the theoretical sex ratio.

The majority of vertebrates have a sex-determining scheme (XX/XY) of male heterogamety or a scheme of female heterogamety (ZW/ZZ). In birds and reptiles, the W chromosome of the heterogametic female (ZW) induces differentiation of the ovary. In fishes and amphibians the male or female of certain species may be heterogametic. Some species of fishes are even *synchronous* or *asynchronous hermaphrodites*, that is, they are able to shed both eggs and sperm at the same time or, alternately, one or the other of the gametes during a particular developmental state. In reptiles all-female parthenogenic (egg development in the absence of activation by a sperm) or gynogenic (activation of the egg by a sperm without any genetic material being contributed) species have been discovered. Although the genetic sex of the species determines the direction in which the gonads initially differentiate, the exogenous administration of sex steroids at a critical time (which differs between species) can induce permanent gonadal sex reversal.

Gonadal Sex is Determined by SRY Gene Expression in the Male, and its Absence in the Female

The undifferentiated gonad has generally been considered to be composed of cortical and medullary regions. In the male, sex differentiation of the gonads involves development of the medullary primordium and suppression of the cortex. In the female, on the other hand, the cortical region develops, whereas medullary differentiation is suppressed. The development of these two anatomical components was for years theorized to be controlled by hypothetical corticomedullary inductive substances, the production of which was related to whether an XX or XY chromosomal complement was present. It is now proposed that the undifferentiated primordium normally tends to develop toward the female in the mammal unless influenced by genes located on the Y chromosome. Mammalian testicular organogenesis is dependent on a product (testis-determining factor, TDF) of the SRY gene (sex-determining region Y gene, denoted as Sry in the mouse and SRY in the human) localized to the short arm of the Y chromosome [19, 29, 32]. TDF, a protein, possesses a DNA-binding sequence known as the HMG (high mobility group) factor that alters the expression of other genes [12]. This suggests a role for TDF as the master switch for other genes downstream in the course of sexual differentiation (Fig. 16.2) [18].

When female mouse embryos carrying the normal pair of X chromosomes are injected with a small fragment of Y chromosome DNA containing the Sry gene, they grow up as males

Figure 16.2   Role of the Sry/SRY antigen in the determination of gonadal sex.

with testes and male behavior. The Y chromosome triggers the genital ridges in the embryo to develop into testes rather than ovaries. Once that happens, all the other changes that make a male animal follow under the influence of hormones produced by the testes. The SRY gene is only a switch; testes can develop in XX women who have no portion of the Y chromosome. Also, in cattle, some genetic females develop testes. These observations suggest that the genes needed to turn the indifferent genital ridge of the embryo into male gonads are also present in the female. However, the gene that normally triggers this change is present only in the male. One important question relates to what switches on the SRY gene. Some XY women appear to have no mutation in the SRY gene [26]. Maybe there is a mutation "upstream" of the SRY gene that regulates its activation [19, 29].

The testes differentiate under the influence of the Y chromosome during the seventh week of gestation in the human, whereas ovarian development usually does not proceed before 13 to 16 weeks. Two X chromosomes appear to be essential for the development of normal ovaries as individuals with a single X chromosome develop gonads that are only partially differentiated.

The presumptive gonadal primordia are composed of coelomic epithelia, underlying mesenchyme, and primordial germ cells. The gonadal anlagen are visible in the 4-week-old human embryo as a pair of genital ridges. The primordial germ cells, the gonocytes, arise in the yolk sac endoderm, move to the mesoderm of the gut, and seed the undifferentiated gonads by migration from the hindgut [6]. The course of migration of the gonocytes may be oriented by some chemotactic substance elaborated by the gonadal anlagen. During the migration of the primordial germ cells, the coelomic epithelium invades to varying degrees the underlying mesenchyme of the presumptive gonads to form the primary sex cords. At this stage, the gonads are *indifferent*, or *bipotential*, in that, depending on the genetic sex of the individual, the gonads will develop into either testes or ovaries. An early sign of sexual differentiation is seen in the distribution pattern of the primordial germ cells. The germ cells of XX embryos remain in the periphery away from the central somatic blastema of the gonad, whereas the germ cells of the XY embryo invade the center of the blastema. Thus, germ cells are attracted not only to the primordial gonads but also to the cortical or medullary regions, depending on whether they are of XX or XY genotype, respectively. Whether these primordial germ cells subsequently undergo spermatogenesis or oogenesis depends on early organizational influences of the SRY gene on gonadal differentiation into either a testis or an ovary. In some nonmammalian vertebrates, although the germ cells normally become spermatocytes or oocytes, *sex reversal* is easily accomplished by early administration of steroids. For example, in the goldfish, presumptive male (XY) embryos can be transformed into phenotypic females by estrogens; they can be subsequently mated to normal males (XY) to produce viable male (YY) offspring [57]. In the medaka (*Oryzias latipes*), in which the presumptive female fish (XX) was converted to a phenotypic male by an androgen, subsequent mating with a normal female (XX) resulted in all-female (XX) progeny.

The primitive gonads of the male and female embryos, which appear morphologically identical, are composed of three components: the primordial germ cells, the mesenchyme of the genital ridge, and a covering layer of epithelium. In the male, the primitive sex cords, which are initially solid, develop into the seminiferous tubules (Fig. 16.3). These ducts subsequently branch and their terminal endings anastomose to form the rete testis, which transports sperm to the epididymis. The seminiferous tubules are lined with epithelial cells that differentiate into *Sertoli cells*; the gonocytes become embedded within these sustentacular cells of Sertoli. The *interstitial cells of Leydig* arise from intertubular elements of the seminiferous tubules; these cells are the source of androgen necessary for development of the accessory sexual organs (e.g., prostate gland), but they disappear shortly after birth and do not become abundant until the onset of adolescence. The developing seminiferous tubules become separated by a connective tissue layer, the tunica albuginea, from the remnant of the coelomic epithelium, which atrophies into the so-called "tunica vaginalis."

In the primitive ovary, the coelomic epithelium undergoes proliferation, and strands of epithelial cells, the primary sex cords, move into the interior of the gonad to form a rete ovarii, which subsequently degenerates and disappears. Later in fetal development, secondary sex cords extend into the underlying mesenchyme (Fig. 16.3). The primordial germ cells are carried along within the proliferating inward migration of the secondary sex (cortical) cords. Some germ cells within the sex cords become isolated and form primordial follicles at about 16 weeks of gestation in the human female.

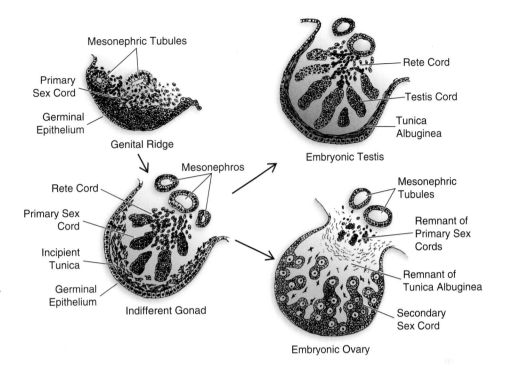

Figure 16.3
Diagrammatic representation of the development of the mammalian ovary and testis from a bipotential primordial gonad. (Prepared by Dr. R. B. Chiasson, University of Arizona.)

Phenotypric Sex of the Genital Ducts Depends on the Presence or Absence of AMH and Androgens

The definitive internal reproductive organs consist of tubular passageways for the exit of gametes produced by the gonads. Glands associated with these structures may contribute various secretions that aid in the dissemination and function of the gametes. During the undifferentiated stage, both Müllerian and Wolffian ducts are present. Development of the female or male accessory sex organs involves differentiation of the Müllerian or Wolffian ducts, respectively, with the concomitant loss of the other. Differentiation of the Müllerian ducts results in formation of the Fallopian tubes, with associated uterus and vagina. Differentiation of the Wolffian ducts, on the other hand, results in the development of the epididymis, ductus deferens, and seminal vesicles.

In the absence of the ovaries or testes, the Müllerian duct system develops and Wolffian ducts atrophy, suggesting that in the former these events are not dependent on any gonadal directive. Atrophy of the Wolffian ducts in the female may represent *programmed cell death (apoptosis)*, a common phenomenon of developmental processes (Chap. 12). In the male fetus, on the other hand, the testes produce a *Müllerian regression factor/inhibitor (MRF/MIF)*, also known as *antiMüllerian hormone* (AMH) [18, 26], which is a glycoprotein consisting of a dimeric structure, a member of the transforming growth factor-β family of peptides (Chap. 12). AMH acts to induce Müllerian duct atrophy [26, 51]. Maintenance and further development of the Wolffian ducts, however, are dependent on the presence of testicular androgen (and possibly, to some minor extent, AMH). AMH is secreted by the Sertoli cells of the fetal testes [26, 41, 43, 51]. It exerts a local effect rather than a systemic one, as unilateral castration in the fetal male rat and rabbit results in female duct development on the side where the testis was removed, and the contralateral duct develops along male lines. The AMH gene is also expressed by granulosa cells of the ovarian follicle, where it may function to regulate the early stages of folliculogenesis.

Occasionally male infants are born with morphologically normal testes but an apparent inability to synthesize androgenic steroids. In these individuals the Müllerian ducts still atrophy, suggesting that AMH is nevertheless still present and not an androgen. In the *persistent Müllerian duct syndrome,* genetic and phenotypic males have Fallopian tubes and a uterus together with male Wolffian duct structures. The underlying defect may be a failure to produce a functional AMH or to an inability of the tissue to respond to the hormone [22]. The development of the male or female urogenital tracts is shown schematically (Fig. 16.4).

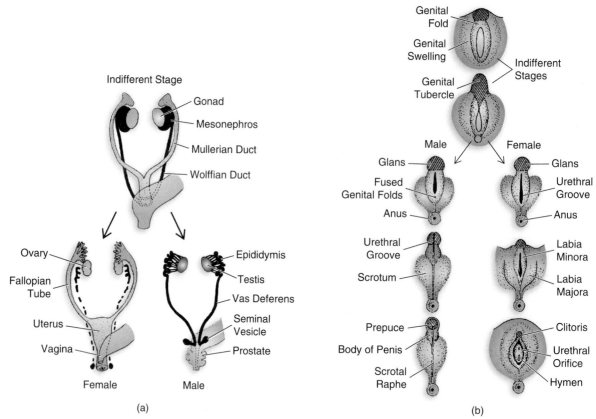

Figure 16.4 Embryogenesis of the male and female phenotypes. (a) Formation of the internal organs of accessory reproduction. (b) Formation of the external genitalia. (From Wilson et al. with permission. "The Hormonal Control of Sexual Development." *Science*, vol. 211, pp. 1278–1284, March 20, 1981. © 1981 by The American Association for the Advancement of Science.)

Phenotypic Sex of the External Genitalia Depends on the Presence or Absence of Androgens

As with the ovary and internal urogenital ducts, the external genitalia develop a female phenotype in the absence of the Y chromosome. Differentiation of the male external genitalia is dependent solely on androgen production by the testes. Development of the penis and scrotum commences shortly after onset of Wolffian duct development. The genital folds elongate and fuse to form the penis and male urethra. The urogenital swellings on each side of the urethral orifice form a bilobed scrotum into which the testes descend (Fig. 16.4). In the female embryo, the genital tubercle becomes the clitoris and the adjacent genital swellings give rise to the labia majora; the genital folds become the labia minora (Fig. 16.4). Removal of the gonads from indifferent embryos of either sex results in development of a female genotype, demonstrating that the male is the induced phenotype.

Of critical importance in development of the external genitalia is the timing of androgen action [54]. In the female fetus, for example, the external genitalia may become masculinized if androgen levels are elevated as in *congenital adrenal hyperplasia* (Chap. 15). Androgens originating from the maternal circulation can also cause genital masculinization in the female fetus; except for clitoral hypertrophy, androgen excess at a later time (eleventh to twelfth week) is without effect. The role of the Y chromosome and gonadal hormones in the differentiation and development of the mammalian reproductive system is shown in Figure 16.5.

Gonadal Steroid Hormone Synthesis and Chemistry

Gonadal steroids are produced by mesodermally derived tissues of the testes and ovaries. The same desmolase system as found in the adrenal is responsible for the first biosynthetic step in steroidogenesis. The nature of the stimulus that activates testosterone biosynthesis in

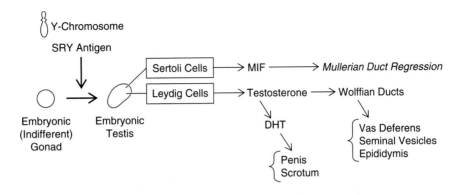

Figure 16.5 The role of the Y chromosome and gonadal hormones in the differentiation and development of the mammalian reproductive system.

the fetal testis is unknown. There is experimental evidence that testes or ovaries of rabbit embryos synthesize testosterone or estradiol, respectively, in media devoid of hormones. It appears, therefore, that differentiation of gonads as endocrine organs is controlled by factors intrinsic to the gonads themselves. It is also possible that during early development the need for gonadotropins, which in the adult normally control conversion of cholesterol to pregnenolone, is circumvented by the presence of C-21 steroids of placental origin.

Unlike the adrenal, 17α-hydroxylase activity is dominant and, through conversion of pregnenolone to 17α-hydroxypregnenolone and 17α-hydroxyprogesterone, provides substrates for androgen biosynthesis. In the testes, testosterone is the major androgen secreted (Fig. 16.6) [23].

Figure 16.6 Biosynthesis of gonadal steroid hormones in the vertebrate testes and ovaries.

Figure 16.7
Cellular conversion
of testosterone to
dihydrotestosterone.

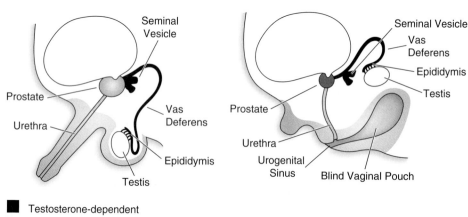

Testosterone

5 α-Reductase

Dihydrotestosterone

In the ovary, androstenedione and testosterone serve as precursors for estrogen formation. Estradiol (E_2) is the major estrogen produced by the ovaries. The key reaction in the ovary is *aromatization* of the A ring of the steroid nucleus. The first step in this reaction involves the hydroxylation of the C-19 carbon followed by removal of the newly formed hydroxymethyl group from the steroid nucleus. The A ring is then aromatized to yield a phenolic hydroxyl group at the C-3 position (Fig. 16.6).

In some tissues, testosterone is converted by 5α-reductase activity to dihydrotestosterone (DHT) (Fig. 16.7). The rudiments of the external genitalia and prostate (the urogenital tubercle and sinus) convert testosterone to DHT, which is then responsible for the development of these organs. The importance of DHT formation in certain tissues for normal virilization is revealed in rare anomalies of male development that are due to the absence of 5α-reductase activity (Fig. 16.8) [7, 21].

Although the ovary differentiates much later than the testes, the enzymatic machinery for estrogen synthesis is developed at the same time as the processes for androgen biosynthesis in the testes. It is unclear whether ovarian estrogen synthesis is important in the development of the human female fetus. Possibly estrogens synthesized by the ovary play a role, as does testosterone in the testes, in the maturation of the ovaries. Sexual differentiation is a sequential, ordered process. During development, the genotype of the zygote determines the nature of the gonad, which then determines the male or female phenotype (primary and secondary sex characteristics). A single treatment of chicken embryos with an aromatase inhibitor (which blocks the synthesis of estrogen from testosterone) at a stage when their gonads are biopotential causes genetic females to develop a permanent male phenotype. These sex-reversed females develop bilateral testes that are capable of complete spermatogenesis and have the physical appearance and behavior of normal males. These results identify aromatase as a key developmental switch in the sex determination of chickens [5, 13, 40].

Whether the male or the female is the heterogametic sex has an important bearing on the role of hormones in gonadal and phenotypic development. In those species that bear young

Seminal
Vesicle

Seminal Vesicle

Vas
Deferens

Epididymis

Testis

Prostate

Vas
Deferens

Prostate

Urethra

Urethra

Epididymis

Urogenital
Sinus

Blind Vaginal Pouch

Testis

■ Testosterone-dependent

☐ Dihydrotestosterone-dependent

Figure 16.8 Illustration of the hypothesis for the role of testosterone and dihydrotestosterone in male sexual differentiation in utero. (From Imperato-McGinley et al., with permission. "Steroid 5 α-reductase deficiency in man: An inherited form of male pseudohermaphroditism." *Science* 186:1213–15. © 1974 by The American Association for the Advancement of Science.)

outside their body (e.g., egg layers), the heterogametic sex may be either male or female. Most mammals, on the other hand, grow and develop in a maternal environment characterized by elevated levels of estrogens. It is likely, therefore, that to protect the genetic male from the influence of estrogens, evolution favored development of the female as the neutral sex. Rather than devising a mechanism of protecting the male from the feminine influence, differentiation toward the male gonadal and body phenotype requires the inductive actions of gonadal androgens. All aspects of human female development, ovarian as well as internal genital ducts and external genitalia, are essentially autonomous processes apparently requiring no hormonally active inductive substances. It has been said that the male mammal is "merely a female that has been subjected to induction by testosterone" [41]. This is not really true since factors other than an androgen (e.g., TDF, MRF) are necessary for normal male sexual development.

Gonadal Steroids and Brain Differentiation

In adult male mammals, there is a tonic (generally uniform) secretion of pituitary gonadotropins, whereas in adult female mammals, secretion of these pituitary hormones is cyclic in nature, that is, the amount of gonadotropins released usually follows a recurrent pattern characteristic of the species. Cyclic *estrous* behavior, the ovarian cycle of ovum maturation and ovulation, as well as the cyclic growth of the uterus, are phenomena dependent on the cyclicity of pituitary gonadotropin secretion (Chap. 18). Questions arise as to the mechanisms controlling such cyclic or noncyclic reproductive events in mammals. Experiments have established that transplantation of the pituitary from a male or female rat to the opposite sex did not alter the normal reproductive processes in either sex. These observations revealed that the pituitaries were equivalent and could not be responsible for the cyclicity or noncyclicity of pituitary gonadotropin secretion. In contrast to the tonic uniform secretion of pituitary gonadotropins in the intact adult male rat, these hormones are released cyclically (as in the female) in adult neonatally castrated male rats. Transplantation of an ovary into adult rats of either sex that had been neonatally castrated did not alter the function of the ovary whether or not it was transplanted into the inappropriate sex. In other words, in the adult (neonatally castrated) male rat, the ovaries cycled (ovulated) normally as in the female. Transplantation of ovaries into male rats castrated as adults produced different results. Ovaries transplanted into these rats failed to cycle. These results suggested that control of pituitary hormone secretion and subsequent gonadal function depends on a system that was programmed early in development and was not localized to the pituitary or gonads.

It was subsequently discovered that a single injection of testosterone into a female rat during a *critical period* (a few days postnatally) resulted in adults that were acyclic. In addition, these ("androgen sterilized") females exhibited male sexual behavior (mounting of other females). These results were consistent with earlier observations that transplanted ovaries only became functional if the transplant was into a neonatally castrated male rat rather than into an intact adult male rat. Apparently, testosterone secreted by the neonatal testes of the male conditioned the animals so that pituitary gonadotropin secretion in the adult animal was tonic rather than cyclic. Similar results were obtained by implantations of testosterone into the hypothalamus (but not other sites), suggesting that the locus of testosterone action was at the level of the hypothalamus, a postulate compatible with the emerging evidence at that time that pituitary hormone secretion is regulated by the brain, particularly the hypothalamus (Chap. 6).

Organizational Effects of Androgens Mediate Male-Type Brain Development

The studies just discussed suggest that deprivation of testosterone in the male animal during his species-specific critical time of brain differentiation will result in a female pattern of sexually dimorphic behavior. Such male animals will assume the female mating posture (lordosis) when administered estrogen but will not mount females even when injected with testosterone. From these studies of androgen effects on the neonatal rodent emerged the hypothesis that testosterone was not only responsible for differentiation of the internal and external genitalia, but was of critical importance for normal differentiation of the brain into the male type (Fig. 16.9). Maximal sensitivity of the hypothalamus to testosterone may be associated with a particular stage of neuronal maturation. Thyroid hormones are known to affect maturation of the central

Figure 16.9 Effects of castration and testosterone administration in the neonatal rat on subsequent adult male and female behavior [33].

nervous system (CNS), and an altered thyroid hormone status such as hyperthyroidism or hypothyroidism shortens or prolongs, respectively, the postnatal period during which the rat brain centers controlling gonadotropin secretion can be differentiated by testosterone. In species that are relatively less mature at birth (e.g., pigeons and many rodents), the critical period extends into postnatal life, whereas in animals more fully developed at birth, the critical period may be predominantly prenatal.

One observation was particularly difficult to reconcile with this hypothesis: estradiol also masculinized the brain of either the male or female rodent. This dilemma was solved when it was discovered that testosterone is aromatized to E_2 within the brain. Several experimental lines of evidence support the hypothesis of androgen-to-estrogen conversion.

1. The effects of testosterone treatment in neonatal female rats are blocked by prior administration of specific estrogen- (but not androgen-) receptor antagonists.

2. The brain possesses the aromatase enzymes required for conversion of testosterone to E_2.

3. Dihydrotestosterone does not mimic the effect of testosterone on neonatal brain differentiation, thus revealing that the actions of testosterone are not mediated through its conversion to DHT. In addition, DHT cannot be converted to E_2.

4. [^{3}H]-labeled testosterone is recovered from the brain mainly as [^{3}H]-labeled estradiol.

5. Aromatase inhibitors impair brain differentiation in response to perinatal testosterone administration.

6. In the Tfm (testicular feminization mutation) mouse, which has greatly reduced levels of androgen receptors, testosterone causes brain differentiations, as it does in normal mice.

7. Targeting of both the estrogen receptor alpha (ERα) and estrogen receptor beta (ERβ) genes eliminates sexual behavior in male mice [25, 36].

Thus, it appears that in addition to its hormonal role on a number of target tissues testosterone serves as a prohormone for DHT biosynthesis in some tissues and for E_2 production within the brain (Fig. 16.10) [33, 34, 45]. If E_2 is indeed responsible for brain differentiation in the male, why is not the brain of the female also masculinized, as E_2 is the major gonadal steroid of the female? First, E_2 production by the fetal ovaries may be minimal. Second, a circulating α-fetoprotein (fetoneonatal estrogen-binding protein, FEBP) is present in high levels within the blood of the fetus and apparently has a specific binding affinity for E_2. Theoretically, therefore, no E_2 is available to reach the brain of the female fetus. The *FEBP protection hypothesis* is supported by the observation that administration of antibodies to the protein produces effects similar to testosterone injections. Synthetic estrogens that exhibit little binding affinity for FEBP also effectively masculinize the fetal brain.

E_2 (derived from testosterone) is available in the male at a critical time in development to regulate the differentiation of the brain, but the mechanisms by which E_2 is able to alter irreversibly the brain and subsequent sexual behavior are unclear. Although the brains of males and females differ physiologically, do they also differ anatomically? It has been discovered

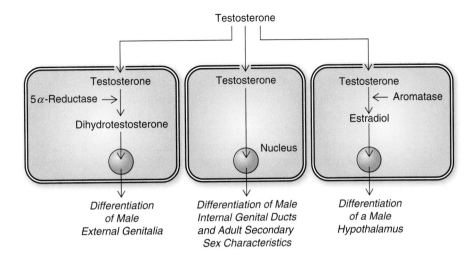

Figure 16.10
Testosterone:
Prohormone for
dihydrotestosterone
and estradiol in certain
target tissues.

that in the rodent there are sex-related differences in the distribution of synaptic connections of nerve cells of the preoptic area (POA) of the brain [38, 47]. The female pattern of synaptic contacts is established if males are castrated before the critical period of fetal development. On the other hand, the male pattern of synaptic distribution is established if newborn female animals are given testosterone. The *sexually dimorphic nucleus* of the preoptic area of the rat is actually visible with the naked eye, and is at least five times larger in the male than in the female. A sexually dimorphic nucleus has also been described for the human brain [1]. The volume of the nucleus is several times as large in men as in women and contains over twice as many cell bodies. This nucleus is located in the preoptic area of the hypothalamus, an area that is essential for gonadotropin release and sexual behavior in other animals. In other areas of the hypothalamus, sexual dimorphisms have been observed where the greater neuronal density is present in the female compared to the male. This is true for the anteroventral periventricular (AVPV) nucleus of the hypothalamus, which is known to be critically important in the neural control of preovulatory gonadotropin surges and ovulatory cyclicity. Thus, a denser neuropil is present in the AVPV of the female, compared to the same neural area in the male. Perinatal testosterone or estrogen injections in female rats can produce the male AVPV phenotype in adulthood. In this case, it is the absence of perinatal androgen that is permissive for the development of an enriched neuronal population, while the presence of androgen during the critical period causes a reduction in cell number.

The cellular mechanisms by which E_2 affects neonatal brain maturation appear similar to those controlling steroid hormone effects on other tissues. Nuclear chromatin binding and subsequent transcriptional and translational events leading to protein synthesis are involved. The ultimate effects of E_2 may involve neuronal growth and neurotransmitter synthesis. By using an in vitro system, it was shown that E_2 and testosterone (but not DHT) enhanced neurite outgrowth from explants of newborn mouse preoptic tissue [49]. These steroid hormone effects are anatomically specific, as other brain regions do not respond similarly. In addition, immunohistochemical studies have revealed that the number and connectivity of certain neurotransmitter-producing neuronal populations, such as basal forebrain dopaminergic neurons, are sexually differentiated in patterns that can be recapitulated in the opposite sex by appropriate treatments during the perinatal critical period [47]. These observations provide clear evidence that there are sex differences in the anatomy, biochemistry, and plasticity of certain regions of the brain and that some of these differences are organized perinatally by testosterone action via aromatization to E_2 [45]. In Chapter 17, we discuss whether the sexually dimorphic nucleus as an anatomical substrate for the action of steroids is responsible for homosexuality. In other words, is homosexuality biological [3]?

Activational Effects of Gonadal Steroids Evoke Acute Neuroendocrine and Behavioral Responses

The permanent actions of gonadal steroid hormones on differentiation and development of the brain led to the proposal that gonadal steroids can have two types of action, either organizational or activational, depending on the developmental state of the CNS [11, 52].

The *organizational effects* of steroids refer to the actual maturation processes leading to development of the dimorphic nuclear center of the POA and possibly other nuclear centers of the brain. The *activational effects* of steroid hormones refer to the actions on acute release of pituitary gonadotropins and to sexual behaviors associated with reproductive processes. In contrast to the organizational effects of gonadal steroids on brain differentiation and function, the activational effects of hormones are reversible, repeatable, and not limited to a critical phase of development. In adult animals, steroid hormones released by the gonads play important roles in regulating behavioral events that relate to reproductive success. Gonadal steroid hormones in the fetus, as discussed, affect the organization of the brain into a sexually dimorphic adult organ. The mechanisms by which the activational effects of steroid hormones are expressed will now be considered.

Control of Pituitary Gonadotropin Secretion. There is evidence, particularly from studies in the female rat, that the AVPV, as well as the preoptic area (POA), are important sites of gonadal steroid hormone action related to the cyclic release of pituitary gonadotropins. The key stimulus for release of the preovulatory surge of gonadotropins is estradiol, and estradiol receptors are abundant in these areas of the brain [39]. It is believed that during the estrous cycle of the female rat, for example, neural stimuli and endocrine signals (estrogen) converge in AVPV neurons, activate them, and they in turn stimulate the GnRH neurons located in the POA and adjacent septal tissues. This stimulation results in a surge of gonadotropin-releasing hormone (GnRH) secretion responsible for the midcycle surge of pituitary gonadotropin (LH) secretion, which, in turn, is then responsible for ovulation. In the male rat, the "masculinized" AVPV is not capable of responding to the neuroendocrine signals that can prompt GnRH surges in females; GnRH release in the male rat thus remains at a continuously basal level.

Testosterone and Behavior in Humans. Although aggressive behavior is a characteristic of violent individuals, it is not consistently related to increased plasma testosterone levels. Individuals with chronic low levels of testosterone, due to genetic abnormalities in steroid biosynthesis, especially if occurring before puberty, exhibit reduced aggression and diminished sexual drive. Exogenously administered testosterone is often effective in restoring sexual interest and overt sexual behavior.

Some synthetic progestins have androgenic activity. In recent decades, millions of pregnant women were treated with progestins and estrogens to prevent miscarriage. It has been discovered that individuals exposed to synthetic progestins during gestation show a significantly higher potential for physical aggression (tomboyism) than their sex-matched unexposed siblings [42]. It would appear that the mechanisms controlling hormone-organized behaviors as reported in laboratory animals may also apply to human behavior.

Gonadal Steroids and Gender Identification. Psychologists in general have argued that although sexual behavior is influenced by hormones, sexual identity is socially determined. In other words, a child will identify with whatever sex he or she is brought up to be as a child. However, pubertal shifts from female to male gender identity in an interrelated group of male pseudohermaphrodites from two rural communities in the Dominican Republic have been described [21]. Feminization of the external genitalia in these males results from a defect or absence of 5α-reductase activity. Although these individuals were brought up initially as girls, they took on male sexual identities at puberty. It was postulated on the basis of these observations that their prenatal exposure to testosterone irreversibly shaped their sexual behavior. According to these investigators, this "experiment of nature" emphasizes the importance of androgens in an organizational as well as activational role (at puberty) in the evolution of male-gender identity [21]. This interpretation has raised the argument of "nature versus nurture" relative to the basis of gender identification in humans. From other studies, however, there is evidence that in male pseudohermaphrodites reared unambiguously as females their postpubertal gender remained consistent with their sex upbringing.

Androgens and Mathematical Ability. A most controversial hypothesis that has been put forward is that math genius may have a hormonal basis [48]. It has been proposed that excess testosterone or an unusual sensitivity to testosterone during fetal life can alter brain anatomy, so that the right hemisphere of the brain becomes dominant; and it is generally thought that mathematical ability is a function of the right side of the brain. It is possible that boys who are exposed to more testosterone than normal in utero would be more likely than girls to be affected. It is also possible, however, that males might have a severe defect in mathematical ability if androgen production during gestation were affected. Uncontrolled social factors inevitably present major confounds in the assessment of any biologically-based sex differences in average mathematical ability, and thus the issue will probably remain unresolved for the foreseeable future.

Activational Roles of Gonadal Steroids in Nonmammalian Vertebrates. Castration eliminates sex behavior in the frog, *Xenopus laevis*; clasping behavior is restored by administration of exogenous testosterone, but not by estradiol. Three distinct populations of gonadal hormone-concentrating cells are present in the brain of *Xenopus*; "testosterone only" cells, "estradiol only" cells, and cells labeled after administration of either hormone. These latter cells may represent neurons where testosterone is converted to estradiol [30]. The regions of hormone uptake are also known to be involved in the neural control of frog sex behavior. Sex behavior in some frogs therefore may depend on testosterone production by the testes and subsequent interaction with one or more nuclear centers within the brain where the hormone may act directly or be converted to E_2. Seasonal initiation of sex behavior would necessitate pituitary gonadotropin secretion to initiate androgen production by the testes.

In birds, the homogametic sex is male, and differentiation of the female CNS phenotype occurs as a result of exposure to ovarian hormones [2, 4]. E_2 appears to be the ovarian product responsible for feminine differentiation. For example, embryonic exposure to an antiestrogen masculinizes behavior in female quail; these birds exhibit the male mating pattern as adults in response to testosterone. Androgens play an important role in the control of song in male birds. Castration abolishes song in some birds; singing can be restored by exogenous testosterone administration. There are specialized brain areas concerned with the production of sound in some birds. In the zebra finch (*Poephila guttata*) all the brain nuclei of the song system are much larger in males than females. Early exposure of the chick to estradiol or dihydrotestosterone influences the establishment of the differences in functional capacity and brain architecture in the zebra finch [9]. When a neonatal female zebra finch is exposed to E_2, her system is subsequently masculinized. Testosterone or dihydrotestosterone then can induce such a female to sing when an adult. These observations suggest that the female zebra finch is the neutral sex with respect to sexual differentiation of the song system [9].

Singing is also a typical behavioral characteristic of the male canary. Ovariectomized adult canaries can be induced to sing by administration of testosterone. Some brain nuclei that compose the efferent pathway for control of song in the canary have been shown to concentrate tritiated androgen. The nucleus robustus archistriatalis (RA) of the forebrain is highly dimorphic in the adult canary, the overall volume being much greater in the male bird. Injections of testosterone into ovariectomized female canaries increase the volume of the RA as well as the length of the dendrites of this nucleus to a state resembling that of the male canary. Although steroid hormones are normally responsible for an organizational effect on the neonatal brain, results reveal that steroid hormones can induce plasticity in the adult brain [30].

In the male canary, two telencephalic nuclei that control song are much larger in the spring when the birds sing than in the fall after several songless months [35]. Such fluctuations may reflect an increase and then a reduction in the numbers of synapses within the brain and may be related to the yearly ability to acquire new motor coordination. According to this hypothesis presented by Nottebohm, "The plastic substrate for vocal learning is renewed once yearly, a growing, then a shedding of synapses, much the way trees grow leaves in the spring and shed them in the fall." This species of bird truly has "a brain for all seasons" [35].

The distribution of gonadal steroid hormone receptors in the brains of members of all vertebrate classes has been determined [30]. Estrophilic neurons are localized predominantly in the medial preoptic area, the mediobasal hypothalamus, and in specific limbic areas of the brain. The distribution of androgen receptors is similar, but not identical between species. Generally, the neural distribution of gonadal steroid receptors, although characteristic of the species, is independent of genetic or phenotypic sex [30]. In the zebra finch, androphilic cells are found exclusively in brain regions that are the control sites of androgen-dependent song. In the spinal cord of the male rat, a group of androgen-concentrating neurons are present in the lumbar region; these neurons, absent in the female, innervate striated muscles of the penis. The existence of gonadal steroid-binding sites in the members of diverse vertebrate groups suggests that binding of these hormones by nerve cells is a general vertebrate phenomenon.

Puberty

Although androgens produced by the fetal testes play a prominent role in the early development of the internal urogenital system and the external genital organs, as well as in brain differentiation, the Leydig cells subsequently become quiescent and remain so until activated much later by gonadotropins from the pituitary. The ovaries of the female also remain relatively inactive during preadolescence. In response to gonadotropin-induced gonadal steroidogenesis, there is a growth spurt and maturation of the gonads. The state at which the gonads come to maturity relative to their endocrine and gametogenic potential for reproductive function is referred to as *puberty*. The average age of puberty is variable between ethnic groups and individuals within any one group, but is about 12.5 to 13 years for the female and 14 years for the male. The timing of puberty in some mammals may be controlled by melatonin, a hormone synthesized and secreted by the pineal gland (Chap. 20) [8]. The adrenal glands of children begin to secrete increased amounts of androgens between 6 and 8 years of age. This change in the preexisting pattern of adrenal steroid secretion occurs before puberty and in the absence of increased ACTH or cortisol secretion. This change in androgen secretion is called the *adrenarche*, and it is accompanied clinically as *pubarche*, the appearance of axillary and pubic hair. There is also a transient acceleration of bone growth and maturation. The biological role and cause of adrenarche is unknown, and puberty can occur in the absence of adrenarche [39, 46].

Advanced maturation of girls may be associated with an accentuation of the abdominal accumulation of subcutaneous fat. Girls with body fat that was predominantly abdominal were found to be more obese and to show increased plasma levels of total E_2 and a lower androgen/estrogen ratio in plasma, possibly due to increased aromatization, especially in abdominal adipose tissue. The findings suggest a reciprocal relationship between body fat distribution, plasma sex hormone levels, and availability of sex steroids in early female puberty.

Critical body weight or a critical amount of body fat is required for first ovulation and menarche. Body fat distribution, rather than body fat mass or body weight, appears to be related to early pubertal endocrine activity. Body fat mass and especially body fat distribution, which are affected by life-style factors such as nutritional intake and physical activities, therefore may be related to hormonal and physical parameters of early puberty [8]. It is believed that the adipocyte-derived hormone leptin, as well as other peripheral metabolic and somatic signals, may function as permissive cues for the activation of GnRH neurosecretion during pubertal maturation. In support of this idea, it has been determined that mutant ob/ob mice, which do not produce leptin, exhibit a failure of puberty that can be reversed by leptin replacement therapy [31].

Among the many physical changes occurring during puberty is a dramatic increase in the overall rate of body growth. There is considerable evidence that this pubertal growth spurt is associated with changes in endogenous growth hormone (GH) levels. Elevated levels in IGF-I concentrations also reflect associated changes in GH concentrations. Enhanced testosterone secretion at puberty may be responsible for enhancing GH secretion, most likely after it is aromatized to E_2. GH and IGF-I levels return to prepubertal levels in early adulthood, whereas sex steroid hormone levels do not decrease [27].

Precocious and Delayed Puberty can have Constitutional or Pathophysiological Origins

Sexual maturity may occur earlier or later than normal; a number of possible factors determine the etiology of such divergent development [17]. *True precocious puberty* is defined as the attainment of sexual maturity at an earlier than normal age. This sexual precociousness may be of a constitutional (genetic) nature, or it may result from disorders of the hypothalamus that result in enhanced GnRH secretion. GnRH analogs can be used to treat precocious puberty due to enhanced gonadotropin secretion. *Precocious pseudopuberty*, on the other hand, characterizes the situation where there is a development of secondary sexual

TABLE 16.1 Endocrine pathophysiology of sexual differentiation and development

Chromosomal disorders (a few examples)
    Gonadal dysgenesis (Turner's syndrome), XO karyotype
        Female phenotype but lack of secondary sexual characteristics (sexual infantilism)
    Seminiferous tubule dysgenesis (Klinefelter's syndrome) XXY karyotype
        Normal male genitalia and male characteristics but seminiferous tubules are abnormal
Hermaphroditism
    True hermaphroditism (mosaicism)
        Both ovarian and testicular components present; equivocal external genitalia
    Male pseudohermaphroditism (testes present but partial or nearly complete female internal and external phenotypes)
        Deficient 17-ketosteroid reductase activity
        Congenital adrenal hyperplasia (due to block in pregnenolone formation)
        Leydig cell agenesis (or hypoplasia)
        Syndromes of androgen resistance
            Testicular feminizing syndrome (absence of target tissue androgen receptors)
            Syndrome of 5α-reductase deficiency (failure to convert testosterone to DHT)
    Female pseudohermaphroditism
        Congenital virilizing adrenal hyperplasia (due to enzyme defect in cortisol biosynthesis)
        Progestogen administration to the mother during fetal development
Sexual precocity (precocious puberty)
    Complete (increased gonadotropin secretion of pituitary or ectopic origin)
    Incomplete (precocious pseudopuberty; development of secondary sex characteristics but lack of gametogenesis)
        Adrenal steroid-secreting tumors (androgens or estrogens)
        Adrenal hyperplasia (e.g., 11β-hydroxylase or 21α-hydroxylase deficiencies; increased adrenal androgen production)
        Early masculinization in the male, masculinization of the female

characteristics without gametogenesis. The problem is that there are excessive levels of circulating steroids, either of gonadal or of adrenal origin. In *congenital adrenal hyperplasia*, excessive amounts of adrenal androgens are produced and may cause early virilization and pseudohermaphroditism (see later discussion) in the female. Interstitial cell tumors of the gonads or sex steroid-secreting tumors of the adrenal glands are also sources of excessive levels of estrogens or androgens (Table 16.1). The high levels of circulating steroids exert a negative feedback inhibition of hypothalamic release of GnRH. In the absence of pituitary gonadotropin secretion, there is a failure of gametogenesis, but the secondary sexual characteristics that normally develop at puberty are well developed. The pubertal process can also be delayed possibly due to panhypopituitarism, where all pituitary hormones, including the gonadotropins, are absent. A defect at the level of the hypothalamus or an isolated deficiency in follicle-stimulating hormone (FSH) or LH secretion could also be responsible for a delayed onset of puberty.

Pubertal Development is Driven by an Activation of the Hypothalamic "GnRH Pulse Generator"

Large fluctuations in blood and urine levels of gonadotropins, androgens, and estrogens occur during development, but lowest levels are present in the preadolescent years. During the prepubertal period, the output of gonadotropins is constant, except for minor fluctuations during the day and night. Surges in gonadotropin secretion occur during sleep in the early stages of puberty, which may indicate that pubertal maturation has begun. By late puberty, there are large fluctuations in gonadotropin secretion that extend throughout the day and night. Gonadotropin secretion in the postpubertal period becomes more uniform again, but at a level about double that of prepubertal individuals.

A number of theories have been put forward to account for the onset of puberty. No one theory provides all the necessary information, but it is likely that there are elements of truth in all the models. The *missing-link hypothesis* suggests that some component of the brain-pituitary-gonadal axis is missing or nonfunctional. The pituitary of immature animals is competent as it secretes normal amounts of gonadotropins when transplanted under the hypothalamus of an adult animal. The ovaries and testes of immature animals are also potentially functional, as they, too, become active when transplanted into adult animals or when stimulated by gonadotropins. These observations reveal that the brain, rather than the pituitary or gonads, is the site that is functionally incompetent prior to puberty.

Another hypothesis suggests that there is a decrease in hypothalamic sensitivity to feedback inhibition by gonadal steroids. Such a change would account for the higher circulating titers of gonadotropins present after puberty. This *gonadostat hypothesis* is supported by the observation that lesions of the hypothalamus often result in enhanced gonadotropin secretion. Also, castration of immature animals leads to an increase in pituitary gonadotropin secretion. Individuals lacking functional ovaries (as in Turner's syndrome) have high circulating levels of FSH and LH long before puberty, which could be evidence that the gonads depress gonadotropic hormone secretion in infancy. The administration of an estrogen elicits the discharge of FSH and LH during puberty, but not in infancy, which suggests that the mechanisms involved in such positive feedback have matured. It is even possible that an increased rate of androgen aromatization in the brain may be responsible for an alteration in hypothalamic sensitivity that results in initiation of the pubertal process.

In the primate, there is convincing evidence that neither adenohypophysial nor ovarian competence is limiting in the initiation of puberty; rather, the process depends on the maturation of the neuroendocrine control system that directs the pulsatile secretion of GnRH from the hypothalamus. For example, normal ovulatory menstrual cycles have been initiated in the prepubertal female rhesus monkey by hourly infusions of GnRH. These animals revert to the immature stage when administration of GnRH is discontinued [55]. Direct measurements of pulsatile GnRH release have been carried out in peripubertal female rhesus monkeys [53], and they confirm that the frequency of pulsatile GnRH neurosecretion is increased in association with the pubertal rise in gonadotropin and gonadal steroid secretions. These findings clearly demonstrate that pubertal maturation is driven by an acceleration of the GnRH pulse generator. However, they also beg the question "What triggers the pubertal acceleration of the hypothalamic GnRH pulse generator?" To a large extent this remains a mystery, although strong cases have been built for a variety of afferent synaptic neurotransmitters, glial cell products, growth factors, and prostaglandins as contributing to the cascade of signals that may activate GnRH pulsatility in pubertal animals [37].

It is also clear that pubertal maturation is linked to the metabolic status of the individual. It has been proposed that puberty occurs in the human female at a critical weight or with a particular body fat composition. In the rat, for example, puberty is reached at a set body size rather than at a specific age [15]. Compelling support derives from the clinical observation that patients with anorexia nervosa and amenorrhea have a prepubertal or early pubertal pattern of gonadotropin secretion, which is reversed to the adult pattern in response to a weight gain. Also, leanness associated with strenuous physical activity is linked with delayed puberty, whereas the *menarche* (time of first menstruation) is usually early in obese individuals. For example, among young ballet dancers, there is a high incidence of primary amenorrhea (failure to initiate the first menstrual cycle), secondary amenorrhea (loss of previously established menstrual cycle), and irregular cycles, which are clearly correlated with excessive thinness [15]. High school and college athletes also have a statistically significant later age of menarche than do nonathletes. A change in the fat/lean ratio may affect metabolism and hormone levels, which may delay menarche and menstrual cycles. It is likely that peripheral metabolic signals, including leptin, insulin, IGF-I, and glucose, collectively provide permissive signals for the activation and maintenance of accelerated GnRH pulsatility during pubertal maturation. Reduction in these metabolic cues may thus explain the failure of puberty, and reversion to the prepubertal neuroendocrine state, in individuals with sustained negative energy balance. The cellular mechanisms mediating these metabolic regulatory effects remain unknown.

Nevertheless, according to the "critical weight hypothesis" (as described before), a young female cannot ovulate for the first time until she has accumulated a critical amount of fat relative to her lean body mass. Likewise, the adult female will cease to ovulate if her fat reserves fall below this critical level. It has been suggested that the evolutionary basis for this hypothetical dependency is the need to delay pregnancy and lactation until the female has accumulated sufficient energy reserves to sustain these activities in the face of food shortage [44].

Pathophysiology of Sex Differentiation and Development

Because of the complexity of the reproductive system, it is no surprise that there are many events that can account for abnormalities in sexual development (Table 16.1). Most defects have a genetic basis, and they may result from a failure of gonadal differentiation, defective steroid hormone biosynthesis or a failure of steroid hormone action on target tissues [10, 17].

Gonadal Dysgenesis is a Failure of Normal Gonadal Differentiation

Disorders of gonadal differentiation include syndromes of *gonadal dysgenesis*, in which a normal 46,XX or 46,XY karyotype is accompanied by a failure of normal gonadal development. In pure gonadal dysgenesis, gonadal development fails before the stage at which they would normally produce AMH and androgens, and thus the individual bears a female sexual phenotype. Gonadal dysgenesis can occur as a result of mutations in the SRY gene. It can also result from mutations in other genes encoding transcription factors, which in turn regulate target genes that are critical for early gonadal development and differentiation.

Pseudohermaphroditism can Result from Defects in Fetal Steroid Synthesis or End-Organ Resistance

In the male or female, gonadal steroid imbalance in the fetus results in *hermaphroditism*. A *true hermaphrodite*, a rare condition, is one who possesses both ovarian as well as testicular tissue. A *male pseudohermaphrodite* is one whose gonads are exclusively testes, but whose genital ducts or external genitalia or both exhibit a female phenotype or that of an incompletely differentiated male. Individuals possessing exclusively ovarian gonadal structures, but whose external genitalia exhibit some masculine characteristics, are considered *female pseudohermaphrodites*.

In those individuals in which female pseudohermaphroditism has an endocrine basis the ambiguity of the external genitalia is due to excess levels of circulating androgens. The degree of virilization depends on the amount and period (developmental time) of exposure to androgens. Female pseudohermaphroditism in most patients is due to *congenital adrenal hyperplasia*. There are several types of congenital adrenal hyperplasia, and the etiology of each relates to a specific defect in steroid biosynthesis, usually a failure in cortisol production. In the absence of cortisol biosynthesis, there is a lack of negative feedback inhibition to the hypothalamus, which results in increased ACTH release and subsequently enhanced stimulation of adrenocortical steroid biosynthesis (Chap. 15). However, the metabolites that accumulate due to enzymatic failure to convert them to cortisol and aldosterone are shunted to pathways of androgen production. The androgens that are now secreted in excess are responsible for virilization of the external genitalia, as well as development of masculine secondary sexual characteristics.

Male pseudohermaphroditism may result from sex chromosomal anomalies, mutant genes, or teratologic factors that lead to defective gonadogenesis. Testosterone is synthesized by the Leydig cells of the testes in response to LH of pituitary origin. There is evidence that male pseudohermaphroditism in some individuals may result from a defect in the LH receptors of fetal Leydig cells. A number of inborn errors of testosterone production can also account for development of hermaphroditism in the male. Three enzymes, which include the cholesterol desmolase complex, 3β-hydroxysteroid dehydrogenase, and 17α-hydroxylase, are present in both the adrenals and testes. Failure of their enzymatic function results in an abnormality of glucocorticoid and mineralocorticoid synthesis, as well as androgen production. These enzyme defects may be partial or complete and are caused by autosomal or X-linked recessive mutations (Table 16.1).

Syndrome of 5α-Reductase Deficiency. Evidence from a familial group of individuals in the Dominican Republic has provided important insights into genetically based male pseudo-hermaphroditism [14, 21]. Failure to virilize certain androgen-dependent structures results from a lack of 5α-reductase activity in these target tissues. The affected individuals had bilateral inguinal or labial testes and a labial-like scrotum at birth; there were no Müllerian structures, but Wolffian structures were well developed. These developmental characteristics clearly reveal the anatomically specific target tissue responses to testosterone and the near absence of DHT-dependent structures. At puberty there was striking virilization of testosterone-dependent secondary sex characteristics: axillary and pubic hair growth, deepening of the voice, increased muscle mass, and an enlargement of the phallus to a near functional size. The enhancement of the phallus mass, which is a developmentally DHT-dependent structure, may have been due to the very high circulating levels of testosterone in these individuals. Affected men had less facial and body hair and less temporal hairline recession than unaffected men from the same families. Acne was absent, and the prostate glands failed to develop. Thus, it appears that the sexual characteristics absent in these individuals are those mainly regulated by DHT. Because of the extreme defect in the development of the external genitalia, male pseudohermaphrodites are usually raised as females [21]. Figure 16.8 depicts the structural changes from the normal male reproductive anatomy that are a consequence of a defect in 5α-reductase.

Syndrome of Testicular Feminization. A number of single gene mutations involve defects in production of androgen-binding protein receptors that lead to the syndrome of testicular feminization. Males with this syndrome have testes and normal (or higher) rates of testosterone secretion, but they are almost completely insensitive to exogenous or endogenous androgen action. These individuals are therefore phenotypic females, often with a truly feminine appearance. Although the external genitalia are unambiguously female and the clitoris normal, the vagina is short and blind ended and the internal genitalia are absent, except for a testis that may be in the abdomen, inguinal canal, or labia majora. Androgen resistance is due to abnormalities of the androgen receptor; the receptor protein is either absent or defective in structure (receptor-negative resistance). That the Wolffian ducts fail to differentiate and external genitalia do not develop indicate that both testosterone and DHT receptors are involved. The absence of Müllerian ducts and their derivatives in the otherwise phenotypic females indicates that the action of MRF has not been compromised. Another type of androgen resistance does not appear to involve either a defect in 5α-reductase activity or cytosolic androgen receptors. The site of the molecular abnormality probably resides at one or more sites distal to the receptor (receptor-positive resistance, see Chap. 17).

Hypogonadism and Hypergonadism can have Gonadal, Pituitary, or Hypothalamic Bases

As noted previously, hermaphroditism may result from a failure in steroid hormone biosynthesis or in end-organ resistance. Defects in the normal development of secondary sex characteristics at puberty may result from defects that reside at the level of the gonads (primary), at the level of the pituitary (secondary), or even at the level of the hypothalamus (tertiary) (Fig. 16.11a). Primary hypogonadism might relate to a failure in production of gonadal steroids due to any one of a number of causes. Failure in a negative feedback inhibition at the pituitary (or hypothalamus) by steroid hormones would lead to enhanced gonadotropin secretion in the face of hypogonadism (hypergonadotropic hypogonadism, Fig. 16.11b). Secondary hypogonadism, on the other hand, could result from a defect in pituitary gonadotropin secretion (hypogonadotropic hypogonadism, Fig. 16.11c). Hypergonadism involving overproduction of gonadal steroids could relate to a primary defect (hypogonadotropic hypergonadism) at the gonads involving a tumorous condition of the steroid-secreting cells (Leydig cells in the male or follicular thecal cells in the female, Fig. 16.11d) or to a secondary defect (hypergonadotropic hypergonadism) involving overproduction of pituitary gonadotropins (Fig. 16.11e).

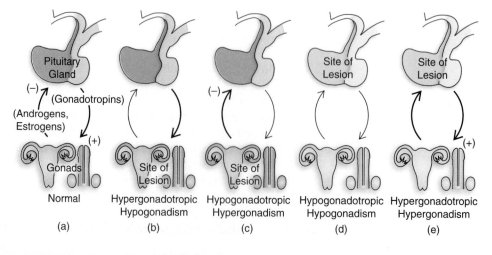

Figure 16.11 Primary (gonadal) or secondary (pituitary) defects causing underproduction or overproduction of gonadal steroids with concomitant effects on pituitary gonadotropin secretion are depicted. The site of the lesion, at either the gonads or the pituitary, is indicated (*).

Normal
(a)

Hypergonadotropic Hypogonadism
(b)

Hypogonadotropic Hypergonadism
(c)

Hypogonadotropic Hypogonadism
(d)

Hypergonadotropic Hypergonadism
(e)

Hypogonadotropic hypogonadism can result from a failure in the normal migration of GnRH neurons from embryonic olfactory placode into the forebrain (Chap. 6), rendering individuals incapable of releasing GnRH into the hypophysial portal vessels. When associated with anosmia, this condition is known as Kallman's syndrome, and it may result from heritable mutations in the KAL gene or other genes that are important in sustaining the GnRH neuronal migratory process. Many cases of hypogonadotropic hypogonadism are not associated with anosmia or other symptoms of Kallman's syndrome, and are likely a result of genetic mutations that are yet to be identified. Recent studies have demonstrated that mutations in a gene encoding a hypothalamic peptide called "kisspeptin," or mutations in the gene encoding its cognate receptor, GPR54, produce a profound hypogonadotropism that is accompanied by a failure of puberty. Experiments in animals have confirmed that this peptide is a critically important transynaptic regulator of GnRH neurosecretion, thereby explaining the absence of pubertal maturation in this subset of hypogonadotropic subjects.

Hypogonadotropic hypogonadism due to a deficiency in GnRH is common in female athletes. Strenuous physical exercise alters the activity of various neuroendocrine systems, and in women, an exercise-induced deficiency of hypothalamic secretion of GnRH results in the syndrome of "hypothalamic amenorrhea" (Chap. 18). Highly trained male athletes, like their female counterparts, may also have a deficiency of GnRH. In habitual athletes of either sex, repeated early increases in stress hormones and gonadal steroids during prolonged periods of intense exercise may eventually cause a suppression of GnRH secretion, leading to hypogonadotropic hypogonadism. The release of GnRH may also be suppressed by the condition of negative energy balance per se, independent of alterations in stress hormone secretions. The mechanisms that mediated these effects remain unclear, but appear to be caused by a reduction in the availability of oxidizable metabolic fuels, a circumstance that is somehow registered by the neuronal circuitries that govern GnRH neurosecretion and transduced into a reduced level of GnRH neuronal activity [44].

GnRH treatment has been used to induce puberty in children with constitutional delay of growth and puberty, and in children with hypogonadotropic hypogonadism. It is possible to mimic the endocrinology, ovarian morphology, secondary sexual characteristics, and growth acceleration of normal puberty. During induction of puberty using pulsatile GnRH treatment, larger doses of GnRH are required in boys than in girls in order to make equivalent progress through puberty. It would appear that girls secrete gonadotropin from the pituitary at a lower threshold of GnRH stimulation than do boys. This may explain why the physical signs of puberty appear slightly earlier in girls than in boys, why idiopathic central precocious puberty is more common in girls, and why constitutional delay of puberty is more common in boys.

Mice homozygous for the hypogonadal (*hpg*) mutation are sexually immature, and germ-cell development is arrested. These mice lack detectable levels of hypothalamic gonadotropin-releasing hormone (GnRH), leading to low levels of LH and FSH. Introduction of a GnRH gene into the genome of these mutant mice resulted in a complete reversal of the hypogonadal state. Transgenic animals homozygous for the *hpg* allele developed fully their reproductive functions. Pituitary and serum levels of LH, FSH, and prolactin were restored to those of normal animals. Immunocytochemistry revealed that GnRH expression was restored in the appropriate hypothalamic neurons of the mice, indicating the neural-specific expression of the introduced gene. The use of gene replacement to rescue the *hpg* mutation illustrates the potential use of gene therapy [28].

Fertility in the hypogonadal mouse has also been restored by transplantation of normal fetal preoptic-area tissue, the major site of GnRH-containing cell bodies, into the third ventricle of adult female hypogonadal mice [16]. Immunocytochemistry revealed GnRH-containing neurons in the grafts and GnRH-containing neuron processes extending to the lateral median eminence of the host brains. These results demonstrate the plasticity of these peptidergic neurons and their functional integration within the brain.

Alcohol and Gonadal Function. There is compelling evidence that ethanol abuse is associated with, and is the most probable cause of, Leydig cell failure in men who are chronic alcoholics. Alcohol abuse is associated with (1) induction of aromatase activity, resulting in an increased androgen-to-estrogen conversion by nonhepatic tissues (e.g., adipose tissue); (2) Leydig cell damage and subsequent diminished binding of gonadotropins to Leydig cell receptors; (3) decreased cAMP levels within Leydig cells; and (4) disturbed steroidogenic enzyme activity within microsomes of these cells. In addition, elevated levels of plasma estrogens may suppress gonadotropin secretion. Enhanced estrogen-to-androgen ratios might then lead to feminization. In rats, there is evidence that prenatal alcohol exposure alters the adult expression of sexually dimorphic behavior.

The endocrine pathophysiology of sexual differentiation and development is summarized in Table 16.1.

MOLECULAR MEDICINE CASE STUDY

"Familial Mutation in the Testis-Determining Gene SRY Shared by an XY Female and Her Normal Father." Jordan et al. *J. Clin. Endocrinol. Metab.* 2002 Jul;87(7):3428–32.

In humans, mutations in the testis-determining gene SRY result in XY sex reversal with pure gonadal dysgenesis (PGD). However, only about 10–15% of the cases of PGD can be explained by mutations within the SRY open reading frame, suggesting the existence of other sex-determining genes. Although SRY is known to bind and bend DNA, its target and mode of action remain elusive. Here, we describe a novel mutation in SRY at codon 127, resulting in a tyrosine (Y) to phenylalanine (F) substitution in the protein. This sequence variant was found not only in the XY female patient but also in her father, who is a phenotypically normal male. However, this Y127F variant was not found in the SRY sequences of 93 other randomly chosen males. This substitution affects a highly conserved tyrosine residue in the HMG box of SRY, in which two de novo mutations have been described previously in XY females with PGD. Furthermore, electromobility shift studies demonstrate that SRY protein harboring the Y127F variant is incapable of binding consensus SRY binding sites in vitro. Taken together, these data suggest that the Y127F variant is a novel mutation with functional consequences and not simply a polymorphism. The allelic variant of SRY transmitted in this family and shared by both a phenotypic female (proband) and a phenotypic male (proband's father) emphasizes the importance of modifier genes in the sex determination pathway.

REVIEW EXERCISES

Match the steroid with its direct steroid precursor:

1. Pregnenolone
2. Progesterone
3. 17α-OH-Progesterone
4. Androstenedione
5. Testosterone
6. Estradiol

A. Progesterone
B. Cholesterol
C. Androstenedione
D. Pregnenolone
E. Testosterone
F. 17α-OH-Progesterone

Think, analyze and discuss:

1. Each individual possesses a genetic sex, gonadal sex, and phenotypic sex.
   a. Describe and compare the defining characteristics of each of these in most male vs. female mammals.
   b. An XX mouse is developed which carries a transgene expressing the TDF protein. Predict the genetic, gonadal, and phenotypic sex of this mouse.
   c. What would be the genetic, gonadal, and phenotypic sex of an XY mouse that bears an inactivating mutation of the SRY gene?

2. Describe the sex phenotype of a male infant who has an inability to synthesize AMH. Which reproductive tissues would be present? Would the same be true for a male infant whose testes lack the ability to synthesize androgens?

3. If a genetic female fetus is exposed to testosterone in utero, would that individual develop a complete male phenotypic sex, a partial male phenotypic sex, or a normal female phenotypic sex? Explain your answer, describing the sex phenotype of the gonads, internal genital ducts, and external genitalia. What would be the developmental outcomes be if the fetus were instead exposed to dihydrotestosterone in utero?

4. Consider an experiment in which rat pups receive the indicated treatments (next page) on the day following their birth. Predict the sexual behavior, pattern of gonadotropin secretions, volume of the SDN, and volume of the AVPV in these animals in adulthood.

Treatments	Sexual behavior (mounting or lordosis)	Gonadotropin secretion (cyclic versus tonic)	Volume of the SDN of the preoptic area (large versus small)	Volume of the AVPV (large versus small)
XY, castration	_____	_____	_____	_____
XX, castration	_____	_____	_____	_____
XX, testosterone 1	_____	_____	_____	_____
XY, castration plus testosterone	_____	_____	_____	_____
XY, castration plus estrogen	_____	_____	_____	_____

5. Why is brain masculinization relatively normal in the XY Tfm mouse, in which androgen receptor expression is deficient? Would it be normal in animals (e.g., rats or mice) perinatally exposed to an aromatase inhibitor? Why or why not?

6. Sex steroids do not affect gonadal sex determination in mammals. Are there effects of sex steroids on gonadal sex determination in birds, amphibians, or fish?

7. Would you expect sex steroids to have organizing effects on behavior in fish that are hermaphrodites? Explain your answer. Do you think that sex steroids would have activational effects on behavior in fish that are hermaphrodites? Explain your answer.

8. When prepubertal female rats are maintained on a stringent, low-calorie diet, they will typically fail to achieve pubertal maturation. Can you explain why this happens? Besides allowing them to feed ad libitum, what treatments might be used to stimulate pubertal development in these food-restricted animals? Propose a hypothesis for the adaptive significance of this mechanism, that is, the tendency for negative energy balance to be accompanied by a suppression of reproductive hormone secretions.

9. Retrospective population studies have suggested that the average age of menarche has declined in developed countries over the past century. Can you provide a reasonable hypothesis that might explain this phenomenon?

10. What are the sexual characteristics of XY individuals who bear a genetic mutation of the 5α-reductase gene? Why are some sexual characteristics affected by the genetic mutation, and not others?

11. In females with congenital adrenal hyperplasia (CAH), a defect in one of the enzymes involved in the production of cortisol can give rise to a partially virilized sex phenotype. Describe how a defect in this steroidogenic pathway can give rise to the characteristics of CAH.

References

[1] Allen, L. S., and R. A. Gorski. 1992. Sexual orientation and the size of the anterior commissure in the human brain. *Proc. Natl. Acad. Sci. USA* 89:7199–202.

[2] Arnold, A. P., et al. 1996. Sexual differentiation of the brain in songbirds. *Dev. Neurosci.* 18:124–36.

[3] Bocklandt, S., and D. H. Hamer. 2003. Beyond hormones: A novel hypothesis for the biological basis of male sexual orientation. *J. Endocrinol. Invest.* 26(3 Suppl.):8–12. Review.

[4] Bottjer, S. W., and A. P. Arnold. 1997. Developmental plasticity in neural circuits for a learned behavior. *Annu. Rev. Neurosci.* 20:459–81.

[5] Bruggeman, V., P. Van As, and E. Decuypere. 2002. Developmental endocrinology of the reproductive axis in the chicken embryo. *Comp. Biochem. Physiol. A Mol. Integr. Physiol.* 131(4):839–46.

[6] Buehr, M. 1997. The primordial germ cells of mammals: Some current perspectives. *Exp. Cell Res.* 232:194–207.

[7] Cai, Li-Q., et al. 1996. 5α-Reductase—2 gene mutations in the Dominican Republic. *J. Clin. Endocrinol. Med.* 81:1730–35.

[8] Clark, P. A., and A. D. Rogol. 1996. Growth hormones and sex steroid interactions at puberty. *Endocrinol. Metab. Clin. North Am.* 25:665–81.

[9] Devoogd, T. J. 1991. Endocrine modulation of the development and adult function of the avian song system. *Psychoneuroendocrinology* 16:41–66.

[10] DiMeglio, L. A., and O. H. Pescovitz. 1997. Disorders of puberty: Inactivating and activating molecular mutations. *J. Pediatr.* 131:58–12.

[11] Doupe, A. J. 1996. Plasticity of a different feather. *Science* 274:1851–53.

[12] Dubin, R. A., and H. Ostrer. 1994. Sry is a transcriptional activator. *Mol. Endocrinol.* 94:1182–92.

[13] Elbrecht, A., and R. G. Smith. 1992. Aromatase enzyme activity and sex determination in chickens. *Science* 255:467–70.

[14] Fratianni, C. M., and J. Imperato-McGinley. 1994. The syndrome of 5α-reductase deficiency. *The Endocrinologist* 4:302–14.

[15] Frisch, R. E., G. Wyshak, and L. Vincent. 1980. Delayed menarche and amenorrhea in ballet dancers. *N. Engl. J. Med.* 303:17–19.

[16] Gibson, M. J., et al. 1984. Mating and pregnancy can occur in genetically hypogonadal mice with preoptic area brain grafts. *Science* 225:949–51.

[17] Grumbach, M. M. 2002. The neuroendocrinology of human puberty revisited. *Horm. Res.* 57(Suppl. 2):2–14.

[18] Haqq, C. M., et al. 1994. Molecular basis of mammalian sexual determination: Activation of Müllerian inhibiting substance gene expression by SRY. *Science* 266:1494–500.

[19] Harley, V. R., M. J. Clarkson, and A. Argentaro. 2003. The molecular action and regulation of the testis-determining factors, SRY (sex-determining region on the Y chromosome) and SOX9 [SRY-related high-mobility group (HMG) box 9]. *Endocr. Rev.* 24(4):466–87.

[20] Hunter, R. H. 1995. *Sex determination, differentiation and intersexuality in placental mammals.* Cambridge: Cambridge University Press.

[21] Imperato-McGinley, J., et al. 1979. Androgens and the evolution of male-gender identity among male pseudohermaphrodites with 5α-reductase deficiency. *N. Engl. J. Med.* 300:1233–37.

[22] Josso, N., et al. 1997. Clinical aspects and molecular genetics of the persistent Müllerian duct syndrome. *Clin. Endocrinol.* 47:137–44.

[23] Labrie, F., et al. 1997. The key role of 17β-hydroxysteroid dehydrogenases in sex steroid biology. *Steroids* 62:148–58.

[24] Lillie, F. R. 1916. The theory of the free-martin. *Science* 43:611–13.

[25] Lindzey, J., and K. S. Korach. 1997. Developmental and physiological effects of estrogen receptor gene disruption in mice. *TEM* 8:137–44.

[26] MacLaughlin, D. T., and P. K. Donahoe. 2004. Sex determination and differentiation. *N. Engl. J. Med.* 350(4):367–78. Review.

[27] Martha, P. M., and E. O. Reiter. 1991. Pubertal growth and growth hormone secretion. *Endocrinol. Metab. Clin. North Am.* 20:165–81.

[28] Mason, A. J., et al. 1986. The hypogonadal mouse: Reproductive functions restored by gene therapy. *Science* 234:1372–8.

[29] Marx, J. 1995. Snaring the genes that divide the sexes for mammals. *Science* 269:1824–25.

[30] McEwen, B. S., and S. E. Alves. 1999. Estrogen actions in the central nervous system. *Endocr. Rev.* 20(3):279–307.

[31] Mounzih, K., R. Lu, and F. F. Chehab. 1997. Leptin treatment rescues the sterility of genetically obese ob/ob males. *Endocrinology* 138(3):1190–3.

[32] Nagai, K. 1996. Molecular basis governing primary sex in mammals. *Jpn. J. Human Genet.* 41:363–79.

[33] Nef, S., and L. F. Parada. 2000. Hormones in male sexual development. *Genes Dev.* 14(24):3075–86.

[34] Negri-Cesi, P., A. Poletti, and F. Celotti. 1996. Metabolism of steroids in the brain: A new insight into the role of 5α-reductase and aromatase in brain differentiation and functions. *J. Steroid Biochem. Mol. Biol.* 58:455–66.

[35] Nottebohm, F. 1981. A brain for all seasons: Cyclical anatomical changes in song control nuclei of the canary brain. *Science* 214:1368–70.

[36] Ogawa, S., et al. 2000. Abolition of male sexual behaviors in mice lacking estrogen receptors alpha and beta (alpha beta ERKO). *Proc. Natl. Acad. Sci. USA* 97(26):14737–41.

[37] Ojeda, S. R., et al. 2006. Minireview: The neuroendocrine regulation of puberty: Is the time ripe for a systems biology approach? *Endocrinology* 147(3):1166–74.

[38] Panzica, G. C., et al. 1995. Structural sex differences in the brain: Influence of gonadal steroids and behavioral correlates. *J. Endocrinol. Invest.* 18:232–52.

[39] Parker, L. N. 1991. Adrenarche. *Endocrinol. Metab. Clin. North Am.* 20:71–83.

[40] Piferrer, F., et al. 1994. Brief treatment with an aromatase inhibitor during sex differentiation causes chromosomally female salmon to develop as normal, functional males. *J. Exp. Zool.* 62:270–255.

[41] Price, D., et al. 1975. Current views on embryonic sex differentiation in reptiles, birds, and mammals. *Am. Zool.* 15(Suppl. 1):173–95.

[42] Reinisch, J. M. 1981. Prenatal exposure to synthetic progestins increases potential for aggression in humans. *Science* 211:1171–3.

[43] Rey, R., and N. Josso. 1996. Regulation of testicular anti-Müllerian hormone secretion. *Eur. J. Endocrinol.* 135:144–52.

[44] Schneider, J. E. 2004. Energy balance and reproduction. *Physiol. Behav.* 81(2):289–317.

[45] Shinoda, K. 1994. Brain aromatization and its associated structures. *Endocrine J.* 41:115–38.

[46] Siegel, S. F., et al. 1992. Premature pubarche: Etiological heterogeneity. *J. Clin. Endocrinol. Metab.* 74:239–47.

[47] Simerly, R. B. 2002. Wired for reproduction: Organization and development of sexually dimorphic circuits in the mammalian forebrain. *Annu. Rev. Neurosci.* 25:507–36.

[48] Spelke, E. S. 2005. Sex differences in intrinsic aptitude for mathematics and science?: a critical review. *Am. Psychol.* 60(9):950–8.

[49] Swaab, D. F., and E. Fliers. 1985. A sexually dimorphic nucleus in the human brain. *Science* 228:1112–14.

[50] Swain, A. and R. Lovell-Badge. 1999. Mammalian sex determination: A molecular drama. *Genes Dev.* 13(7):755–67.

[51] Teixeira, J., S. Maheswaran, and P. K. Donahoe. 2001. Mullerian inhibiting substance: An instructive developmental hormone with diagnostic and possible therapeutic applications. *Endocr. Rev.* 22(5):657–74.

[52] Tobet, S. A., and I. K. Hanna. 1997. Ontogeny of sex differences in the mammalian hypothalamus and preoptic area. *Cell. Mol. Neurobiol.* 17:565–601.

[53] Watanabe, G., and E. Terasawa. 1989. In vivo release of luteinizing hormone releasing hormone increases with puberty in the female rhesus monkey. *Endocrinology* 125(1):92–9.

[54] Wiener, J. S., et al. 1997. Molecular biology and function of the androgen receptor in genital development. *J. Urol.* 157:1377–85.

[55] Wildt, L., G. Marshall, and E. Knobil. 1980. Experimental induction of puberty in the infantile female rhesus monkey. *Science* 207:1373–5.

[56] Wolf, U. 1995. The molecular genetics of human sex determination. *J. Mol. Med.* 73:325–31.

[57] Yamamoto, T. 1975. A YY male goldfish from mating estrone-induced XY female and normal male. *J. Hered.* 66:2–4.

Hormones and Male Reproductive Physiology

*C*astration of young males to provide eunuchs was a custom of some earlier societies. Eunuchs fail to develop the secondary sex characteristics that typify postadolescent development of the normal male. The physiological basis for this atypical male development was not understood, but it was undoubtedly obvious that the testes must have provided some stimulus to normal male development. As early as 1771, Hunter was able to induce male characteristics in the hen by transplantation of testes from a rooster; spontaneous sex reversal in the hen had been noted to be associated with conversion of an ovary to a testis. In 1849, Berthold showed that transplantation of the gonads into castrated roosters prevented loss of male secondary sex characteristics and sexual behavior (Chap. 1). In 1889, Brown-Séquard popularized the notion of the role of testes in the maintenance of virility by his claim that testicular extracts administered to himself restored vigor.

An active androgenic substance (androsterone) was first isolated from the urine of men by Butenandt in 1931. Testicular extracts were prepared in 1927 and the major androgenic principle was soon isolated in crystalline form. The chemical structure of this testicular androgenic principle was elucidated and synthesized by Ruzicka and Wettstein in 1935, and appropriately named **testosterone**. The role of testosterone and other hormones in the control of normal and abnormal sexual development in humans and other vertebrates is the topic of this chapter.

Anatomy of the Male Reproductive System

In the human fetus, the indifferent gonads of the genetic male are induced to differentiate into testes. The fetal testes, in turn, produce testosterone, which is responsible for differentiation and development of the urogenital system characteristic of the male. The testes become quiescent until puberty when they are activated by pituitary gonadotropins (see Chap. 16).

The development of the male phenotype involves at least two distinct sets of genes. The first comprises those genes that must be expressed for the undifferentiated gonad to form a testis and includes the SRY gene on the Y chromosome encoding the testis-determining factor. Somatic cells of the developing testis express anti-Müllerian hormone (AMH) causing regression of the Müllerian ducts that would otherwise form female reproductive tract structures. Development of male reproductive tract structures and secondary sexual characteristics are, however, androgen-dependent. Thus, not only must the undifferentiated gonad form a testis, but the fetal testis must begin to synthesize androgens at a critical time during testicular differentiation. Complete development of the male phenotype, therefore, requires expression of a second set of genes encoding the enzymes required for conversion of cholesterol to the male sex steroid hormones testosterone and 5α-dihydrotestosterone.

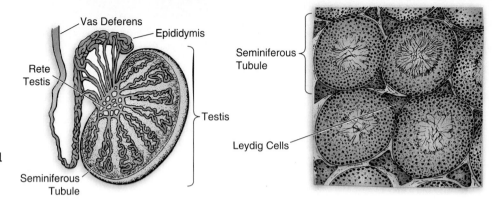

Figure 17.1 Gross and microscopic anatomy of the human testis.

The Major Functions of the Testes are Spermatogenesis and Steroidogenesis

The two primary physiological functions of the adult testes are to provide an environment for spermatogenesis and to secrete testosterone to regulate a variety of bodily functions related to male reproductive function. In the human adult male, the testes are located within the scrotum; each testis is ovoid in shape and is about 4 to 6 cm in length and 2 to 3 cm in diameter. A connective tissue sheath, the tunica albuginea, encapsulates each testis. The testis consists of convoluted *seminiferous tubules* within which sperms are produced. These tubules converge into the rete testis, which opens to efferential ductules to the *epididymis*. The epididymis is composed of a head (caput), body (corpus), and the tail, which connects directly with the vas deferens (Fig. 17.1). The outer sheet of the seminiferous tubules is made up of connective tissue and smooth muscle; the inner lining is composed of Sertoli cells within which are embedded the spermatogonia and various stages of immature as well as mature sperms. The suggestion that the Sertoli cells provide nutrients and other factors necessary for sperm maturation is compatible with the observation that the germ cells are, indeed, embedded deeply amongst the Sertoli cells. The fully matured spermatozoa, spermatids, are released into the lumen of the seminiferous tubules and subsequently advance slowly to the rete testis and epididymis where they are stored within the tail. Between the seminiferous tubules are found the interstitial cells of Leydig, the cellular source of androgen production within the testes (Fig. 17.1).

Source, Synthesis, Chemistry, and Metabolism of Androgens

As in adrenal steroidogenic tissue, cholesterol serves as the substrate for pregnenolone biosynthesis in the Leydig cells. Extracellular low-density lipoproteins are the major substrate for androgen production by Leydig cells. Unlike in the adrenal, however, conversion of pregnenolone to 17-hydroxylated steroids provides the predominant steroidogenic pathway in testicular interstitial tissue. The conversion of pregnenolone to progesterone with subsequent 17-hydroxylation appears not to provide an important pathway in humans. The 17-hydroxysteroids are converted by side-chain cleavage to 17-ketosteroids, and these, in turn, are converted to testosterone. Testosterone is the principal steroid produced by Leydig cells of the testis (Fig. 17.2). Androstenedione and dehydroepiandrosterone are also produced, but the physiological potencies of these androgens are so low that they will not substitute for normal Leydig cell function. Although some androgens are 17-ketosteroids, not all 17-ketosteroids are androgens and not all androgens are 17-ketosteroids. For example, etiocholanolone has no androgenic action and testosterone is not a 17-ketosteroid. An oxygen atom at the C-3 position and a 17-hydroxyl or keto group are required for androgenic activity. In some tissues, testosterone is converted to either dihydrotestosterone (DHT) or estradiol (E_2), which are the biologically active steroids affecting these tissues (see Fig. 16.10).

Almost 100% of the testosterone in the blood is bound to protein: about 40% is bound to a β-globulin called gonadal steroid-binding globulin, about 40% is bound to albumin, and 17% to other proteins. Inactivation of testosterone, which occurs primarily in the liver, involves the following metabolism: oxidation of the 17-OH group, reduction of the A ring,

Figure 17.2   Testicular biosynthesis and hepatic metabolism of testosterone.

and reduction of the 3-keto group (Fig. 17.2). The primary urinary products of androgens in humans are androsterone and etiocholanolone, which are excreted in the form of glucuronide and sulfate conjugates.

Endocrine Control of Testicular Function

The testis has two major functions: androgen production and spermatogenesis. The control of these diverse functions requires the coordinated activity of a number of pituitary hormones, which are, in turn, regulated by a complex of neurohumoral inputs from the hypothalamus.

Male Reproductive Function is Maintained by a "Hypothalamic-Pituitary-Testicular Axis" of Hormones

Early experiments established that hypophysectomy led to testicular atrophy (Chap. 5). Restoration of testicular function followed administration of pituitary extracts or, after further purification, of pituitary gonadotropins. These classical observations revealed that the pituitary gonadotropins, LH and FSH, control both the steroidogenic and spermatogenic functions of the testes. Subsequent experiments established that secretions of the gonadotropins are, in turn, controlled by release of gonadotropin-releasing hormone (GnRH) into the hypophysial portal vasculature. Thus, the hypothalamic-pituitary-gonadal axis in males was determined to operate as a three-tiered functional hierarchy: GnRH neurons secrete the decapeptide into the hypophysial portal vessels from axon terminals in the median eminence; GnRH is conveyed to the anterior pituitary, where it can bind and activate GnRH receptors on gonadotropes, thereby stimulating synthesis and secretion of the gonadotropins; the gonadotropins, LH and FSH, circulate and bind their receptors in Leydig cells and Sertoli cells, respectively; LH is the primary stimulus for steroidogenesis and testosterone secretion from the Leydig cells, and FSH supports the development and spermatogenic activities of Sertoli cells.

Pituitary gonadotropin secretion is enhanced after orchidectomy, whereas gonadotropin secretion is diminished after administration of exogenous androgens. These observations established that testicular androgens exert a negative feedback on pituitary gonadotropin secretion. Part of this feedback is at the level of the hypothalamus, since castration has been shown to result in an acceleration of GnRH release, while testosterone implants prevent or reverse this effect. Testosterone also has direct inhibitory effects on pituitary responsiveness to GnRH stimulation, indicating that feedback suppression is also exerted at the level of the pituitary gonadotrope. It is likely that feedback mechanisms operate at both hypothalamic and pituitary levels to provide integrated homeostatic feedback control within the male reproductive axis.

The neurosecretion of GnRH occurs in an intermittent, or "pulsatile" pattern in both males and females, and in virtually all physiological circumstances [10, 46]. The cellular mechanisms that maintain this pulsatile GnRH release pattern remain unknown, and are therefore collectively referred to as the "GnRH pulse generator," the pulsatile release pattern is necessary to maintain responsiveness to GnRH by preventing gonadotropes from becoming refractory (down-regulated) to continued GnRH stimulation [4]. Changes in the frequency of GnRH pulses are believed to mediate physiological changes in gonadotropin secretions. Thus, frequency coding of GnRH release appears to be involved in the activation of the male reproductive axis during pubertal maturation [24], in transitions between reproductive states in seasonally breeding animals [50], and in other physiologically important changes in gonadotropin secretions. The negative feedback actions of testosterone in the hypothalamus are likewise manifest as a deceleration of GnRH pulsatility [49]. In the adult human male, pulsatile GnRH secretion, as deduced from pulsatile LH release patterns in peripheral blood, occurs with a frequency of approximately 1 pulse/90 minutes. Pulsatile GnRH replacement therapies in hypogonadotropic hypogonadal men have been used with great success to elevate gonadotropin levels into the normal range, and thereby induce or restore fertility [57].

In a number of mammals, LH is released on exposure of a male to a female. Successive presentation of the same female to a male mouse may lead to habituation, where LH secretion is diminished on subsequent presentations of the female. Introduction of a novel female, on the other hand, will initiate a burst of LH secretion [2]. This adaptive neuroendocrine response may be important in providing a stimulus to courtship and copulatory behavior in some species.

The following evidence clearly establishes the individual roles of pituitary gonadotropins in regulating testicular function [58]. Radiolabeled LH specifically binds to Leydig cells, whereas radiolabeled FSH binds only to Sertoli cells. LH increases cAMP levels in the interstitial cells of the testes, but not the seminiferous tubules. FSH, on the other hand, does not increase cAMP levels in the Leydig cells, but does stimulate production of the cyclic nucleotide in seminiferous tubules devoid of germ cells or in enriched fractions of Sertoli cells. Although the Sertoli cell is the major site of FSH action, there is evidence that FSH enhances the number of Leydig cell LH receptors (Chap. 16). Although FSH does not by itself stimulate steroid biosynthesis within purified testis interstitial tissue, in combination with LH it causes a dramatic increase (synergism) in 3β-hydroxysteroid dehydrogenase-isomerase activity. These latter observations are difficult to reconcile with data suggesting a lack of Leydig cell FSH receptors. The actions of FSH may be indirect.

Inhibin Exerts Negative Feedback Actions on Pituitary FSH Secretion

The Sertoli cells of the testes produce a peptide hormone, inhibin, whose major physiological role in the adult is to exert feedback control over the secretion of pituitary FSH. Inhibin itself is stimulated by FSH. Thus, a reciprocal relationship between FSH and inhibin secretions exists, where alterations in either hormone are self-limiting as they produces compensatory changes in the other. This specific feedback loop permits differential feedback control over FSH secretion, in the absence of any alterations in LH secretion. This control mechanism may contribute to the divergent FSH and LH secretory rates that occur in certain physiological states.

Inhibin is a heterodimeric protein hormone that is a member of the TGFβ family of growth factors. It is composed of two polypeptides, one α subunit and one β subunit, connected by disulfide bonds. Two forms of the inhibin β subunit exist, called inhibin βA and inhibin βB. The inhibin α subunit combines with βA to form inhibin A, and with βB to form inhibin B. The inhibin B molecule is the predominant inhibin form in men and other male mammals. While inhibin specifically inhibits FSH secretion, an additional member of the TGFβ family, *activin*, was also identified on the basis of its potency in *stimulating* FSH secretion. Activin is composed of dimerized inhibin β subunits, combined as βA-βA in activin A, βB-βB in activin B, and βA-βB in activin AB. An activin-binding protein called *follistatin* has also been identified, and it appears to neutralize the stimulatory actions of activin on FSH synthesis and secretion.

Interestingly, high levels of FSH and normal levels of LH are present in the plasma of oligospermic (low sperm count) males and in males after testicular irradiation and cytotoxic chemotherapy. Sertoli cells alone are not capable of reducing FSH levels in the absence of spermatogenesis. It is postulated that inhibin production by Sertoli cells in adult men may be regulated by influences deriving from maturing sperms. By contrast, inhibin production by Sertoli cells can occur normally in children, apparently independent of any influence of maturing germ cells.

Granulosa cells from the ovarian follicle also secrete a substance during culture, presumably inhibin, that acts directly on pituitary cell cultures derived from the male or female to preferentially suppress FSH secretion. Administration of anti-inhibin antisera to rats of either sex causes a rise in serum FSH levels; LH levels, in contrast, remain unchanged. A summary scheme of the roles of FSH and inhibin in the control of testicular (and ovarian) function is provided (Fig. 17.3).

Prolactin can Regulate LH Receptor Number in Leydig Cells

Hypophysectomy of the male rat results in a loss of testicular LH receptors; administration of FSH or LH does not, however, re-establish testicular LH receptor concentration. Inhibition of pituitary FSH and LH secretion from the rat pituitary by administration of anti-GnRH or by estradiol or testosterone treatment does not result in a loss of testicular LH receptors. These results suggest that one or more pituitary hormones other than the gonadotropins might be responsible for maintenance of testicular receptors. Inhibition of pituitary prolactin (PRL) secretion by ergot alkaloids results in a decrease in testicular LH receptors, whereas PRL treatment prevents loss of LH receptors in hypophysectomized animals. These observations suggest that PRL may play a role in the control of testicular Leydig cell LH receptor number.

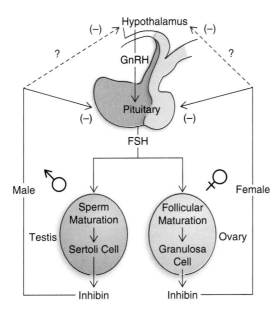

Figure 17.3 A summary scheme of the roles of FSH and inhibin in the control of testicular (and ovarian) function.

Physiological Roles of Androgens

Testicular androgens are responsible for the growth and development of those tissues and organs that characterize the male (Table 17.1). The role of gonadal androgens in the differentiation and development of the male urogenital system, the accessory sex organs, and the external genitalia has already been described (Chap. 16). Although many target tissues respond directly to testosterone, this androgen must be first converted either to DHT or E_2 in some other tissues to mediate its actions (see Fig. 16.10). After the initial actions of testosterone in early fetal development, the gonads remain quiescent until puberty when gonadal activity is increased in response to secretion of pituitary gonadotropins. The elevated circulating levels of androgens that ensue are responsible for initiating spermatogenesis (gametogenesis) and for growth and development of the secondary sex characteristics that first become evident during the pubertal process. Some of the established roles of androgens in the male are discussed in what follows.

Spermatogenesis Depends on Both FSH and Testosterone

FSH and testosterone are required for the initiation of spermatogenesis during sexual maturation [61]. Administration of FSH to immature or mature hypophysectomized rats markedly increases the size of the testes but does not accelerate the appearance of mature sperm or increase the secretory activity of the Leydig cells. For completion of spermatogenesis, an androgenic influence is needed, which can be provided by the administration of testosterone. Spermatogenesis can be maintained in hypophysectomized adult animals by testosterone in the absence of gonadotropins, but its initiation at puberty requires FSH. Resumption of spermatogenesis in regressed testes following hypophysectomy also requires administration of FSH. In immature animals, FSH increases the number of Sertoli cells, which accounts for the testicular hypertrophy that follows hemicastration. FSH is required for the normal reinitiation of sperm production during the breeding season of monkeys. Although LH alone stimulates sperm production in some patients with deficiencies in LH and FSH production, others have required a combination of FSH and LH to initiate spermatogenesis. FSH alone has never been reported to initiate or maintain spermatogenesis in human males.

Although the details of the individual roles of FSH and testosterone in spermatogenesis remain unresolved, the following model has been proposed. FSH interaction with Sertoli cell plasmalemmal receptors results in cAMP production and the synthesis of an androgen-binding protein (ABP). Presumably, cAMP activates a protein kinase that leads to the genomic production of a mRNA coding for ABP. The ABP is then secreted into the lumen of the seminiferous tubules. Testicular receptors for LH are specifically localized to the Leydig

TABLE 17.1 Biological effects and roles of testicular androgens in the human male

Primary locus of action	Physiological response
Prepubertal	
Accessory sex glands	Wolffian duct differentiation and growth
External genitalia	Growth and differentiation (scrotum and penis)
Pubertal	
Skeletal muscle (enhanced protein synthesis)	Masculine body growth and physique (Na^+, K^+, H_2O retention)
Bone (bone formation)	Epiphyseal closure ($Ca^{2+}, SO_4^{-2}, PO_4^{-3}$ retention)
Vocal cords	Voice change
Skin	Hair growth (beard, axilla, chest, pubic, and general body surface)
	Hair loss (e.g., forehead)
	Sebaceous gland growth and sebum production
Testis	Sertoli cell maturation and androgen-binding protein synthesis
	Spermatogenesis
External genitalia	Penile and scrotal growth
Accessory sex glands	Prostate gland, seminal vesicle, bulbourethral gland growth and secretion
Central nervous system	Sexual activity (libido increased)
Hypothalamo-pituitary axis	Inhibition of LH secretion

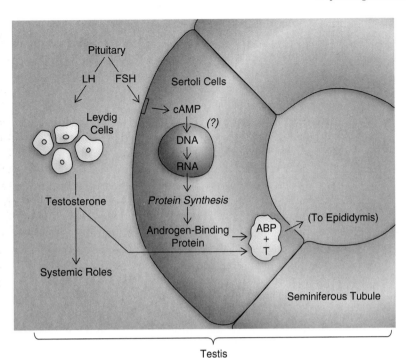

Figure 17.4 Model of FSH and LH action on Sertoli and Leydig cells.

cells. In response to LH, cAMP is produced which then causes Leydig cell testosterone production (Fig. 17.4). At least part of this LH effect is mediated by a stimulation of steroidogenic acute regulatory protein (StAR) synthesis, which mediates cholesterol transfer from the outer to inner mitochondrial membrane in the Leydig cell, the rate-limiting step in steroidogenesis. Testosterone is released from the Leydig cells and finds its way into the systemic circulation and to the adjacent seminiferous tubules. Because Sertoli cells are connected by tight junctions, they apparently provide a barrier (blood–testis) to most large molecules. Testosterone may be taken up by the Sertoli cells by an active transport mechanism or by facilitated diffusion. The blood–testis barrier first appears at puberty and may function to create some special environment for spermatogenesis. The barrier may also protect the germ cells from the immunological system. Within the Sertoli cells, testosterone is bound to ABP. This binding protein may provide a mechanism for testosterone sequestration close to the spermatocytes whose maturation is androgen dependent. Because germ cells lacking androgen receptors develop into fertile spermatozoa in the presence of normal Sertoli cells, it is presumed that the hormonal effects of testosterone on spermatogenesis are mediated via the Sertoli cells.

Androgen-binding protein may also provide a mechanism for the accumulation of androgen within Sertoli cells, which then can be released (via vesicular exocytosis) into the lumen of the seminiferous tubules. Within the lumen, ABP may function to transport testosterone to the epididymis. The spermatozoa mature in the caput and corpus regions of the epididymis where they develop the potential for fertilization and motility. These characteristics of mature sperm within the epididymis are soon lost in castrated animals, but can be maintained by testosterone administration.

Testosterone Acts at Several Neural Loci to Modulate Reproductive Behavior and Sexual Function

Unlike in the female, gonadal steroids do not exert positive feedback actions in the pituitary or hypothalamus of the male to stimulate cyclic release of pituitary hormone surges. Nevertheless, pituitary gonadotropin secretion is increased after gonadectomy, and exogenous androgens depress the elevation of gonadotropin secretion in the castrated animal. Therefore, testicular androgens exert a tonic inhibitory feedback action on pituitary gonadotropin secretion. These negative feedback actions are mediated by testosterone's actions in preoptic, hypothalamic, and anterior pituitary cells, through the activation of nuclear androgen receptors or via the aromatization of testosterone to estrogen, and subsequent activation of estrogen receptors. Nuclear androgen- and estrogen-binding sites at these sites, as well as those present in septal, limbic, and several other brain structures of vertebrates, also represent loci of androgen activation of sexually related behaviors (Chap. 16). For example, implantation of androgen within specific areas of the brain can induce copulatory behavior in fowl.

In the dove, *Streptopelia risoria*, male courtship depends on the action of androgen on the preoptic-anterior hypothalamus (AHPOA) of the brain [17]. The aggressive components of courtship, as well as perch calling, are specifically testosterone-dependent, whereas nest-oriented courtship activity and nest soliciting appear to be mediated by estrogens (derived from testosterone) acting on the AHPOA.

A sexually dimorphic nucleus is present in the fifth and sixth lumbar segments of the male rat spinal cord [7]. This nucleus contains motor neurons that innervate the perineal striated muscle of the penis. This nucleus is diminished or absent in the normal female and in males who are genetically insensitive to androgens. The cell bodies of these motor neurons accumulate androgens but not E_2. These motor neurons probably represent a site of androgen action modifying penile reflexes during copulatory behavior.

The spinal nucleus of the bulbocavernosus (SNB) contains many more motor neurons in adult male rats than in females. Androgens establish this sex difference during a critical prenatal period that coincides with normally occurring cell death in the SNB region. The sex difference in SNB motor neuron number arises primarily because motor neuron loss is greater in females than in males during the early postnatal period. Prenatal androgen treatment in females attenuates cell death in the SNB region, reducing motor neuron loss to levels typical of males. These observations suggest that steroid hormones determine sex differences in neuron numbers by regulating normally occurring cell death (apoptosis) and that the timing of this cell death may therefore define critical periods for steroid hormone effects on neuron number.

In androgen-sensitive motor neurons that mediate male copulatory functions, decreases in androgen levels after castration of adult rats result in a decrease in both the dendritic length and soma size of the neurons. The changes could be reversed by androgen replacement. These results indicate a high degree of synaptic plasticity in adult motor neurons and suggest that normal changes in androgen levels in adulthood are associated with significant alterations in the structure and function of these neurons [41].

In the male frog, *Xenopus laevis*, spinal neurons projecting to muscles primarily involved in the clasp reflex during amplexus accumulate [³H]dihydrotestosterone. DHT added to an isolated spinal cord preparation containing these neurons changes the firing patterns of the neurons. Androgens or their metabolites therefore may regulate mating behavior in these animals by an initial action within specific spinal neurons that control muscle activity during mating.

Gonadal hormones alter the level of spontaneous electrical activity of anatomically defined populations of neurons within the brain and change the responses of peripheral and central neuronal pathways to sensory stimulation in some vertebrate species. For example, testosterone alters preoptic neuron responses to electrical stimulation of the olfactory bulb and to natural sexual odors. Therefore, in the adult animal, androgens may be significant in the interception and interpretation of olfactory cues important to reproductive success.

Gonadal androgens are essential for establishment and maintenance of male dominance and aggressive behavior in most birds (e.g., domestic fowl, mallards). Sexual aggressiveness is diminished after castration but can be reestablished by administration of androgens. In phalaropes (*Steganopes tricolor*), however, the female is more active than the male in courtship behavior. During the breeding cycle, female phalaropes produce more gonadal androgens than males [26]. In females, the nuptial plumage is also more brilliant than that of males. Administration of testosterone (but not E_2 or PRL) to phalaropes of either sex in the dull juvenile or adult nonbreeding plumage results in formation of the full plumage pattern that normally develops only in the female [31]. These results clearly establish that androgens in the female phalarope are responsible for inducing nuptial plumage and dominant mating behavior during the breeding season.

Hormone Actions in the Fetal Brain may Program Sexual Orientation

The preoptic area and anterior hypothalamus of the brain participates in the regulation of male-typical sexual behavior [16, 23, 44, 45, 55]. The volumes of four cell groups in this region (interstitial nuclei of the anterior hypothalamus (INAH) 1, 2, 3, and 4) were measured in postmortem tissue from three subject groups: women, men who were presumed to be heterosexual, and homosexual men. No differences were found between the groups in the volumes of INAH 1, 2, or 4. As has been reported previously, INAH 3 was, however, more than twice as large in the heterosexual men as in the women. It was also more than twice as large in the heterosexual men as in the homosexual men. This finding indicates that INAH 3 is dimorphic with sexual orientation, at least in men, and suggests that sexual orientation has a biological substrate. Further interpretation of the results of this study must be considered speculative. In particular, the results do not allow one to decide if the size of INAH 3 in an individual is the cause or consequence of that individual's sexual orientation, or if the size of INAH 3 and sexual orientation covary under the influence of some third, unidentified variable. Although the validity of the comparison between species is uncertain, it seems more likely that in humans, too, the size of INAH 3 is established early in life under the organizational effects of androgens, and the neuronal group later influences sexual behavior, rather than the reverse [23, 44, 45, 52].

Studies in domestic ram populations have provided additional clues in this regard [55]. As many as 8–10% of rams exhibit a sexual partner preference for other males. Recent work has demonstrated that a sexually dimorphic nucleus (oSDN) exists in the ovine preoptic-anterior hypothalamic tissues, and that the oSDN is larger in female-oriented rams than in male-oriented rams or in ewes. Moreover, levels of mRNA encoding aromatase were also found to be higher in the oSDN of female-oriented rams versus male-oriented rams or ewes, which were similar to each other. These data suggest that aromatase activity, and hence the level of estrogen produced in the oSDN during fetal development, are correlated with sexual partner preference in rams. It remains to be determined if these variables are causally linked, and whether this developmental relationship holds any relevance to a biologically deterministic model of human sexual orientation [6].

Testosterone Stimulates Development of Male Secondary Sex Characteristics

Puberty is the last phase of the complex process of sexual maturation, a process by which an individual acquires reproductive competency. The dramatic developmental and behavioral changes in the male at puberty result from enhanced testosterone secretion by the testes and the actions of testosterone or one of its metabolites on specific target tissues. Dimorphic secondary sex characteristics are typical of all vertebrates. These differences are most often modifications of the integument or underlying tissues: skin coloration; hair color, distribution, and coarseness; development of specialized integumental structures such as horns, antlers, beaks, claws, and spines [14]. In the male, androgens profoundly affect such courtship behaviors as aggression, bodily movements and display, and even vocalization. Only a few representative examples of the role of androgens among the major groups of vertebrates are discussed here.

Sex Organs. The accessory reproductive glands are dependent on testosterone to enable them to contribute secretory products to the semen. Androgens increase the content of endoplasmic reticulum within the cells of the prostate, seminal vesicles, and bulbourethral glands. The spermatozoa contain only a relatively small amount of cytoplasm and apparently must be nourished by constituents of the seminal fluid. Fructose, a source of metabolic energy for the spermatozoa, is secreted by the seminal vesicles. The effects of testosterone on the prostate gland are greatly augmented by PRL, which is without effect on this gland in the castrated animal. The penis and scrotum also enlarge in response to testosterone or DHT.

Skin. Sebaceous gland activity is stimulated by androgens most likely derived from testosterone. The acne often present in the male during the pubertal process is due to the increased activity of these glands in response to elevated plasma levels of androgens. The coarseness of hair in some animals is increased by androgens, and the pattern of hair growth is also affected. Androgens are stimulatory to hair growth in the axilla, the pubic area, and on the chin. In contrast, androgens cause recession of the male hairline. Androgens may even cause baldness (alopecia) in individuals with such a genetic predisposition. Castration of males who are becoming alopecic prevents further extension of the bald areas but does not promote general regrowth of hair. In females with adrenal virilism the excessive levels of androgens may induce baldness; loss of hair ceases when the abnormal masculinization ends.

The response of a tissue to an androgen depends on the presence of a specific androgen receptor, and enzymes such as 5α-reductase or aromatase that metabolize testosterone to DHT and estrogen, respectively. The derived DHT has increased potency at the androgen receptor, and the estrogen produced by aromatase elicits responses through estrogen receptors, if present in the target tissue. The abundance of other steroidogenic enzymes may also determine the characteristics of a target tissue response. Studies have demonstrated the conversion of dehydroepiandrosterone into androstenedione, testosterone, and DHT in human sebaceous glands, and the greater enzymic activity of Δ^5-3β-hydroxysteroid dehydrogenase (3β-HSD) in sebaceous glands of bald scalp than in hairy scalp. Greater 3β-HSD activity and increased androgen-binding capacity may provide a biochemical explanation for the disease mechanism of androgenic alopecia. Furthermore, such studies may provide new insight into the mechanism of skin diseases caused by hyperandrogenization, such as acne, hirsutism, and seborrhea, besides male pattern baldness [1, 56].

In most vertebrates, skin, hair, and feather coloration differ between the sexes and can be striking in some teleosts and birds [26, 31]. Often the color of the skin changes during the breeding season. These pigmentary changes are usually androgen dependent and involve increases or decreases in the number of pigment cells and the amount and kind of pigment within integumental chromatophores (Chap. 8). In some birds, such as the weaver finch, the bill becomes melanized in response to androgens during the breeding season.

The Sexually Dimorphic Kidney. In Chapter 16, it was noted that gonadal steroids affect sexual dimorphic differentiation and development of nuclear centers within the vertebrate central nervous system. Other organs and tissues are also differentially affected by gonadal steroids. The proximal tubules of the kidneys of male mice, for example, contain mitochondria and lysosomes that are ultrastructurally different from those of females. Males also have higher kidney activities of mitochondrial cytochrome C oxidase and lysosomal hydroxylases. The female pattern of organellar structure develops after orchidectomy. Testosterone administration induces the male pattern of cellular structure and function in castrated male mice or in female mice [37]. Sex differences in kidney function and metabolism, as well as pathophysiology, have been documented and may relate to differences in the hormonal milieu between the two sexes.

Submaxillary Glands of Mice. As noted in Chapter 12, submaxillary gland production of nerve growth factor (NGF) and epidermal growth factor (EGF) in the mouse is acutely controlled by androgens. Several enzymes are more abundant in the male submaxillary gland than in the female. The cellular synthesis of these enzymes is androgen-dependent and can be induced in the female by administration of an androgen. In boars, salivary glands use nonandrogenic steroids of testicular origin and secrete them into the saliva where they may function as sex attractants (e.g., musk).

Brood Patches. Some birds develop a brood patch on the abdomen during the breeding season. Feathers are lost from this area and the skin becomes thick and hypervascularized so that warmth can be imparted to the incubating eggs. In female passerine birds, where the female develops a patch, estrogen and PRL synergize to cause brood patch development [32]. In those species in which both sexes develop a patch (e.g., quail), estrogens or androgens synergize with PRL to initiate patch development. In the phalarope, in which only the male develops a patch, patch development is regulated by the synergistic actions of PRL and androgens.

Epidermal Cornifications. In many amphibians, black, cornified structures may occur on the forelimbs or hindlimbs. These nuptial pads, as they are designated, assist the male in grasping the female during amplexus. These are androgen-dependent structures that regress after castration but can be reinstated following androgen-replacement therapy. In the newt, nuptial pads develop in response to androgens, but only if prolactin and thyroid hormone are also present [14, 30].

Antlers. A vast array of morphological outgrowths of the integument characterize the male of the species and are often enlarged or otherwise exaggerated during the breeding season. The growth of antlers in some species of deer might be considered the most conspicuous of integumental growths. The antlers are solid bony outgrowths that arise from the frontal bones and are borne usually by the male. The growth and shedding of antlers is under the control of androgens, except in caribou where both the male and female possess antlers. In the red deer stag (*Cervus elaphus*), the cycle of testosterone secretion is responsible for the redevelopment of the secondary sexual characteristics each year; the animal undergoes a type of "annual puberty and senescence" [48]. Testosterone stimulates development of the neck mane and rutting odor and is responsible for loss of velvet from the antlers. Changes in photoperiod affect testicular androgenesis. Increasing day length is inhibitory to testicular androgenic activity in the Sitka deer (*Cervus nippon*) [22]. Testicular activity resumes at the summer solstice when the hours of daylight stabilize.

Breeding Tubercles. Androgens increase the skin thickness of the salmon and also increase integumental mucus production. In some fishes, breeding tubercles develop on the head of the male. These structures apparently evolved to enable breeding individuals to maintain close contact during spawning and may be particularly important in fishes that spawn in fast-moving water [60, 66].

Androgens Exert Anabolic Actions in Muscle, Cartilage and other Target Tissues

The major extragenital site of androgen action is skeletal muscle, which may account for part of the body-weight difference between males and females of many species. Growth of the musculature and cartilage of the larynx of the human causes a permanent deepening of the voice. Because skeletal muscle cannot convert testosterone to DHT, it is likely that testosterone has a direct anabolic action on muscle. The myotropic actions of androgens result from their ability to increase retention of dietary nitrogen through protein synthesis. A great many derivatives of testosterone have been prepared with the hope that they might be of practical use in promoting general body growth without concomitantly producing masculinizing effects. These compounds are referred to as *anabolic steroids*.

Anabolic steroids are synthetic molecules developed in the hope of obtaining a complete separation of the androgenic and myotropic (anabolic) actions of testosterone. Such a goal has never been fully achieved. However, some synthetic steroids present a partial dissociation between these two activities. Since a single hormonal receptor apparently mediates the androgenic as well as the anabolic actions of testosterone, differences in patterns of androgen metabolization in the muscles and the accessory sex organs have been proposed as a possible cause of the phenomenon.

It remains unclear, however, which molecular mechanisms mediate the anabolic effects of androgens in skeletal muscle [9, 67]. Most likely androgens act via nuclear androgen receptors expressed in "satellite cells" which are quiescent precursors of myoblasts, the committed myogenic cells. It is postulated that androgens stimulate satellite cell proliferation and differentiation into myoblasts, which then fuse with existing myofibers that comprise new muscle tissue. It has also been proposed that the anabolic actions of androgens (at least in pharmacological doses) in skeletal muscle may derive from competitive antagonism of glucocorticoid receptors (which enhance protein catabolism).

The abuse potential of anabolic steroids has been evident for many years, particularly among individuals looking to enhance their athletic abilities in competitive sports. Most professional sports organizations now ban the use of these substances, and require regular blood tests to screen for the presence of anabolic steroids and other illicit performance-enhancing drugs. Unfortunately, many amateur athletes who wish to improve performance, as well as those seeking to achieve an increase in lean body mass for cosmetic reasons, continue to abuse these drugs without an appreciation of their side effects and health risks. These include acne, hair growth and loss, liver and adrenal gland damage, atrophy of the testes, infertility, and virilization in women. Of great concern is the ability of high doses of anabolic steroids to induce increases in aggression and hostility, and other mood disturbances that can ultimately lead to severe depression, hypomania, or psychotic features.

Serum Testosterone Levels Decline in Aging Men

It is now generally accepted that there is an age-associated decrease in serum testosterone levels in healthy men. Testosterone is clearly necessary to maintain libido; the hormone is responsible for men's secondary sexual characteristics—the beard, muscles, skin thickness, and aggressive behavior. Young men with abnormally low testosterone levels, a condition known as hypogonadism, often suffer a loss of bone, muscle, energy, and libido. Testosterone therapy can reverse their symptoms. So, it is currently debated if testosterone might reduce some of the effects of aging [11, 35].

Muscle mass is increased in elderly men taking testosterone [63, 35]. There is worry, however, that testosterone replacement therapy might enhance the growth of prostate cancer. And, since androgens increase the production of red cells, they might thicken the blood, thus raising the risk of stroke [11, 35]. Other areas of concern include: water retention, hepatotoxicity, exacerbation of sleep apnea, development of polycythemia or gynecomastia [35, 63].

Physiological Roles of Estrogens

Most interesting has been the discovery that estrogens as well as androgens are necessary for normal reproductive function in the male [25, 33, 38, 40]. The use of gene knockout techniques involving a mutant mouse line without a functional estrogen receptor provided information on estrogen functions in the male [38].

Fertility. In estrogen receptor knockout (ERKO) mice, the testes undergo progressive atrophy associated with decreased epididymal sperm counts and motility, and viability. Estrogen regulates the reabsorption of luminal fluid in the head of the epididymis. Disruption of estrogen function therefore causes sperm to enter the epididymis diluted rather than concentrated, resulting in infertility [38]. Are reported declines in human sperm counts possibly due to potential effects of environmental estrogens?

Male Sexual Behavior. ERKO mice exhibit deficits in mating behavior such as decreased intromissions and ejaculations. As in rats (Chap. 16), the conversion of testosterone to estradiol is critical for masculinization of hypothalamic nuclei that control sex and aggressive behaviors. It remains to be determined whether the observed intromission/ejaculation defects are due to differences in the organization or differentiation of central (preoptic area-anterior hypothalamic nuclei or spinal nucleus of the bulbocavernosus) or peripheral (muscles involved in the penile reflexes) mechanisms involved in male sexual behavior [38, 47].

Epiphyseal Fusion. Several "experiments of nature" have provided information on the role of estrogens and androgens in mediating epiphyseal fusion in men. Smith and colleagues described a 28-year-old man with complete estrogen resistance because of a nonsense mutation in the estrogen receptor gene [19, 59]. Despite normal virilization and adult male testosterone levels for more than a decade after the completion of puberty, this man had unfused epiphyses, a bone age of 15, and a height of 6 ft, 8 in (204 cm). A 24-year-old man with aromatase deficiency because of a homozygous missense mutation in the aromatase gene was also discovered. Again there were unfused epiphyses, a bone age of 14, and a height of 6 ft, 8 in (204 cm) even in the presence of supraphysiological levels of testosterone. These remarkable cases provide a clear demonstration that estrogens regulate epiphyseal growth and normal bone growth in the male.

Cardiovascular Function. Premenopausal women have a lower risk of coronary heart disease than men or postmenopausal women and estrogens are thought to contribute to this lower risk. There is experimental evidence that physiological levels of E_2 are important in maintaining plasma levels of HDL cholesterol, especially the HDL_2 fraction. E_2 in the amount normally produced in men may offer some degree of protection against cardiovascular disease in males, as it does in women [3]. Other evidence supports a role for estrogen function/therapy in cardiovascular physiology [18]:

1. Long-term estrogen therapy improves vascular function in male to female transsexuals.
2. Arterial reactivity (elasticity) is enhanced in genetic males taking high-dose estrogens.
3. Androgen deprivation is associated with improved endothelium-dependent dilation in adult men.
4. Decreased mortality is seen in users of estrogen replacement therapy.

Mechanisms of Androgen Action

Androgens mediate their actions through the classical scheme of steroid hormone action (see Fig. 13.15). They interact with cytoplasmic and nuclear receptors, a two-step mechanism, to stimulate transcriptional and translational processes related to protein synthesis.

Androgen Receptors. The androgen receptor belongs to the subfamily of steroid hormone receptors within a larger family of nuclear proteins that likely evolved from a common ancestral gene. The androgen receptor has been cloned and its sequence determined. The receptor has highest sequence identity with the progesterone receptor. The gene for the receptor is localized on the human X chromosome. The androgen receptor gene is comprised of eight exons (A–H), coding for three specific functionalities of the receptor (Fig. 17.5). The N-terminal segment is coded by exon A. The function of this "transactivator segment" at present is not clearly defined, but may (1) optimize the transactivation capability of the receptor

Figure 17.5 Schematic structure of the androgen receptor. The steroid hormone receptor is comprised of eight exons. The role of the amino terminal exon (A) is undetermined, but like similar receptors, provides specificity for binding the receptor to its substrate, DNA. The DNA-binding domain (66 amino acids in length), encoded by exons B and C, interacts with the hormone-responsive element of the DNA. The androgen-binding domain (about 252 amino acids) at the C-terminal end is encoded by exons D-H [28].

and (2) specify gene recognition in the transcriptional regulation. The DNA-binding domain, a 66–68-amino-acid sequence, is encoded by exons B and C, which code the first and second (C-terminal) zinc finger motifs, respectively. The first zinc finger specifies the receptor's DNA recognition, and the second is mainly responsible for dimerization of two receptor molecules during their association with DNA [5, 20, 28]. The androgen-binding C-terminal domain consists of about 252 amino acids and is encoded by exons D–H (Fig. 17.5). A model for androgen activation of the cognate receptors is depicted in Figure 17.6.

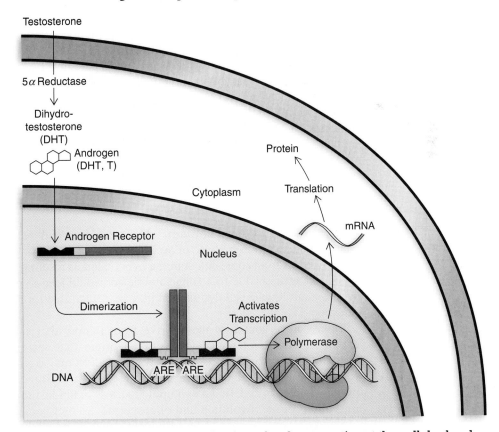

Figure 17.6 Diagram of the mechanism of androgen action at the cellular level. The androgen enters the cell by passive diffusion. It binds to the androgen-binding domain of the receptor. This binding is hypothesized to result in a conformational change exposing the receptor's DNA-binding domain and enabling it to bind to the nuclear chromatin. This binding to DNA initiates transcription of mRNA and, ultimately, translation into androgen-specific proteins. (From Imperato-McGinley and Canovatchel [28]. Reprinted by permission of the publisher from *Trends in Endocrinology and Metabolism* 3:75–81, 1992. ©1992 by Elsevier Science Inc.)

Cyproterone Acetate

Figure 17.7 Structure of cyproterone acetate, an antiandrogen.

Antiandrogens. Some of the most potent antiandrogens are derivatives of progesterone. Although they may possess weak androgenic activity, they are inhibitory to the actions of testosterone because of their receptor occupancy [21]. Cyproterone acetate is one of the most potent antiandrogens (Fig. 17.7). For example, treatment of the pregnant rat with cyproterone acetate results in male fetuses that are morphologically feminized, and the adult behavior of these rats is that of the female. Administration of the antiandrogen in the mature male causes atrophy of the seminal vesicles, prostate, and other androgen-responsive target organs. Pituitary gonadotropin secretion is enhanced after antiandrogen treatment, as after castration, and in the human male cyproterone acetate causes a loss of libido. In the female, on the other hand, this antiandrogen has been used successfully to treat hirsutism and virilization. In the male, acne and the development of baldness are reversed by antiandrogen treatment. Although cyproterone acetate has been used with some success to treat (delay) precocious puberty, its inhibition of the anabolic actions of androgens may preclude its use in the treatment of sexual precocity.

Pathophysiology

Mutations that impair male reproductive function (e.g., androgen action) appear to be relatively common. The comparative frequency may stem in part from the fact that sexual development is essential for reproduction, but not for the life of an individual. Mutations that block androgen action completely do not affect life span, whereas mutations that severely impair the action of hormones essential for life (e.g., insulin, cortisol, thyroxine) are probably lethal in utero.

Familial Male Precocious Puberty. True precocious puberty (Chap. 16) is characterized by early sexual development involving both spermatogenesis as well as development of secondary sexual characteristics. Early secretion of pituitary gonadotropins can account for some forms of precocious puberty. Constitutively active forms of the lutropin/choriogonadotropin receptor (LHR) resulting from mutations in the LHR have been shown to cause gonadotropin-independent precocious puberty in boys [43]. Mutations in G-protein-coupled receptors (GPCRs) can lead to either loss or gain of signaling function. Gain of function mutations promote agonist-independent activation (constitutive activity) of GPCRs, presumably by mimicking the agonist-induced conformational state of the seven transmembrane helical bundle/receptor.

Leydig cell hypoplasia leading to male pseudohermatophroditism, the physiological counterpart of familial male precocious puberty, may also be caused by point mutations or deletions of the LHR gene that result in truncated or dysfunctional receptor protein with resulting resistance to LH action [39, 64].

Hypogonadism/Hypergonadism. Hypogonadism may result from a failure in pituitary gonadotropin secretion because of an isolated defect in one or the other of the gonadotropes or it may result from some defect in the hypothalamus resulting in a failure to secrete GnRH. Leydig cell agenesis due to a congenital defect would lead to male pseudohermaphroditism, whereas adult Leydig cell dysfunction may be responsible for the climacteric experienced by some men [11].

Primary hypergonadism may derive from tumors that secrete excess androgens [51]. Feminizing tumors of gonadal or adrenal origin that secrete estrogens have also been documented in the male. Secondary hypergonadism may result from any factors leading to excessive pituitary gonadotropin secretion. Gonadal dysfunction in hyperprolactinemia is now widely recognized. In males, impotence, loss of libido, reduced androgen secretion with testes and prostate involution and oligospermia are not commonly involved with galactorrhea and/or gynecomastia. The pathogenic role of hyperprolactinemia in hypogonadism is confirmed in men and women by its reversal when PRL is lowered either by surgically ablating a prolactinoma or by the use of drugs. Some examples of endocrine disorders are outlined in Table 17.2 and discussed below.

Syndromes of Androgen Resistance. Various genetic defects can result in the synthesis of an abnormal androgen receptor with loss or impairment of its ability to function. In general, mutations in the androgen-binding domain result in an androgen receptor that is unable to bind androgen, that is, the "receptor-negative" androgen insensitivity syndrome, or one that

TABLE 17.2 Endocrine pathophysiology of the human male reproductive system

Hypogonadism
Primary
    Leydig cell deficiency (Leydig cell agenesis)
    Adult Leydig cell failure (male climacteric phase)
    Germinal cell aplasia (Sertoli-cell-only syndrome)
Secondary
    Gonadotropin deficiency (hypogonadotropic hypogonadism)
    Hypothalamic hypogonadism (defect in GnRH secretion)
Hypergonadism
Primary (steroid-secreting testicular tumors)
    Virilizing (androgen-secreting) Leydig (interstitial) cell tumors (macrogenitosomia in
      the prepubertal male)
    Feminizing (estrogen-secreting) Leydig (interstitial) cell tumors
Secondary
    Hypothalamic origin (enhanced GnRH secretion)
    Pituitary origin (hypergonadotropic hypergonadism)
Syndromes of androgen resistance
Testicular feminizing syndrome (absence or defect of androgen receptors)
Syndrome of 5α-reductase deficiency (failure to convert testosterone to DHT)
Gynecomastia (breast enlargement)

has altered or impaired binding affinity (Fig. 17.8). In the "receptor-positive" form of complete androgen insensitivity, there is normal binding to the androgen receptor. However, the androgen-receptor complex is incapable of interacting with androgen-responsive DNA sequences. A single nucleotide substitution in exon C of the DNA-binding domain of the androgen receptor (Fig. 17.9) has been determined to cause at least one form of receptor-positive complete androgen insensitivity [5, 29]. It is expected that other deletions, substitutions, and so on, will be found in other subjects with the syndrome [5, 28].

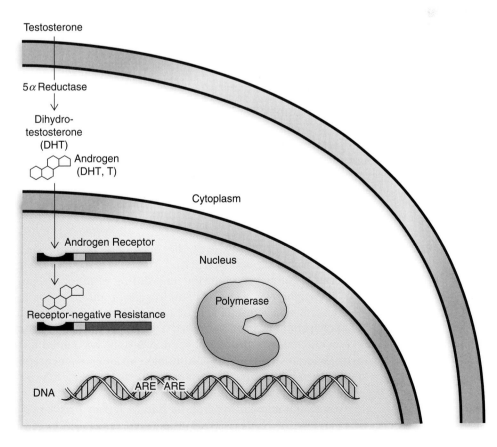

Figure 17.8 Diagram depicting the inability of the androgen receptor to bind to the ligand owing to mutations in the androgen-binding domain of the androgen-receptor genome (receptor-negative resistance). Consequently, no binding to nuclear chromatin occurs. (From Imperato-McGinley and Canovatchel [28]. Reprinted by permission of the publisher from *Trends in Endocrinology and Metabolism* 3:75–81, 1992. ©1992 by Elsevier Science Inc.)

Figure 17.9 Diagram showing the inability of the androgen-receptor complex to bind to nuclear DNA (receptor-positive resistance), secondary to mutations in the DNA-binding domain of the androgen-receptor genome. (From Imperato-McGinley and Canovatchel [28]. Reprinted by permission of the publisher from *Trends in Endocrinology and Metabolism* 3:75–81, 1992. ©1992 by Elsevier Science Inc.)

Male Pseudohermaphroditism. Male pseudohermaphroditism traditionally implies female or intersexual genital development in individuals with histologically normal or almost normal testes. As noted in Chapter 16, male pseudohermaphroditism may be classified into three broad categories related to defects in the following: (1) testosterone synthesis, (2) androgen-receptor synthesis or function, and (3) absent or defective activity of Müllerian regression factor. In addition, an isolated deficiency of Leydig cells and a defect in any one of the five or more enzymes required for testosterone biosynthesis will individually lead to male pseudohermaphroditism [34, 54].

A lack of LH production and secretion or an LH receptor defect would also result in failure of testosterone production and, therefore, defects in normal genital development. In sex-reversed XY females, several de novo mutations or deletions in the SRY gene have been described. Testis determination depends on the inheritance of the Y chromosome-encoded testis-determining factor (TDF). In the absence of the Y chromosome, the testis-determining pathway fails to be initiated or is blocked so that the gonads follow the pathway of ovarian development. Dihydrotestosterone (DHT), the product of testosterone metabolism by the testicular enzyme 5α-reductase, virilizes the urogenital sinus and external genitalia. Both steroids exert their androgenic effects by interacting with an androgen receptor protein, whose affinity for DHT is much greater than for testosterone, hence the poor virilization of patients who lack 5α-reductase [28] (see Fig. 17.7).

Gynecomastia. Growth of the mammary tissue of the male, gynecomastia, may be common during the neonatal period. This enlargement of the breasts is generally attributed to maternal hormones reaching the fetus during gestation. Prepubertal gynecomastia may result from a peripheral conversion of androgens produced by the testes and adrenals to estrogens. Adolescent gynecomastia may be associated with a decreased testosterone/estradiol ratio of unknown etiology. The slow increase in the prevalence of gynecomastia in adult males, which is accentuated over the age of 45, may also be accounted for by the age-related increase of estrogen/testosterone levels. Although uncommon, gynecomastia may occur unilaterally rather than bilaterally. If gynecomastia is accompanied by galactorrhea, the possibility of a PRL-secreting tumor should be considered.

Congenital adrenal hyperplasia due to 11β-hydroxylase deficiency has a high incidence among Jews of North African origin and results in the development of gynecomastia in untreated patients. Estrogen production is high as a result of increased steroidal substrates for aromatization. Estrogens are formed predominantly from extraglandular aromatization of adrenal androgens (e.g., androstenedione) [47].

An interesting clinical report described how a 70-year-old man developed gynecomastia. The etiology of the breast enlargement could not be immediately determined. It was then realized that his wife had been using a vaginal cream containing an estrogen. In fact, the cream was also used as a lubricant to facilitate intercourse two to three times a week. When the exposure to estrogen was terminated, gynecomastia disappeared over the subsequent three months [15]. Gynecomastia in males exposed to other sources of estrogens (as well as marihuana smoke) has been reported.

Premature Adrenarche/Pubarche.   Premature pubarche refers to the isolated development of sexual hair at an early age due to increased levels of adrenal androgens (adrenarche). In the female, it is known that adrenal androgens are responsible for growth of sexual hair. In the male, the penis is of normal size; therefore, it is believed that adrenal androgens, rather than testosterone (which can be converted to DHT), are responsible for early sexual hair growth.

Adult Leydig Cell Failure (Male Climacteric Phase).   In some men, Leydig cell function may decline with age; the fall in serum testosterone levels may produce symptoms similar to those of the postmenopausal woman. The age of onset is variable and may be caused by a variety of factors (e.g., as a result of mumps). Although androgen therapy may not improve sexual function, muscle function may be restored, thus counteracting the negative nitrogen balance that is a sequel of androgen deficiency.

Feminizing Adrenocortical Carcinoma.   Increased estrogen production by an adrenal tumor may inhibit pituitary-hypothalamic function, resulting in decreased pituitary gonadotropin secretion, which, as expected, leads to testicular atrophy.

Sertoli-Cell-Only Syndrome (Germinal Cell Aplasia).   This syndrome may arise from a congenital absence of germ cells. The seminiferous tubules are therefore populated only by Sertoli cells. FSH levels may be preferentially elevated (absence of inhibin?) in this syndrome.

Benign Prostatic Hyperplasia.   Prostatic hyperplasia is a common occurrence in aging men. Dihydrotestosterone accumulation within the prostate serves as the humoral mediator of hyperplasia of the gland. An enhanced uptake of DHT in the gland may be due in part to enhanced intracellular binding of the androgen. The process is accelerated, however, by estrogens, which enhance the level of androgen receptors in the gland. Thus, an increase in androgen receptors allows for androgen-mediated growth even in the face of declining androgen production in advanced age. Both gynecomastia, as discussed earlier, and prostate hyperplasia may relate to the declining ratio of androgens to estrogens, which is common in the aging process of men.

Prostate Carcinoma.   Several hundred thousand new cases of prostatic carcinoma, of which about 80% are androgen-dependent, are diagnosed each year in the United States. Surgical castration and administration of pharmacological amounts of estrogen are treatments that have been employed to lower androgen levels in the management of the cancer. Castration is generally not acceptable to many men, and cardiovascular disease may ensue from the use of high doses of estrogens. "Medical castration" using analogs of gonadotropin-releasing hormone (GnRH) appear useful in the clinical treatment of the cancer. Inhibitors of 5α-reductase also show some success in the treatment of prostate neoplasia [36, 42, 62].

Impotence.   The physiologic basis for the control of penile erection is not totally understood. In the flaccid state, the penile vascular and cavernous smooth muscle are tonically contacted. Sexual stimulation causes release of neurotransmitters that result in relaxation of these smooth muscle cells, producing the vascular events mediating penile erection. The relaxation of the smooth muscle cells is not mediated by adrenergic or cholinergic mechanisms. Instead, nitric oxide and (NO) vasoactive intestinal peptide (VIP, see Chap. 10) [53] and prostaglandin E_1 have been implicated as neurotransmitters (NO, VIP) or paracrine mediators (PGE_1) that mediate the relaxation response that causes erection [13].

Nitric oxide (NO) is a cytotoxic agent of macrophages, a messenger molecule of neurons, and a vasodilator produced by endothelial cells. Its production is catalyzed by the enzymes neuronal nitric oxide synthase (nNOS) in neurons and epithelial nitric oxide synthase (eNOS) in epithelial cells. NOS has been localized to rat penile neurons innervating the corporal cavernosa and to neuronal plexuses in the adventitial layer of penile arteries. Small doses of NO synthase inhibitors abolish electrically-induced penile erections. These results establish NO as a physiologic mediator of erectile function [8, 27]. In the smooth muscle cell, NO stimulates the production of cGMP, while PGE_1 stimulates the cAMP accumulation. Both second messengers activate their corresponding protein kinases, which leads to Ca^{2+} channel closure and sequestration of intracellular Ca^{2+}. Lowered intracellular Ca^{2+} concentrations produce a relaxation of the smooth muscle cell. Drugs such as Viagra (Pfizer), the "pill for impotence," work by inhibiting the phosphodiesterase 5 (PDE5) that metabolizes cGMP to $5'GMP$. Thus, elevations in cGMP caused by NO are enhanced, producing a more pronounced and prolonged relaxation of the smooth muscle cells.

Pharmacological Considerations. Cannabinoids (substances present in marihuana, e.g., Δ^9-tetrahydrocannabinol, Δ^9-THC) inhibit testicular function in all vertebrate species studied. Testicular testosterone synthesis is decreased, which is correlated with lowered plasma levels of testosterone and involution of the prostate, seminal vesicles, and epididymis. Prolonged cannabinoid intake also leads to diminished spermatogenesis. The immediate effects of cannabinoids on the male reproductive system appear to be reversible. In humans, marihuana smoking decreases plasma testosterone levels and the sperm count. In mice cannabinoids reduce fertility and increase the incidence of chromosomal abnormalities, not only in the treated mice, but also in their untreated male offspring. The occurrence of congenital birth defects indicates that cannabinoids are capable of inducing genetic mutations that are transmissible to offspring [12]. Alcoholism may also lead to gonadal dysfunction, possibly by diminishing the number of gonadotropin receptors possessed by Leydig cells. Smoking of tobacco is now clearly implicated in the etiology of erectile dysfunction [65].

MOLECULAR MEDICINE CASE STUDY

"Pituitary function in a man with congenital aromatase deficiency: effect of different doses of transdermal E2 on basal and stimulated pituitary hormones." Rochira V et al., *J. Clin. Endocrinol. Metab.* 2002 Jun;87(6):2857–62.

To clarify the role of estrogen on male pituitary function, the effects of different doses of transdermal E_2 on pituitary secretion were evaluated in a man with aromatase deficiency. The study protocol was divided into the following three phases: no E_2 treatment (phase 1); 25 microg transdermal E_2 twice weekly for 9 months (phase 2); 12.5 microg transdermal E_2 twice weekly for 9 months (phase 3). Pituitary function was studied in detail during each phase of the study protocol by measuring hormone levels in basal conditions and after dynamic testing (GnRH, insulin tolerance test, GHRH plus arginine, TRH, and corticotropin-releasing factor; tests). Basal and GnRH-stimulated gonadotropin levels were inversely related to E_2 serum levels, according to the dosage of estrogen administered. Basal and stimulated

GH, PRL, and TSH serum levels did not change during the protocol study. The secretory pituitary reserve of GH was clearly impaired. Basal and stimulated ACTH and cortisol serum levels were not modified by estrogen administration. This study demonstrated that in the human male E_2 is required at the pituitary level for normal functioning of gonadotropin feedback both in basal and stimulated conditions. In this patient GH deficiency seems to be an adult-onset event since he reached a tall stature. However, the finding of a severe impairment in GH response to potent provocative stimuli together with the insensitivity of the GH/IGF-I axis to circulating estrogens strongly suggest a possible involvement of estrogens on both the development and maturation of the somatotrophic axis. Finally, the congenital lack of estrogen activity seems to be associated with a slightly impaired secretion of PRL and TSH, suggesting a possible role of estrogens on the pituitary secretion of these hormones in the human male.

REVIEW EXERCISES

Match the exons of the androgen receptor with their function:

1. Exon A
2. Exon D
3. Exon C
4. Exon E
5. Exon B
6. Exon F

A. Androgen-binding domain
B. DNA-binding domain
C. Transcriptional transactivation

Match the molecule with the cell type:

1. GnRH receptor
2. LH receptor
3. FSH receptor
4. inhibin receptor
5. inhibin
6. LHβ subunit
7. androgen binding protein
8. testosterone
9. activin receptor
10. androgen receptor

a. Sertoli cell
b. Gonadotrope
c. Leydig cell
d. Sperm cell
e. Neurons in the SNB
f. Satellite cells

Think, analyze and discuss:

1. Anabolic steroid abuse can produce a significant reduction in the size of the testes. Provide a plausible explanation for this phenomenon. Discontinuing anabolic steroid abuse may permit the testes to reattain their original size. Describe the probable sequence of events that may underlie this regrowth.

2. Precocious puberty can occur as a consequence of premature activation of gonadotropin secretion. In many cases, administration of a potent GnRH agonist has proven to be effective in reducing gonadotropin secretion in these boys. Why would a GnRH agonist be expected to down-regulate gonadotropin secretion? Would this treatment be effective in cases of precocious puberty that arise from mutations in the LH receptor that are constitutively active? If not, then what alternative therapy might be considered?

3. What physical and endocrine characteristics would you expect to be evident in a man with a complete ERα deficiency? An aromatase deficiency? What treatment would you recommend for men with an aromatase deficiency? Would the same treatment regimen be effective in the man with the ERα deficiency?

4. How do drugs such as Viagra (Pfizer) act to treat erectile dysfunction? Considering the cellular actions of drugs such as Viagra, why are these drugs not recommended for use by individuals who are taking nitroglycerine tablets for angina? Can you think of any other potential pharmacological strategies that might be used? Which molecules might be targeted for stimulation or inhibition in the arterial or cavernous smooth muscle cells?

5. Explain how androgens, LH, and FSH control spermatogenesis. Would testosterone treatment be potentially useful as a male contraceptive strategy? How might it work?

6. Gynecomastia can occur in neonates, prepubertal boys, adolescent boys, and adult men. However, the underlying bases for the condition differs for each of these stages of development. Provide a plausible explanation for the occurrence of gynecomastia in males at all of these ages.

7. What causes alopecia? Why do some females develop this condition?

8. Only males have antlers in most species of deer. Provide a mechanistic hypothesis that would explain why male and female caribou both have antlers.

9. What might cause microphallus (abnormally small penis size in adulthood)?

10. Describe "receptor-negative" and "receptor-positive" androgen resistance. What experimental methods could be used to determine if a patient who exhibits androgen resistance has one or the other type? (You may assume that the nucleotide sequence of the gene in an individual with a mutation would be known, the AR amino acid sequence in this individual would be deduced, and that the mutant AR could be expressed in cells). What would be the results of your experiments be in either case?

References

[1] Alonso, L. C., and R. L. Rosenfield. 2003. Molecular genetic and endocrine mechanisms of hair growth. *Horm. Res.* 60(1):1–13.

[2] Anand, S., et al. 2002. Differential regulation of luteinizing hormone and follicle-stimulating hormone in male Siberian hamsters by exposure to females and photoperiod. *Endocrinology* 143(6):2178–88.

[3] Bagatell, C. J., et al. 1994. Physiological levels of estradiol stimulate plasma high density lipoprotein$_2$ cholesterol levels in normal men. *J. Clin. Endocrinol. Metab.* 78:855–61.

[4] Belchetz, P. E., et al. 1978. Hypophysial responses to continuous and intermittent delivery of hypothalamic gonadotropin-releasing hormone. *Science* 202(4368):631–3.

[5] Black, B. E., and B. M. Paschal. 2004. Intranuclear organization and function of the androgen receptor. *Trends Endocrinol Metab.* 15(9):411–17.

[6] Bocklandt, S., and D. H. Hamer. 2003. Beyond hormones: a novel hypothesis for the biological basis of male sexual orientation. *J. Endocrinol. Invest.* 26(3 Suppl.):8–12.

[7] Breedlove, S. M., and A. P. Arnold. 1980. Hormone accumulation in a sexually dimorphic motor nucleus of the rat spinal cord. *Science* 210:564–6.

[8] Burnett, A. L., et al. 1992. Nitric oxide: A physiologic mediator of penile erection. *Science* 257:401–3.

[9] Celotti, F., and N. Cesi. 1992. Anabolic steroids: A review of their effects on the muscles, of their possible mechanisms of action and of their use in athletics. *J. Steroid Biochem. Mol. Biol.* 43:469–77.

[10] Clarke, I. J., and J. T. Cummins. 1982. The temporal relationship between gonadotropin releasing hormone (GnRH) and luteinizing hormone (LH) secretion in ovariectomized ewes. *Endocrinology* 111(5):1737–9.

[11] Cowley, G. 1996. Testosterone and other hormone treatments offer new hope for staying youthful, sexy and strong. *Newsweek*, Sept. 16:67–75.

[12] Dalterio, S., et al. 1982. Cannabinoids in male mice: Effects on fertility and spermatogenesis. *Science* 216:315–16.

[13] Dean, R. C., and T. F. Lue. 2005 Physiology of penile erection and pathophysiology of erectile dysfunction. *Urol. Clin. North Am.* 32(4):379–203.

[14] Dent, J. N. 1975. Integumentary effects of prolactin in the lower vertebrates. *Am. Zool.* 15:923–35.

[15] DiRaimondo, C. V., A. C. Roach, and C. K. Meador. 1980. Gynecomastia from exposure to vaginal estrogen cream. *N. Engl. J. Med.* 302:1089–90.

[16] Dominguez, J. M., and E. M. Hull. 2005. Dopamine, the medial preoptic area, and male sexual behavior. *Physiol. Behav.* 86(3):356–68.

[17] Doupe, A. J. 1994. Songbirds and adult neurogenesis: A new role for hormones. *Proc. Natl. Acad. Sci. USA* 91:7836–8.

[18] Eung, A. C. 1997. Estrogen for men: Reversal of cardiovascular misfortune *J. Am. Coll. Cardiol.* 29:1445–6.

[19] Frank, G. R. 1995. The role of estrogen in pubertal skeletal physiology: Epiphyseal maturation and mineralization of the skeleton. *Acta Paediatr.* 84:627–30.

[20] Gast, A., et al. 1995. A single amino acid exchange abolishes dimerization of the androgen receptor and causes Reifenstein syndrome. *Mol. Cell. Endocrinol.* 111:93–8.

[21] Gormley, G. J. 1995. Finasteride: A clinical review. *Biomed. Pharmacother.* 49:319–24.

[22] Goss, R. J. 1968. Inhibition of growth and shedding of antlers by sex hormones. *Nature* 220:83–5.

[23] Hamer, D. H., et al. 1993. A linkage between DNA markers on the X chromosome and male sexual orientation. *Science* 261:321–7.

[24] Harris, G. C., and J. E. Levine. 2003. Pubertal acceleration of pulsatile gonadotropin-releasing hormone release in male rats as revealed by microdialysis. *Endocrinology* 144(1):163–71.

[25] Hess, R. A., et al. 1997. A role for estrogens in the male reproductive system. *Nature* 390:509–12.

[26] Höhn, E. O., and S. C. Cheng. 1967. Gonadal hormones on Wilson's phalarope (*Steganopus tricolor*) and other birds in relation to plumage and sex behavior. *Gen. Comp. Endocrinol.* 8:1–11.

[27] Ignarro, L. J. 1992. Nitric oxide as the physiological mediator of penile erection. *J. NIH Res.* 4:59–62.

[28] Imperato-McGinley, J., and W. J. Canovatchel. 1992. Complete androgen insensitivity. Pathophysiology, diagnosis, and management. *TEM* 3:75–81.

[29] Janne, O. A., et al. 1993. Androgen receptor and mechanism of androgen action. *Ann. Med.* 25:83–89.

[30] Jannini, E. A., S. Ulisse, and M. D'Armiento. 1995. Thyroid hormone and male gonadal function. *Endocr. Rev.* 16:443–59.

[31] Johns, J. E. 1964. Testosterone induced nuptial feathers in phalaropes. *Condor* 66:449–54.

[32] Jones, R. E. 1971. The incubation patch of birds. *Biol. Rev.* 46:315–39.

[33] Jones, M. E., et al. 2006. Of mice and men: The evolving phenotype of aromatase deficiency. *Trends Endocrinol. Metab.* 17(2):55–64.

[34] Josso, N., and N. Clemente. 2003. Transduction pathway of anti-Mullerian hormone, a sex-specific member of the TGF-beta family. *Trends Endocrinol. Metab.* 14(2):91–7.

[35] Kaufman, J. M., and A. Vermeulen. 2005. The decline of androgen levels in elderly men and its clinical and therapeutic implications. *Endocr. Rev.* 26(6):833–76.

[36] Kenny, B., et al. 1997. Pharmacological options in the treatment of benign prostate hyperplasia. *J. Med. Chem.* 40:1293–315.

[37] Koenig, H., et al. 1980. Testosterone-mediated sexual dimorphism of mitochondria and lysosomes in mouse kidney proximal tubules. *Science* 209:1023–6.

[38] Korach, K. S. 1994. Insights from the study of animals lacking functional estrogen receptor. *Science* 266:1524–6.

[39] Kremer, H., et al. 1995. Male pseudohermaphroditism due to a homozygous missense mutation of the luteinizing hormone receptor gene. *Nature Genet.* 9:160–4.

[40] Kudwa, A. E., et al. 2006. Roles of estrogen receptors alpha and beta in differentiation of mouse sexual behavior. *Neuroscience* 138(3):921–8.

[41] Kurz, E. M., D. R. Sengelaub, and A. P. Arnold. 1986. Androgens regulate the dendritic length of mammalian motoneurons in adulthood. *Science* 232:395–8.

[42] Lalani, E.-N., M. E. Laniado, and P. D. Abel. 1997. Molecular and cellular biology of prostate cancer. *Cancer Metastasis Rev.* 16:29–66.

[43] Latronico, A. C., et al. 1995. A novel mutation of the luteinizing hormone receptor gene causing male gonadotropin-independent precocious puberty. *J. Clin. Endocrinol. Metab.* 80:2490–4.

[44] LeVay, S., and D. H. Hamer. 1994. Evidence for a biological influence in male homosexuality. *Sci. Am.* 270(5):44–9.

[45] LeVay, S. 1991. A difference in hypothalamic structure between heterosexual and homosexual men. *Science* 253(5023):1034–7.

[46] Levine, J. E., et al. 1982. Simultaneous measurement of luteinizing hormone-releasing hormone and luteinizing hormone release in unanesthetized, ovariectomized sheep. *Endocrinology* 111(5):1449–55.

[47] Lindzey, J., and K. S. Korach. 1997. Developmental and physiological effects of estrogen receptor gene disruption in mice. *TEM* 8:137–44.

[48] Lincoln, G. A. 1971. The seasonal reproductive changes in the Red Deer stag (Cervus elaphus). *J. Zool. Lond.* 163:105–23.

[49] Matsumoto, A. M., and W. J. Bremner. 1984. Modulation of pulsatile gonadotropin secretion by testosterone in men. *J. Clin. Endocrinol. Metab.* 58:609–14.

[50] Meredith, J. M., F. W. Turek, and J. E. Levine. 1998. Effects of gonadotropin-releasing hormone pulse frequency modulation on the reproductive axis of photoinhibited male Siberian hamsters. *Biol. Reprod.* 59(4):813–19.

[51] Miller, W. L., 1997. Pathophysiology, genetics, and treatment of hypergonadism. *Pediatr. Endocrinol.* 44:375–95.

[52] Mustanski, B. S., et al. 2005. A genomewide scan of male sexual orientation. *Hum. Genet.* 116(4):272–8.

[53] Ottesen, B., et al. 1984. Penile erection: Possible role for vasoactive intestinal polypeptide as a neurotransmitter. *Br. Med. J.* 288:9–11.

[54] Rey, R., et al. 1994. Anti-Müllerian hormone in children with androgen insensitivity. *J. Clin. Endocrinol. Metabol.* 79:960–4.

[55] Roselli, C. E., et al. 2004. Sexual partner preference, hypothalamic morphology and aromatase in rams. *Physiol. Behav.* 83(2):233–45.

[56] Sawaya, M. E., L. S. Honig, and S. L. Hsia. 1989. Increased androgen binding capacity in sebaceous glands in scalp of male-pattern baldness. *J. Invest. Dermatol.* 92:91–5.

[57] Seminara, S. B., F. J. Hayes, and W. F. Crowley, Jr. 1998. Gonadotropin-releasing hormone deficiency in the human (idiopathic hypogonadotropic hypogonadism and Kallmann's syndrome): Pathophysiological and genetic considerations. *Endocr. Rev.* 19(5):521–39.

[58] Simmoni, M., J. Gromoll, and E. Nieschlag. 1997. The follicle-stimulating hormone receptor: Biochemistry, molecular biology, physiology, and pathophysiology. *Endocr. Rev.* 739–73.

[59] Smith, E. P., et al. 1994. Estrogen resistance caused by a mutation in the estrogen-receptor gene in a man. *N. Engl. J. Med.* 331:1056–61.

[60] Smith, R. J. F. 1974. Effects of 17β-methyltestosterone on the dorsal pad and tubercles of flathead minnows (*Pimephales promelas*). *Can. J. Zool.* 52:1031–8.

[61] Spiteri-Grech, J., and E. Nieschlag. 1993. Paracrine factors relevant to the regulation of spermatogenesis—A review. *J. Reprod. Fert.* 98:1–14.

[62] Stoner, E. 1996. 5α-reductase inhibitors/Finasteride. *The Prostate 6 (Supplement)*:82–7.

[63] Tenover, J. L. 1997. Testosterone and the aging male. *J. Androl.* 18:103–6.

[64] Themmen, A. P. N., and H. G. Brunner. 1996. Luteinizing hormone receptor mutations and sex differentiation. *Eur. J. Endocrinol.* 134:533–40.

[65] Vine, M. R. 1996. Smoking and male reproduction: A review. *Intern. J. Androl.* 19:323–37.

[66] Wiley, M. L., and B. B. Collette. 1970. Breeding tubercles and contact organs in fishes, their occurrence, structure and significance. *Am. Mus. Natur. Hist. Bull.* 143:147–53.

[67] Yue, C., J. D. Zajac, and H. E. MacLean. 2005. Androgen regulation of satellite cell function. *J. Endocrinol.* 186:21–31.

Hormones and Female Reproductive Physiology

I t was noted earlier that in mammals, the female phenotype develops sponta-neously, apparently in the absence of any gonadal hormone directive. At puberty, however, ovarian steroid hormone secretion is essential for development of female secondary sex characteristics. In addition, gonadal hormone production regu-lates the cyclic pattern of pituitary gonadotropin secretion characteristic of the female and is responsible for other cyclic phenomena as egg maturation, ovulation, and the menstrual cycle.

It has long been known that ovariectomy results in uterine atrophy and the loss of sexual activity and reproduction. The role of the ovaries in the control of reproduc-tive function was established in 1900 by Knauer, who found that ovarian transplants prevented the atrophic symptoms of gonadectomy. Ovarian extracts were then found to maintain the integrity of reproductive structures following ovariectomy. Allen and Doisy identified the Graafian follicle as a major source of estrogenic activity [4]. A putative female sex hormone was then discovered in the blood of a number of ani-mals, and it was further observed that the concentration of the substance varied with the phase of the menstrual cycle in the human female. An important discovery was the finding that this substance, a steroid, was present in the urine in large amounts during pregnancy. Chemists were able to isolate the active substance from urine in crystalline form and to determine its chemical structure. This steroid hormone, **estradiol**, plays an essential role in the control of secondary sex characteristics in the female of most vertebrate species. It was also established that the corpus luteum of the ovary secreted a steroid hormone that is necessary for normal reproductive func-tion during pregnancy. This hormone, **progesterone**, was isolated and subsequently synthesized in 1934.

Although ovarian estrogens and progestins play pivotal roles in the regulation of female reproductive physiology, it is now realized that many other hormones of neural, placental-uterine, and adrenal origin are also essential for normal reproductive function in the female.

Anatomy of the Female Reproductive System

Like the testes in the male, the ovaries serve both a gametogenic and an endocrine function (Fig. 18.1). The female gametes, ova, are released (ovulated) from the ovary into the abdom-inal cavity where they find their way into the closely adherent uterine tubes (Fallopian tubes, oviducts). The eggs may become fertilized en route down the oviducts by spermatozoa pre-viously introduced into the vagina by the male ejaculate. If fertilization occurs, the fertilized egg, the *zygote*, may then become embedded within the lining of the uterus and through embryogenesis develop into a fetus. The general morphological and functional features of the human female reproductive system will be described.

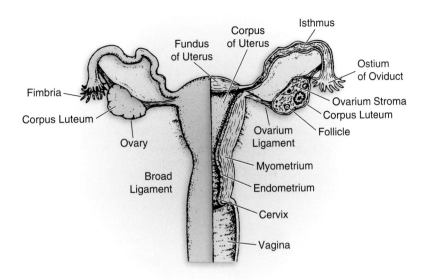

Figure 18.1
Reproductive organs
of the human female.

The Major Physiological Activities of the Ovary are Hormonogenesis and Gametogenesis

The ovary has two functional roles that are distinct but intertwined. The first is hormonogenesis, and the second is gametogenesis. The gonad in the homogametic species develops in the absence of any apparent endocrine influence (Chap. 16). In the human female, the gametogenic potential of the ovary is established early in fetal development, but the endocrine role of the ovary is not realized until puberty. Each of the embryonic ovaries is initially populated by about one thousand to two thousand *primordial germ cells*, which, through rapid proliferation, give rise in each ovary to about 3 million oocytes. At birth, this number is reduced through cell death (apoptosis) to about 1 million oocytes in each ovary, and by puberty, each ovary may only be populated by about 250,000 oocytes. Only an exceedingly small fraction of these viable oocytes will develop fully into mature egg cells. Indeed, because a single ovum is usually ovulated during each human reproductive cycle, a total of only 400 to 500 oocytes are released from the ovaries; the remaining 99.9% are destined for atresia during the years of ovarian activity (puberty to menopause) [28].

The ovary consists of both epithelial and mesenchymal components. The mesenchymal tissue differentiates into *interstitial tissue*, which will be the primary source of estrogen production by the ovary. The epithelial tissue will become closely associated with the germinal elements of the ovary and, in addition to providing a nutritive environment for the oocytes, will also provide an important source of hormones during particular phases of the female cycle.

At birth, each oocyte is surrounded by a single layer of flattened epithelial-derived *granulosa cells*; the combined structure is called a *primordial follicle* (Fig. 18.2). These primordial follicles lie mostly near the periphery (cortex) of the ovary but are separated from each other by stromal (connective) and interstitial tissue. Most primordial follicles remain in an arrested state, which may last until puberty or even menopause, if they are not selected for further differentiation and development. Within the embryonic ovary, the primordial follicles begin the reduction division of meiosis, but when meiotic division is delayed in the late prophase, the follicles and their primary oocytes may continue to increase greatly in size. Further development of a primordial follicle involves transformation of the follicular epithelial cells into a single layer of cuboidal cells surrounding the oocyte; the composite structure is referred to as a *primary follicle* (Fig. 18.2).

Under endocrine stimulation once during each ovarian cycle after puberty, 6 to 12 primary follicles develop into *secondary follicles*. This process involves an increase in the size of the oocyte and in the number of granulosa cell layers that surround each oocyte (Fig. 18.2). During the development of these secondary follicles, the granulosa cells secrete a mucoid material that forms the *zona pellucida* around the oocyte (Fig. 18.2). The granulosa cells develop protoplasmic processes that penetrate the zona pellucida and make contact with the plasmalemma of the oocyte. Although a number of primary follicles may be selected for further development into secondary follicles during each menstrual cycle, usually only one

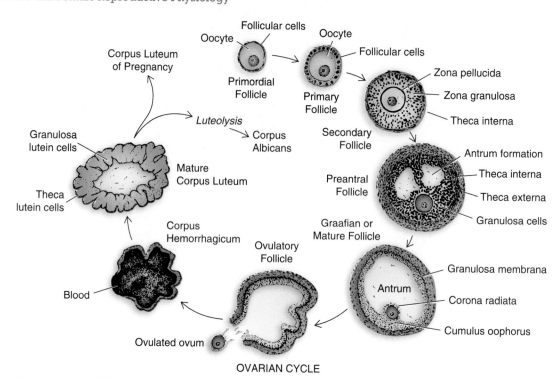

Figure 18.2 The primate ovarian follicular cycle.

is destined to develop into a mature follicle. The others, by mechanisms that are not fully understood, become atretic and disappear with time.

During each ovarian cycle, selected primary oocytes complete the first meiotic division with resulting extrusion of the first polar body and formation of the *secondary oocyte*, which contains most of the cytoplasm. The first meiotic division is completed shortly before ovulation. The secondary oocyte immediately enters the second reduction division of meiosis, a process that is arrested in metaphase unless fertilization occurs subsequent to ovulation. The second polar body is extruded if the oocyte is penetrated by a sperm. The diploid state of the transiently haploid oocyte is therefore reconstituted by the haploid chromosomal contribution of the sperm to the zygote.

The granulosa cells of follicles destined for further maturation continue to increase in number. At the same time, interstitial tissue adjacent to the follicle becomes arranged concentrically around it to form the *theca* (theca folliculi). Those thecal cells adjacent to the follicle, the *theca interna*, are surrounded by an additional outer layer of interstitial cells, the *theca externa*, which merges somewhat imperceptibly with the ovarian stroma. The theca interna remains separated from the granulosa cells by a basement lamella. Although the theca is penetrated by vascular elements, no capillaries penetrate into the zona granulosa.

Continued proliferation of granulosa cells and the incorporation of surrounding interstitial cells into the theca are accompanied by the accumulation of fluid in spaces or clefts within the granulosa cells. As the follicle enlarges, a single large vesicle or antrum is formed. Those granulosa cells that remain adherent to the ovum comprise the coronal granulosa cells; those granulosa cells that remain in contact with the surrounding theca constitute the *membrana granulosa*. A bridge of granulosa cells connects those cells adherent to the ovum with the membrana granulosa and constitutes the *cumulus oophorus*. During ovulation, this connection is severed and the ovum is ejected with its surrounding layer of granulosa cells, the *corona radiata*. The fully developed mature follicle, shown in Figure 18.3, is known as a *Graafian follicle*.

"Mammalian ovulation is a unique biological phenomenon in that it requires the physical disruption of healthy tissue at the surface of the ovary. There is no conspicuous change in the appearance of a mature ovarian follicle during the first several hours after it is stimulated by an ovulatory surge in pituitary gonadotropins. However, 4 to 6 hours into the ovulatory process, the follicle begins to blush. There is clear evidence that the capillaries in the follicle wall dilate, and the tissue becomes hyperemic. There is negligible other macroscopic, or microscopic, evidence of pending rupture until 1 to 2 hours before the follicle wall actually

Figure 18.3 Scanning electron micrograph of the human Graafian follicle. (From P. Bagavadoss. The Reproductive Endocrinology Program, Department of Anatomy, The University of Michigan.)

bursts. As the time of rupture nears, the apex of a mature follicle protrudes more and more above the surface of the ovary and the follicle wall itself gradually becomes thinner. Eventually, the apical most portion of the follicle becomes translucent and rapidly balloons above the normal curvature of the follicle wall to form a stigma. This nipple-like blob may not form in all species of mammals, and will not occur if the vascular supply to the ovary has been impaired. However, a follicle will usually rupture within several minutes after the stigma forms. The eventual rupture of a follicle is dependent on adequate degradation of the collagenous connective tissue in the thecal layers of the follicle wall and on a modest, but essential, intrafollicular pressure of about 20 mmHg that arises from capillary hydrostatic pressure. After the follicle wall bursts, the oocyte and surrounding cumulus cells are usually extruded within 1 to 2 minutes. Ovulation is complete when the egg-bearing cumulus mass is expelled from the ovary.

Current information from biochemical data indicate that the ovulatory surge in luteinizing hormone (LH; or exogenous hCG) initiates acute changes in steroid and eicosanoid metabolism in the granulosa cells of mature follicles. The ensuing increases in local prostaglandins, lipoxins, kinins, platelet-activating factor, and other vasoactive agents collectively cause substantial dilation of the capillaries in the theca interna of the follicle wall. This significant change in the capillaries of ovulatory follicles results in a fourfold increase in the volume of the ovarian vascular compartment. Concomitant with this hyperemic response, the permeability of the thecal capillaries increases to the extent that serum proteins are exuded into the interstitial spaces of the follicle in a manner characteristic of inflamed tissues. Since blood serum is well known for its ability to activate fibroblasts, it has been hypothesized that the exuded serum stimulates the quiescent fibroblasts in the theca externa and tunica albuginea of an ovulatory follicle and causes the resting fibroblasts to transform into proliferating cells. These activated thecal cells begin secreting a metalloproteinase that degrades the extracellular matrix of collagenous connective tissue in the follicle wall. Ultimately, the follicle wall loses its tensile strength and eventually ruptures under the force of a modest, but effective, intrafollicular pressure" [18].

Significant progress has been made in the delineation of molecular events mediating induction of ovulation by the LH surge [47, 48]. The rate-limiting enzyme in the formation of prostaglandins, cyclooxygenase-2 (COX-2) is induced in cumulus cells by the LH surge, and in mice null for COX-2 [13], or the prostaglandin E_2 receptor EP2 [58], ovulation fails to occur in response to LH. However, PGE_2 can restore cumulus expansion and ovulation in the COX-2 deficient mice. These observations demonstrate that the induction of COX-2 expression and PGE_2 actions in the cumulus–oocyte complex are obligatory in LH-induced

Folliculogenesis

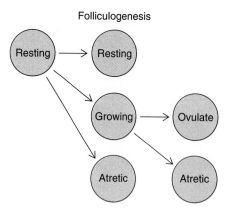

Figure 18.4   Ovarian follicles may be found in four basic conditions: at rest, growing, atretic, or ready to ovulate. (From Irianni and Hogden [28], with permission. *Endocrinology and Metabolism Clinics of North America* 21:19–38, 1992.)

ovulation. The progesterone receptor (PR) expressed in mural granulosa cells has also been identified as a critically important component of the ovulatory process. Mice null for the PR also fail to ovulate in response to hormonal stimulation [37]. Two "downstream" targets of the activated PR are proteases that may be involved in follicular rupture, "a disintegrin and metalloproteinase, with thrombospondin-like motifs" (ADAMTS-1) [47, 48], and the lysosomal protease, cathepsin L [47, 48].

The Dominant Ovarian Follicle.   Although many follicles may begin to mature during each ovarian/menstrual cycle, typically, only a single follicle sustains its inherent gametogenic potential, whereas the others become atretic. Any ovarian follicle destined to ovulate is derived from a group of growing follicles drawn, in turn, from a pool of nonproliferating primordial follicles formed during fetal development (Fig. 18.4). Pituitary gonadotropins support this progression of follicular maturation, but about 99.9% of all ovarian follicles are lost spontaneously to atresia; only a few achieve ovulation. Depending on the species, usually only a few, or even just one, of these follicles of a given group escape atresia at various stages of development and finally reach maturity, culminating in ovulation of a fertilizable oocyte. This successive reduction of potentially ovulatory follicles during each ovarian cycle to a number characteristic of the species suggests some sort of selection. This process is especially evident in the higher primates, including women, where typically the process of folliculogenesis leading to the elaboration of a single mature gamete in each menstrual cycle is regulated with a high degree of precision [28].

The follicle that eventually matures and ovulates is thought to be the one whose granulosa cells most rapidly acquire high levels of aromatase and LH receptor in response to the intercycle follicle-stimulating hormone (FSH) rise, that is, the one with the lowest FSH "threshold." During the midfollicular phase, this follicle begins to increase estradiol (E$_2$) secretion and the steroid feeds back to regulate pituitary FSH secretion negatively. This causes a progressive reduction in the circulating FSH level and thereby limits FSH-dependent development of other follicles with relatively high FSH thresholds. Thus, only one follicle becomes fully mature, being protected against the fall in circulating FSH by the relatively high responsiveness of its granulosa cells to both FSH and LH. Follicular selection thus appears to be dependent upon the delicate interplay between gonadotropin secretions, ovarian steroid production, and maturation-specific alterations in the responsiveness of the ovary to gonadotropins [62]. At the cellular level, it is likely that follicular selection involves the induction of genes by FSH that promote granulosa cell proliferation and survival. Follicular development is also associated with increasingly dense capillaries surrounding the mature follicle. These capillaries may permit increased delivery of gonadotropin to the mature follicle and thereby selectively enhance its development. Paracrine factors such as vascular endothelial growth factor (VEGF) appear to be involved in this maturation-related angiogenesis.

It has been stated that "The purposes of the ovarian follicle are to (1) preserve the resident oocyte; (2) mature the oocyte at the optimal time; (3) produce a hormonal milieu that will develop a lush proliferative endometrium; (4) yield well-timed release of the oocyte; (5) provide for a high-quality corpus luteum function, leading to implantation; and (6) preserve the hormonal conditions required for gestation until the fetoplacental metabolism is adequate—a formidable sequence designed by nature" [39].

The Corpus Luteum. After rupture of the mature follicle and liberation of the ovum during ovulation, the follicle promptly fills up with blood, forming what is called a *corpus hemorrhagicum*. The granulosa and thecal cells rapidly increase in number and the clotted blood is absorbed. Vascular elements from the theca now penetrate the granulosa cells. The granulosa cells begin to accumulate large quantities of cholesterol; this luteinization process leads to formation of the *corpus luteum* [50]. The mature corpus luteum of some species appears to contain a number of distinct cell types. Cells derived from the theca interna migrate into granulosa-derived areas of the luteal tissue soon after ovulation to give rise to small luteal cells, theca lutein cells, and fibroblasts. The large luteal cells apparently differentiate from the membrana granulosa. Although luteal cell heterogeneity is commonly accepted, the definitive origin of each cell type and its individual functions within the corpus luteum of pregnancy remain unclear.

Fallopian Tubes Convey Ova Towards the Uterus

In the human female, these paired oviducts are about 10 cm long and are closely adherent to the superiolateral aspects of the uterus (see Fig. 18.1). The ostium tubae, the fimbriated ovarian extremity of the oviduct, spread over most of the medial surface of the ovary, and the undulatory movements of the fimbriae assist ova transport into the lumen of the Fallopian tubes. The oviducts proper are composed of longitudinal and circular muscular layers covered by a simple columnar epithelium that comprises the luminal mucosa. The ciliated mucosal cells beat toward the uterus and thus rapidly convey the ova toward the uterus. Fertilization of the egg takes place within the oviducts.

The Uterus is the Site of Implantation of a Fertilized Egg and Fetal Development

The uterus, connected to the oviducts at superiolateral angles, is a thick-walled, muscular organ that serves as a site for fetal development and as an endocrine organ during pregnancy. The bulk of the uterus is composed of smooth muscle, the *myometrium* (see Fig. 18.1). An *endometrium* covers the mucosal aspect of the myometrium and is composed of connective tissue and an extensive vascular network. The endometrium, in turn, is covered by a simple epithelium. The thickness of the endometrium varies dramatically throughout the menstrual cycle in response to ovarian hormones. The myometrium is also similarly variable in thickness, most profoundly during pregnancy.

Ovarian Steroid Hormones

The ovarian follicle is the source of three types of steroid hormones: progestogens (progestins), androgens, and estrogens [4]. The relative amounts of each class of steroid vary throughout the menstrual cycle and drastically change in the pregnant state. During the follicular phase of the menstrual cycle, estradiol is the major steroid hormone secreted by the ovary, whereas during the luteal phase and during pregnancy, progesterone is the major steroid hormone secreted.

Estrogen Biosynthesis Requires Androgen Production in Thecal Cells and Aromatization in Granulosa Cells

The *two-cell theory* of estrogen production suggests that the thecal cells produce C_{19} androgens that are then delivered to the granulosa cells wherein they are aromatized to estrogens (Fig. 18.5) [26, 27]. This theory is supported by the observation that granulosa cells from several species secrete estrogens if given an androgen substrate. In addition, thecal cells produce large amounts of androgens. The CYP17 gene that encodes 17-hydroxylase/C_{17-20} lyase is actively regulated by LH. Granulosa cells, on the other hand, have little or no capacity for producing C_{19} androgens from C_{21} steroids, but do have an active aromatase system. As follicular maturation progresses, the ability of granulosa cells to aromatize androgens increases. Estrogen production increases within the follicle during the preovulatory phase and is highest at the time of the LH/FSH surge. Before exposure to a high level of LH, androgen and estrogen levels predominate; after the LH surge and during the luteal phase of the cycle, however, progesterone is the major steroid produced.

Figure 18.5 Two-cell, two-gonadotropin hypothesis of estrogen synthesis.

Figure 18.6   Biosynthesis and metabolism of estradiol.

A modified version of the two-cell theory suggests that LH stimulates androgen production within the thecal cells. The androgens are then aromatized within the thecal cells but are also made available to the granulosa cells for aromatization to estrogens. The estrogens produced by the thecal cells would be the major source of circulating levels of the steroid, whereas estrogens synthesized by the granulosa cells would serve a local role, possibly related to ovum maturation. The granulosa cells are regulated through FSH stimulation of cAMP production and subsequent induction and activation of aromatase activity.

Estradiol (E_2) is readily oxidized to *estrone* within the liver (Fig. 18.6); estrone may be further hydrated to *estriol* (E_3). These three estrogens are excreted in the urine as glucuronides and sulfates. During pregnancy, the placenta is an additional source of estrogens. Indeed, the formation of estrogens is not limited to the ovaries, placenta, or adrenals, as some peripheral tissues (e.g., adipose tissue) can produce significant quantities of estrogens from steroid precursors. Aromatization of androstenedione and testosterone within tissues is a major source of estrogens in the male and postmenopausal female.

Progesterone Biosynthesis Occurs Primarily in Luteal Cells

The growth of the preovulatory follicles is dependent on both FSH and LH acting in concert. FSH promotes the growth of the follicle by acting through receptors on the granulosa cells and inducing the aromatase enzyme required to convert androgens to estrogens. The androgens originate from the theca under the control of LH (Fig. 18.5). Whereas FSH receptors are only present on granulosa cells in the latter stages of preovulatory development, LH receptors, present initially only in the theca, appear in the antral granulosa cells and are probably coupled to the same second-messenger (cAMP) system as FSH receptors. These cells have little 17,20-lyase activity, and thus they synthesize and secrete progesterone, and not androgens or estrogens, in response to LH. During the preovulatory surge, LH acting directly on the granulosa cells initiates luteinization, and the enhancement of progesterone synthesis and secretion as the luteinized granulosa cells transform to become the corpus luteum.

Progesterone synthesis is an early step in the biosynthesis of androgen and estrogen production within the thecal cell. Thecal cell progesterone production is not, however, considered an important source of vascular levels of progesterone. The corpus luteum is the major source of circulating progesterone. During the follicular phase of the cycle these cells, which are essentially devoid of a smooth endoplasmic reticulum characteristic of steroid-secreting cells, may use an androgen substrate for aromatization to estrogens as discussed before. Just prior to the LH/FSH surge in some species, progesterone biosynthesis is initiated within the granulosa cells. The fact that granulosa cells from large follicles spontaneously luteinize in culture, but fail to do so in the presence of follicular fluid obtained from small follicles, suggests that a luteinization inhibitor may be present and may function to keep granulosa cells from secreting prematurely. Luteinized cells contain large quantities of cholesterol; it has been shown that rat luteal cells preferentially use, and are acutely dependent on, plasma low-density lipoprotein complexes (Chap. 15). Luteal cells are the major source of circulating progesterone following the luteinization process.

Androgens May Support some Aspects of Female Pubertal Maturation

With the commencement of ovarian estrogen synthesis at puberty, androstenedione and testosterone, precursors of estrogens, are secreted by the ovaries [53]. The development of secondary sex characteristics during the pubertal process appears to be almost totally accounted for by the actions of estrogens. Nevertheless, it is possible that the growth spurt that occurs at puberty may, in part, be influenced by androgens of ovarian origin. In addition, acne, common to many females at puberty, results from sebaceous gland activation by ovarian androgens. Pubic and axillary hair growth are also attributed to androgens of ovarian and/or adrenal origin.

Adrenarche leads to the development of sexual (pubic or axillary) hair (pubarche). It is associated with an increase in serum levels of dehydroepiandrosterone sulfate (DHEAS) and changes in the adrenal response to ACTH. These changes in adrenal androgen production are referred to as biochemical adrenarche and result from maturational changes in the activities of the adrenal enzymes 3β-hydroxysteroid dehydrogenase (3β-HSD), 17-hydroxylase, and 17,20-desmolase. The consequence of these changes in enzyme activity is increased production of adrenal androgens.

Paracrine-Acting Growth Factors Regulate Ovarian Function

The roles of insulin-like growth factors (IGFs), especially IGF-I, in regulating the ovarian cycle, folliculogenesis, and granulosa cell steroidogenesis have been documented [2]. Studies from several laboratories demonstrated that IGFs promote both replication and differentiation of cultured granulosa cells. IGFs affect FSH-induced enhancement of progesterone, estrogen, and cAMP production, as well as LH receptor induction. In porcine thecal cells, IGFs increase basal and gonadotropin-induced progesterone secretion. In addition, hCG-induced synthesis of thecal androstenedione and testosterone are enhanced when estradiol synthesis is decreased. Porcine theca and granulosa cells contain receptors for IGF-I. The possible involvement of ovarian IGFs in follicular development in vivo was also suggested by measurements of IGF-I in porcine follicular fluid and culture media from porcine granulosa cells. Indeed, gonadotropin, estrogen, as well as cAMP (the presumed mediator of gonadotropin action), enhance the secretion of immunoreactive IGF-I by porcine granulosa cells. Estrogen receptor activation in granulosa cells also leads to an increase in IGF-receptor expression [47]. Thus, the hormone-induced secretion of growth factors and increases in sensitivity to growth factors appears to serve an important autocrine mechanism by which follicular growth and differentiation occur (Fig. 18.7). Additionally, growth factors of the epidermal growth factor (EGF) family appear to mediate the effects of LH, particularly during the preovulatory period in which cumulus expansion and oocyte maturation occur.

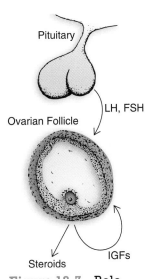

Figure 18.7 Role of IGFs in ovarian steroidogenesis.

Physiological Roles of Ovarian Steroid Hormones

There is no evidence that the fetal or preadolescent human ovary produces significant quantities of estrogens or other gonadal steroids. At puberty, however, ovarian steroidogenesis is activated by pituitary gonadotropins. During the follicular phase of the ensuing menstrual cycles, estrogens are the main steroidal products of the ovary, whereas during the luteal phase of each cycle, progesterone is the hormonally important steroidal product of the postovulatory follicle.

Estrogens. Estrogens produced during pubertal maturation in the human female are responsible for growth and development of the vagina, uterus, and oviducts, organs essential to ovum transport, zygote maturation, and implantation of the conceptus. Estrogens affect the distribution of fat deposition, a process that occurs in the postadolescent female. Mammary growth and development is also initiated by the actions of estrogens in concert with other hormones. Estrogen is a key endocrine component of the menstrual cycle in the adult, with actions in the brain, pituitary gland, and ovary to control ovulatory cyclicity. Other physiological actions of estrogens are summarized in Table 18.1.

TABLE 18.1 Some physiological effects and roles of ovarian steroid hormones in mammals

Primary site of action	Physiological action
Estradiol	
CNS	Maintains libido and sexual behavior
	Facilitates maternal behavior
	Has negative and positive feedback effects on GnRH release
	Stabilizes thermoregulatory systems
	Provides neuroprotection
Pituitary	Has negative and positive feedback effects on gonadotropin secretion
	Increases pituitary GnRH receptor number
	Increases oxytocin production
	Increases prolactin production
Ovary	Is required for ovum maturation (is luteolytic in some mammalian species)
Vagina	Causes proliferation and cornification of the mucosa
Oviducts	Causes growth and development in preparation for gamete transport
Uterus	
Cervix	Increases mucus secretion
Endometrium	Increases blood flow
	Increases prostaglandin biosynthesis at term
	Increases number of oxytocin receptors at term
	Causes decidualization response (increases the number of estrogen receptors in the decidua)
Myometrium	Synthesizes contractile proteins of smooth muscle cells
	Increases membrane excitability (increases sensitivity to oxytocin)
Mammary glands	Causes ductule and stromal growth and development, fat accretion
Skin	Induces sebaceous gland secretion (thinner fluid)
	Stimulates axillary and pubic hair growth (possibly in concert with gonadal and adrenal androgens)
General body effects	Causes H_2O and Na^+ retention, weight gain (anabolic action), and female type of fat distribution
	Maintains bone mineral deposition
Liver	Causes hepatic angiotensinogen production
	Causes hepatic production of thyroid-binding globulin
Blood	Decreases plasma cholesterol formation
Progesterone	
CNS	Increases sexual receptivity in estrogen-primed animals (at least in some mammalian species)
	Inhibits basal GnRH and gonadotropin secretion during the ovarian luteal phase
	Blocks release of preovulatory GnRH and gonadotropin surges during pregnancy
Oviducts	Causes growth and development for gamete transport
Uterus	
Endometrium	Stimulates growth and development in preparation for blastocyst implantation
	Decreases estrogen receptor number (at least, in the rat)
Cervix	Increases mucus consistency
Myometrium	Causes antiestrogen effects (myometrial hyperpolarization, decreased sensitivity to oxytocin, decreased estrogen receptor number, maintenance of pregnancy)
Vagina	Inhibits estrogen-induced vaginal cornification
Mammary glands	Is necessary for lobular-alveolar development (in some species)
	Inhibits prepartum prolactin-induced lactogenesis by decreasing PRL receptor number
General body effects	Causes thermogenic action (rise in basal metabolic rate)

Progesterone. Progesterone is the ovarian hormone of pregnancy and is responsible for preparing the reproductive tract for zygote implantation and the subsequent maintenance of the pregnant state. It has been speculated that preovulatory plasma levels of progesterone may trigger sexual behavior in some species. In some rodents, for example, progesterone appears necessary for induction of sexual receptivity. Progesterone may also play a role in the initiation of nest-building activity and brooding behavior in some avian species. It must be emphasized that many actions of progesterone are often, but not always (e.g. in the ovary) on estrogen-primed tissue. Table 18.1 summarizes the known physiological roles of progesterone in the human female.

Androgens. The role of gonadal hormones in modulating human female sexual interest remains a controversial issue. In the hypoactive sexual desire disorder (HSD), women's gonadal hormones fluctuated normally over the menstrual cycle, were within normal limits for each cycle phase, and were never significantly different from those of controls. Testosterone, non-SHBG (steroid hormone binding globulin) bound testosterone, and prolactin (PRL) did not differ between the HSD women with the most and least severe HSD parameters (e.g., frequency of fantasy, masturbation, or female-initiated coitus), or between women with lifelong and acquired HSD. These findings provide no evidence that reproductive hormones are important determinants of individual differences in the sexual desire of these eugonadal women [52].

It has been reported that women prisoners with higher levels of testosterone, like their male counterparts, are more likely jailed for violent behavior and tend toward aggressive, dominant behavior behind bars as well. A study of 87 female inmates in a maximum security prison found that the higher a woman's testosterone levels, the more violent her crimes and overbearing her behavior in prison. Testosterone levels generally decline with age in both men and women, as does criminal behavior.

Mechanisms of Action of Ovarian Steroid Hormones

Ovarian steroid hormones, E_2 and progesterone, manifest their actions as described for the general actions of steroid hormones (see Chaps 4, 17).

Two Estrogen Receptor Isoforms (ERα, ERβ) Mediate Genomic Actions of Estrogen

Similar to the actions of other steroid hormones, estrogen regulates the transcription of target genes by activating its receptors in the nuclei of target cells. Two distinct ER genes encode the ERα and ERβ proteins, which are homologous molecules that share a molecular domain structure (DNA binding, ligand binding, and activation function domains) that is common to all of the steroid receptor superfamily members. Binding of estrogen to either ER prompts dissociation of the receptor from heat shock protein chaperones. These "activated" receptors then dimerize, recruit co-activator proteins, and regulate gene transcription via binding to palindromic estrogen response element (ERE) sequences in the promoter regions of target genes. The activation function (AF) domains of the receptors interact with transcriptional co-regulators, and complex together with enzymes and factors as the "transcriptional machinery" that controls RNA polymerase II and initiation of gene transcription. In addition to the foregoing "classical" mechanism of ER function, "non-classical" mechanisms have also been documented, in which ER can regulate the expression of genes independently of binding to EREs. In these cases ERs appear to be involved in protein–protein interactions with other transcription factors, thereby enhancing or repressing their actions at non-ERE transcriptional response elements, or at ERE half-sites associated with other response elements.

It is believed that the specific responses of a given cell to estrogen, in large part, depend upon the amount and type of ER present, the complement of co-activator proteins expressed in that cell, and the properties of the target gene promoters. The expression patterns of ERα and ERβ are overlapping in some tissues and cell types, but in others either may predominate. In the ovary, both ERs are expressed but ERα is localized to the thecal and interstitial cells, while ERβ is primarily expressed in granulosa cells. Studies of ER gene deletion mutant mice, the ERα and ERβ "knockout" mice (αERKO and βERKO), have revealed that ERα plays a predominant role in mediating estrogen's actions in classical target tissues, such as uterus, hypothalamus, pituitary, breast, and skeleton. However, clear roles for ERβ have been demonstrated in estrogen's effects in the ovary, where it mediates effects on folliculogenesis, and in other tissues, including the cardiovascular system and extra-hypothalamic brain regions [25, 31].

Cellular Localization of Estrogen Receptors.   There has been continued debate as to whether the steroid hormone receptor is initially localized to the cytoplasm to then be translocated to the nucleus following ligand activation or whether the receptor is localized exclusively to the nucleoplasm. In Figure 18.8, it is clearly shown that the receptor may be initially localized to either compartment depending on the particular cell type and/or ligand.

Nonsteroidal Estrogens and Antiestrogens.   A number of nonsteroidal compounds possess estrogenic activity, the most potent of which is diethylstilbestrol (DES). The similarity between the structures of DES and the natural steroids is illustrated (Fig. 18.9). DES is highly active when given orally, apparently because it is degraded more slowly in the gastrointestinal tract. Anti-estrogens, such as clomiphene and tamoxifen (Fig. 18.9), are nonsteroidal compounds that, through competition with estrogen receptors, prevent actions of endogenous estrogens from expressing their full effects on their target tissues. By this action, they antagonize a variety of estrogen-dependent processes, such as uterine growth and negative feedback to the hypothalamus. Interest in these drugs derives from the hope that they might prove useful in preventing the growth of estrogen-dependent mammary tumors (Chap. 19). Development of new selective estrogen receptor modulators (SERMs) is likewise of intense interest, given their potential for treatment of osteoporosis and menopausal symptoms with minimized risk of deleterious side effects.

Progesterone's Genomic Actions are Mediated by Progesterone Receptors A and B (PR$_A$, PR$_B$)

Progesterone also regulates gene transcription by activating one or both of two receptor proteins, PR$_A$ and PR$_B$. The two proteins are expressed from a single gene as a consequence of transcriptional regulation at two alternative promoter sequences, and translation initiation at two alternative translational start sites. The PR$_A$ is thus an N-terminally truncated version of PR$_B$. In vitro studies have demonstrated that the transcriptional activities of the two receptor isoforms are partially overlapping but can also be distinct. To dissect the possible physiological roles of the two PRs, a complete PR gene knockout (PRKO) mouse was developed [37], as well as two isoform-specific deletion mutant mice that specifically lack the ability to produce PR$_A$ or PR$_B$, respectively [43]. Analyses of their phenotypes have revealed that female PRKO mice are infertile, with profound deficits in ovulation, uterine development and function, mammary gland development, neuroendocrine function, and reproductive behavior. Selective ablation of PR$_A$ resulted in normal mammary gland responses to progesterone but severe uterine hyperplasia and impaired ovulation. By contrast, loss of PR$_B$ was accompanied by normal responses to progesterone in uterus and ovary but impaired breast development during pregnancy. Thus PR$_A$ plays a most important role in uterine and ovarian function, while PR$_B$ appears to be of greater importance in mediating progesterone's effects on the mammary glands.

Neuroendocrine Control of Ovarian Function

Activation and maintenance of normal follicular function is dependent on gonadotropins secreted by the adenohypophysis (Chap. 5). Both FSH and LH are required to stimulate ovarian changes leading to ovulation [32, 33]. Treatment of hypophysectomized, immature, female animals with LH causes thecal cell stimulation, but no follicular growth and, depending on the species, no significant estrogen production. When injections of purified FSH are given, follicular development proceeds only to antrum formation and only minimal amounts of estrogens are produced. Normal follicular development occurs only when both FSH and LH are administered to an animal. These observations support the two-cell, two-gonadotropin scheme of follicular development and steroid hormone production.

Pituitary gonadotropin secretion is initiated during pubertal development and, indeed, secretion of gonadotropins at this time is responsible for the development of secondary sex

-ligand   +ligand

Figure 18.8 Steroid hormone modulation of steroid receptor activity visualized in cultured living cells. Steroid receptors are ligand-dependent transcription factors in which steroid hormones play an important role in modulating receptor activity. The four panels show an optical section of cells from a human mammary epithelial cancer cell line expressing the glucocorticoid receptor (GR; top two panels) or estrogen-receptor alpha (ER; bottom two panels) tagged to a naturally fluorescent protein, the green fluorescent protein (GFP), from the jellyfish *Aequorea victoria.* Presence of the GFP tag allows these two steroid receptors to be directly visualized by fluorescent microscopy, such as a confocal laser-scanning microscope used to obtain the images shown here. In the absence of ligand, GR exists in the cytoplasm (top left panel) and is excluded from the nucleus (the large dark area in the center of the panel). In contrast, the unliganded ER exists in the nucleus and is barely detectable in the cytoplasm (bottom left panel). Note that the ER is excluded from the nucleoli (dark areas) within these nuclei. Steroid hormone causes a biochemical transformation or activation of the receptor and its regulation of hormone-responsive genes, as proposed in the two-step mechanism of steroid hormone action. As seen here, presence of the synthetic ligand, dexamethasone (dex), causes GR to translocate from the cytoplasm to the nucleus and to concentrate at discrete foci, giving a punctate nuclear appearance (top right panel). Although not proven, these foci might reflect the accumulation of the receptor at hormone-responsive genes. Similarly, exposure of the ER-expressing cells to its hormone, 17β-estradiol (E_2), causes a redistribution of the receptor and concentration at discrete foci (bottom right panel). Unlike GR where the redistribution involves translocation from the cytoplasm to the nucleus, the redistribution of ER occurs entirely within the nuclear compartment. Thus, the importance of steroid hormones in modulating steroid receptor activity is evident from the direct visualization of steroid receptors in cultured living cells. Scale bar equals 10 microns. (Courtesy of Dr. Han Htun, Departments of Ob/Gyn & Molecular and Medical Pharmacology, UCLA School of Medicine, Los Angeles.) (See *Molecular Biology of the Cell* 10:471–86, 1999.)

Figure 18.9 Diethylstilbestrol (DES) is an example of a synthetic nonsteroidal estrogen. Note the partial structural similarity of two antiestrogens, clomiphene and tamoxifen, to DES.

characteristics typical of the adult female. It has been documented in the female primate [57] and rodent [54] that the activation of gonadotropin secretion during pubertal maturation is mediated by an acceleration of pulsatile GnRH neurosecretion. The central nervous system (CNS) organizational basis for cyclic release of pituitary gonadotropins in the adult female is established early in fetal development (Chap. 16). The detailed mechanisms controlling pituitary gonadotropin secretion are best understood in the primate [32, 33, 36, 45] and rodent [36]; this text will primarily discuss the former.

A Neural "GnRH Pulse Generator" Directs Pituitary Gonadotropin Secretion

Elegant studies on the rhesus monkey established the role of the brain and pituitary in the control of ovarian function in the primate [32]. Pituitary gonadotropin secretion is critically dependent on hypothalamic GnRH release. Administration of antisera to GnRH causes an abrupt reduction in plasma gonadotropin concentrations. Discrete lesions within the medial basal hypothalamus of the female monkey result in a sudden decrease in plasma gonadotropin levels. There is a pulsatile pattern of gonadotropin secretion with a frequency of approximately one pulse per hour (circhoral) [32, 33]. The concentration of GnRH in pituitary stalk blood of ovariectomized monkeys fluctuates with a frequency similar to that of pituitary gonadotropin secretion. The circhoral rhythm of gonadotropin secretion is abolished by α-adrenoceptor antagonists, confirming that pulsatile GnRH release is regulated by neural elements.

The neuronal mechanisms that are responsible for generating the pulsatile rhythm of GnRH release have been collectively referred to as the "GnRH pulse generator" [32]. In primates, the neuroendocrine elements that comprise the GnRH pulse generator appear to be largely restricted to the medial basal hypothalamus, where the bulk of the GnRH neurons reside. While the cellular basis of GnRH pulsatility remains unclear, it has been demonstrated that fetal GnRH neurons, when removed during their migration to the hypothalamus and cultured in vitro, exhibit pulsatile GnRH release activity despite their isolation from most other cell types. Thus, GnRH neurons themselves appear to be endowed with the capability of releasing GnRH in a coordinated, pulsatile pattern, and this intrinsic activity may function as the basic GnRH pulse generating mechanism in vivo. This basal pulsatile GnRH rhythm, in turn, is physiologically regulated both neural and endocrine signals, conveyed through afferent neuronal circuitries or by direct hormonal effects on GnRH neurons. These modulatory effects are most often manifest as an increase or decrease in the frequency of GnRH pulsatility. For example, stress or undernutrition can inhibit the activity of the reproductive axis, most likely through the retardation of the GnRH pulse generator. The cellular mechanisms by which stress, metabolic cues such as leptin [7], or other environmental variables such as photoperiod can regulate the activity of the GnRH pulse generator remain to be fully understood.

Clinical trials have demonstrated that pulses of unchanging doses and frequency of GnRH result in normal pituitary and ovarian function in women with hypothalamic amenorrhea. Such trials have established pulsatile GnRH as the treatment of choice for induction of ovulation in hypogonadotropic hypogonadism [24, 32].

Menstrual Cyclicity is Maintained by Ovarian Feedback Mechanisms

Negative Feedback.   Both estrogen and progesterone exert a negative feedback suppression of gonadotropin secretions during the menstrual cycle. These feedback effects maintain a low and slow "basal" pulsatile LH secretion pattern throughout the follicular and luteal phases of the cycle. Experimentally, this negative feedback loop has been demonstrated in studies showing that removal of the ovaries results in a dramatic rise in LH secretion, and replacement with estrogen and progesterone can return LH to basal levels. The negative feedback actions of both steroids are exerted at the hypothalamic level, to suppress GnRH pulse generator activity, and at the level of the anterior pituitary gland to suppress responsiveness to GnRH stimulation. The relative importance of the hypothalamic and pituitary feedback effects may vary among species, and has been the subject of much debate in the case of rhesus monkeys and women. Classic studies have suggested that the pituitary mechanism predominates in primates [32], although direct measurements of pulsatile GnRH release in female rhesus macaques have revealed that GnRH release is diminished by estrogen treatment [41], implicating the hypothalamic mechanism as well.

Progesterone also exerts negative feedback control over pulsatile LH secretion, particularly during the luteal phase of the cycle. Feedback suppression by progesterone likewise inhibits release of estrogen-induced gonadotropin surges, probably by means of a CNS mechanism. This same inhibitory mechanism operates during pregnancy and lactation as a result of suckling-induced PRL secretion. It appears to involve a reduction of the frequency of GnRH pulse generation [32].

Positive feedback.   In spontaneously ovulating animals, the maturing follicle secretes high levels of estrogen that stimulate the abrupt release of a mid-cycle preovulatory LH surge. This stimulatory action of estrogen is referred to as "positive feedback," and it is mediated by cellular level by mechanisms that differ from those mediating its negative feedback effects. In ovariectomized animals, the administration of an estrogen dose of sufficient magnitude will trigger release of a preovulatory-like surge of gonadotropins. Estrogen clearly acts on the pituitary gland where it stimulates LH secretion, at least in part by priming pituitary gonadotropes to the stimulatory actions of GnRH. It may also exert some of its positive feedback effect at the hypothalamic level, by evoking a GnRH surge into the hypophysial portal vessels, which would in turn stimulate the LH surge. The relative importance of these hypothalamic and pituitary positive feedback mechanisms has also been the subject of controversy. In rats [10], sheep [42], and other animals it is clear that the release of mid-cycle gonadotropin surges is stimulated by the neurosecretion of a GnRH surge into the hypophysial portal vessels, which triggers release of an LH surge from the estrogen-primed pituitary gland. In primates, however, the pituitary feedback mechanism may be sufficient to drive the release of the LH surge. Supporting this idea is the following observation: If the hypothalamic source of GnRH is removed by discrete hypothalamic lesions and GnRH is administered by chronic, intermittent intravenous infusion, the pituitary responds by pulsatile release of gonadotropins. Remarkably, these animals then go through "normal" menstrual cycles, including a preovulatory surge of LH/FSH and typical follicular and luteal phase levels of plasma E_2 and progesterone [33]. This implies that the stimulation of the preovulatory gonadotropin surge does not *require* release of a GnRH surge by the hypothalamus. However, GnRH surges have been documented in estrogen-treated, ovariectomized monkeys, and in ovary-intact animals during the preovulatory period [37, 46]. It may be the case that these two positive feedback actions—one in the hypothalamus and one at the anterior pituitary—are physiologically redundant, ensuring the successful completion of this critically important endocrine event.

The course and duration of the primate menstrual cycle is determined not by the brain, but rather by the ovary itself, through its negative and positive feedback signals to the hypothalamus and pituitary gland. Thus, low levels of estrogen during the early follicular phase of the menstrual cycle exert a negative feedback action that maintains a basal level of gonadotropin secretion. By the late follicular phase, the maturing follicle produces increasing amounts of estrogen. After estrogen levels rise and remain above a critical level for at least 36 hours, the negative feedback effect is reversed and a positive feedback ensues, which results in the release of the preovulatory gonadotropin surge. Luteal progesterone secretion then reestablishes negative feedback until the demise of the corpus luteum (luteolysis). Thus, the duration of the ovarian cycle, at least in the rhesus monkey, is determined by the characteristic duration of follicular development, as well as the functional lifespan of the corpus luteum. The sum of both processes is approximately 28 days [32].

Intrafollicular Polypeptides Regulate Folliculogenesis and Oocyte Maturation

Several peptides have been isolated from ovarian follicles and have been claimed to function as putative hormones in the regulation of oocyte maturation.

Oocyte Maturation Factors. Oocytes obtained from middle and late antral follicles of mice resume meiosis when removed from the follicle and cultured in vitro. In contrast, oocytes cultured with granulosa cells do not mature. These observations indicate that granulosa cells hold the oocyte in meiotic arrest, although the mechanisms mediating this arrest remain a mystery. It has been established that the maintenance of high levels of cAMP in the oocyte prevents meiotic maturation. Recent studies have demonstrated that the activation of a G_s-coupled receptor, GPR3, may be responsible for this sustained cAMP elevation in the oocyte [40]. There is no known endogenous ligand for GPR3, and it exhibits a high level of constitutive (intrinsic) activation. It has been suggested that a ligand present in cumulus cells stimulates GPR3, perhaps in the regions of contact between these cells and the oocyte. The putative ligand—a potential oocyte maturation inhibiting factor—may be a lipid present in the membranes of cumulus cells [39, 40].

Meiosis resumes in response to stimulation by the preovulatory LH surge. In vitro experiments have demonstrated that the inhibitory action of granulosa cells on oocyte maturation is reversed by addition of LH to the medium. LH is not effective, however, in overcoming the inhibitory activity of granulosa cell-conditioned medium on oocyte maturation. These results suggest that LH may mediate its effect through an action on the granulosa cells. Recent studies suggest that LH activates its receptors in mural granulosa cells, stimulating production of epidermal growth factor-like proteins that in turn act on the cumulus cells to stimulate oocyte maturation. The oocyte maturation factors that may mediate the actions of the cumulus cells on the oocyte remain unknown. Such a meiosis-inducing factor may mediate its effects by reducing GPR3 activity, inactivating G_s, activating G_i, raising intracellular Ca^{2+} levels, or stimulating phosphodiesterase activity in the oocyte. Each of these possible actions would result in a reduction in cAMP levels in the oocyte and a resumption of meiosis.

Ovarian Growth Factors. Induction of LH receptors is a critical aspect of granulosa cell differentiation and ovarian follicular development. By this process, the follicle acquires the responsiveness to LH and the subsequent capacity to ovulate and luteinize. Pituitary FSH functions as the inducer of granulosa cell LH-receptor acquisition. This FSH-dependent LH receptor induction is inhibited by epidermal and fibroblast growth factors (Chap. 12). These and other growth factors therefore regulate follicle development as well as oocyte maturation.

Inhibins. Evidence supporting the existence of the gonadal polypeptide peptide, inhibin, inhibitory to pituitary FSH secretion in the male was reviewed (Chap. 17) [12, 46]. Equally compelling evidence for a granulosa-derived peptide in the female was marshaled. Inhibin is present in follicular fluid, ovarian and granulosa cell extracts, granulosa cell-conditioned media, and ovarian venous plasma [17, 21]. Inhibin exerts a suppressive action on both basal and GnRH-stimulated pituitary FSH secretion. The precise cellular localization and factors that may regulate the synthesis and secretion of inhibin remain to be clarified. A model for the role of inhibin in the control of pituitary FSH secretion was shown (see Fig. 17.3).

Inhibin has been isolated from follicular fluid from several species of animals [6, 21, 29, 38]. The peptide is composed of two subunits that are linked by disulfide bridges. The two subunits are, however, encoded by separate genes (Fig. 18.10). Antibodies to inhibin confirm its presence in the plasma of men and women. The half-lives of inhibin mRNAs in the rat are very short. This is consistent with inhibin production being tightly regulated in response to transient conditions during the estrous cycle and that the control of inhibin biosynthesis is at the level of transcription.

FSH stimulation induces inhibin secretion, and inhibin acts to suppress FSH secretion, completing the negative feedback loop. For example, inhibin is increased in the plasma of women given FSH, but not in castrated subjects. Cultured granulosa cells secrete inhibin when exposed to FSH. Inhibin levels in the plasma of women undergoing induced ovulation by FSH rise and are correlated with E_2 levels. Similarly, in the male, inhibin is decreased in

Figure 18.10
Structural relationships between inhibins and activins.

the testis following hypophysectomy and becomes elevated in response to FSH. These observations support the view of a feedback loop between the release of ovarian and testicular inhibin and FSH secretion. During the ovulatory cycle, the production of inhibin drops dramatically as a consequence of the preovulatory LH surge [8]. The LH-induced suppression of inhibin secretion is accompanied by a periovulatory FSH surge in some species, which functions to select a crop of follicles for development in the upcoming cycle.

Activins.   During the initial steps of inhibin purification, purified fractions of follicular fluid exhibited stimulatory rather than inhibitory effects on FSH release from pituitaries in vitro. When the amino acid sequence of inhibin was identified, it was found that the β subunits of inhibin and transforming growth factor β (TGFβ) were similar. As TGFβ can enhance FSH release in vitro, it was initially suggested that this stimulatory effect might be due to TGFβ or a protein similar to TGFβ. It was then discovered that the stimulatory activity was due to dimers of the β subunits of inhibin, $\beta_A\beta_B$, $\beta_A\beta_A$, and $\beta_B\beta_B$. These peptides were named activin AB, activin-A, and activin-B, respectively (Fig. 18.10). Activins can enhance basal secretion of FSH in a dose-dependent manner in vitro without affecting the secretion of LH [6, 17].

Follistatin.   Follistatin is a single peptide chain of molecular weight 32,000–35,000 isolated from porcine follicular fluid, which is distinct from inhibin and can inhibit the release of FSH, but not LH, from cultures of pituitary cells. It has since been determined that follistatin is produced in abundance in the pituitary, where it may inhibit FSH by a paracrine or autocrine mechanism [34]. Follistatin inhibits FSH release indirectly, by binding activins with high affinity and thereby neutralizing their ability to stimulate FSH production [6].

Mammalian Reproductive Cycles

Females of most vertebrate species are subject to cyclic changes in reproductive activity [5]. Most often these changes are integrated with seasonal environmental changes so that the young are born under more favorable conditions of climate and food availability. In many mammals other than primates, females experience recurring periods of sexual excitement referred to as *estrus* (from the Greek *oistros*, meaning mad desire or heat), during which time they are psychologically as well as physically receptive to the male. The female primate does not go through an *estrous cycle*, but eggs are nevertheless matured within the ovaries during a precise follicular cycle of events, and the genital tract is also cyclically prepared for passage and implantation of the zygote. The monthly cycle of uterine maturation and sloughing is therefore a characteristic feature of the primate *menstrual cycle*.

The Primate Menstrual Cycle is Orchestrated by Cyclic Secretions of Pituitary and Gonadal Hormones

Ovarian Cycle.   The production and secretion of pituitary gonadotropins in the primate are controlled by cyclic ovarian follicular events; the duration of the cycle appears to be dependent on the genetic program that is read out to completion once follicular maturation is initiated. FSH levels are elevated at the beginning of the cycle, but they become diminished through most of the early and middle follicular phases. Follicular selection and early maturation beyond the preantral stage may be dependent on the initially elevated plasma levels of FSH. Follicular development beyond the early antral stage may additionally be dependent upon LH. Increased estrogen (and inhibin) secretion by the maturing follicles exerts a negative feedback inhibition of pituitary gonadotrope FSH secretion. Luteinizing hormone levels also remain low during most of this follicular phase due to the negative feedback actions of estrogens on the hypothalamus and pituitary. With continued follicular maturation, estrogen levels become increasingly elevated to a peak at mid-cycle. The prolonged action of the higher concentrations of estrogens is the stimulus to the mid-cycle FSH/LH surge. The subsequently elevated plasma levels of LH provide the stimulus to ovum release from the mature Graafian follicle. The granulosa cells, which have now become responsive to LH, initiate progesterone biosynthesis and secretion. At this stage, the postovulatory follicle has become an endocrine gland in the classical sense. During the follicular phase plasma progesterone levels are low, but with commencement of the luteal phase they become elevated.

Progesterone levels are elevated just prior to the LH/FSH surge, apparently in response to increasing levels of LH, which is also secreted at that time. The action of progesterone on the hypothalamus results in postovulatory decreases in both LH and FSH secretion. Under conditions of low circulating levels of these gonadotropins, there is no stimulus to folliculogenesis, and estrogen levels therefore remain only minimally elevated during the luteal phase. As the corpus luteum matures during the subsequent week following ovulation, progesterone levels become increasingly elevated to a midluteal peak. Afterward, they level off and decline unless the ovulated ovum is fertilized and takes up residence within the uterine lining. With the demise of the corpus luteum in the nonpregnant female and the sharp decline in plasma progesterone levels, pituitary gonadotropins are again secreted at higher levels, which leads to the initiation of the next round of ovarian folliculogenesis and steroid hormone production. The cyclic pattern of pituitary gonadotropin and gonadal steroid hormone secretion in the rhesus monkey is illustrated in Figure 18.11 [14].

Uterine Cycle. The menstrual cycle of the human female is approximately 28 days long and is numbered from the first day of the menses. Menstruation is the process in which the lining of the uterus is shed once during each cycle, a process that in most women takes 4 to 5 days. Under the influence of increasing titers of plasma estrogens, the endometrium of the uterus increases in thickness, reaching a maximal width of 3 to 5 mm just prior to ovulation (Fig. 18.12). Stromal connective tissue cells proliferate and extracellular collagen deposits are increased. In response to luteal phase progesterone levels, uterine glands increase in complexity from simple tubular elements during the follicular phase of the cycle to thick, coiled structures with a glandular lumen containing abundant secretory material. Spiral arteries within the endometrium become thickened and engorged with blood, particularly in response to luteal levels of progesterone. If implantation of a zygote fails to occur, then by about 11 days following ovulation lymphocytes begin to invade the endometrium, and by day 14 (day 1 of the cycle), sloughing of the endometrium occurs due to loss of ovarian steroid hormone support. In the absence of a hormonal directive, the spiral arteries become constricted and the blood lost from these arteries along with stromal debris composes the bulk of the menstrual flow [19].

The nature of the cervical mucus is also characteristically altered during the menstrual cycle. During the follicular phase, the mucus is rather thin and watery. In response to periovulatory levels of progesterone, the mucus becomes thickened and is composed of innumerable tiny channels that apparently provide access for the sperm through the cervical os.

Vaginal Cycle. In prepubertal and postmenopausal females, the vaginal epithelium is thin, being composed of a few layers of epithelial cells. In response to estrogens, this epithelium proliferates and subsequently consists of many more layers of epithelial cells. The histological features of the vaginal epithelium change in a characteristic manner during the menstrual cycle. Early in the cycle, the epithelium consists mainly of rounded basal cells that stain intensely with certain dyes. Maximal growth of the epithelium occurs during the periovulatory period. At this time, the basal cells are overlain with layers of more flattened cells; the outermost cells are very flat and keratinized (cornified), and they fail to stain, thus indicating that they are dead. Toward the end of the luteal phase, the vaginal epithelium becomes invaded with leukocytes, and by the initiation of the next cycle, cells of the outer layers of the epithelium are lost.

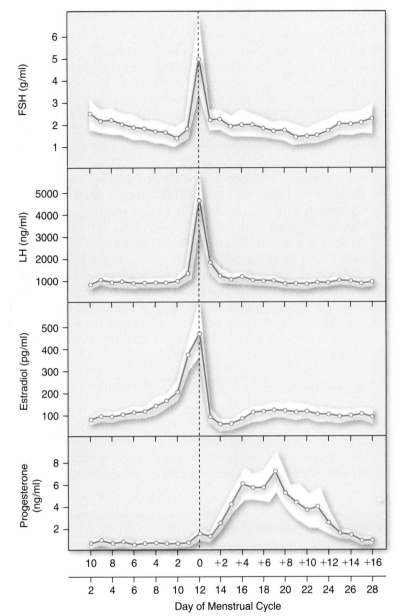

Figure 18.11 Serum concentrations of mFSH, mLH, estradiol, and progesterone in 20 rhesus monkeys during ovulatory menstrual cycles. (From DiZerega and Hodgen [14], with permission.)

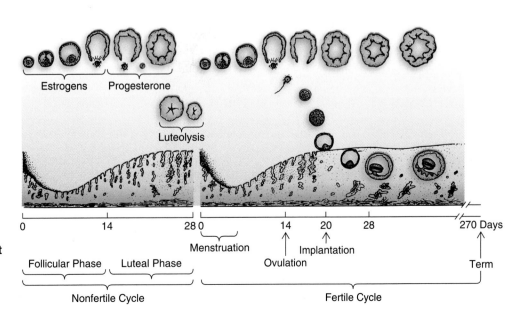

Figure 18.12 Cycle of uterine endometrial growth and development during nonfertile and fertile cycles in the human female.

Females of Various Animal Species may be Induced or Spontaneous Ovulators

Most mammals (e.g., primates, hamsters, mice, rats) ovulate at the end of a follicular phase and then initiate development of corpora lutea. In contrast to these *spontaneous ovulators*, certain animals (domestic cats, rabbits, minks) go through a follicular phase, but then remain in a state of sexual receptivity where the follicles mature and are usually released after copulation. These *induced* or *reflex ovulators* generally mate during estrus. During mating there is a reflex release of LH from the pituitary that leads to ovulation usually 12 to 48 hours later (Table 18.2). Some animals exhibit a *constant estrus* (e.g., rabbits), whereas estrus in other species is a seasonal phenomenon with a long anestrous period between cycles, where ovaries and follicles remain small.

Spontaneous ovulators can be divided into two major groups: (1) animals with nonfunctional corpora lutea and short (4- to 5-day) ovarian cycles (e.g., rats, mice, hamsters); and (2) animals with functional corpora lutea and long estrous cycles (e.g., pigs, cows, horses). The spontaneous ovulators with long cycles can be further subdivided into two groups: (1) animals with but one estrous cycle (monestrous) in a mating season; and (2) animals that have two or more estrous cycles (polyestrous) in the mating season. In some spontaneous ovulators, such as rats, the biological circadian clock times the release of the preovulatory GnRH and gonadotropin surges to occur only within a restricted period on the afternoon of proestrus, the day immediately preceding estrus. The timing of the surge ensures that ovulation will occur 6–12 hours later, coinciding with the period of behavioral estrous. The coordination of these neuroendocrine events maximizes the chances of fertilization and successful reproduction.

Delayed Implantation is an Adaptive Mechanism that Permits Optimal Timing of Birth

In some species the fertilized egg, the zygote, may reside within the uterine cavity for a considerable time. This *delayed implantation* allows flexibility between mating and birth. Most often, all reproductive events must be crowded into a short time interval. Of fundamental importance is that the young be born at the optimum season of the year for survival and growth [60]. In colonial animals, such as certain seals, the sexes are usually together only for

TABLE 18.2   The estrous cycle of various mammalian species[a]

Species	Length of cycle (days)	Duration of estrus	Ovulation Type	Time
Cow (*Bos taurus*)	21	13–14 hours	Spontaneous	12–16 hours after end of estrus
Goat (*Capra hircus*)	20–21	1–3 days	Spontaneous	30–36 hours after onset of estrus
Sheep (*Ovis aries*)	16	20–48 hours	Spontaneous	12–24 hours before end of estrus
Pig (*Sus scrofa*)	21	2–3 days	Spontaneous	35 hours after onset of estrus
Horse (*Equus caballus*)	19–23	4–7 days	Spontaneous	1–2 days before end of estrus
Dog (*Canis familiaris*)	60	7–9 days	Spontaneous	1–3 days after start of estrus
Cat (*Felis catus*)	–	4 days with male; 9–10 days without male	Induced	20–30 hours after mating
Ferret (*Mustela furo*)	–	Continuous	Induced	30 hours after mating
Mink (*Mustela vison*)	8–9	2 days	Induced	40–50 hours after mating
Fox (*Vulpes vulpes*)	90	1–5 days	Spontaneous	1–2 days after onset of estrus
Ground squirrel (*Citellus tridecemlineatus*)	16	6–11 hours	Induced	8–12 hours after mating
Guinea pig (*Cavia porcellus*)	16	20 hours	Spontaneous	10 hours after start of estrus
Golden hamster (*Mesocricetus auratus*)	4	10 hours	Spontaneous	8–12 hours after start of estrus
Mouse (*Mus musculus*)	4	10 hours	Spontaneous	2–3 hours after start of estrus
Rat (*Rattus norvegicus*)	4–5	13–15 hours	Spontaneous	8–10 hours after start of estrus
Rabbit (*Orcytolagus cuniculus*)	No cycle	Continuous	Induced	10 hours after mating
Rhesus monkey (*Macaca mulatta*)	28[b]	None	Spontaneous	14 days prior to onset of menstrual bleeding
Human (*Homo sapiens*)	28[b]	None	Spontaneous	14 days prior to onset of menstrual bleeding

[a]From van Tienhoven [59], with permission.
[b]Menstrual cycle.

a short time each year and must breed, give birth, and rear their young during this critical interval. In certain marsupials, the suckling young may be lost due to harsh environmental conditions. The loss of the suckling stimulus (absence of prolactin) causes an unimplanted blastocyst to break diapause (from the Greek *dia*, through, completely, and *pausa*, pause; arrested embryonic development). Within each species, the length of the implanted gestation period is rigidly fixed, but in some species of bats the young may experience a delayed development. The hormonal requirements for implantation of a delayed blastocyst are poorly understood. In the European badger, there is a fertile postpartum coitus in February, but the fertilized eggs remain in the blastocyst stage until December when implantation occurs [59].

Environmental Cues can Regulate the Timing of Reproduction

Reproductive success depends on successful mating, fetal growth and development, and the birth and rearing of young under appropriate environmental conditions. Success in these sequential events requires that eggs be ovulated at the right time, eggs become fertilized, and the nutritional state of the mother be adequate to provide for the needs of the growing offspring, whether in utero or postpartum. Environmental cues play important roles in synchronizing mating behavior in animals and provide signals indicative of when food sources may become available. For example, some desert species are opportunistic breeders and mate following rainfall. In many small rodents, reproductive activity is restricted to the spring and the fall; within the confines of the laboratory, however, these animals become continuous breeders.

A variety of exogenous factors—auditory, visual, tactile, and odoriferous—serve as signals to initiate reproductive behavior in some species. Lighting conditions as well as species-specific odors play particularly important roles.

Light. The most universal environmental synchronizing cue is light. Seasonal and daily changes in light duration and intensity are cyclic phenomena that usually directly or indirectly relate to other environmental factors such as the abundance of water and food. Light information must be received (sensed), transcribed (a neural processing mechanism), and translated into a physiological response. In vertebrates, a neural sensory system, or "eye" must monitor the presence or absence of light and transmit this information by neural afferents to the central nervous system, which then directly or indirectly affects pituitary gonadotropin secretion. In either case, neurohormones released from the hypothalamus provide the initial input to pituitary hormone secretion. The important role of the pineal gland in the control of reproductive processes in vertebrates is discussed in Chapter 20.

Olfaction. Smell is particularly crucial in eliciting mating behavior in many animals [44]. Chemical messengers released by one member of a species may be received by a second member of the same species and produce a physiological response. These *pheromones* are volatile hydrocarbons (see Fig. 2.5), which, in mammals at least, interact with receptors of olfactory epithelial cells of the recipient animal. Nervous afferents to the CNS then cause either a rapid behavioral response or slower physiological response involving the release of pituitary gonadotropins. Again, as for light stimuli, hypothalamic neurosecretory neurons provide the final common pathway linking sensory perception to pituitary-gonadal activation.

In the mouse, a number of effects ascribed to pheromones have been noted. Female mice housed with four or more other female mice may become *pseudopregnant*; that is, the corpora lutea are maintained in the absence of mating (*Lee-Boot effect*). If female mice are housed in very large groups, the incidence of anestrus increases. These observations suggest that female mice secrete one or more pheromones that affect the estrous cycle. The presence of a male mouse may cause shortening and synchronization of the estrous cycle of grouped female mice (*Whitten effect*). Bedding or urine from a male mouse is equally effective, suggesting that odor is the stimulus to synchronization and shortening of the estrous cycle. When prepubertal female mice are reared in the presence of a male (or his urine), they attain first estrus several weeks earlier than if reared in the absence of the male (*Vandenbergh effect*). An additional observation made by Vandenbergh was that the odor of an adult female caused precocious testicular development of young males. In contrast, testes development is markedly retarded when young males are reared with adult males. If a recently impregnated female mouse is exposed to a strange male, pregnancy may be blocked; she will return to estrus within one week. The bedding or urine of the strange male is equally effective in terminating pregnancy (*Bruce effect*). Females made anosmic by destruction of the olfactory bulbs are unaffected by the presence of the "strange" male. The source of the male odor is unknown but may be derived from the preputial glands.

Pheromones and other stimuli that activate reproductive behavior fall into two broad categories: *releaser effects* and *primer effects*. Releaser effects resulting from a visual or odoriferous signal involve an immediate behavioral response on the part of the recipient. This often involves activation of a stereotyped mating behavior in the female, such as assuming a posture (lordosis) conducive to copulatory activity by the male. Primer effects also involve activation of CNS afferents, but in addition, pituitary gonadotropin secretion is enhanced or inhibited, most likely due to increases or decreases in hypothalamic secretion of GnRH. The Bruce effect appears to involve an inhibition of pituitary PRL secretion as the hormone is required for maintenance of the corpus luteum and can repair the block to pregnancy induced by the strange male if administered to the female. It has been speculated that the block to pregnancy involves the reestablishment of PRL-inhibiting factor (dopamine) secretion by the hypothalamus.

A study was made of the female stimuli that induce male gonadotropin (GtH) surge during spawning in the goldfish. In the presence of ovulatory females, olfactory tract sectioned (OTX) males failed to show sexual behavior or the GtH surge, whereas sham-operated (sham) males spawned and showed a GtH surge. When OTX and sham males were separated from ovulatory females with an opaque partition, but with water circulating between male and female compartments, the GtH surge occurred only in sham males, although they could not court with the females. These results indicate that an olfactory stimulus (pheromone) from ovulatory females is essential for the occurrence of male GtH surge. Pheromone(s) from ovulatory female goldfish thus function both as a releaser stimulating sexual behavior and as a primer inducing GtH surge in males [30].

Scientists have obtained data suggesting that human beings produce pheromones that affect sexual physiology [11]. Animals have long been known to secrete pheromones that typically function as sex attractants, but the existence of such substances in humans has only been speculated. However, research suggests their existence in humans. Women who had sex with men at least once a week were found to be more likely to have normal-length menstrual cycles, fewer infertility problems, and a milder menopause than women who were celibate or who had sex in a sporadic "feast-or-famine" pattern [11].

The pheromone findings indicate that an essential factor, aside from sexual intercourse itself, is exposure to specific aromatic chemicals exuded in a man's normal body odors. When a women receives these chemicals, by smell or skin absorption, even though she may not consciously notice them, they automatically improve her physiological functioning. The evidence suggests that the male chemicals, which are secreted by special sweat glands in the armpits and possibly around the nipples and in the genital region, are not effectively transmitted except in the intimate contact ordinarily associated with sex. Researchers have been able to duplicate some of the male pheromone's effects by exposing women who had no current sexual relationship to male pheromones in the form of what they dubbed "male essence." This contained substances extracted with alcohol from absorbent pads that male volunteers wore under their arms. The study was done with female volunteers whose menstrual cycles were longer than 33 days or shorter than 26 days, deviations from the normal average of 29.5 days. Three times a week the women came to the clinic to have male essence rubbed under their noses. The women said they could smell only the alcohol. After about 12 to 14 weeks, their menstrual cycles changed, slowing in some cases and speeding up in others, to approximately 29.5 days. A control group of similar women who were dosed with plain alcohol only showed no significant change in cycle length [11].

In a related experiment, scientists found that women produce another pheromone that can cause other women's menstrual cycles to shift into synchrony [60]. The researchers used a similarly obtained "female essence," which was collected at measured intervals during the donor's menstrual cycle and administered in the same sequence. Within a few menstrual cycles, the recipients shifted their cycles to synchronize with those of the donor. This finding confirms widely reported anecdotes that women who live (e.g., dormitories) or work together eventually develop synchronized menstrual cycles [11].

Pathophysiology

Amenorrhea. The term designates a relatively common disturbance in the human female characterized by an absence of the monthly menstrual flow. The etiology relates to a deficiency in estrogen production and a failure, therefore, in the monthly proliferative growth of the endometrium resulting in an absence of monthly sloughing of the uterine lining. The failure of the menses to be initiated at puberty is referred to as *primary amenorrhea*. The etiology may relate to a genetic defect, resulting in a failure of gonadal maturation (or total gonadal dysgenesis), or more specifically to a defect in estrogen biosynthesis. *Secondary amenorrhea* refers to a failure to menstruate after regular menses have been initiated. Pregnancy and the menopause are, of course, examples of normal physiological bases for failure to resume the menses. Failure of pituitary gonadotropin secretion or hyperprolactinemia are defects that result in amenorrhea.

Disturbances of the menstrual cycle are a frequent symptom in patients with eating disorders. Amenorrhea develops early in anorexia nervosa. A disturbed hypothalamic regulation of gonadotropin secretion causes amenorrhea. In bulimia (binge eating), amenorrhea is less frequent, occurring in about half the patients. The pulsatile, intravenous administration of GnRH is a highly successful method of inducing ovulation in patients suffering from amenorrhea secondary to hypothalamic dysfunction.

Altered Gonadotropin Secretion in Female Athletes. Secondary amenorrhea may be a consequence of strenuous exercise in some female athletes. Menstrual alterations have been noted in women participating in a variety of athletic endeavors. Studies have linked menstrual disturbances to weight loss and decreased body fat-to-lean ratios (Chap. 16), but the discrete disturbances in the brain pituitary-ovarian axis have not been pinpointed. Pulsatile gonadotropin secretion is critical to maintaining normal cyclical function of the pituitary-gonadal axis. It has now been shown that some long-distance runners with secondary amenorrhea or severe oligomenorrhea have unambiguously decreased spontaneous LH pulse frequencies. Generally, the effect is reversible with weight gain.

Isolated Gonadotropin Deficiency. This defect is characterized by a bihormonal deficiency of FSH and LH. In patients with isolated gonadotropin deficiency (IGD) administration of GnRH enhances FSH and LH secretion, thus restoring normal gonadal function [29]. It is likely that IGD may relate to a suprapituitary etiology involving an impaired synthesis and secretion of endogenous GnRH [61].

Premature Ovarian Failure. Premature ovarian failure has been usually assumed to represent one extreme of the temporal spectrum of menopause and has been a subject of neglect. Premature ovarian failure may be secondary to hypothalamic or pituitary failure (hypogonadotropic hypogonadism) or to a primary ovarian unresponsiveness to gonadotropins (hypergonadotrophic hypogonadism). The latter condition has been defined as secondary amenorrhea with persistently elevated gonadotropin levels before the age of 35 years [20]. Within this definition, there are two subsets of patients. In one, there has been a true premature menopause with a total depletion of ovarian follicles and therefore a permanent loss of ovarian function. In the other group, follicles are still present but apparently unresponsive to circulatory gonadotropins [3]. In the case of "follicular ovarian failure," there are numerous primordial follicles, and gonadotropin levels are elevated. A follicular ovarian failure may be due to genetic abnormalities, radiation injury, or chemotherapy. The defect could also relate to an FSH receptor defect, or to an autoimmune disease with production of anti-FSH receptor antibodies. The etiology of this condition is clearly speculative [20].

Polycystic Ovarian Disease. The polycystic ovarian syndrome (PCOS) is one of the most common causes of infertility in women, as it has been estimated that 5–8% of women exhibit one or more symptoms of the condition. The reproductive symptoms of PCOS can include some or all of the following: polycystic ovaries, hyperandrogenemia, excess LH secretion, impaired follicular development, and anovulation. Metabolic features of the syndrome can include insulin resistance, hyperinsulinemia, hirsutism, and obesity. It has been theorized that PCOS is an inherited syndrome in which one or more gene mutations gives rise to the core characteristic of the syndrome, functional hyperandrogenemia [15, 49]. The exposure of the female fetus to excess androgens is believed to reprogram the development of multiple tissues [1], such that they exhibit the reproductive and metabolic PCOS pathophysiologies, beginning in adolescence and prevailing throughout the adult reproductive lifespan.

Premenstrual Syndrome and Premenstrual Dysphoric Disorder.   Premenstrual syndrome (PMS) has been defined as "the cyclic recurrence, in the luteal phase of the menstrual cycle, of a combination of distressing physical, psychological, and/or behavioral changes of sufficient severity to result in deterioration of interpersonal relationships and/or interference with normal activities" [56]. Premenstrual dysphoria (PMD) is considered a severe form of PMS that can occur in 2% of women of reproductive age. It is characterized by an array of debilitating symptoms that include major depression, anxiety, irritability, anger dyscontrol, impaired concentration and energy, and physical symptoms such as bloating and breast tenderness. The hallmark feature of PMD is the intermittent manifestation of symptoms, appearing during the luteal phase of the menstrual cycle and remitting after the onset of menses [16, 22]. Symptoms also remain stable from cycle to cycle [22, 56]. No diagnosis-related differences in gonadal steroids, gonadotropins, or sex hormone-binding globulin have been consistently observed in patients with PMS or PMD, compared with controls. Thus, both the levels of reproductive hormones (including estradiol, progesterone, follicle-stimulating hormone, luteinizing hormone, and ovarian and adrenal androgens) and their pattern of secretion over the menstrual cycle do not appear to be disturbed in PMS. Rather, PMS and PMD may occur as a result of an abnormal response of the CNS to normal cyclic hormone secretions. Supporting this idea is a study which showed that suppression of ovarian steroid secretions in women with PMS significantly reduced their symptoms, but replacement with physiological estrogen and progesterone treatments caused the symptoms to reoccur. The same treatments had no effect on mood in women without PMS [51]. Recent clinical studies have shown that certain antidepressant medications, selective serotonin reuptake inhibitors (SSRIs), are effective in the treatment of PMD when given intermittently during the luteal phase of the menstrual cycle [22, 23].

Hirsutism and Virilization.   Hirsutism is defined as the presence of hair in women on areas of the body where hair usually is not present [9]. Chief locations include the face, chest, areola of the breasts, or the abdomen above the symphysis pubis (male escutcheon). The underlying endocrine etiology of hirsutism is increased androgen production by the ovary and/or the adrenal gland. The presence of excess unbound testosterone leads to the development of hirsutism. Approximately 10% of women in the United States exhibit hirsutism during their reproductive years, and the incidence is even greater in menopausal women. Measurement of circulating androgens in these women has revealed that 80–90% are hyperandrogenic. Enzymatic defects in adrenal cortisol metabolism that lead to excess androgen secretion (Chap. 15) or excess androgen production by an adrenal or ovarian tumor may cause hirsutism. Increased facial and body hair growth, increased muscle mass, and clitoral enlargement are manifestations of excessive adrenal or gonadal androgen production (adult adrenogenital syndrome). Cyproterone acetate (see Fig. 17.7), an androgen antagonist, has been used successfully in the treatment of hirsutism and masculinization.

Hirsutism is only one manifestation of hyperandrogenic conditions. The degree of hirsutism does not correlate with the degree of androgen production or the circulating levels of serum testosterone; rather, the severity of hirsutism depends on the availability and metabolism of testosterone by the skin and its appendages. The skin of hirsute women is highly sensitive to available testosterone owing to increased activity of 5α-reductase, as compared with nonhirsute women. The peripheral effects of testosterone, in addition to hirsutism, include increased sebum secretion from sebaceous glands. This leads to oily skin. Infection of these active sebaceous glands with resident microorganisms leads to the aciniform eruptions, which are a common feature of this condition.

MOLECULAR MEDICINE CASE STUDIES

Infertility can result from disrupted hormone actions in the hypothalamus, pituitary, and gonad. Described below are three different cases of receptor mutations that impair (1) the actions of kisspeptin (Chap. 17) on GnRH neurons, (2) GnRH's actions on gonadotropes, and (3) FSH actions in the ovary, respectively.

"Hypogonadotropic hypogonadism due to loss of function of the KiSS1-derived peptide receptor GPR54." de Roux et al., *Proc. Natl. Acad. Sci. USA.* 100(19):10972–6, 2003. "Hypogonadotropic hypogonadism is defined as a deficiency of the pituitary secretion of follicle-stimulating hormone and luteinizing hormone, which results in the impairment of pubertal maturation and of reproductive function. In the absence of pituitary or hypothalamic anatomical lesions and of anosmia (Kallmann syndrome), hypogonadotropic hypogonadism is referred to as isolated hypogonadotropic hypogonadism (IHH). A limited number of IHH cases are due to loss-of-function mutations of the gonadotropin-releasing hormone receptor. To identify additional gene defects leading to IHH, a large consanguineous family with five affected siblings and with a normal gonadotropin-releasing hormone receptor coding sequence was studied. Homozygosity whole-genome mapping allowed the localization of a new locus within the short arm of chromosome 19 (19p13). Sequencing of several genes localized within this region showed that all affected siblings of the family carried a homozygous deletion of 155 nucleotides in the GPR54 gene. This deletion encompassed the splicing acceptor site of intron 4-exon 5 junction and part of exon 5. The deletion was absent or present on only one allele in unaffected family members. GPR54 has been initially identified as an orphan G protein-coupled receptor with 40% homology to galanin receptors. Recently, a 54-aa peptide derived from the KiSS1 protein was identified as a ligand of GPR54. The present study shows that loss of function of GPR54 is a cause of IHH, and it identifies GPR54 and possibly KiSS1 protein-derived peptide as playing a major and previously unsuspected role in the physiology of the gonadotropic axis."

"Mutation Ala(171)Thr stabilizes the gonadotropin-releasing hormone receptor in its inactive conformation, causing familial hypogonadotropic hypogonadism." Karges et al., *J. Clin. Endocrinol. Metab.* 88:1873–9, 2003. "Mutations of the GnRH receptor have been recognized as a cause of familial gonadotropin deficiency. We here identify and functionally characterize a novel human GnRH receptor variant bearing an Ala(171)Thr substitution located at transmembrane helix 4 (TMH4). The affected kindred displays severe hypogonadotropic hypogonadism. After in vitro expression in human embryonic kidney 293T cells, the Ala(171)Thr mutant GnRH receptor exhibited a lack of phospholipase C activity in signal transduction. Specific receptor binding of (125)I-labeled GnRH ligand was undetectable in Ala(171)Thr GnRH receptor-transfected cells. Molecular modeling and dynamic simulation of the Ala(171)Thr GnRH receptor suggests the introduction of a stable hydrogen bond between residue Thr(171) and Tyr(119) side-chains at a distance of 2 A. Although spatially distant from the GnRH ligand-binding site, this hydrogen bond impedes conformational mobility of the TMH3 and TMH4 domains required for sequential ligand binding and receptor activation, thus stabilizing the GnRH receptor in its inactive conformation. Receptor structure modeling and functional data provide a comprehensive molecular view of how mutation Ala(171)Thr causes a complete loss of GnRH receptor function" (Fig. 18.13).

"A mutation in the follicle-stimulating hormone receptor as a cause of familial spontaneous ovarian hyperstimulation syndrome." Montanelli et al., *J. Clin. Endocrinol. Metab.* 89:1255–8, 2004. "Ovarian hyperstimulation syndrome (OHSS) occurs mainly after excessive stimulation of the ovaries by exogenous gonadotropins administrated in the context of in vitro fertilization procedures (iatrogenic OHSS). Recently, spontaneous and recurrent occurrence of the disease (spontaneous OHSS) was shown in two families to be caused by mutations affecting the follitropin receptor (FSHr). The two mutant FSHr (T449I, D567N) harbor aminoacid substitutions in the serpentine portion of the receptor and display abnormally high sensitivity to the pregnancy hormone hCG, thus providing a satisfactory explanation to the phenotype. In addition, mutant D567N also showed increased sensitivity to thyrotropin (TSH) and displayed increase in basal (ligand-independent) activity. In this report, we describe a new familial case of recurrent OHSS. The affected women were heterozygous for a different mutation involving codon 449, where an alanine was substituted for threonine. Similar to D567N, the T449A FSHr mutant shows an increase of its sensitivity to both hCG and TSH, together with an increase in basal activity. Together with the two previous studies, this report shows that inappropriate stimulation of the FSHr by hCG is a cause of spontaneous OHSS."

(Continued)

(Continued)

Figure 18.13 Clinical and genetic characteristics of patients with GnRHR mutation. (a) Family pedigree, illustrating autosomal recessive mode of inheritance. *Squares,* Males; *circles,* females. (b) Original DNA sequencing graphs, showing compound heterozygous mutations Ala^{171}Thr/Gln^{106}Arg (subjects II-1 and II-2) and monoallelic mutations Ala^{171}Thr (subject I-1) and Gln^{106}Ala (subject I-2). Nucleotide exchanges are indicated by *arrows.* (c) Phenotype in terms of basal hormone values. Abnormal findings are in *bold.* Normal values: males: LH, 1.0–10.5 mU/ml; FSH, 1.5–9.7 mU/ml; testosterone, 300–1,000 ng/dl; estradiol, 6–44 pg/ml; females, midluteal phase: LH, 0.83–15.5 mU/ml; FSH, 1.3–9.5 mU/ml; testosterone, 20–80 ng/dl, estradiol, 15–115 pg/ml. (From Karges et al. 2003 Mutation Ala(171)Thr stabilizes the gonadotropin-releasing hormone receptor in its inactive conformation, causing familial hypogonadotropic hypogonadism. *J. Clin. Endocrinol. Metab.* 88:1873–9.)

REVIEW EXERCISES

Match the terms:

1. Graafian follicle
2. Atretic follicle
3. Primordial follicle
4. Egg
5. Interstitial tissue
6. Epithelial tissue

A. Resting follicle
B. Mature follicle
C. Granulosa cells
D. Expiring follicle
E. Ovum
F. Theca folliculi

Think, analyze and discuss:

1. The two-cell, two-gonadotropin hypothesis states that the stimulation of estrogen production requires the coordinated actions of two cells and the two gonadotropins.

a. Name the two ovarian cell types, the two gonadotropins, and the specific roles that each cell and each gonadotropin play in the synthesis of estrogen.
b. What effect would an aromatase enzyme inhibitor have on ovarian estrogen production? On ovarian androgen levels?

2. In recent studies, mutant mice null for the FSH receptor gene have been developed. The female FSH receptor knockout (FSHrKO) mice are infertile and have undeveloped gonads and accessory sex organs.

a. Predict how serum estrogen levels might be altered in FSHrKO mice, compared to wild-type (normal) animals. Explain your answer.

b. Predict how serum androgen levels might be altered in the FSHrKO animals, and explain your answer.

c. Predict how serum inhibin levels might be altered in the FSHrKO animals, and explain your answer.

d. Predict how serum LH and FSH levels might be altered in the FSHrKO animals, and explain your answer.

e. What effect would estrogen treatment have on serum LH and FSH levels in the FSHrKO animals? Explain your answer for each gonadotropin.

f. Predict how folliculogenesis would be impacted by the deficiency of FSH receptors in the FSHrKO mice. At what stage of follicular development would the process be affected?

3. Gene targeting was also used in recent studies to produce LH receptor knockout (LuRKO) mice. At birth, the LuRKO mice were found to develop with ovaries and genital structures indistinguishable from their wild-type counterparts. Postnatally the LuRKO females displayed underdeveloped uteri and external genitalia, and ovaries of reduced size compared to wild-type mice. The LuRKO mice were found to be infertile.

a. Predict how the levels of estrogen, progesterone, LH, and FSH might be altered in the serum of adult female LuRKO mice. For each hormone, explain your answer.

b. Predict how folliculogenesis would be impacted by the deficiency of FSH receptors in the FSHrKO mice. At what stage of follicular development would the process be affected?

4. Clomiphene citrate is an anti-estrogen that is used clinically to induce follicular maturation and ovulation in women who are anovulatory. It is taken by women over a period of 4 days during the mid-follicular phase of the menstrual cycle.

a. Formulate an hypothesis as to how clomiphene citrate may induce follicular maturation, and how this may then lead to ovulation induction. How might the use of clomiphene citrate affect the uterus?

b. Another option for ovulation induction is letrozole, an aromatase inhibitor. Why would this drug also be effective?

5. In ewes, ovulatory cycles and mating behavior occurs only when the animals enter into estrous during the late fall or winter months, i.e. during "short-day" photoperiods.

a. What is the adaptive significance of a breeding season that occurs during this annual period?

b. Why is it that in some rodents, such as hamsters, estrous cycles and mating behavior occur during "long-day" photoperiods?

6. Oocytes obtained from middle and late antral follicles of mice resume meiosis when removed from the follicle and cultured in vitro. In contrast, oocytes cultured with granulosa cells do not mature. Which of the following treatments would result in oocyte maturation in cultures containing both oocytes and granulosa cells? Which would stimulate maturation? Provide an explanation for each of your responses:

a. Inhibition of GPR3 expression with anti-sense oligonucleotides.

b. LH.

c. Inhibitor of adenylate cyclase.

d. Inhibitor of adenylate cyclase with 8-bromo-cAMP, a diffusible cAMP analog.

e. A phosphodiesterase inhibitor.

f. Removal of granulosa cells and addition of 8-bromo-cAMP.

7. Levonorgestrel (Norplant) is a hormone-based contraceptive method in which capsules containing this progestin are implanted subcutaneously. Release from these capsules continuously delivers progestin and thereby provides contraception on a continuous basis. What is the endocrine basis of its effectiveness?

8. Congenital adrenal hyperplasia is an inherited condition which leads to excess androgen production in prenatal and postnatal life. What would be the likely reproductive abnormalities in women with this condition?

References

[1] Abbott, D. H., et al. 2005. Androgen excess fetal programming of female reproduction: A developmental aetiology for polycystic ovary syndrome? *Hum. Reprod. Update* 11(4):357–74.

[2] Adashi, E. Y. 1998. The IGF family and folliculogenesis. *J. Reprod. Immunol.* 39(1–2):13–19.

[3] Aillomäki, K., et al. 1996. Clinical features of primary ovarian failure caused by a point mutation in the follicle-stimulating hormone receptor gene. *J. Clin. Endocrinol. Metab.* 81:3722–6.

[4] Allen, E., and E. A. Doisy. 1923. An ovarian hormone: Preliminary report on its localization, extraction, and partial purification and action in test animals. *JAMA* 81:819–21.

[5] Bennett, L. L. 1991. The Long and Evans monograph on the estrous cycle in the rat. *Endocrinology* 129:2812–14.

[6] Bilezikjian, L. M., et al. 2004. Autocrine/paracrine regulation of pituitary function by activin, inhibin and follistatin. *Mol. Cell. Endocrinol.* 225(1–2):29–36.

[7] Brann, D. W., et al. 2002. Leptin and reproduction. *Steroids* 67(2):95–104.

[8] Burkart, A. D., et al. 2005. Repression of the inhibin alpha-subunit gene by the transcription factor CCAAT/enhancer-binding protein-beta. *Endocrinology* 146(4):1909–21.

[9] Carmina, E., and R. A. Lobo. 1997. Gonadotrophin-releasing hormone agonist therapy for hirsutism is as effective as high dose cyproterone acetate but results in a longer remission. *Hum. Reprod.* 12:663–6.

[10] Chappell, P. E., and J. E. Levine. 2000. Stimulation of gonadotropin-releasing hormone surges by estrogen. I. Role of hypothalamic progesterone receptors. *Endocrinology.* 141(4):1477–85.

[11] Cutler, W. B., et al. 1986. Human axillary secretions influence women's menstrual cycles: The role of donor extract from men. *Horm. Behav.* 20:463–73.

[12] de Kretser, D. M., et al. 2004. The role of activin, follistatin and inhibin in testicular physiology. *Mol. Cell. Endocrinol.* 225:57–64.

[13] Dinchuk, J. E., et al. 1995. Renal abnormalities and an altered inflammatory response in mice lacking cyclooxygenase II. *Nature* 378:406–9.

[14] DiZerega, G. S., and G. D. Hodgen. 1980. Changing functional status of the monkey corpus luteum. *Biol. Reprod.* 23:253–63.

[15] Ehrmann, D. A., R. B. Barnes, and R. L. Rosenfield. 1995. Polycystic ovary syndrome as a form of functional ovarian

hyperandrogenism due to dysregulation of androgen secretion. *Endocr. Rev.* 16:322–53.

[16] Endicott, J., et al. 1999. Is premenstrual dysphoric disorder a distinct entity? *J. Womens Health Gend. Based Med.* 8:663–79.

[17] Eramada, M. K., et al. 1993. Inhibin/activin subunit mRNA expression in human granulosa-luteal cells. *Mol. Cell. Endocrinol.* 92:R15–20.

[18] Espey, L. L., and H. Lipner. 1994. Ovulation. In: E. Knobil and J. Neill, eds., *The physiology of reproduction,* 2nd edn. New York: Raven Press, pp. 725–80.

[19] Ferenczy, A. 1993. Ultrastructure of the normal menstrual cycle: A review. *Microscop. Res. Tech.* 25:91–105.

[20] Fox, H. 1992. The pathology of premature ovarian failure. *J. Pathol.* 167:357–63.

[21] Grady, R. R., M. C. Charlesworth, and N. B. Schwartz. 1982. Characterization of the FSH-suppressing activity in follicular fluid. *Recent Prog. Horm. Res.* 38:409–56.

[22] Grady-Weliky, T. A. 2003. Premenstrual dysphoric disorder. *N. Eng. J. Med.* 348:433–8.

[23] Halbreich, U., et al. 2002. Efficacy of intermittent, luteal phase sertraline treatment of premenstrual dysphoric disorder. *Obstet. Gynecol.* 100:1219–29.

[24] Henzl, M. R. 1993. Gonadotropin-releasing hormone and its analogues: From laboratory to bedside. *Clin. Obstet. Gynecol.* 36:617–35.

[25] Hewitt, S. C., J. C. Harrell, and K. S. Korach. 2005. Lessons in estrogen biology from knockout and transgenic animals. *Annu. Rev. Physiol.* 67:285–308.

[26] Hillier, J. G., P. E. Whitelaw, and C. D. Smyth. 1994. Follicular oestrogen synthesis: The "two-cell, two-gonadotrophin" model revisited. *Mol. Cell. Endocrinol.* 100:51–4.

[27] Hillier, S. G., et al. 1995. Gonadotropin control of follicular function. *Horm. Res.* 43:216–23.

[28] Irianni, F., and G. D. Hodgen. 1992. Mechanism of ovulation. *Reprod. Endocrinol.* 21:19–38.

[29] Knight, P. G. 1996. Roles of inhibins, activins, and follistatin in the female reproductive system. *Front. Neuroendocrinol.* 17:476–509.

[30] Kobayashi, M., K. Aida, and I. Hanyu. 1986. Pheromone from ovulatory female goldfish induces gonadotropin surge during spawning in male goldfish. *Gen. Comp. Endocrinol.* 62:70–9.

[31] Koehler, K. F., et al. 2005. Reflections on the discovery and significance of estrogen receptor beta. *Endocr. Rev.* 26(3):465–78.

[32] Knobil, E. 1980. Neuroendocrine control of the menstrual cycle. *Recent Prog. Horm. Res.* 36:53–88.

[33] Knobil, E., et al. 1980. Control of the rhesus monkey menstrual cycle: Permissive role of hypothalamic gonadotropin-releasing hormone. *Science* 207(4437):1371–3.

[34] Lee, B. L., G. Unabia, and G. Childs. 1993. Expression of follistatin mRNA by somatotropes and mammotropes early in the rat estrous cycle. *J. Histochem. Cytochem.* 41:955–60.

[35] Levine, J. E. 1997. New concepts of the neuroendocrine regulation of gonadotropin surges in rats. *Biol. Reprod.* 56(2):293–302.

[36] Levine, J. E., et al. 1985. In vivo gonadotropin-releasing hormone release and serum luteinizing hormone

measurements in ovariectomized, estrogen-treated rhesus macaques. *Endocrinology* 117(2):711–21.

[37] Lydon, J. P., et al. 1995. Mice lacking progesterone receptor exhibit pleiotropic reproductive abnormalities. *Genes Dev.* 9(18):2266–78.

[38] Mather, J. P., A. Moore, and R.-H. Li. 1997. Activins, inhibins, and follistatins: Further thoughts on a growing family of regulators. *Soc. Exp. Biol. Med.* 215:209–22.

[39] Mehlmann, L. M. 2005. Stops and starts in mammalian oocytes: Recent advances in understanding the regulation of meiotic arrest and oocyte maturation. *Reproduction* 130:791–9.

[40] Mehlmann, L. M., et al. 2004. The Gs-linked receptor GPR3 maintains meiotic arrest in mammalian oocytes. *Science* 306:1947–50.

[41] Mizuno, M., and E. Terasawa. 2005. Search for neural substrates mediating inhibitory effects of oestrogen on pulsatile luteinising hormone-releasing hormone release in vivo in ovariectomized female rhesus monkeys (*Macaca mulatta*). *J. Neuroendocrinol.* 17(4):238–45.

[42] Moenter, S. M., R. C. Brand, and F. J. Karsch. 1992. Dynamics of gonadotropin-releasing hormone (GnRH) secretion during the GnRH surge: Insights into the mechanism of GnRH surge induction. *Endocrinology* 130(5):2978–84.

[43] Mulac-Jericevic, B., and O. M. Conneely. 2004. Reproductive tissue selective actions of progesterone receptors. *Reproduction* 128(2):139–46.

[44] Parkes, A. S., and H. M. Bruce. 1961. Olfactory stimuli in mammalian reproduction. *Science* 134:1049–54.

[45] Pau, K. Y., et al. 1993. Preovulatory gonadotropin-releasing hormone surge in ovarian-intact rhesus macaques. *Endocrinology* 133(4):1650–6.

[46] Phillips, D. J., and T. K. Woodruff. 2004. Inhibin: Actions and signalling. *Growth Factors* 22(1):13–18.

[47] Richards, J. S., et al. 2002. Novel signaling pathways that control ovarian follicular development, ovulation, and luteinization. *Recent Prog. Horm. Res.* 57:195–220.

[48] Robker, R. L., et al. 2000. Progesterone-regulated genes in the ovulation process: ADAMTS-1 and cathepsin L proteases. *Proc. Natl. Acad. Sci. USA* 97:4689–94.

[49] Rosenfield, R. L., and R. B. Barnes. 1993. Menstrual disorders in adolescence. *Endocrinol. Metab. Clin. North Am.* 22:491–505.

[50] Rossmanith, W. G. 1993. Contemporary insights into the control of the corpus luteum function. *Horm. Metab. Res.* 25:192–8.

[51] Schmidt, P. J., et al. 1998. Differential behavioral effects of gonadal steroids in women with and in those without premenstrual syndrome. *N. Engl. J. Med.* 228:209–16.

[52] Schreiner-Engel, P., et al. 1989. Low sexual desire in women: The role of reproductive hormones. *Horm. Behav.* 23:221–34.

[53] Simone, D. A., and V. B. Mahesh. 1993. An autoregulatory process for androgen production in rat thecal and interstitial cells. *Biol. Rep.* 48:46–56.

[54] Sisk, C. L., et al. 2001. In vivo gonadotropin-releasing hormone secretion in female rats during peripubertal development and on proestrus. *Endocrinology* 142(7):2929–36.

[55] Sluyser, M. 1995. Mutations in the estrogen receptor gene. *Hum. Mutat.* 6:97–103.

[56] Steiner, M. 1997. Premenstrual syndromes. *Annu. Rev. Med.* 48:447–55.

[57] Terasawa, E., and D. L. Fernandez. 2001. Neurobiological mechanisms of the onset of puberty in primates. *Endocr. Rev.* 22(1):111–51.

[58] Tilly, S. L., et al. 1999. Reproductive failure and reduced blood pressure in mice lacking the EP2 prostaglandin E2 receptor. *J. Clin. Inv.* 103:1539–45.

[59] Van Tienhoven, A. 1968. *Reproductive physiology.* Philadelphia: W. B. Saunders.

[60] Weller, L., and A. Weller. 1997. Menstrual variability and the measurement of menstrual synchrony. *Psychoneuroendocrinology* 22:115–28.

[61] Yen, S. S. 1993. Female hypogonadotropic hypogonadism. Hypothalamic amenorrhea syndrome. *Endocrinol. Metab. Clin. North Am.* 22:29–58.

[62] Zeleznik, A. J. 2001. Follicle selection in primates: "many are called but few are chosen". *Biol. Reprod.* 65:655–9.

Endocrinology of Pregnancy, Parturition, and Lactation

The ovulated egg has two possible fates: (1) if it fails to become fertilized, it undergoes lysis; (2) if, on the other hand, the ovum becomes fertilized, it (the zygote) may develop into an offspring of the species. If such an event is to be successful, a complex number of integrated neuroendocrine events between both conceptus and mother must transpire. For example, pregnancy, parturition, and lactation are unique female reproductive events that require the participation of a number of new hormones not previously involved in either female or male physiological functions.

Oviparity, Ovoviparity, and Viviparity

*After fertilization embryonic development in **oviparous** species (all birds) takes place outside the body in eggs that are covered with one or more protective membranes (shell, jelly). In **ovoviparous** species (e.g., reptiles), the mother gives birth to live young, which are nevertheless developed within a protective egg retained within the oviduct but receive no nutrition from the mother. In **viviparous** animals, the young develop within the mother and receive nourishment through vascular connections between embryo and mother. Except for the duckbilled platypus and spiny anteater, all mammals are viviparous.*

Hormones play essential roles in the processes of fetal growth and development, parturition at term, and, in most mammals, the control of lactation. Due to the introductory nature of this book, only a few details of this complex topic can be discussed and these are limited mostly to the primate.

Pregnancy

Fertilization of the Egg and Implantation of the Blastocyst Initiates Development of the Fetal-Placental Unit

In the primate, usually a single egg is ovulated approximately midway through the menstrual cycle. During coitus, spermatozoa released by the male into the vagina travel via the uterus to the oviducts where the ovum may become fertilized [50]. Many spermatozoa may penetrate the corona radiata surrounding the ovum and, although more than one sperm can penetrate the zona pellucida, usually only one enters the ovum. In response to the sperm, the oocyte completes the second meiotic division and expels the second polar body. The resulting female pronucleus comes in contact with the male pronucleus that has been formed after loss of the sperm tail. Fusion of the male and female pronuclei, to form the zygote, reestablishes the diploid chromosomal number of the egg. During passage down the uterine tube, which takes about 2 days, the zygote undergoes rapid mitotic divisions, and the resulting cells are referred to as *blastomeres*. By about 3 days, a compact mass of cells,

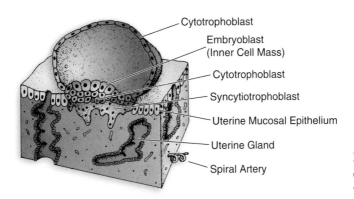

- Cytotrophoblast
- Embryoblast (Inner Cell Mass)
- Cytotrophoblast
- Syncytiotrophoblast
- Uterine Mucosal Epithelium
- Uterine Gland
- Spiral Artery

Figure 19.1 Implantation of the blastocyst within the uterus.

the *morula*, enters the uterus. Continued cell division produces a hollow sphere, the early *blastocyst*, which is composed of a single layer of cells, the *trophoblast*, and an inner cell mass, the *embryoblast*, which is attached to the trophoblastic wall at the embryonic pole of the blastocyst. The inner cell mass, through differentiation and growth, will form the embryo, whereas the trophoblast will establish contact with the maternal circulation to provide the initial mechanism for the exchange of nutrients, oxygen, and waste products between fetus and mother. After residing within the uterus for about 2 days, the embryonic pole of the blastocyst becomes implanted in the endometrial epithelium on about day 6 (Fig. 19.1). In response to the blastocyst, the underlying epithelium and endometrium undergo cellular changes, a so-called *decidualization process*. As a result, the endometrial tissue enlarges to form an implantation chamber, the *decidua*, to accommodate the growing embryo. The trophoblastic cells in contact with the uterine epithelium proliferate into an invasive *syncytiotrophoblast*, which consists of a multinucleated protoplasmic mass (Fig. 19.1). By 10 days, the conceptus is completely embedded within the endometrium. The syncytiotrophoblast forms lacunar networks that establish contact with the endometrial capillaries to form the primitive uteroplacental circulation.

Gonadal steroids appear to be required for implantation. There is evidence that the blastocyst synthesizes estrogens, and it has been proposed that steroids synthesized or accumulated by the blastocyst may play a role in implantation through a local action on the adjacent endometrium. Indeed, in the rat uterus, the concentrations of nuclear receptors for both estradiol (E_2) and progesterone are higher in implantation sites than in nonimplantation regions of the endometrium.

hCG Rescues the Corpus Luteum

The corpus luteum normally regresses about 12 days after ovulation during an infertile cycle in the primate. If, however, the ovum is fertilized and subsequently implants within the uterus, then by 10 days after ovulation a glycoprotein molecule unique to pregnancy is now present within the blood. This protein is secreted by the syncytiotrophoblast and, in humans, is referred to as *human chorionic gonadotropin* (hCG) or choriogonadotropin [26, 34]. Detection of this protein in the urine provides the basis for the most common test for pregnancy.

The role of hCG is to stimulate progesterone biosynthesis by the luteal cells of the corpus luteum. Initially, luteinizing hormone (LH) of pituitary origin is stimulatory to progesterone production by the corpus luteum. But LH levels drop precipitously after the midcycle LH/FSH surge. During the menstrual cycle, progesterone secretion by the corpus luteum reaches a peak about 8 days after its formation. If the egg is not fertilized, progesterone levels decline rapidly and menstruation follows. The role of hCG is to rescue the corpus luteum, thereby prolonging its life span by converting it into a *corpus luteum of pregnancy*. Plasma levels of hCG rise to their highest between about the ninth and fourteenth weeks of pregnancy and then begin to decline gradually, reaching a nadir at approximately twenty weeks of gestation. Luteal function begins to decline while circulating levels of hCG are at their peak, suggesting that failure of luteal activity is not related to declining levels of hCG.

Luteal cell hCG receptors are identical to LH receptors; therefore they are often referred to as LH/hCG receptors, and either hormone may be used to study activation of cAMP formation and progesterone synthesis by luteal cells. The β subunits of LH and hCG are closely

Figure 19.2 Hypothetical structural features of the LH/CG receptor. (From McFarland et al. 1989. Lutropin-choriogonadotropin receptor: An unusual member of the G protein-coupled receptor family. *Science* 245:494–9, with permission. Copyright 1989 by the American Association for the Advancement of Science.)

related in sequence, and these two hormones bind to the same receptor and elicit identical biological responses [26]. The immediate response of target cells to the binding of LH or hCG is an increase in adenylate cyclase activity mediated by intracellular, membrane-associated G proteins. The receptor protein displays the structural features of both a leucine-rich proteoglycan (extracellular domain) and of a G-protein-coupled receptor. The other members of the G-protein-coupled receptor family bind small ligands (such as serotonin or acetylcholine). Whereas binding of such ligands is thought to occur at sites formed by the assembly of the seven transmembrane helices, LH and hCG are thought to bind to a site on the extracellular part of this receptor. Thus the large extracellular domain and the specific mechanism of hormone-mediated signal transduction set the LH/CG-R apart from other G-protein-coupled receptors (Fig. 19.2) [23].

In many mammals (e.g., rats, rabbits, but not primates), the pituitary gland is essential for the initial development as well as the survival of the corpora lutea in the pregnant female [33]. Hypophysectomy in these animals results in atrophy of the corpus lutea, which can, however, be maintained by administration of pituitary extracts. The pituitary hormone responsible for luteotropic action in these species is prolactin (PRL). In the rat, transplantation of the adenohypophysis to an ectopic site, such as the kidney, shortly after ovulation will allow development of the corpora lutea to an active state and at the same time keep the female in a state of pseudopregnancy. In the absence of an inhibitory hypothalamic control, the ectopically transplanted adenohypophysis autonomously secretes PRL [33]. Implantation of fertilized ova within the uterus is apparently perceived by sensory neural elements, which, through spinal afferents, convey this information to the hypothalamus. This is believed to result in an inhibition of hypothalamic dopaminergic neurons and, in the absence of dopamine secretion into the hypophysial portal system, PRL is secreted autonomously.

The Placenta Assumes the Role of an Endocrine Organ

With the demise of the corpus luteum in the primate, E_2 and progesterone production is taken over by the placenta. However, the placenta is not capable of producing these steroid hormones without a supply of precursors from both the fetus and the maternal compartment.

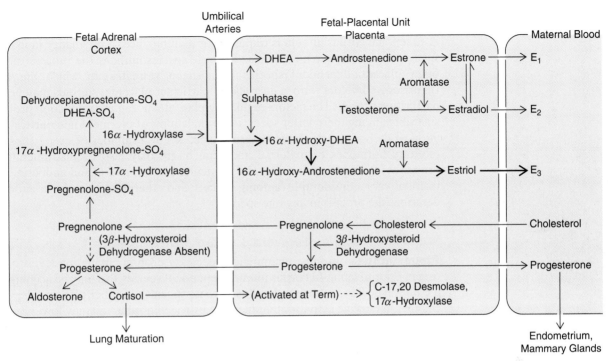

Figure 19.3 The fetal-placental unit.

Progesterone. The placenta, incapable of de novo progesterone biosynthesis, is dependent on cholesterol derived from the maternal blood supply [36] (Fig. 19.3). The progesterone produced by the placenta is released into the maternal circulation to serve a multitude of functions related to pregnancy: maintenance of uterine structure and function, mammary growth and development, and inhibition of pituitary gonadotropin secretion. In addition, placental progesterone is used as a substrate for corticoid production by the fetal adrenals that lack an active 3β-hydroxysteroid dehydrogenase.

Estrogens. Pregnenolone of placental origin is also used by the fetal adrenals in the production of precursors for estrogen production within the placenta. The placenta itself has only a limited capability for estrogen synthesis due to minimal 17α-hydroxylase activity. Within the fetal adrenal cortex, however, this enzyme is responsible for production of dehydroepiandrosterone sulfate (DHEA-SO$_4$). This steroid metabolite serves as a precursor substrate for estrone (E$_1$) and E$_2$ synthesis by the placenta. Much of the substrate is, however, converted by a fetal adrenal 16α-hydroxylase to precursors that lead to copious estriol (E$_3$) production. Measurements of E$_3$ levels in the maternal plasma or urine as a means of evaluating fetal well-being have been undertaken, but their usefulness is questionable. It is obvious from the preceding discussion that the fetal adrenals and the placenta, with respect to steroid hormone production, are incomplete endocrine organs. There is a circular flow of steroid metabolites that passes from the maternal compartment to the placenta, to the fetal adrenals, and then back through the placental compartment to the maternal bloodstream (Fig. 19.3).

Placental Lactogens. Several proteins are made by the placenta that are closely related in structure to prolactin and growth hormone. In rats, two of these, placental lactogen I and II (PL-I and PL-II) were identified as prolactin-like molecules that can bind to the prolactin receptor with high affinity and mimic the actions of prolactin. A single PL is expressed in humans. The structure and functions of PLs have been discussed in detail (Chap. 12). In general, the placental lactogens exert a variety of effects on maternal tissues, such as lactogenesis, and luteal maintenance and progesterone production (at least in rats) during the latter stages of gestation. In humans, PL-I may be important in stimulating mammary cell proliferation, and in stimulating some of the adaptations of the maternal lipid and carbohydrate metabolism that occur during the third trimester of pregnancy. Other placental prolactin-like hormones, such as proliferin, have been implicated in the alterations in angiogenesis, hematopoiesis, and lymphocyte function that occur during pregnancy [20].

Parturition

A functional corpus luteum is required for maintenance of pregnancy in many mammalian species (e.g., goat, sow); its demise in these species initiates the process of parturition. In other placenta-dependent species (e.g., sheep, primates) in which the corpus luteum regresses well before term, a decrease in particular placental steroids may be the key to the parturition process. The factors regulating placental hormone production probably vary considerably among these latter species. Prostaglandins of uterine origin participate in the initiation of delivery of the fetus at term by actions at a number of target sites. One or more pituitary hormones of maternal and fetal origin may also be instrumental in activating processes leading to parturition. The particular roles of neural and endocrine factors in parturition vary considerably among species and, therefore, no single model adequately describes the process in any one species.

Neural and Endocrine Mechanisms Control Parturition

Progesterone.   In most mammalian species, a drop in circulating levels of progesterone occurs prior to labor. In corpus luteum-dependent species, this may be accomplished by uterine luteolytic factors (prostaglandins in some species). In other placenta-dependent species, changes in enzyme activities that increase estrogen production may lower progesterone levels. Progesterone is directly antagonistic to uterine smooth muscle contraction induced by either oxytocin or prostaglandins. The *progesterone block hypothesis* was formulated to provide a theoretically relevant mechanism by which the uterus might be protected from premature contraction and expulsion of the fetus. In this model a lowering of progesterone levels at term would be the stimulus to parturition.

Estrogens.   Estrogens increase myometrial excitability, possibly by lowering the membrane potential of uterine smooth muscle. The actions of estrogens on the myometrium are, however, antagonized by the action of progesterone. In the rat, the number of uterine estrogen receptors increases as progesterone levels decline. Estrogens enhance uterine excitability by a number of mechanisms: increasing endometrial PG synthetase activity, increasing myometrial and endometrial oxytocin receptors, and increasing oxytocin production and secretion by the neurohypophysis (Chap. 7).

Prostaglandins.   There is evidence that in most species studied, PGs play an important role in parturition. In many species, increased synthesis and release of PGs precede labor. In some large animals (e.g., goat, sow) that depend on the corpus luteum as a source of progesterone, $PGF_{2\alpha}$ released from the endometrium may be the luteolytic factor responsible for luteal regression. The resulting drop in luteal progesterone production is followed by uterine contractions and parturition. As noted, uterine PG synthesis may be dependent on stimulation by placental estrogens.

Placental Prolactin.   Levels of PRL increase in the human fetus during late gestation. PRL levels are very high in amniotic fluid, and synthesis of PRL by choriondecidual tissue has been demonstrated. This placental PRL is immunologically similar to pituitary PRL and should not be confused with placental lactogen (PL), which differs considerably in primary structure. Increased levels of PRL coincide with a stage in development during which major changes in organ growth occur in the fetus and may be responsible for increased growth and function of the fetal adrenal cortex (Chap. 12).

Autonomic Motor Innervation.   The female reproductive tract is richly innervated by adrenergic neurons. The role, if any, of such innervation in parturition is unresolved. Both estrogens and progestins affect the norepinephrine (NE) content of these nerves, as well as the turnover of NE, the activity of enzymes related to catecholamine biosynthesis, and the release of NE from nerve terminals. In the progesterone-dominated uterus catecholamine stimulation of myometrial smooth muscle β-adrenoceptors causes relaxation of the uterus. During the latter stages of pregnancy in some species, stretch-induced hypertrophy of the uterus causes degeneration of the nerves in the uterine corpus. Withdrawal of this neural inhibitory influence to the corpus may allow spontaneous myogenic contractions to intensify [21].

It has been noted that gap junctions (nexuses, low-resistance electrical pathways) are present between the uterine muscle cells of a number of species (including the human) immediately before, during, and immediately after delivery [9]. These junctions are absent at all other times during pregnancy and are also lacking in immature or nonpregnant animals. Ovariectomy of pregnant animals at midterm causes the rapid appearance of gap junctions, and the appearance of gap junctions at term is prevented by progesterone administration. The absence of gap junctions throughout the gestation period may be important in preventing electrical communication between uterine muscle cells. The acquisition of gap junctions at term may be an essential element in synchronizing uterine contractility for effective expulsion of the fetus [9]. Because gap junction formation may be initiated by progesterone withdrawal, this could provide the morphological and functional bases for the progesterone block hypothesis formulated much earlier by Csapo.

Oxytocin. Oxytocin (OT), a neurohypophysial hormone, has a direct uterine-contracting (oxytocic) action (Chap. 7). Fetal movements monitored by the uterine cervix and relayed by spinal afferents are stimulatory to OT release during labor in the human. The sensitivity of the myometrium to OT is enhanced by estrogens and depressed by progesterone. In the human female, maternal plasma OT levels increase with advancing gestation. It is not clear, however, whether OT is an initiating factor or only facilitative to human labor. Plasma estrogen concentrations increase during gestation and in the rat are known to increase the affinity and number of uterine OT receptors. The actions of OT on the uterus could be mediated indirectly through stimulation of endometrial and myometrial $PGF_{2\alpha}$ production. $PGF_{2\alpha}$ might then stimulate uterine smooth muscle cells, leading to contraction of the uterus and expulsion of the fetus.

The Fetal Adrenal Cortex. There is compelling evidence, particularly in sheep but also in other large mammals, that the onset of parturition is initiated by the activation of the fetal pituitary-adrenal axis. The fetal adrenal gland increases in weight rapidly during the last 2 weeks of gestation. This growth is primarily due to hypertrophy and hyperplasia of adrenal cortical cells. Premature delivery can be induced in the pregnant ewe by infusion of ACTH or glucocorticoids (but not mineralocorticoids) and can be prevented by fetal adrenalectomy or hypophysectomy. There is evidence that the fetal brain signals the precise "time for birth." The paraventricular nucleus (PVN) (in sheep) apparently acts as a computer assessing signals from various organs. When the organs have reached the proper degree of development, the PVN sends a hormonal signal (CRH?) to the pituitary to start producing ACTH, thereby initiating labor [30, 51, 57].

Increased fetal glucocorticoid production in sheep is stimulatory to placental production of estrogen from progesterone; this, therefore, leads to a subsequent fall in maternal plasma and tissue progesterone concentrations and a consequent rise in estrogen concentrations. The actions of fetal adrenal glucocorticoids may be to induce synthesis of 17,20-desmolase and 17α-hydroxylase within the placenta (Fig. 19.3). The resulting change in estrogen-progesterone levels may provide the stimulus to uterine production of PGs or related hormones (prostacyclins) and to an increase in uterine OT receptor number.

Corticotropin-Releasing Hormone (CRH). CRH is produced by intrauterine tissues and has been proposed to play a role in the regulation of human pregnancy and parturition. Pro-CRH mRNA is expressed in placental tissue and decidua in increasing amounts during pregnancy, and this increase is associated with a steep rise in maternal serum CRH concentrations. In tissue culture, CRH release from placental and chorion trophoblast cells is inhibited by progesterone and stimulated by catecholamines, oxytocin, and glucocorticoids. Moreover, CRH can stimulate prostaglandin production from fetal membranes and maternal deciduas, suggesting that this might function to enhance myometrial contractility. CRH can also synergize with prostaglandin F2α, oxytocin, and other factors to directly induce myometrial contractility, although it produces little effect on its own. Increased CRH levels have been observed in the serum of women who present with preterm labor, suggesting that a rise in CRH may be involved in the induction of labor itself. The putative roles of CRH in the maintenance of pregnancy and the initiation of labor remain to be clarified [3].

Relaxin. In 1926, Hisaw reported that an aqueous extract of the corpora lutea of the pregnant sow "relaxes" the pubic symphysis of the guinea pig. This biologically active substance was purified and named *relaxin* [42, 43]. Because of difficulties in isolating this factor, the chemical structure was not determined until much later. The development of a reliable radioimmunoassay (RIA) made possible the determination of the blood levels of the peptide throughout pregnancy, the production sites of the hormone, and the factors that may regulate relaxin secretion [44]. Most interesting was the discovery that the primary structures of relaxin and insulin are similar. Although there is only about 40% homology between the residues, the conformations of the two peptides are comparable. The cross-linking pattern of the two hormones strongly suggests that they have come into existence by gene duplication. It has been concluded, *a posteriori*, that relaxin, like insulin, is synthesized as a prohormone in a single chain to facilitate the correct folding of the protein. The remarkable molecular phylogenetics and evolution of the relaxins has been provided [42].

Studies on a variety of species, including humans, leave little doubt that the corpus luteum is the source of relaxin [43]. The source of luteal relaxin may be the granules observed in the granulosa lutein cells. Relaxin may also be produced and stored within granulocytes localized to the endometrium of rhesus monkeys and adult human females. In other species, such as the guinea pig, cat, rabbit, and horse, immunoreactive or bioactive relaxin levels in plasma or serum appear to be derived primarily from the placenta or uterus. Relaxin concentrations in luteal and other tissues are highest during pregnancy (Fig. 19.4). In the human, relaxin concentrations are four times higher in the ovarian vein draining the ovary containing the corpus luteum of pregnancy, than in either peripheral plasma or the contralateral ovarian vein. Immunoreactive relaxin is present in the serum as early as the fourth week of pregnancy; it is detectable throughout the course of gestation but is only rarely detected in the plasma of nonpregnant women. Plasma levels of immunoreactive relaxin rise to a peak shortly before parturition in rodents and pigs, which is correlated with the increase in cervical dilatability and the formation of an interpubic ligament (Fig. 19.5). Plasma RIA relaxin is also markedly elevated in late pregnancy in the dog, rhesus and Java monkey, and humans. Immunoreactive relaxin was found in the decidua, the placenta, and the myometrium of a pregnant baboon in which the corpus luteum had been removed much earlier. This observation suggests that these tissues have the ability to synthesize relaxin and may function in primate pregnancy during late gestation. Relaxin has also been found in the testes of armadillos and roosters, but is undetectable in the testis and serum of a number of male mammals, including humans. The role, if any, of relaxin in the male is therefore unknown.

The biological effects of relaxin are associated with pregnancy and parturition. Relaxin acts on the pubic symphysis to transform the connective tissues from a compact cartilaginous type

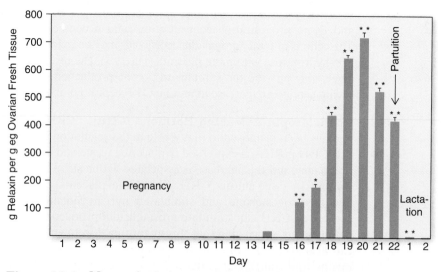

Figure 19.4 Mean relaxin immunoreactivity levels (± SEM) in ovarian extracts from pregnant and lactating rats. Ovaries obtained from two animals were pooled for each day shown. Asterisks denote those mean relaxin concentrations that differ significantly from those of the preceding observation (*P < 0.01). (From Sherwood, O. D. and V. E. Crnekovic. 1979. Development of a homologous radioimmunoassay for rat relaxin. *Endocrinology* 104:893–7, with permission.)

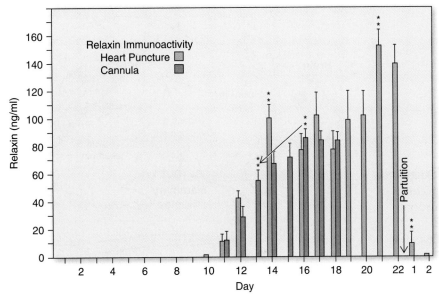

Figure 19.5 Relaxin immunoreactivity levels (± SEM) in the peripheral sera of anesthetized (heart puncture) and unanesthetized (cannula) rats. Asterisks denote those mean values that differ significantly (*P < 0.01) from those using the same end point that precede or are indicated with an arrow. (From Sherwood, O. D., et al. 1980. Radioimmunoassay of relaxin throughout pregnancy and during parturition in the rat. *Endocrinology* 107:691–8, with permission.)

to a more fluid, flexible structure. This results, in some species, in the formation of a ligament between the pubic bones. This increased flexibility and enlargement of the birth canal is important to successful parturition in a number of species.

Relaxin may be present within the endometrium of the uterus; in the rhesus monkey the peptide may function as a local hormone to control endothelioid cytomorphosis. This response involves hypertrophy and proliferation of the endothelial cells of the blood vessels just below the implanted embryo. This vascular response to relaxin could provide increased blood flow to the fetus. Relaxin also inhibits uterine motility by relaxing the myometrium. It has been speculated that because of its myometrium-inhibiting activity, relaxin may play a role in maintenance of pregnancy. Other effects of relaxin on the collagen framework and distensibility of the uterus, as well as similar effects on the uterine cervix, have been described.

Relaxin increases the secretion of two key collagenolytic enzymes, collagenase and plasminogen activator, from dispersed amnion and chorion cell cultures in vitro. These results support a possible localized action of relaxin on collagen degradation in fetal membranes, leading to their eventual rupture at the time of parturition. Relaxin and growth hormone may act synergistically in stimulating mammary gland growth. Relaxin promotes development of the mammary nipples and thereby enables normal lactational performance [43]. Endogenous relaxin promotes growth of the vagina in pregnant rats [43]. The evidence is convincing that relaxin subserves a multifunctional role in preparing the female for parturition and possibly other roles related to pregnancy (Fig. 19.6).

A Mechanistic Understanding of Labor Initiation in Humans Remains Elusive

While many factors are known to be involved in the process of labor, as described above, the sequence of events that induces and temporally organizes labor and parturition remains unclear. One model for the initiation of labor in the human suggests that, as a result of the rising estrogen levels during gestation, the concentration of uterine OT receptors increases [29]. Rapid fetal growth near term increases uterine distension, which may also contribute to the increase in uterine OT receptors near term, as shown in rats (Chap. 7). The increased numbers of OT receptors probably lower the threshold of the uterus to a level where

Figure 19.6 Postulated physiological roles of relaxin in the rodent. (From O. David Sherwood, with permission.)

myometrial contractions are initiated. Oxytocin may bind to decidual receptors and stimulate PG biosynthesis. The coupling of OT receptor activation and PG biosynthesis may be the crucial event in the initiation of labor. During spontaneous labor there is an increase in plasma OT levels in the fetal umbilical artery compared to the umbilical vein, indicating a flow of OT from the fetus toward the maternal compartment. Oxytocin derived from the fetus may provide the stimulus for the increased production of PGs at the onset of labor. Hypothalamoneurohypophysial maturation within the fetus, leading to fetal-adrenal activation and a decline in progesterone biosynthesis, as well as increased neurohypophysial hormone secretion (by the neurohypophysis as well as the uterus), may provide the final essential directive for the induction of parturition.

Lactation

In mammals, two ectodermal ridges (so-called "milk lines") appear on either side of the ventral midline early in fetal life. Localized thickenings become the mammary buds, which, in the female, grow into the underlying dermis to form the primary mammary cords, the precursors of the duct systems. In the human male, early mammary gland development is suppressed by gonadal androgens and, although there is an initial hypertrophy of the primary ducts and the secretion of a colostrum-like "witch's milk," caused by the maternal hormones of pregnancy, these glands soon become inactive. Further growth of the undeveloped mammae in the human female is not initiated until ovarian cycles begin. At puberty, further growth and branching of the ducts occurs and a lobular system is developed. Most of the size increase of the mammary glands is due to interlobular fat deposition. Mammary growth and development at puberty is mainly in response to gonadal estrogens, but adrenal glucocorticoids and growth hormone (GH) may also be involved (Fig. 19.7).

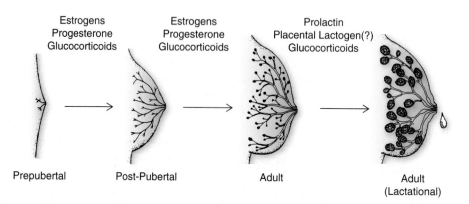

Figure 19.7 Hormonal regulation of mammary gland growth and development.

Estrogens
Progesterone
Glucocorticoids

Estrogens
Progesterone
Glucocorticoids

Prolactin
Placental Lactogen(?)
Glucocorticoids

Prepubertal

Post-Pubertal

Adult

Adult
(Lactational)

Proliferation of a lobular-alveolar system is initiated at pregnancy. Besides the requirement for estrogens and possibly glucocorticoids and GH for continued duct growth, progesterone and prolactin are required for full development of the ductule system (Fig. 19.7). Placental lactogen may also be required for full development of the breasts in the pregnant human female. Milk production in the mature mammary gland occurs near parturition. The following hormones have been implicated as essential to mammary growth and lactogenesis in some species: estrogen, progesterone, glucocorticoids, GH, insulin, placental lactogen, relaxin, and PRL [31].

Although milk constituents begin to appear before parturition in most species, high rates of synthesis do not usually occur until after birth. Milk is synthesized within the cells lining the mammary gland alveoli. Milk is a complex nutrient consisting mainly of milk sugar (lactose) lipids, milk proteins (casein and whey), as well as monovalent and divalent cations, and most interesting, immune antibodies. These products are released by macrovesicular exocytosis into the alveolar lumen, where they are stored until ejected by the action of OT on the myoepithelial cells covering the contraluminal surface of the alveolus (see Fig. 7.4). Many hormones of unknown function are found in milk [18].

Milk secretion is regulated by PRL through an action on plasmalemmal receptors of mammary gland alveolar secretory cells [11, 35]. In the rabbit an increase in PRL receptors, synchronous with the onset of lactation, occurs at the same time as the major rise in serum PRL levels at parturition. Estradiol increases the number of mammary gland PRL receptors, whereas progesterone suppresses this increase. PRL also up-regulates its own receptors. The dramatic increase in lactogenesis that follows parturition can be partly explained, therefore, by the removal of the inhibitory action of progesterone on the mammary gland coupled to the positive actions of PRL on the stimulation and production of its own receptors. Suckling-induced PRL secretion is required for maintenance of postpartum lactogenesis in some animals, such as the human, but not in others, such as the cow.

Fatty acids derived from dietary fat intake are converted within mammary gland epithelial cells to triglycerides (milk fats). These fatty acids are made available to mammary gland epithelial cells by activation of membrane-bound lipoprotein lipase. The activity of this enzyme is negligible in nonlactating animals but is enhanced 2 to 3 days before parturition, apparently in response to rising levels of PRL. Prolactin activation of lipoprotein lipase is blocked by simultaneous administration of actinomycin D, indicating that synthesis or activation of the enzyme requires mRNA-directed protein synthesis. Fatty acids are also synthesized within mammary gland epithelial cells in response to PRL.

In certain fishes, PRL stimulates renal Na^+/K^+-activated ATPase and controls salt excretion by the nasal salt gland of some marine birds. Prolactin also activates the transport of Na^+ and K^+ in mammary tissue apparently through an action on a Na^+/K^+ pump, which is localized almost exclusively to the basolateral membranes of mammary epithelial cells. Control of transepithelial Na^+ transport may be the underlying and most basic action of PRL on mammary gland milk production.

The secretion of PRL from the pituitary is under an inhibitory control by the hypothalamus (Chap. 6). A PRL release-inhibiting hormone, most probably dopamine, is released from hypothalamic dopaminergic neurons into the hypophysial portal system where the catecholamine is carried to the lactotrophs of the pars distalis. Inhibition of hypothalamic dopamine release or inhibition of dopamine interaction with lactotroph receptors (by ergot alkaloids, e.g., ergocryptine) results in PRL secretion.

Lactotroph hyperplasia is a prominent finding in the adenohypophyses of pregnant women. The increase in the amount of PRL mRNA is paralleled by lactotroph hyperplasia. The presence of mitoses in PRL-immunoreactive cells provides evidence that proliferation of preexisting lactotrophs contributes to lactotroph accumulation. Growth hormone immunoreactive cells show a marked reduction in GH mRNA, indicating that GH synthesis is inhibited. In many GH-immunoreactive cells, PRL mRNA becomes apparent. These findings demonstrate that GH is stored following discontinuation of GH synthesis. It appears that when PRL is secreted in excess during pregnancy, somatotrophs are recruited to produce PRL. These somatotrophs begin to express PRL mRNA, transform to bihormonal mammosomatotrophs, and possibly later to lactotrophs, contributing to PRL production. Mature somatotrophs may be regarded as reserve cells in the adenohypophysis, having the potential to switch hormone synthesis and to convert to mammosomatotrophs and possibly lactotrophs [49].

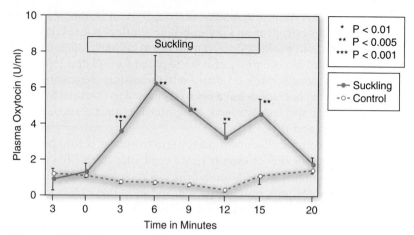

Figure 19.8 Mean (± SEM) plasma oxytocin concentrations for six nursing and six control subjects. Asterisks indicate significance relative to control subjects. (From Fuchs et al. 1984. Release of oxytocin and prolactin by suckling in rabbits throughout lactation. *Endocrinology* 114:462–9, with permission.)

The stimulus to PRL secretion is a neuroendocrine reflex involving neural afferents from the teats to the hypothalamus. A suckling-induced neuroendocrine reflex mechanism is also responsible for secretion of OT from the neurohypophysis (Fig. 19.8) [29]. Blood concentrations of PRL increase progressively throughout pregnancy; apparently due to the influence of increasing concentrations of placental steroids, particularly estrogens. Nevertheless, milk secretion is inhibited by a direct action of progesterone on the mammary glands. At parturition, blood levels of PRL are about 20 times greater than normal, but the level of the hormone remains elevated for only about a week postpartum in the absence of suckling. Blood concentrations of PRL remain high for the duration of lactation in breast-feeding women, and PRL is also released during each suckling episode in response to tactile stimulation of the nipple. Estrogens exert a profound action on pituitary mammotroph PRL production. Indeed, the elevated plasma levels of estrogens just prior to parturition may be important in stimulating lactogenesis through stimulation of PRL secretion. Estrogens appear to enhance lactotroph PRL secretion (at least in rats) by increasing prolactin production as, well as the number of thyrotropin-releasing hormone (TRH) receptors (TRH stimulates PRL secretion) present in these cells, an action that is blocked by the estrogen receptor antagonist tamoxifen (Fig. 19.9) [10].

Figure 19.9 Effect of tamoxifen, an estrogen antagonist, on pituitary TRH receptor number. (From Gershengorn, M. C., et al. 1979. Estrogens increase the number of thyrotropin-releasing hormone receptors on mammotropic cells in culture. *Endocrinology* 105:171–6, with permission.)

The placenta secretes large amounts of estrogens and progesterone, hormones inhibitory to follicle-stimulating hormone (FSH) secretion during pregnancy. Therefore, plasma FSH levels are normally suppressed during pregnancy and, at term, are low or undetectable. Blood levels of FSH increase postpartum to normal follicular phase levels. Both pituitary and plasma levels of LH are also extremely low during pregnancy, apparently also due to a negative feedback inhibition by placental steroid hormones. Inhibition of pituitary gonadotropin production during pregnancy may provide an adaptive mechanism whereby further egg maturation and release is inhibited so that the nutritive needs of the nursing infant are sustained. In nonlactating women, LH concentrations may remain low during the early puerperium (state of the woman after childbirth) but return to normal cyclic levels within 3 to 5 weeks, when the PRL concentration returns to its normal low levels.

In lactating women, blood E_2 concentrations are significantly lower than those of nonlactating women, and no ovarian follicular development occurs during the period of lactation as long as PRL levels remain high. Plasma levels of LH and E_2 increase soon after weaning, concomitant with a drop in PRL secretion, indicating the resumption of ovarian activity. Because the return of menstruation and fertility is usually delayed in women who breast-feed, it has been suggested that breast-feeding acts as a natural birth spacer or "nature's own contraceptive" [45]. In those societies where breast-feeding is the sole source of nutrition for the baby, lactational amenorrhea (postpartum infertility) may last for 2 to 3 years [24]. The duration of the period between birth and the onset of a menstrual cycle in the mother is probably a function of the frequency and duration of suckling. Although breast-feeding usually delays conception, it cannot do so indefinitely and women can become pregnant before the breast-feeding infant is weaned.

Breast-feeding is associated with a very significant prevention of infant morbidity and mortality throughout the world, and yet the duration, if not the incidence of breast-feeding, continues to decline worldwide. Nevertheless, the contraceptive effect of breast-feeding continues to make a substantial impact on fertility control worldwide [11].

Hormonal Contraception

The common contraceptive drugs in clinical use for women contain estrogens or progestogens, either singly or in a variety of combinations and concentrations. The estrogens are usually synthetic derivatives of ethinyl estradiol (Fig. 19.10). The progestogens are usually 19-nortestosterone or 17-hydroxyprogesterone derivatives such as norethindrone (Fig. 19.10). The *combination contraceptive preparations* contain an estrogen and a progestogen and are often administered daily for 21 days and stopped for 7 days, during which time withdrawal uterine bleeding (menses) occurs. Through a combined negative feedback to the hypothalamus (and pituitary?), LH and FSH secretions are suppressed. There is an absence of an LH/FSH surge, and the failure of a follicular phase rise in FSH secretion results in lack of ovarian follicular development. Endogenous blood levels of E_2 remain low due to suppression of LH and FSH secretion.

Progestogens administered alone have complex effects that relate to the dosage. Besides suppression of gonadotropin secretion and inhibition of follicular development, cervical mucus composition is modified, which may prevent sperm entry into the uterine cavity. In addition, endometrial histology may be altered and thus interfere with implantation of the ovum should fertilization occur.

Some contraceptive steroid regimes consist of estrogens administered alone for a number of days (usually 15) followed by a progestogen for several days (usually 5). These *sequential contraceptive preparations* simulate to some degree the normal sequence of ovarian steroid secretion. A dose of a progestin, e.g. "Plan B" (Duramed Pharmaceuticals), has been used with success as a "morning-after pill," often as an emergency postcoital contraceptive [37, 53]. Silastic steroid-impregnated devices that provide a slow delivery of a steroid are available as contraceptive depot preparations. Even intrauterine devices (IUDs) impregnated with progestogens have been reported to provide significant contraceptive action.

Superactive agonist analogs of gonadotropin-releasing hormone (GnRH) have been developed for potential use in hypogonadal men and women. These stimulatory analogs have been discovered to exert paradoxical inhibitory effects on pituitary-gonadal function in both sexes, probably because they down-regulate pituitary responsiveness to GnRH

Ethinyl Estradiol

Norethindrone

Figure 19.10
Examples of structures of two common contraceptive steroids, an estrogen, ethinyl estradiol, and a progestogen, norethindrone.

Anti-hormone
RU 486

Figure 19.11 Structure of RU 486, a synthetic progesterone antagonist.

stimulation. Postovulatory administration of these stimulatory analogs may have a luteolytic effect in women. The effects of these GnRH analogs may be mediated at the level of the pituitary, to cause a down-regulation of GnRH receptors, and also at the level of the gonad through some unknown action. Antibodies to choriogonadotropin may provide a novel method of contraception.

Pregnancy Termination. Increased plasma progesterone concentrations are responsible for the lack of ovulation during pregnancy, presumably operating, via negative feedback, on the hypothalamus-pituitary LH-release system. This inhibitory effect of progesterone is the basis of current oral contraceptives, which contain a synthetic progesterone analog (a progestin). RU 486, a steroid with high affinity for the progesterone receptor, is the first available active antiprogesterone (Fig. 19.11). It has been used successfully as a medical alternative for early pregnancy interruption, and it also has other potential applications in medicine [2].

When progesterone enters the target cell, it binds to a nuclear protein receptor and, in the process, it changes the shape of the receptor and frees an associated heat shock protein (Chap. 3). This allows the receptor–hormone complex to bind to the hormone response elements on the DNA. That step, in turn, alters the DNA so that the genes controlled by progesterone can be transcribed. RU 486, like progesterone, binds to the receptor but does not

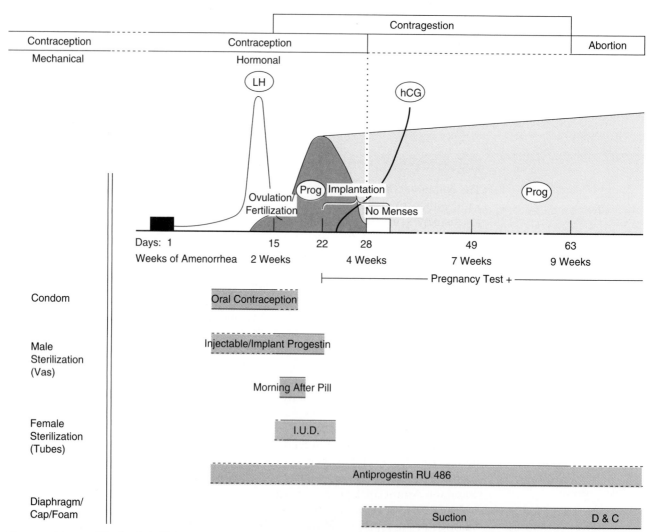

Figure 19.12 Methods of birth control. Techniques are shown in shaded bars. Solid lines indicate the times when a method is most efficient; for mechanical conception no time dependency is indicated. Dotted lines show when the method might also have some effect. LH = luteinizing hormone; hCG = human chorionic gonadotropin; prog = progesterone; IUD = intrauterine device; D & C = dilatation and curettage. (From Etienne-Emile Baulieu, with permission. "RU486: A Compound That Gets Itself talked About." *Human Reproduction,* vol. 9 (Suppl. 1), pp. 1–6, 1994.)

release the heat shock protein. Indeed, the heat shock protein may become even more tightly bound to the receptor. As a result, the receptor is unable to bind to the hormone-response elements, and no transcription of the DNA takes place. In addition, since RU 486 occupies the receptors, it prevents progesterone from binding to them, and therefore prevents any physiological events that depend on progesterone, such as the maintenance of pregnancy (Fig. 19.11) [2].

Birth control techniques range from methods preventing fertilization to the interruption of pregnancy at various stages. Figure 19.12 shows the overlapping categories of several methods (classified as contraception, contragestion, and abortion) and their periods of efficacy, measured from the last menses. Common terms can be ambiguous. Contraception is usually understood to mean preventing fertilization, but specialists also use it to mean the period of time lasting until implantation is complete. To some biologists and theologians, abortion might mean any maneuver after fertilization; to practitioners, it takes place only after implantation. Most birth control techniques can work in several ways. Even some oral contraceptives do not always block ovulation; for example, they can alter the endometrium and may prevent implantation, which is a postovulatory effect. The figure shows contragestion from day 15, when fertilization takes place, and it spans the time of other postovulatory methods.

Menopause

The onset of menopause results from a loss in the cyclic activity of the ovary, which is believed to be caused by a failure at the level of the ovary to respond to gonadotropins. It has been proposed that this is due to an exhaustion of the postmitotic pool of ovarian follicles that is established during embryonic development [17]. Others have argued, however, that reproductive senescence has a neuroendocrine basis in women [55, 56], as it clearly does in rats [55], whereby subtle changes in neural signals begin to occur in middle age that may precede and accelerate the loss of follicles, leading to menopause.

Fertility begins to decline about 10 years before the menopause, and by age 50, most primary follicles have been lost. There appears to be no relationship between the age of onset of menopause and the age of onset of menarche. Also, the number of children born or the age at the time of birth of the first child does not appear to be related to the age of menopause [27]. The nutritional status of the individual may, however, influence the onset of menopause. The age of menopause may have increased during the last century [12, 15] and may now average about 52 years, being lower in some less developed countries: 44 or younger in the Punjab, New Guinea, and Central Africa. It appears that the onset of menopause is getting later.

As women approach menopause, there may be a striking increase in serum FSH levels, relative to those of LH. Eventually, as estradiol secretion falls to low levels, both FSH and LH concentrations rise and remain elevated, apparently due to the removal of the negative steroid feedback mechanism characteristic of active ovarian function. The premenopausal rise in FSH secretion may relate to the progressive loss of inhibin, whose role is postulated to exert a negative feedback control of pituitary FSH secretion. Progressive loss of ovarian follicles and their maturation would be expected to reduce the production of inhibin.

Many studies in animals have shown how the declining activity of the ovary is the primary cause of a reduced fertility in older females. Rising hypothalamic thresholds to the feedback actions of steroids are also age-related in rats. Similar situations might arise in women at the onset of the menopause, but it is not easy to design studies to clarify this situation. One such analysis of hypothalamic GnRH function was conducted in 12 women of various ages between 27 and 64, who had been previously oophorectomized [1]. Oophorectomy had been done between 10 months and several years before the study, and none of the women had taken oral steroids or injected estrogens for 30 days or more before the onset of the analysis. Plasma samples were collected every 10 minutes between 08.00 and 13.00 hours for assays of PRL, E_2, FSH, and LH. Estradiol levels were low, and mean levels of gonadotropins, together with their pulse frequency and pulse amplitude, did not differ in two groups of women between 27 and 49 years of age and 52 and 64 years of age, respectively. The calculations were the same whether chronological age or age after menarche was used for comparisons and despite varying intervals after the oophorectomy was performed.

The pattern of GnRH release in the absence of gonadal feedback thus appears to be similar in the hypothalamus of young or aging women, and therefore the inherent hypothalamic GnRH pulse generating mechanism does not seem to be affected by age. It was concluded, therefore, that ovarian failure is the main consequence of reproductive aging in women [1], and that an acceleration of GnRH pulse generator activity and gonadotropin secretions occur secondarily to the loss of ovarian hormone feedback. There is, indeed, an increase in GnRH gene expression in the medial basal hypothalamus of postmenopausal women [38]. While this idea is generally accepted, there is nevertheless some evidence to suggest that hypothalamic GnRH pulse generation may undergo subtle changes prior to the menopause. Another study [22], for example, showed that in middle-aged, regularly menstruating women (presumably approaching menopause), the frequency of LH pulses is decreased. It therefore remains a possibility that an initial decline in GnRH pulsatility may precede the onset of menopause, and perhaps contribute to the irregularity of menstrual cycles that leads up to menopause [38].

In the absence of gonadal estrogens in the body during menopause, it is not unexpected that a number of physiological changes take place. The uterus, an estrogen-dependent organ, becomes smaller and the endometrium atrophic. Atrophic vaginitis as well as vaginal dryness may occur, but these changes can be reversed by exogenous estrogens applied locally or given systemically. There is an increased risk of coronary thrombosis in postmenopausal women, reaching a level of risk similar to that of men.

During the *climacterium*, that period preceding termination of the reproductive period, some women experience episodic sensations of menopausal "hot flashes" (menopausal flushes/flashes), usually involving the face and neck and upper part of the chest, which may be associated with profuse sweating. The subjective sensation of heat is associated with objective signs of cutaneous vasodilation and a consequent drop in core body temperature. Other symptoms may include flushing, palpitations, anxiety, and night sweats. Hot flashes occur in about two-thirds of postmenopausal women. They usually last about 4 minutes, and can occur several times a week or even many times per day [48]. It is likely that hot flashes are a result of the withdrawal of estrogen's effects on preoptic and hypothalamic thermoregulatory circuitries. However, their molecular and cellular basis are poorly understood. There have been some reports of a synchrony between these menopausal flushes and pulses of LH secretion, suggesting a common hypothalamic mechanism. Hormone replacement therapy (HRT; estrogen, or estrogen plus progesterone) is effective in reducing or preventing hot flashes. However, many women have been discouraged from using HRT following the Women's Health Initiative (WHI) clinical trials, which determined that HRT may increase the risk of breast cancer and cardiovascular complications (coronary heart disease, stroke, and venous thromboembolism) [41]. Since relief from hot flashes represents a major impetus for many women to use HRT, the search for viable non-steroidal substitute treatments are now of intense interest.

After the menopause, there is a reduction in the cortical thickness and the tensile strength of bones, resulting from an increase in loss of mineral content. *Postmenopausal osteoporosis* can be prevented by estrogen administration, but this depends on how soon after menopause estrogen replacement therapy begins [39, 40]. Estrogens prevent osteoporosis and its most serious medical consequence, hip fracture. Many epidemiological studies have also suggested that estrogens significantly lower the risk of cardiovascular disease and stroke [5, 47], although this belief was not supported by the findings of the WHI clinical trials, as noted above. However, the WHI studies were performed on women who were an average of 12 years postmenopausal, while most epidemiological studies have focused on women who begin HRT at menopause [28]. The beneficial effects of estrogen may thus be evident when HRT is started at menopausal onset, a possibility that will require further study [52, 54].

Unopposed long-term estrogen therapy increases the risk of developing endometrial hyperplasia, endometrial cancer, and possibly breast cancer as well [13, 41]. The risk of developing endometrial cancer has been reduced by combining a progestin with the estrogen. Although some progestins may reverse the cardioprotective effect of estrogens, those with minimal androgenicity appear less likely to do so. Hormone replacement therapy that combines estrogen with a progestin of minimal androgenicity is thus a rational alternative to unopposed estrogen therapy [13, 14, 19].

Menopause and Libido. Women appear to show a decline in libido after the menopause, but there is considerable debate whether such changes are intrinsic or due to influences of the sexual partner or society. Changes in the female reproductive tract such as reduction in the thickness of the vaginal epithelium and decreases in vaginal secretions due to reductions in estrogen secretion might also be expected to affect female sexual responses. Although there have been many clinical trials of postmenopausal estrogen replacement, very few studies have assessed sexual function objectively. Contradictory results exist in behavior studies that have been published. It has been reported that estrogen replacement enhanced libido, sexual activity, and orgasmic capacity but also that estrogen replacement did not change coital frequency, coital satisfaction, or frequency of masturbation. The data are even more difficult to interpret because it is not possible to determine whether the effects of estrogen replacement are being mediated at the level of the reproductive tract or the central nervous system.

Pathophysiology

Because of the complexity of the female reproductive system, the cyclic nature of ovarian hormone production and secretion, and the fact that the growth and development of a number of organs, in particular the uterus and mammary glands, are dependent on ovarian hormone secretion, it is not surprising that a large number of pathological states are attributable to endocrine dysfunctions. The pregnant state, dependent on a multitude of hormonal events unique to the female, is vulnerable to endocrine dysfunctions that can endanger the life of both the fetus and mother.

Hyperprolactinemia. The most common example of pituitary hypersecretion of a hormone involves PRL [4]. Not only does hyperprolactinemia lead to *galactorrhea* (excess milk production), but amenorrhea and anovulation are complicating sequelae of excessive PRL secretion. Breast engorgement due to excessive lactogenesis usually results from excessive PRL secretion from a pituitary adenoma (prolactinoma). The etiology of the prolactinoma is uncertain but could result from a failure of hypothalamic release of the PRL-inhibiting factor, dopamine, thus leading to lactotroph hyperplasia and eventual adenoma formation. The onset of galactorrhea may date to a normal postpartum lactation that fails to be discontinued (Chiari–Frommel syndrome).

Suckling of the breasts is the normal stimulus to PRL secretion. It appears that stimuli that increase afferent impulses in the neuroendocrine reflex pathway leading to PRL secretion, such as surgery, trauma, tight-fitting garments, or continued breast manipulation, may lead to galactorrhea (neurogenic galactorrhea-amenorrhea). The amenorrhea that accompanies the galactorrhea probably results from PRL inhibition of hypothalamic GnRH secretion and a subsequent block of the ovulatory surge of gonadotropins. In addition, elevated plasma PRL levels are directly inhibitory to ovarian estrogen production, which may also be, in part, responsible for the accompanying amenorrhea. Women with increased PRL levels and a resulting decreased estrogen production may experience bone demineralization and associated incidence of clinical bone fractures. Bromocriptine, a dopamine-receptor agonist, is effective in establishing normal estrogen levels and ovulatory menstrual cycles in most hyperprolactinemic women.

Hormones and Breast Cancer. The early observation that oophorectomy may effect a rapid remission of advanced breast cancer in some premenopausal women provided evidence that some human breast cancers may depend on sex steroids for their continued proliferation [6, 8, 46]. Hypophysectomy and adrenalectomy are a means of hormone deprivation through endocrine ablation, but unfortunately not all women respond favorably to such radical treatment. This is because only 50–60% of human breast cancers are hormone-dependent and therefore responsive to endocrine manipulation. Patients with hormone-dependent cancers, however, may be favorable candidates for endocrine therapy. It is important therefore to distinguish those women with such hormone-responsive cancers. It has been demonstrated that the quantitative determination of the estrogen-receptor (ER) content of an excised tumor specimen often provides useful information as to the best type of therapy for the patient with advanced breast cancer. Tumors that contain low or negligible amounts of ER rarely respond to endocrine ablation or other hormone therapy (e.g., antiestrogen administration), whereas patients with receptor-rich cancers often benefit from endocrine treatment. Tamoxifen, an antiestrogen in breast cancer cells, is prescribed for premenopausal women with ER-positive tumors. Aromatase inhibitors, which reduce estrogen synthesis, are often prescribed for post-menopausal women with ER-positive breast cancer.

Early onset, long-lasting, ovulatory cycle function seems to increase the risk of breast cancer [6, 25]. Several studies on a number of populations and different ethnic groups have shown that women who have had an early menarche are at a greater risk of developing breast cancer than those who have had a late menarche. There has been, and in some countries still is, a secular trend in an earlier age at menarche, being most evident in countries in which the age at menarche has been high. In these countries, also, the breast cancer risk has been relatively low and is now increasing. There is a reduction in the risk of breast cancer among premenopausal women who have lactated [32].

The response of some breast cancer patients to endocrine therapy is limited due to the development of hormone-independent tumors, secondary to the emergence of autonomous cell clones that achieve dominance in the tumor mass. The loss of hormone dependency could be due to mutated or truncated estrogen receptors that act constitutively, i.e., enhance transcriptional activity in the absence of the hormone. Somatically generated mutations in the estrogen receptor have, indeed, been found at the mRNA/cDNA level in human breast cancer biopsies and in established breast cancer cell lines.

It has been reported that a physiological way to reduce breast cancer risk might exist. Subjects who had participated in organized athletic activity while in college had a lower lifetime occurrence rate of breast cancer than their nonathletic classmates. It was suggested that this might be dependent on endocrine mechanisms. The athletes in all age groups had a later age of menarche than the reference nonathlete group in this study. In a number of studies, it has been shown that strenuous physical activity may lead to extensive delay in the onset of menarche.

Cigarette smoking is associated with several diseases of major importance in women. Notably, smokers appear to have an increased risk of cardiovascular disease and osteoporosis and a decreased risk of breast and endometrial cancer. Hormonal mechanisms, particularly an antiestrogenic effect of smoking in women, have been postulated as mediators of these differences in risk. This hypothesis is supported by the observation in several studies that cigarette smoking is also associated with changes in fertility and earlier menopause. In one study, cigarette smokers had significantly higher mean plasma levels of the adrenal androgens dehydroepiandrosterone sulfate and androstenedione than nonsmokers. These results suggest that the possible decreased risk of breast and endometrial cancer associated with cigarette smoking may not be mediated solely through lower levels of endogenous estrogen, at least in postmenopausal women, and they raise questions about the role of androgens in disease mechanisms in older populations. The higher levels of adrenal androgens and their consistent relation to smoking in both men and women suggested that more attention should be focused on the role of the androgens, or at least of the androgen–estrogen balance, in older populations [16].

REVIEW EXERCISES

Match the terms with their description:

1. Zygote   **A.** Unfertilized egg
2. Morula   **B.** A hollow sphere of cells
3. Blastocyst   **C.** An embryo
4. Ovum   **D.** Compact mass of cells
5. Neonate   **E.** The cell that results from fertilization
6. Fetus   **F.** Newly born offspring

Think, analyze and discuss:

1. Different reptiles display all three modes of embryonic development. What factors might have favored the evolution of viviparity from ovoviviparity in certain species?

2. Synthetic estrogens used in contraceptives, like ethinyl estradiol, are excreted intact in the urine. What effects might this source of estrogen have on wildlife?
3. Most home pregnancy tests indicate the presence or absence of hCG in a woman's urine.
   a. Why is this an accurate indicator of pregnancy?
   b. What is the function of hCG?
   c. Would a pregnancy test that is based on the detection of hCG be useful within the first week following fertilization? Why or why not? Would it still be likely to indicate the presence of hCG during the third trimester of pregnancy? Why or why not?
   d. hCG is often used in hormone regimens that are designed to induce ovulation. Why would hCG be effective in this regard? How does it work?

4. The cessation of menstrual cycles during lactation, called lactational amenorrhea, has been referred to as "nature's own contraception." Provide an hypothesis as to the possible mechanisms that mediate the inhibitory effects of nursing on menstrual cyclicity. Design an experiment that could be used to test your hypothesis in experimental animals.

5. Predict the pattern of prolactin secretion that would most likely be evident in the serum of a women throughout the third trimester of pregnancy. What is the endocrine stimulus for this pattern? Make the same prediction for a woman who nurses her baby, and for a woman who does not. Provide a mechanistic explanation for the likely difference in prolactin levels between these two women.

6. Approximately 20% of all deliveries are preceded by some form of labor induction, usually given to women who experience prolonged pregnancy or hypertensive disorders. Pitocin and other oxytocic compounds are commonly used at term to induce or strengthen uterine contractions. How do these drugs work? If oxytocin were given prior to term, would it be expected to produce as pronounced effects on labor? Why or why not?

7. Pulsatile GnRH therapy can be used to treat women who present with hypothalamic hypogonadotropic hypogonadism. Potent GnRH analogs, however, are used to treat children for certain types of precocious puberty, in which secretions of pituitary gonadotropins are prematurely elevated. Why is it that GnRH and GnRH agonists can be used to raise gonadotropins in one case, and to depress gonadotropins in another? Provide a mechanistic explanation for this apparent paradox.

8. As a woman enters the perimenopausal period, hormone levels are altered as the ovaries are depleted of viable follicles. Which hormone would be measured as the earliest indicator that a woman is entering menopause? Provide an explanation for your answer.

9. Aromatase inhibitors are often prescribed for postmenopausal women to treat ER-positive breast cancer. Why are these compounds less likely to be prescribed for ER-positive breast cancer patients who are premenopausal, and have normal menstrual cycles?

References

[1] Alexander, S. E., et al. 1990. The effect of aging on hypothalamic function in oophorectomized women. *Am. J. Obstet. Gynecol.* 162:446–9.

[2] Baulieu, E.-E. 1989. Contragestion and other clinical applications of RU486, an antiprogesteron at the receptor. *Science* 245:1351–7.

[3] Challis, J. R. G., et al. 2000. Endocrine and paracrine regulation of birth at term and preterm. *Endocr. Rev.* 21:514–50.

[4] Davis, J. R. 2004. Prolactin and reproductive medicine. *Curr. Opin. Obstet. Gynecol.* 16(4):331–7.

[5] Ettinger, B. 1998. Overview of estrogen replacement therapy: A historical perspective. *Proc. Soc. Exp. Biol. Med.* 217:2–5.

[6] Feigelson, H. S., and Henderson, B. E. 2000. Future possibilities in the prevention of breast cancer: Role of genetic variation in breast cancer prevention. *Breast Cancer Res.* 2(4):277–82.

[7] Fevold, H., F. L. Hisaw, and R. K. Meyer. 1930. The relaxative hormone of the corpus luteum. Its purification and concentration. *J. Am. Chem. Soc.* 52:3340–8.

[8] Gadducci, A., et al. 2005. Breast cancer and sex steroids: Critical review of epidemiological, experimental and clinical investigations on etiopathogenesis, chemoprevention and endocrine treatment of breast cancer. *Gynecol. Endocrinol.* 20(6):343–60.

[9] Garfield, R. E., S. Sims, and E. E. Daniel. 1977. Gap junctions: Their presence and necessity in myometrium during parturition. *Science* 198:958–9.

[10] Gershengorn, M. C., B. E. Marcus-Samuels, and E. Geras. 1979. Estrogens increase the number of thyrotropin-releasing hormone receptors on mammotropic cells in culture. *Endocrinology* 105:171–6.

[11] Goffin, V., et al. 2002. Prolactin: The new biology of an old hormone. *Annu. Rev. Physiol.* 64:47–67.

[12] Greendale, G. A., and M. Sowers. 1997. The menopause transition. *Endocrinol. Metab. Clin. North Am.* 26:261–75.

[13] Grodstein, F., et al. 1996. Postmenopausal estrogen and progestin use and the risk of cardiovascular disease. *N. Engl. J. Med.* 335:453–61.

[14] Grodstein, F., et al. 1997. Postmenopausal hormone therapy and mortality. *N. Engl. J. Med.* 336:1769–75.

[15] Hill, K. 1996. The demography of menopause. *Maturitas* 23:113–27.

[16] Khaw, K. T., S. Tazuke, and E. Barrett-Connor. 1988. Cigarette smoking levels of adrenal androgens in postmenopausal women. *N. Engl. J. Med.* 318:1705–9.

[17] Knobil, E., and S. S. Yen. 1996. The advent of menopause. *Science* 274:18–20.

[18] Koldovsky, O., and W. Thornburg. 1987. Hormones in milk. *J. Pediatr. Gastroenter. Nutr.* 6:172–96.

[19] Linsay, R., et al. 1996. Estrogen replacement in menopause. *J. Clin. Endocrinol. Metab.* 81:3829–38.

[20] Linzer, D. I., and S. J. Fisher. 1999. The placenta and the prolactin family of hormones: Regulation of the physiology of pregnancy. *Mol. Endocrinol.* 13(6):837–40.

[21] Marshall, J. M. 1981. Effects of ovarian steroids and pregnancy of adrenergic nerves of uterus and oviduct. *Am. J. Physiol.* 240:C165–74.

[22] Matt, D. W., et al. 1998. Characteristics of luteinizing hormone secretion in younger versus older premenopausal women. *Am. J. Obstet. Gynecol.* 178:504–10.

[23] McFarland, K. C., et al. 1989. Lutropin-choriogonadotropin receptor: An unusual member of the G protein-coupled receptor family. *Science* 245:494–9.

[24] McNeilly, A. S. 2001. Lactational control of reproduction. *Reprod. Fertil. Dev.* 13(7–8):583–90.

[25] Melbye, M., et al. 1997. Induced abortion and the risk of breast cancer. *N. Engl. J. Med.* 336:81–5.

[26] Menon, K. M., et al. 2004. Regulation of luteinizing hormone/human chorionic gonadotropin receptor expression: a perspective. *Biol. Reprod.* 70(4):861–6.

[27] Merzenich, H., H. Boeing, and J. Wahrendorf. 1993. Dietary fat and sports activity as determinants for age at menarche. *Am. J. Epidemiol.* 138:217–24.

[28] Mitchell, S., et al. 2005. Is the estrogen controversy over? Deconstructing the Women's Health Initiative Study: A critical evaluation of the evidence. *Ann. N.Y. Acad. Sci.* 1052:43–56.

[29] Murata, T., et al. 2000. Oxytocin receptor gene expression in rat uterus: Regulation by ovarian steroids. *J. Endocrinol.* 166(1):45–52.

[30] Nathanielsz, P. W. 1996. The timing of birth. *Am. Sci.* 84:562–69.

[31] Neville, M. C., T. B. McFadden, and I. Forsyth. 2002. Hormonal regulation of mammary differentiation and milk secretion. *J. Mammary Gland Biol. Neoplasia* 7(1):49–66.

[32] Newcomb, P. A., et al. 1994. Lactation and a reduced risk of premenopausal breast cancer. *N. Engl. J. Med.* 330:81–7.

[33] Nikitovitch-Winer, M. B., and J. W. Everett. 1959. Histologic changes in grafts of rat pituitary on the kidney and upon retransplantation under the diencephalon. *Endocrinology* 65:357.

[34] O'Connor, J. F., et al. 1994. Recent advances in the chemistry and immunochemistry of human chorionic gonadotropin: Impact on clinical measurements. *Endocr. Rev.* 15:650–83.

[35] Ormandy, C. J., and R. S. Sutherland. 1993. Mechanisms of prolactin receptor regulation in mammary gland. *Mol. Cell. Endocrinol.* 9:C1–6.

[36] Pepe, G. J., and E. D. Albrecht. 1995. Actions of placental and fetal adrenal steroid hormones in primate pregnancy. *Endocr. Rev.* 16:608–48.

[37] Practice Committee, American Society for Reproductive Medicine. 2004. Hormonal contraception: Recent advances and controversies. *Fertil. Steril.* 82(2):520–6.

[38] Rance, N. E., and S. V. Uswandi. 1996. Gonadotropin-releasing hormone gene expression is increased in the medial basal hypothalamus of postmenopausal women. *J. Clin. Endocrinol. Metab.* 81:3540–6.

[39] Reid, I. R. 1997. The role of calcium in the prevention and treatment of osteoporosis. *The Endocrinologist* 7:294–9.

[40] Rosen, C. J., and C. R. Kiessenich. 1997. The pathophysiology and treatment of postmenopausal osteoporosis. *Endocrinol. Metab. Clin. North Am.* 26:295–311.

[41] Rossouw, J. E., et al. 2002. Writing Group for the Women's Health Initiative Investigators. Risks and benefits of estrogen plus progestin in healthy postmenopausal women: Principal results From the Women's Health Initiative randomized controlled trial. *JAMA* 288(3):321–33.

[42] Sherwood, O. D. 2004. Relaxin's physiological roles and other diverse actions. *Endocr. Rev.* 25(2):205–34.

[43] Sherwood, O. D. 1994. Relaxin. In: E. Seid, E. Knobil, and J. Neill, eds. *The physiology of reproduction,* vol. 1. New York: Raven Press, pp. 861–1009.

[44] Sherwood, O. D., et al. 1980. Radioimmunoassay of relaxin throughout pregnancy and during parturition in the rat. *Endocrinology* 107:691–8.

[45] Short, R. V. 1993. Lactational infertility in family planning. *Ann. Med.* 25(2):175–80.

[46] Simpson, E. R., et al. 2005. Estrogen—the good, the bad, and the unexpected. *Endocr. Rev.* 26(3):322–30.

[47] Skafar, D. F., et al. 1997. Female sex hormones and cardiovascular disease in women. *J. Clin. Endocrinol. Metab.* 82:3913–18.

[48] Stearns, V. 2002. Hot flushes. *The Lancet* 360:1851–61.

[49] Stefaneanu, L., et al. 1992. Pituitary lactotrophs and somatotrophs in pregnancy: A correlative in situ hybridization and immunocytochemical study. *Virchows Archiv. B Cell Pathol.* 62:291–6.

[50] Snell, W. J., and J. M. White. 1996. The molecules of mammalian fertilization. *Cell* 85:629–37.

[51] Thorburn, G. D., S. A. Hollingworth, and S. B. Hooper. 1991. The trigger for parturition in sheep: Fetal hypothalamus or placenta? *J. Dev. Physiol.* 15:71–9.

[52] Turgeon, J. L., et al. 2004. Hormone therapy: Physiological complexity belies therapeutic simplicity. *Science* 304:1269–73.

[53] Van Look, P. F. A., and H. von Hertzen. 1993. Emergency contraception. *Br. Med. Bull.* 49:158–70.

[54] Wickelgren, I. 1997. Estrogen stakes claim to cognition. *Science* 276:675–8.

[55] Wise, P., et al. 2002. Neuroendocrine modulation and repercussions of female reproductive aging. *Recent Prog. Horm. Res.* 57:235–56.

[56] Wise, P., et al. 1996. Menopause: The aging of multiple pacemakers. *Science* 273:67–70.

[57] Wood, C. E. 2005. Estrogen/hypothalamus-pituitary-adrenal axis interactions in the fetus: The interplay between placenta and fetal brain. *J. Soc. Gynecol. Investig.* 12(2):67–76.

CHAPTER 20

Endocrine Role of the Pineal Gland

Once described as an obscure and vestigial organ, the pineal gland is now believed to influence many physiological processes. Its primary role is to transduce the sensory information associated with the presence of light or dark into an endocrine signal of darkness. The functional significance of this signal varies with the life history of each species. It was originally believed that the pineal secretes a hormone that has antigonadotropic properties; however, a vast amount of experimental data implicates melatonin, an indoleamine, as a pineal hormone that can regulate many physiological functions. In addition to having both inhibitory and stimulatory affects on reproduction, melatonin influences immune function, metabolism, and facilitates the entrainment of circadian rhythms [2, 37, 55]. Clinical evidence reveals that children with parenchymal pinealomas may be delayed in their sexual development, whereas destructive (nonparenchymal) pinealomas are often associated with precocious puberty [16]. However, the detailed mechanisms by which the pineal affects many physiological and behavioral processes are unclear. Circulating melatonin levels are elevated at night in essentially all vertebrates as a result of increased synthesis and release from the pineal gland. This increase serves as the "hormonal signal of night" and is used to coordinate daily and seasonal rhythms with the day/night cycle. The melatonin signal therefore is essential for survival in many seasonally breeding animals.

This chapter summarizes the vast but sometimes conflicting literature on the role of the pineal in mammalian reproductive physiology and biological rhythmicity. In addition, the pineal as an endocrine organ controlling other physiological processes is discussed. A number of monographs are available that provide further information on the anatomy, biochemistry, and physiology of this intriguing endocrine organ and its hormone, melatonin [16, 40, 50, 52].

Pineal Development and Morphology

The human pineal gland arises as a median evagination of the diencephalic roof of the embryonic brain. In most mammals, the pineal gland moves away from the roof of the third ventricle and loses connection with the brain, except for a thin stalk. The adult human pineal (epiphysis) is a pine-cone-shaped organ, a shape that suggested the organ's name (Fig. 20.1). The pineal is innervated by postganglionic fibers originating from the *superior cervical ganglia*; the pineal is therefore an effector organ of the autonomic nervous system [55]. The pineal parenchymal cells, pinealocytes, are derived from the ependymal lining of the epithalamus; both light and dark parenchymal cells can be distinguished in the mammalian pineal. The dark cells contain pigment granules of an unknown nature, as well as glycogen deposits of undefined physiological significance. Since distinction is based only on a difference in electron density of the cytoplasm, the "light" and "dark" pinealocytes may only reflect differences in the functional stage of the same cell type that may be manifested as a differential

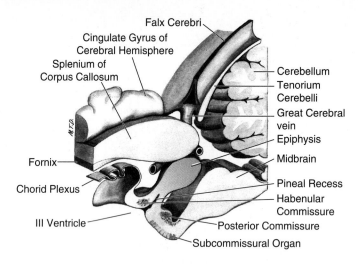

Figure 20.1 The human pineal gland (epiphysis) and its anatomical relation to the diencephalic roof. (From Wurtman, Axelrod, and Kelly, 1966. Evidence for a nonretinal pathway of light in the pineal gland of newborn rats. *Proc. Natl. Acad. Sci. USA* 56:515–20, with permission).

susceptibility to the fixative. Fibroblasts and glial cells make up the rest of the glandular mass, which, in humans, is about 170 to 175 mg in average weight. Calcification of the human pineal begins during the second decade of life, and by 60 years, 70% of all pineal glands may be at least partly calcified. Nevertheless, there is no evidence that calcification signals a loss of function; on the contrary, biochemical studies indicate no change in biochemical activity of the pineal with age.

The Melatonin Hypothesis

Early anatomists held various views on the physiological function of the pineal in the human. This unique unpaired structure that lies deeply recessed under the cerebral hemispheres of the brain drew their attention and speculation. The philosopher Descartes considered it as the "seat of the soul."

Early Observations Suggested that the Pineal can Influence Reproductive Function

The possible physiological significance of the pineal was first recognized by Heubner who noted precocious sexual maturity in a young boy whose pineal was destroyed by a tumor. Holmgren noted that the cells of the pineal gland of an elasmobranch were sensory-like in nature: the pinealocytes resembled the sensory cells of the retina. Because some reptiles possess a prominent "third eye," the pineal of mammals, including humans, was considered a vestige of this primitive visual organ. The observation that the human pineal may become calcified at an early age further consolidated thought that the pineal, indeed, was a vestigial organ and therefore of little physiological consequence. A monograph by Kitay and Altschule [21] described, however, some remarkable clinical correlations with pineal dysfunction. The evidence clearly revealed that the pineal might in some way be related to reproductive function in humans.

McCord and Allen made the interesting observation that bovine pineal extracts added to the water in which tadpoles swam caused the larvae to blanch, that is, to become very light in color or even transparent [28]. This interesting pigmentary effect was duly appreciated by the dermatologist Aaron Lerner, who was searching for a factor that might be responsible for vitiligo (white patches of skin) in humans. He was able to isolate and determine the structure of a pineal substance, an indoleamine, which he named melatonin. This was a momentous event in the history of pineal research as this unique molecule of pineal origin could now be readily synthesized and made available for a variety of physiological studies. Melatonin, *N*-acetyl-5-methoxytryptamine (Fig. 20.2), proved to have potent effects on integumental pigmentation in some animals, but not humans, as will be discussed. Most important, however, this indoleamine was shown to have antigonadal effects on the mammalian reproductive system.

Profound changes in gonadal function are observed in many animals when they are exposed to continuous light or darkness. Maturation of the gonads of rodents, for example, is delayed when these animals are maintained under conditions of continuous darkness. This

Figure 20.2   The structure of melatonin (*N*-acetyl-5-methoxytryptamine).

effect can be prevented by pinealectomy (epiphysectomy). In contrast, continuous light leads to the early onset of sexual development and to a more rapid increase in gonadal weight; constant light also causes a reduction in size and function of the pineal gland. Pineal ablation in young rodents usually leads to accelerated gonadal maturation, and these developmental effects can be reduced by injections of pineal extracts. Melatonin, like pineal extracts, administered to young rodents also results in a delay of gonadal maturation. These observations are consistent with a hypothesis that photic cues received by an animal in some way affect pineal release of melatonin, which then exerts modulatory effects on reproductive hormone secretions. The "melatonin hypothesis" thus emerged.

While melatonin was originally regarded as an antigonadotropic hormone, it is now known that melatonin can have both stimulatory and inhibitory effects on the reproductive axis, as well as at other target organs, depending upon the physiological and species-specific *context* in which it is released, and the *pattern* of release that occurs under those circumstances. For example, the short duration of nocturnal melatonin secretion that occurs in the summer months stimulates the hamster reproductive axis, but inhibits the sheep reproductive axis. By contrast, the long duration of nocturnal melatonin secretion that occurs in the winter months produces the reverse effects—reproductive inhibition in the hamster and stimulation in the sheep. These opposite responses to melatonin reflect specific adaptations of these seasonally breeding animals to accommodate their differing gestational periods, ensuring that young in both cases are delivered during an environmentally hospitable time of year.

Studies in Hamsters have Provided Important Information on Pineal Function

From studies on the Syrian or Golden hamster (*Mesocricetus auratus*) and Siberian hamster (*Phodopus sungorus*) the role of the pineal in mammalian reproductive processes has been further elucidated. Changes in length of the daily photoperiod are especially important in controlling gonadal activity in the hamster, which in their natural habitats breed seasonally and undergo seasonal changes in metabolism and other physiological functions. The Golden hamster hibernates; the Siberian hamster remains active all year around, but exhibits periods of daily torpor when photoperiods are short. The reproductive organs of the hamster are extremely sensitive to the influence of environmental lighting and to the activity of the pineal gland. In the male, short photoperiods or blinding lead to gonadal atrophy with complete loss of testicular spermatogenic activity. The gonads may be reduced to only 20% of their normal size. The accessory organs (seminal vesicles and coagulating glands) also atrophy, indicating a loss of support by gonadal androgens. These atrophic effects result from decreased secretion of follicle-stimulating hormone (FSH) and luteinizing hormone (LH) from the pituitary. Pinealectomy prevents gonadal regression in hamsters maintained on nonstimulatory short days. In the female, the data are less clear, but there is a decrease in uterine weight, apparently due to decreased estrogen production in response to short photoperiods or blinding. Plasma gonadotropin levels of female golden hamsters on short days are decreased relative to that of females exposed to long days.

There is a daily rhythm of pineal melatonin synthesis in the hamster, a rhythm influenced by environmental lighting. Superior cervical ganglionectomy, however, abolishes the rhythm of pineal melatonin production. The mechanism by which melatonin influences physiological function has been partially elucidated through some ingenious experiments which used testicular gonadotropin secretion as an endpoint. There appear to be both a short day-induced alteration in the neural drive on gonadotropin secretion and an increase in the sensitivity of the hypothalamopituitary axis to the negative feedback effect of steroid hormones. These effects are referred to as the steroid-independent and steroid-dependent effects of photoperiod. On short days, castrated male hamsters are much more sensitive to the negative feedback effects of exogenous testosterone than are animals exposed to long days. This increased sensitivity is blocked or reduced by pinealectomy. Thus, the short-day-induced increase in sensitivity of the hamster hypothalamo-hypophysial axis to testosterone feedback is mediated, at least in part, by the pineal gland.

In photoperiodic species, i.e., species in which the annual cycle is driven by changes in day length, there is a spontaneous recrudescence of the gonads to the normal adult condition in hamsters that have been exposed to the inhibitory photoperiod for about 27 weeks. These animals have become photorefractory or insensitive to the effects of the inhibitory photoperiod. This could help explain what normally happens under hibernating conditions. Hamsters are reproductively competent when they emerge from their burrows in the spring. The spontaneous onset of the gonadal refractory condition appears to be a single occurrence, not a cyclical phenomenon, as the animals must be exposed to a stimulatory photoperiod for several weeks to break the photorefractory condition and permit additional responses to the inhibitory conditions. Failure to break the refractory state results in the maintenance of the recrudesced gonads indefinitely. In other species (ewe, starling), however, there is evidence for both a spontaneous onset and termination of reproductive activity that occurs cyclically with a period of about a year (i.e., circannually). These animals are thought to possess a circannual clock that may be entrained by melatonin or other factors.

It is unclear why the gonads of blinded or hibernating hamsters spontaneously become activated. The hypothalamo-hypophysial-gonadal axis may become refractory to the pineal antigonadotropic hormone. It has been shown that exogenous melatonin injections cause testicular regression in pinealectomized hamsters regardless of the photoperiod. Injections of melatonin during the early part of the day, however, are often ineffective in causing gonadal atrophy in intact hamsters. Also, in the presence of continuously elevated levels of melatonin (in animals carrying implants of melatonin), pinealectomized animals are rendered insensitive to daily injections of the hormone. Thus, the continuous exposure to melatonin renders the target tissue relatively unresponsive to this hormone. It may therefore be important that melatonin be released rhythmically from the pineal, rather than continuously, to be physiologically effective.

These observations leave little doubt that the pineal, through the action of its antigonadotropic hormone melatonin, is a key component in the control of reproductive processes in this mammal (Fig. 20.3). There is evidence that the pineal functions in a similar role in some other mammals and some nonmammalian species.

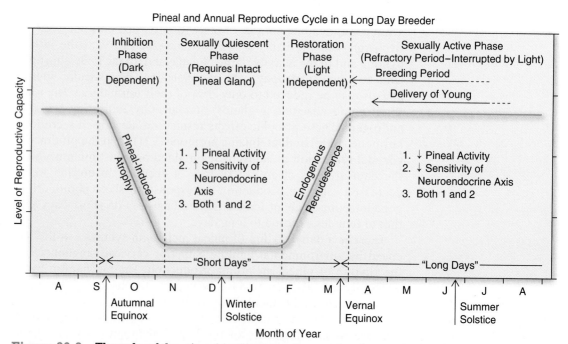

Figure 20.3 The role of the pineal in the annual reproduction cycle of a long-day breeder, the hamster. (From Reiter, R. 1978. *Progress in Reproductive Biology* 4:169–90, with permission).

Pineal Indoleamine Biosynthesis

The biochemistry of pineal indoleamine biosynthesis is well documented [22, 49, 55]. Indoleamine biosynthesis involves use of the amino acid tryptophan, which is converted to 5-hydroxytryptophan by the enzyme tryptophan hydroxylase (Fig. 20.4). The enzyme 5-hydroxytryptophan decarboxylase acts on 5-hydroxytryptophan to form 5-hydroxytryptamine (5-HT, *serotonin*), which is converted to *N*-acetylserotonin by the action of *N*-acetyltransferase. The *N*-acetylserotonin produced is *O*-methylated by hydroxyindole-*O*-methyltransferase (HIOMT) to form *N*-acetyl-5-methoxytryptamine (melatonin). It is believed that the increase in *N*-acetylserotonin concentration acts by a mass action effect to enhance the production of melatonin. Pineal melatonin biosynthesis is mainly controlled by *N*-acetyltransferase activity, which may be the rate-limiting event in the production of this indoleamine. Others argue, however, that HIOMT activity may be of prime importance to melatonin biosynthesis. Melatonin is then metabolized in the liver to 6-hydroxymelatonin by melatonin hydroxylase and converted to a sulfate or to a glucuronide for urinary excretion.

Although acetylation to *N*-acetylserotonin is a necessary step in the biosynthesis of melatonin, deamination of serotonin by monoamine oxidase can also occur in the pineal. The deaminated product may be either oxidized to 5-hydroxyindoleacetic acid or reduced to 5-hydroxytryptophol. The latter compounds then can become *O*-methylated by HIOMT to give 5-methoxyindole acetic acid and 5-methoxytryptophol.

The Rhythm of Melatonin Production is Affected by Light

The production of melatonin is under the control of the circadian system; however, the locus of the control varies among species. In mammals, output from the suprachiasmatic nucleus provides the circadian timing signals, but in some species of birds and many other species the pineal gland itself contains a circadian clock capable of generating a rhythm of melatonin. Melatonin synthesis within the rat pineal is dramatically affected by photic cues received by the eyes. At night there is an increase in the activity of *N*-acetyltransferase, which is 10- to nearly 100-fold greater than values in the light. The concentration of *N*-acetylserotonin is subsequently increased to values 10 to 30 times greater than those observed under day conditions. HIOMT activity is also increased, which results in elevated levels of pineal melatonin. Pineal enzyme activities are rapidly depressed by light. Pineal serotonin levels reveal marked diurnal changes, with highest levels noted during the daylight hours. Serotonin levels are depressed after darkness, probably because serotonin is the substrate for *N*-acetyltransferase action and is therefore converted to *N*-acetylserotonin. Reversal of external lighting conditions reverses the rhythm of pineal enzyme activity and indoleamine biosynthesis. Thus, a daily diurnal rhythm of pineal biosynthetic activity is observed and is controlled by the normal day-to-day changes in natural lighting. This diurnal fluctuation of pineal enzyme activity and melatonin synthesis is lost under conditions of continuous illumination. The rhythm is maintained, however, though diminished, in animals kept in the dark. A central nervous system (CNS) site is thus responsible for producing a cyclic signal that is responsible

Figure 20.4 Pathway of melatonin biosynthesis and metabolism within the pineal gland.

Figure 20.5 Pathway for serotonin conversion to melatonin in the pineal gland. Daily measurements over a 24-hour period of serotonin content, *N*-acetyltransferase activity (NAT), hydroxyindole-*O*-methyltransferase activity (HIOMT), and melatonin content in chick pineals were made. The bar at the top of the graph represents the 24-hour lighting regimen in which the birds were held (L:D 12:12 hours of light in alternation with 12 hours of dark). The daily change in melatonin is believed to be a consequence of the daily change in NAT. The numbers (x-fold) on the graph are the ratio of peak to nadir values. (From Binkley, S. A. 1979. Pineal rhythms in vivo and in vitro. *Comp. Biochem. Physiol.* 64A:201–6, with permission.)

for the persistence of pineal rhythmicity. The daily rhythm of pineal indoleamine biosynthesis in the bird is depicted in Figure 20.5 and has also been carefully documented in the rat.

The Suprachiasmatic Nucleus Controls Pineal Melatonin Release through a Multi-Synaptic Pathway

The role of the CNS in the control of pineal indoleamine biosynthesis in mammals has been determined by a variety of surgical techniques. Melatonin is synthesized in response to norepinephrine released from postganglionic neurons from the superior cervical ganglia. Thus the pineal gland is considered to be a *neuroendocrine transducer*, like the adrenal chromaffin tissue, as neural input to these organs is converted into an endocrine output [56]. Postganglionic stimulation of pinealocytes depends on the absence of light activation of the retina of the eyes. The pineal gland, in essence, is the intermediary between the external photoperiod and internal milieu. The pineal gland is the site at which information about light and dark is translated, or transduced, into a chemical messenger [37]. There is also a suggestion that pineal melatonin biosynthesis may be affected by the electromagnetic spectrum [40].

Light information is registered by melanopsin-containing photoreceptors in the ganglion cell layer of the retina [52, 53]. From there it is conveyed to the suprachiasmatic nuclei (SCN) of the brain by way of a retinohypothalamic pathway [30]. While the visual pathways convey signals related to image formation and processing, the retinohypothalamic pathway is a separate system concerned with transmitting information about the presence and intensity of light [52, 53]. Neuronal circuits from the suprachiasmatic nuclei convey information via the medial forebrain bundle to the upper thoracic spinal cord and then out to the superior cervical ganglia. From these ganglia, the postganglionic neurons proceed to innervate the pineal. Disruption of this neural pathway anywhere between the lateral eyes and the suprachiasmatic nuclei stimulates pineal indoleamine biosynthesis. Removal of the superior cervical ganglia (ganglionectomy) or decentralization of the ganglia, on the other hand,

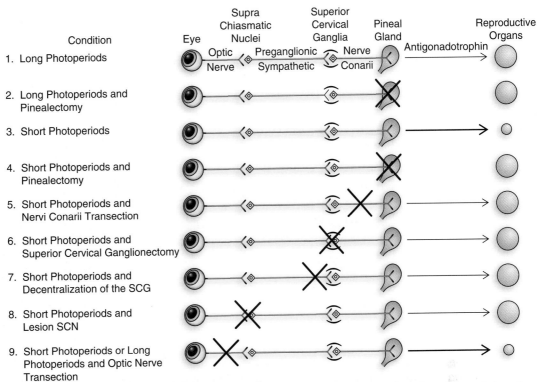

Condition	Eye	Supra Chiasmatic Nuclei	Superior Cervical Ganglia	Pineal Gland	Reproductive Organs

Figure 20.6 Surgical procedures that eliminate or exaggerate pineal antigonadotropic activity in mammals. The X's represent removal of the organ or surgical transection of a fiber tract. The thickness of the arrows indicates the antigonadotropic capability of the pineal gland. The phrase preganglionic sympathetic fibers refers to a multitude of neurons that intervene between the suprachiasmatic nuclei (SCN) and the superior cervical ganglia (SCG). Decentralization of the SCG refers to separating the SCG from their connections with the central nervous system. (From Reiter, J. 1978 *Recent Progress in Reproductive Biology* 4:169–90, with permission.)

abolishes the rhythms of indoleamine biosynthesis. Lesions of the medial forebrain bundle also block pineal *N*-acetyltransferase rhythms, as do lesions of the suprachiasmatic nuclei. A summary of the surgical procedures is provided (Fig. 20.6). These data suggest that the suprachiasmatic nuclei is the CNS site responsible for generation of the nocturnal activity of pineal indoleamine biosynthesis in mammals. The circadian oscillatory activity of the cells of the suprachiasmatic nuclei may be entrained to the daily photoperiod.

Norepinephrine Regulates Melatonin Biosynthesis via β₁-Adrenergic Receptors

Norepinephrine released from superior cervical postganglionic neurons interacts with pinealocyte β₁-adrenoceptors, which leads to an increase in pineal cAMP production [44]. Elevation of this intracellular second messenger results in conversion of tryptophan to serotonin and then serotonin to *N*-acetylserotonin. This response is mimicked by (Bu)₂cAMP or theophylline, a phosphodiesterase inhibitor, which elevates pineal cAMP levels. Norepinephrine, but not (Bu)₂cAMP, increases uptake of tryptophan into pinealocytes. The neurotransmitter therefore has a twofold effect: it increases intracellular levels of the substrate, tryptophan, as well as cAMP, whose action is to enhance enzymatic utilization of the substrate for melatonin biosynthesis. Injection of propranolol, a β-adrenoceptor antagonist, just before the onset of darkness, inhibits the nighttime rise in pineal *N*-acetyltransferase activity, as does reserpine, a drug that depletes adrenergic neurons of catecholamines. A single dose of isoproterenol, a β-adrenoceptor agonist, administered during the day causes an immediate increase in pineal *N*-acetyltransferase activity. Electrical stimulation of the superior cervical ganglia causes a rapid increase in the concentration of cAMP in the pineal gland of rats. These experimental manipulations clearly reveal the role of noradrenergic postganglionic neurons in the control of pineal biosynthetic activity. A summary depicting the CNS pathways and mechanisms controlling pineal function is given (Fig. 20.7).

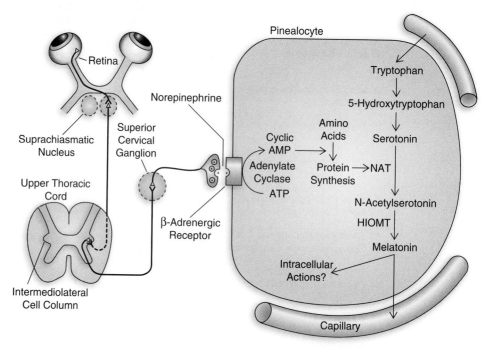

Figure 20.7 CNS pathway and mechanisms controlling pineal indole metabolism in mammals. (From Karasak and Reiter, "Morpho-functional aspects of the mammalian pineal gland." *Microscopy Res. Tech.* 21:136–57. ©1992 John Wiley & Sons, Inc. Used by permission of Wiley-Liss, Inc., a subsidiary of John Wiley & Sons, Inc.)

Melatonin Secretion and Circulation

Melatonin is present in the plasma and urine of all animals studied, including humans, and pinealectomy reduces the circulating levels of the indoleamine in experimental animals. As for pineal melatonin, plasma levels of melatonin of humans and other animals (sheep, pig, rat, cow, donkey, camel, chicken, salmon, lizard) are highest at middark and lowest at midlight periods (Fig. 20.8). In addition to the daily melatonin rhythm in blood and urine of primates, there is a diurnal melatonin rhythm in primate cerebrospinal fluid (CSF). Night peak values are 2 to 15 times higher than day values. This increase occurs soon after lights are turned off, and the decrease toward day values occurs rapidly after lights are turned on again (Fig. 20.9). The changes in CSF melatonin concentrations appear to reflect daily changes in plasma melatonin concentrations. It is not clear, however, whether melatonin is secreted into the CSF only, into the plasma only, or into both. A 24-hour rhythm in the concentration of CSF melatonin suggests the possibility that the CSF may be an important route of communication between the pineal gland and other parts of the brain.

HIOMT activity is present in some blood cells, the Harderian gland, and the retina, and melatonin may also be synthesized in other extrapineal sites, such as the hypothalamus, retina, and gastrointestinal tract. These sites may theoretically assume some functional significance following pinealectomy.

Site of Action of Melatonin

There is evidence for brain, pituitary, and peripheral antigonadotropic actions of melatonin [30]. The evidence for a CNS effect is derived from the following information. Pinealectomy leads to increased motor and EEG activity, whereas melatonin administration reduces spontaneous motor activity, promotes sleep with slow EEG activity, and prolongs the duration of barbiturate-induced sleep. Melatonin may modify CNS neurotransmitter function as increased levels of gamma-aminobutyric acid (GABA) and serotonin have been noted in the brain after melatonin administration. Melatonin implants into the medial preoptic and suprachiasmatic

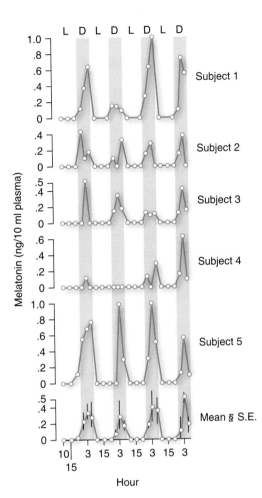

Figure 20.8 Diurnal plasma melatonin levels in humans. Note the nocturnal elevation during four consecutive cycles in five adult male subjects. (From Vaughan, Meyer, and Reiter, *Journal of Clinical Endocrinology and Metabolism,* vol. 42, pp. 752–64. ©1976 J. B. Lippincott Publishing Company, used by permission.)

and retrochiasmatic areas of the mouse brain elicit complete gonadal regression. Using in vitro autoradiography, in combination with a high-affinity radioligand (2-[^{125}I]melatonin), melatonin binding sites have been reliably and repeatedly identified in the SCN and, as originally reported, in the median eminence region of the mammalian hypothalamus. The pars tuberalis of the pituitary gland contains an abundance of gonadotrophs. The density of these immunoreactive cells is sufficient to discriminate the zona tuberalis from the pars distalis. In all species studied, the pars tuberalis contains high-affinity melatonin binding sites. This phylogenetically conserved melatonin-binding region may be the site of action of this indoleamine in controlling gonadotropin secretion and sexual function.

Figure 20.9 Diurnal pattern of CSF melatonin in the rhesus monkey. An individual animal was studied for 6 consecutive days and CSF was collected every 90 minutes. (From Reppert et al., with permission. *Endocrinology* 104:295–301, 1979. ©1979 American Roentgen Ray Society. Williams & Wilkins Company.)

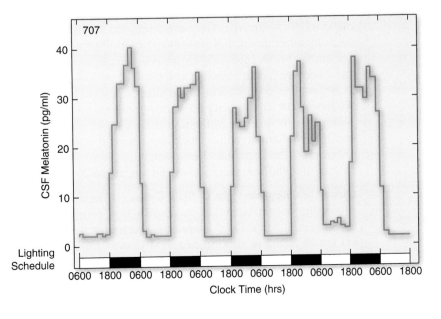

"A family of high-affinity, G-protein-coupled receptors for the pineal hormone melatonin has been cloned from vertebrates. These recombinant receptors exhibit similar affinity and pharmacological characteristics to each other and to endogenous receptors, as defined with the melatonin agonist 2-[^{125}I]iodomelatonin (^{125}I-Mel). Two mammalian melatonin receptor subtypes have been identified by molecular cloning studies. The mammalian Mel_{1a} melatonin receptor is expressed in most sites containing ^{125}I-Mel binding. This includes the hypothalamic suprachiasmatic nucleus and hypophysial pars tuberalis, presumed sites of the circadian and some of the reproductive actions of melatonin, respectively. The mammalian Mel_{1b} melatonin receptor is expressed in retina and brain and may mediate the reported effects of melatonin on retinal physiology in some mammals. A third receptor subtype, the Mel_{1c} melatonin receptor, has been cloned from zebra fish, *Xenopus*, and chickens but not from mammals" [41, 42]. The Mel_{1a} and Mel_{1b} receptors are now known as the MT_1 and MT_2 receptors, respectively. Gene targeting methods have been used to generate melatonin receptor-deficient mice, and to analyze the physiological role(s) of each receptor subtype [20]. Studies in MT_1 and MT_2 null animals has revealed that the MT_1 receptor mediates the acute effect of melatonin on electrical activity in SCN neurons, while MT_2 receptors appear to be of greater importance in mediating the ability of melatonin to phase shift the SCN circadian clock [20, 25].

Pineal Rhythms and Biological Clocks

The pineal gland synthesizes melatonin in response to photic information received from the eyes [31, 32]. Because of the rapid response of the epiphysial-synthesizing machinery and the short half-life of the released product, melatonin, circulating levels of the indoleamine may be an accurate reflection of the amount of photic input to the eyes. The pineal therefore provides a mechanism for the measurement of the duration of the dark and light periods. Thus in animals whose reproductive patterns fit into a specific seasonal scheme, the pineal may play a pivotal role in the control of their gonadal function. Indeed, it is the pineal gland, an end organ of the photoperiodic input system, that translates the photic message into a chemical signal. The pineal gland, in essence, is the intermediary between the external photoperiod and internal milieu. The pineal gland is the site at which light and dark information is translated, or transduced, into a chemical messenger. Melatonin is the "chemical expression of darkness" [40].

In mammals, light information is first perceived by photoreceptor elements of the eyes; this information is then relayed through the retinohypothalamic pathway to the SCN. A rhythm of *N*-acetyltransferase activity, however, is maintained in blinded animals kept in constant lighting or in normal animals in continuous darkness. The signal generator is a neural oscillator (*biological clock*) with a period of about 24 hours that only transmits a signal to the pineal gland periodically. The pineal rhythm is truly circadian in nature. Circadian rhythms have, by definition, periods of about 24 hours. They persist ("free-run") under constant conditions, with respect to principal environmental time cues (Zeitgebers), and are thus endogenous rhythms rather than driven ones (e.g., those that are repeatedly stimulated by a cyclically changing environment). They are entrained by light and temperature cycles and, in some cases, by other less prominent time cues. Entrainment normally serves to synchronize these not-quite-24-hour biological rhythms to the precise daily rhythm of the environment. Biological clocks are synchronized or entrained by periodically recurring environmental stimuli. The SCN contains an endogenous circadian clock that generates a rhythm of pineal melatonin synthesis with a periodicity of slightly greater than 24 hours; restricting the cycle to precisely 24 hours is the function of the prevailing light to dark environment [37]. Although more than one mammalian circadian clock may exist, the SCN is considered the master oscillatory system. It is the circadian clock mechanism, intrinsic to the cells of the SCN, that directs the pattern of melatonin secretion by the pineal gland.

Circadian Rhythmicity in SCN Cells.   Classic studies demonstrated that the SCN is the site of the master circadian pacemaker that drives most, if not all of the major circadian rhythms in mammals and many other vertebrate species. These include demonstrations that (1) the SCN shows striking circadian glucose utilization, (2) SCN ablation eliminates most overt physiological, behavioral, and metabolic circadian rhythms, (3) tissue explants containing the SCN continue to exhibit circadian electrophysiological activity rhythms in vitro, and (4) circadian rhythmicity can be restored to SCN-lesioned arrhythmic hosts by implantation of fetal brain tissue containing SCN cells. The pacemaker role of the SCN in a mammalian circadian system was also tested by neural transplantation from a mutant strain of hamster that shows a short circadian period. Small neural grafts from the suprachiasmatic region restored circadian rhythms to arrhythmic animals whose own nucleus had been ablated. The restored rhythms always exhibited the circadian period of the donor genotype regardless of the direction of the transplant, mutant to wild type (or vice versa), or genotype of the host. Rhythmicity was apparent 6 to 7 days after transplantation. Immunocytochemical analysis indicated that neural connections had been made between graft and host brain. The basic period of the overt circadian rhythm, therefore, is determined by cells of the suprachiasmatic region [22, 36].

In female rats blinded early in pregnancy, the circadian rhythms remain as they were at the time the rats were blinded. It was discovered that rat fetuses show their mothers' extrinsic day–night cycles [17, 19, 23]. These observations indicate that animal fetuses have functioning biological clocks that are set by their mother. The fetal clock is unaffected when the mother rat's pineal is removed, suggesting that melatonin of pineal origin does not set the fetal biological clock.

Molecular Basis of Circadian Rhythmicity.   Within the past decade, tremendous progress has been made in characterizing the molecular mechanisms that function as core functional components of cellular circadian oscillators [33, 43, 51]. This molecular clock machinery operates in the ~10,000 cells of each of the paired SCN nuclei. Clock mechanisms also appear to function in many peripheral tissues, where they may subserve timing mechanisms controlled by the output of the SCN, or operate independently. The core clock mechanism has been found to consist of overlapping transcriptional feedback loops, resulting in 24-hour rhythmic patterns of gene expression. In the positive regulatory loop, two basic "helix-loop-helix" transcriptional activators, *Clock* and *BMal1*, heterodimerize and bind recognition sequences called "E-boxes" in the promoter regions of the genes Period (*Per*) and Cryptochrome (*Cry*), thereby activating transcription of these genes. Once translated, the *Per* and *Cry* proteins then function as negative regulators of *Clock/BMal1* activity, thus forming the major circadian autoregulatory feedback loop. This cycle of molecular events produces a synchronized rhythmic output from the SCN, conveyed both synaptically and humorally to other brain regions and peripheral tissues. The concerted output of the SCN clock confers circadian rhythmicity to a multitude of physiological control systems, including pineal melatonin secretion. As mentioned in several chapters of this book, the circadian clock also controls secretion patterns of several hypothalamic, pituitary, and peripheral hormones. Circadian rhythms in ACTH, for example, occur under the influence of the SCN neural oscillator. The stimulation of GnRH and gonadotropin surges in female rodents is also timed within the circadian cycle by an SCN directive [12, 14].

Other Circadian Clocks.   In non-mammalian species the pineal gland itself possesses a circadian pacemaker. A 24-hour circadian clock has also been found in the mammalian retina and that of other species. Cultured retinas produced melatonin on a 24-hour cycle that peaks at night. Thus, mammals have a second timepiece that "ticks independently of the SCN" [31, 32]. The test-tube retinas, unlike the cultured SCN clock, can be reset, or entrained, with light, which should help scientists hone in on the light-absorbing molecules underlying the rhythm of the circadian clocks [31, 32]. The significance of clock protein expression in a variety of other CNS and peripheral tissues is currently under investigation. However, current thinking revolves around the developing concept of a photo-neuroendocrine axis in which many of the components interact to maintain the temporal synchrony of the body.

Chronobiology: Rhythms of Life.   Chronobiology deals with the rhythmic patterns that occur in all forms of life. Virtually all organisms exhibit approximately daily (circadian) cycles. In human beings, prominent rhythms are found in blood pressure, circulatory pulse, body core temperature, and surface temperature, and in chemical variables of blood, urine, and tissues. For medicine, this new science may clarify the relationships of rhythms to prediction, prevention, diagnosis, and treatment of diseases. Several decades of research worldwide have established that medical diagnoses can be subject to a much higher proportion of false positives (e.g., office hypertension) and false negatives (e.g., odd-hour hypertension) when only single samples are taken at arbitrary times of the day, instead of taking rhythms into account. Radiation, chemotherapy, and other treatments have been shown to have markedly different efficacy and safety depending on the pattern of administration within the day [48].

These phenomena are now being clarified at the molecular level; for example, a direct relationship between drug toxicity and the status of the *Clock/BMal1* complex has been demonstrated [1].

Melatonin for the Control of Seasonal Reproductive Cycles. Manipulating the reproductive cycle of photoperiodic species in the laboratory can be accomplished by turning on and off a light switch at the desired time of day. In those photoperiodic species in which the breeding season in nature is confined to only a very limited time of year, reproductive activity in the laboratory can be initiated in any month by careful control of the light cycle prior to and during the induction of reproductive function.

Following confirmation of the link between pineal function and seasonality, coupled with the availability of sufficient quantities of melatonin for experimental procedures, melatonin was routinely administered to many mammalian species with a view to manipulating seasonal rhythms. Research groups from Australia, the United States, and Britain simultaneously demonstrated that daily (late afternoon) administration of supplementary melatonin to ewes in midsummer substituted for short photoperiodic conditions and advanced the onset of breeding activity. It was shown that continuous melatonin treatment by implant methods also simulated short day length to induce early reproductive activity in both ewes and rams. Such sustained elevations of plasma melatonin might be physiologically perceived as a "super-short" day. If melatonin treatment can effectively induce those seasonal responses associated with short photoperiod, it has an obvious commercial application in all sheep-producing countries, whether its primary intention is for early lambing, improved fecundity, or a combination of both [24, 39].

Pathophysiology

Two contrasting types of pinealoma are associated with precocious or delayed sexual maturation [11, 13]. Parenchymal pinealomas, which consist of an enlarged mass of pinealocytes, are associated with delayed puberty. Destructive pinealomas, which consist of nonparenchymal tissue (e.g., connective tissue), are associated with enhanced precocious development of sexual maturation. The interpretation of these clinical observations is as follows. An overactive pineal (parenchymal pinealoma) secretes an excess of a factor that is inhibitory to gonadal development. In the absence of this factor, because of destruction of the pineal, the antigonadotropin is absent and the individual experiences a precocious development of the gonads. Pineal tumors are rare in the female, but about one-third of all males below the age of sexual maturation who have pineal tumors undergo precocious puberty [21].

Hypogonadism in Humans. Although the association has not been unequivocally established, a number of recent reports suggest that melatonin may influence human reproductive function [26]. Some patients with hypothalamic hypogonadism have unusually high plasma melatonin concentrations, suggesting that increased pineal activity may be involved in the pathogenesis of this condition. Some boys with delayed puberty have elevated daytime plasma melatonin concentrations, and more than half of the children with precocious sexual development have plasma melatonin concentrations lower than those of age-matched normal children. These data suggest that melatonin may be responsible for pathologic conditions of the human reproductive system [27].

There are at least two reports showing that women suffering from hypothalamic amenorrhea have abnormally high nocturnal melatonin levels. These subjects are characterized by decreased GnRH pulsatility, a change readily induced by melatonin. Likewise, women with this condition are typically anovulatory, a condition that could also be mediated by melatonin since it is known to be capable of suppressing the ovulatory hormone surges required for the rupture of ovarian follicles and shedding of the ova. In addition to an augmented melatonin secretion at night, the duration of elevated nocturnal melatonin is also prolonged in women with hypothalamic amenorrhea. Either the higher levels or the increased duration of elevated melatonin levels could account for the suppression of reproductive physiology in these women [37].

The Pineal Gland (Melatonin) and Aging. Because of its exclusive nighttime synthesis, melatonin has come to be known as the "chemical expression of darkness" and as the "Dracula of the endocrine system." At birth, the circadian melatonin rhythm in mammals is absent. In the rodent pineal, the cycle becomes apparent postnatally shortly after the post-ganglionic sympathetic nerves grow into the developing gland. In newborn humans, a melatonin rhythm in the blood is not discernible until 3 to 4 months of age, after which it seems to develop rapidly until one year of age. Prepubertal mammals exhibit a robust circadian melatonin rhythm. As humans undergo sexual maturation, there is claimed to be a significant drop in nocturnal melatonin levels, a change that may be permissive to pubertal development. After adulthood is achieved, virtually all mammals continue to exhibit a 24-hour melatonin rhythm with low and high values being associated with day and night, respectively [37].

In recent years, melatonin has been implicated as an anti-aging hormone [34]. Indeed, the hypothesis has been put forward that "aging is secondary to pineal failure." According to this hypothesis, aging is a syndrome of a relative melatonin deficiency accompanied by a diminished melatonin/5-HT ratio, which is detrimental to neurophysiology and causally related to the aging process. Dietary restriction clearly increases the life span of a variety of animals; likewise, the procedure also tends to preserve pineal melatonin rhythm. The conservation of the melatonin rhythm in food-restricted animals is particularly interesting since, typically, prolonged food restriction depresses the function of virtually every other endocrine organ; yet the melatonin cycle responds in an opposite manner, that is, it is maintained. The question then arises, is the prolonged life span experienced by food-restricted animals related to greater melatonin availability? Only a few data relate to the ability of melatonin to influence the duration of survival, but the correlations are positive. When mice were given melatonin in their drinking water, they lived noticeably longer (20%), that is, from a mean of 752 ± 80 days in nonmelatonin-treated mice to a mean of 931 ± 80 days in mice given melatonin every night. The contrary expectation would be that pinealectomized animals, with the resulting melatonin deficiency, would die at an earlier age than pineal intact animals; such studies have not been performed [38].

Thus, the pineal gland, via its hormone melatonin, may somehow, either directly or indirectly, delay aging itself or inhibit age-related disease processes. Because of these findings, melatonin has been classified as an anti-aging hormone and as a juvenile hormone. If, in fact, these well-based predictions are finally unequivocally verified, the pineal gland could be known as the veritable "fountain of youth." The data accumulated to date might justify serious consideration that supplemental melatonin intake may be beneficial in delaying the aging process [38].

The Pineal Gland and Cancer.   Melatonin alters the firing rate of the gonadotropin-releasing hormone (GnRH) pulse frequency generator in the hypothalamus, thus reducing pituitary secretion of gonadotropins and prolactin (PRL) and, indirectly, the secretion of estrogens by the gonads. In mammals, melatonin has been shown to delay puberty, suppress ovulation, and reduce gonadal steroidogenesis. The incidence of estrogen-related cancers in the female is directly correlated with the age of menarche (first menstruation). In other words, the earlier the onset of menstrual cycles, the more years a woman is exposed to estrogens (which are known to be carcinogenic). The hypothesis has been advanced that blind women, particularly those blind since childhood, may have a low risk of breast cancer due to increased melatonin secretion from the pineal gland [35].

Melatonin Effects on Humans

Melatonin has been injected into humans on and off over the last 20 years to determine the effects, if any, of the indoleamine on bodily function [29]. It is hoped that therapeutic applications directed toward correcting abnormalities of circadian rhythms will be discovered [2–4, 45]. Melatonin administered orally may advance the time of self-rated "fatigue" or actual sleep. Melatonin may also cause an advance in the endogenous rhythm of melatonin secretion. Based on these observations, melatonin has been administered to attempt to alleviate jet-lag following long transmeridian flights [4, 6]. It has been claimed that the results support the concept that melatonin secretion works as an endogenous synchronizer, preventing loss of synchrony among the multitude of bodily rhythms.

Although the phase-shifting effect of melatonin was improved sleep in subjects whose circadian system is desynchronized, this effect is considered separate from the more immediate hypnotic effects reported for melatonin. Melatonin can produce short-term hypnotic effects without concurrent shifts in the circadian system. Thus, it is unlikely that the short-term hypnotic effects of melatonin are related to immediate phase shifts of the circadian system. Current research suggests that melatonin administration increases the likelihood of sleep when the inclination for sleep is low, but not when it is high. This can be interpreted as a mild hypnotic effect or, alternatively, as evidence that melatonin functions as a sleep propensity modulator [9, 54].

Although melatonin can be shown to improve the sleep–wake pattern in free-running blind subjects, it is still not clear whether this effect is mediated by an hypnotic or circadian mechanism [46, 47]. Experimental studies of the phase-shifting effects of melatonin suggest a phase–response curve consistent with the proposition outlined above. There is evidence that melatonin can produce significant phase advances when administered in the late afternoon and early evening at doses that will be largely eliminated prior to the subsequent sleep period. This suggests that the improvement in sleep following evening administration may reflect the hypnotic effects, while afternoon melatonin administration is more likely to be related to circadian effects.

Melatonin and Photpheriodism in Humans.   Humans exhibit seasonal alterations in several physiological and behavior processes, and therefore it has been hypothesized that melatonin may mediate sensitivity to photoperiod in humans as it does in many other mammals [8]. Studies that have sought to establish the role of melatonin in seasonal human phenomena, however, have provided largely inconsistent results. It is possible that some individuals may possess sensitivity to photoperiod, while others do not, owing to genetic and/or experiential factors that have yet to be ascertained. This possibility may explain some of the inconsistent results obtained in human studies, where investigators have examined the potential relationships between photoperiod and birthrate or reproductive hormone secretions [8]. Some psychiatric disorders, such as seasonal affective disorder (SAD), develop and remit in a seasonal pattern, and there has been much interest in the role that pineal melatonin secretion may play in these conditions [54].

Melatonin Supplements.   Numerous articles lauding the benefits derived from taking melatonin have been published. A number of pharmaceutical preparations are available (Fig. 20.10). It has been suggested, however, that "if unusual melatonin rhythms can harm the eye" then "it may not be wise to take melatonin supplements" [31, 32]. Also, jet-lagged travelers have been advised to lay off melatonin pills, since too much melatonin may "numb" the SCN. Again, melatonin may have as yet unknown reproductive effects in humans [2, 3, 6]. Melatonin may mediate some actions intracellularly on calmodulin to then affect microtubular function in some cells (see below). Given its lipophilicity and probable easy access to all cells (e.g., sperm), there should again be some concern relative to its long-term use in humans. However, pharmaceutical firms recently have developed, patented, and begun marketing melatonin analogs as sleeping pills.

Figure 20.10 Example of a melatonin supplement that is commercially available. (Courtesy of Christopher B. Heward, Emerald Pharmaceuticals.)

Other Proposed Roles of the Pineal

The pineal has been suggested to affect almost every endocrine gland in the body, as well as many other physiological activities [10]. The pineal like its diencephalic hypothalamic counterpart, the pituitary, may function in the control of a large number of physiological processes. A few of the more recognized roles of the pineal will be described.

Ocular Melatonin.   Melatonin is present in the retina of many animals as are the enzymes N-acetyltransferase (NAT) and HIOMT, and serotonin is converted to melatonin in the eye in vitro. Like the pineal, ocular NAT activity shows a daily light–dark cycle that can be modified by environmental lighting. Ocular melatonin probably gets into the bloodstream, as rhythms of circulating melatonin are often still present after pinealectomy.

Melatonin synthesis by the eye might serve some endocrine role, or melatonin may act locally to regulate some ocular function. For example, the normal cyclic shedding of the outer retinal segment of the rat is blocked by reserpine treatment that also abolishes the circadian rhythm of indoleamine biosynthesis. Melatonin therefore may regulate the cyclic metabolism of photoreceptor cells. In addition, the photoreceptors of some poikilotherms are retracted during periods of bright illumination, an event facilitated by melatonin. Pigment migration within retinal melanocytes also occurs in response to photic cues in some species. Pinealectomy abolishes this response, whereas melatonin has the opposite effect. Melatonin therefore may play an important role in retinal light sensitivity and visual acuity in some vertebrates.

The Pineal Gland in Birds is Directly Light-Sensitive

In birds, as in mammals, the activity of the enzymes responsible for melatonin synthesis (NAT and HIOMT) and the amount of melatonin in the pineal gland are enhanced in darkness and depressed in light. Serum levels of melatonin are increased in birds during dark periods. Even after blinding, changes in pineal indoleamine biosynthesis occur in response to environmental lighting. The thin skull of birds may allow light to penetrate directly to the pineal. In addition a circadian rhythm of pineal melatonin synthesis occurs in isolated pineals maintained in organ culture in the absence of light; these isolated pineals are directly light-sensitive (Fig. 20.5).

In the sparrow, *Passer domesticus*, the pineal gland is essential for persistence of the circadian locomotor rhythm under conditions of constant darkness. Removal of the pineal results in arrhythmic locomotor activity. Pinealectomized sparrows will nevertheless still entrain to light–dark cycles and reveal other signs that are partially indicative of a circadian system. The free-running rhythm of locomotor activity is not abolished by disruption of the neural input to the pineal or its neural output. Most interestingly, rhythmicity can be restored to pinealectomized birds by the implantation of a donor pineal to the anterior chamber of the eye. The transplanted pineal transfers the phase of the donor bird's rhythm to the host. The avian pineal therefore seems to be coupled to other components of the circadian system by an endocrine, rather than a neural, mechanism.

It has been suggested that the avian pineal contains a self-sustained oscillator that produces a rhythmic hormonal output. Furthermore, it is believed that circadian fluctuations of this hormone entrain a damped oscillator located elsewhere in the body, which in turn drives the locomotor activity. In this model, each oscillator would have separate access to environmental light cycles. Locomotor and other behaviors of pinealectomized birds would be determined exclusively by the damped oscillator, but would be unable to free run (in the absence of light cues) because the self-sustained oscillator is lacking. Restoration of the damped oscillator to its normal state can be reestablished by cyclic hormonal output from a transplanted pineal.

The continuous administration of melatonin reduces the total amount of perch-hopping activity in sparrows, an effect reversed to normal after cessation of melatonin treatment. The evidence suggests that the pineal, through its product melatonin, may play a role in both the timing and the amount of activity expressed throughout the active and resting cycle in birds. Pinealectomy abolishes the normal circadian rhythm of body temperature in constant darkness and also alters significantly the amplitude of body temperature rhythms entrained to light cycles. There is evidence that the pineal gland may influence thermoregulatory behavior and physiology in some reptiles and mammals. In some birds, reproductive activity is clearly related to photoperiodic events, but the pineal gland and melatonin have not been implicated in the control of such activity.

The Pineal Glands of Poikilotherms are also Photosensitive

In the mammal, light information is received through the eyes and conveyed through the CNS to control pineal melatonin synthesis. As discussed at the outset of this chapter, cells of the pineal of certain poikilotherms of amphibians, reptiles, and teleosts were shown to be sensory in structure and function (Fig. 20.11). The morphology of these cells resembles that of the retinal photoreceptors of the eyes. In addition, electrophysiological recordings indicate that these pineal sensory elements are directly photosensitive and are apparently activated in the absence of light to synthesize and release melatonin. As in mammals, there is a diurnal rhythm of plasma melatonin in poikilotherms (fishes, lizards) that is totally or partially abolished by pinealectomy, but other sources of melatonin may also exist.

Infant rats do not require the eyes for the cyclic nocturnal fall in their pineal serotonin levels [56]. This drop in pineal serotonin, however, can be inhibited by continuous illumination. Thus, these young rodents appear to see even though their eyelids are closed. If, however, the heads of these animals are completely covered with black hoods, there is a decrease in pineal 5-HT levels. There is evidence that the pinealocytes of newborn rats contain photoreceptor organelles as do poikilothermic vertebrates. Thus, in their ontogeny, these cells recapitulate their phylogeny relative to the structure of these elements.

From a comparative evolutionary standpoint, it is interesting that the earliest pineal systems (cyclostomes, elasmobranch and teleost fishes, amphibians, reptiles, and birds) are

Figure 20.11 The lizard pineal gland and its anatomical relation to the diencephalic roof. (From Wurtman, Axelrod, and Kelly, 1966. Evidence for a nonretinal pathway of light in the pineal gland of newborn rats. *Proc. Natl. Acad. Sci. USA* 56:515–20, with permission.)

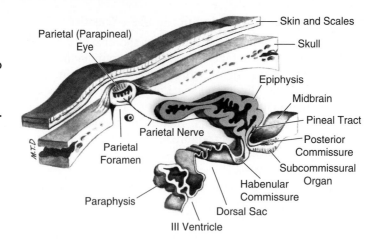

directly photosensitive. In all these vertebrates, the pineal synthesizes and releases melatonin in the absence of light. There is also evidence that the pineal glands of these animals are not directly controlled by nervous input. In adult mammals, on the other hand, the same biochemical events take place in the pineal cells in the absence of light, but the pinealocytes are regulated via photic cues received initially by the eyes. Photostimulation of the eyes results in neural information that is then conveyed to the pinealocytes. Even in their ontogeny, the pinealocytes of both birds and mammals, at least in those few studied, possess photosensitive sensory cells. Thus, there has been a gradual transformation from a directly photosensitive sensory system to an indirectly regulated system (in mammals), controlled through the nervous system by information received from the lateral eyes. Nevertheless, the evidence is clear that the pineal glands of all vertebrates, whether directly photoreceptive or not, are actively engaged in the biosynthesis of indoleamines.

The Pineal Gland and Melatonin Release Control Chromatophores in Poikilothermic Vertebrates

The discovery of McCord and Allen [28] that bovine pineal glands contain a factor that causes tadpoles to lighten in color was ultimately responsible for the search and elucidation of the structure of melatonin. There is now evidence that melatonin controls color change in certain poikilothermic vertebrates, at least at certain developmental stages. When amphibian larvae are placed in the dark, they rapidly become lighter in color. This body-blanching response is eliminated by pinealectomy but is mimicked when melatonin is added to the water in which larvae swim. Melatonin-induced lightening of amphibian larvae is due to the direct effect of the indoleamine on melanosome aggregation within dermal melanophores (Chap. 8). There is strong experimental evidence that the body-blanching response of larval amphibians, as well as that of cyclostomes to darkness, is due to melatonin release from the pineal [5].

The normal background response of larval and adult amphibians to a light- or dark-colored background is controlled by the presence or absence of circulating levels of melanocyte-stimulating hormone (MSH) and is not under the control of the pineal gland [5]. The control of chromatic responses by the pineal gland and melatonin in other vertebrates has not been studied in depth. Melanophores of certain species of fishes and reptiles do respond to melatonin, but this need not necessarily imply that the indoleamine plays any normal role in the control of chromatic behavior in these vertebrates.

Melatonin Mechanisms of Action

The receptor for melatonin has now been cloned from the pigment cells (melanophores) of the skin of frogs [15]. The membrane receptor is a member of the G-protein-linked receptor superfamily.

There is evidence that melatonin mediates its cytoskeletal actions by intracellular interactions with calmodulin (CaM) [7]. The high-affinity binding of melatonin to CaM suggests that the hormone is able to modulate all activity by intracellularly binding to CaM at physiological concentrations. Antagonism of CaM by melatonin affects microtubular polymerization and thus cytoskeletal structure. Since the structures of melatonin and CaM are

Figure 20.12
Schematic representation of the melatonin receptor based on structure–function studies of melatonin-related analogs. (Reprinted with permission from Heward and Hadley *Life Sciences,* vol. 17, pp. 1167–78. ©1975 Pergamon Press, Ltd.)

phylogenetically well preserved, CaM-melatonin interaction probably represents a major mechanism for cellular synchronization in animal physiology [7].

The fact that melatonin is extraordinarily effective in reversing the darkening (melanosome-dispersing) action of MSH is of broader significance than melatonin's immediate chromatic effect. Although there is strong evidence that melatonin is the mammalian pineal antigonadotropin, less information exists as to its locus of action. There is only meager information relative to the putative hypothalamic neurons, pituitary cells, or gonadal cells on which the indoleamine may mediate its action. Thus, because the cellular site of action is unknown, the mechanism of melatonin action has not been easily studied. The melanophores of some frogs, lizards, and fishes, however, provide model systems for deriving some information on melatonin mechanisms of action and have been used as a bioassay for the indoleamine. The cellular mechanisms by which chemical messengers work are generally similar between species. Therefore, it might be expected that studies of melatonin actions on integumental melanophores may be applicable to other cellular systems including those of humans. From a study of many structural analogs of melatonin, it was determined that a methoxy group on the fifth carbon atom of the indole nucleus is necessary for melanosome aggregation (skin lightening) within melanophores [18]. The *N*-acetyl group, on the other hand, is necessary for binding of melatonin to its receptor. This can be demonstrated by the use of *N*-acetyltryptamine, which lacks intrinsic agonistic (lightening) activity but is competitively inhibitory to the actions of melatonin. The tryptamine nucleus and the 5-methoxy and *N*-acetyl groups are therefore essential for complete activity of melatonin. The proposed structural requirements of the melatonin receptor of frog skin melanophores in terms of binding site affinity and intrinsic agonistic activity are shown (Fig. 20.12).

REVIEW EXERCISES

Match the manipulation with its effect on plasma melatonin levels:

1. Decreased day length
2. Increased day length
3. Pinealectomy
4. Blinding
5. Inhibition of *N*-acetyl-transferase
6. Stimulation of the superior cervical ganglion

A. Increased melatonin
B. Decreased melatonin

Think, analyze and discuss:

1. What sort of daily pattern would you expect melatonin synthesis/secretion to exhibit in nocturnal species? Would it differ from the pattern in other species? Why or why not?
2. Why might the intake of foods high in tryptophan make an individual feel sleepy? At the cellular and biochemical level, how would this work?
3. In humans, melatonin release does not become rhythmic until 3 to 4 months of age. How might this observation explain the intermittent sleep pattern of newborns?

4. The role of the pineal gland in regulating gonadal development is perhaps most easily demonstrated in rodents. What would be the likely gonadal response in a prepubertal rodent to:
   a. Continuous darkness.
   b. Continuous light.
   c. Removal of the pineal gland.
   d. Removal of the pineal gland and infusions of melatonin.
   e. Denervation of the pineal gland.

5. Plot the likely 24-hour pattern of circulating melatonin levels in seasonally breeding hamsters housed in (a) short-day photoperiod or (b) long-day photoperiod. In either photoperiod, what effect would electrical stimulation of the superior cervical ganglia during the daytime have on melatonin secretion? What effect would be seen following injection of a β-adrenergic receptor antagonist just prior to the onset of the dark period? What effect would be seen following injection of a β-adrenergic receptor agonist during the daytime?

6. In a seasonally breeding hamster species, what would be the likely gonadal response in males to:
   a. Short-day photoperiod.
   b. Long-day photoperiod.
   c. Blinding.
   d. Pinealectomy.

7. In male hamsters, what would be the relative levels of LH and FSH in animals under each of the conditions listed in 5 a–d? If male hamsters were castrated and maintained in either a short-day or long-day photoperiod, which group would exhibit a greater gonadotropin response to testosterone treatment? What effect would pinealectomy have on the gonadotropin response to testosterone?

8. In the *Clock* mouse, a loss-of-function genetic mutation in the *Clock* gene is responsible for an impaired molecular clock mechanism. Predict the phenotypes that might be exhibited by these animals in terms of the following physiological or behavioral activities:
   a. ACTH secretion.
   b. Pineal melatonin secretion.
   c. Gonadotropin secretions in females.
   d. Locomotor activity.
   e. Feeding behavior.

9. The pineal gland synthesizes and releases melatonin in the absence of light in virtually all vertebrate animals studied. For the following animals, predict what effect removal of neural inputs to the pineal gland would have on melatonin secretions:
   a. Birds.
   b. Infant rat pups.
   c. Frogs.
   d. Adult rats.

References

[1] Antoch, M. P., R. V. Kondratov, and J. S. Takahashi. 2005. Circadian clock genes as modulators of sensitivity to genotoxic stress. *Cell Cycle* 4:901–7.

[2] Arendt, J. 2005. Melatonin: Characteristics, concerns, and prospects. *J. Biol. Rhythms* 20(4):291–303.

[3] Arendt, J. 1997. Safety of melatonin in long-term use (?). *J. Biol. Rhythms* 12:673–81.

[4] Arendt, J., et al. 1997. Efficacy of melatonin treatment in jet lag, shift work, and blindness. *J. Biol. Rhythms* 12:604–17.

[5] Bagnara, J. T., and M. E. Hadley, 1970. Endocrinology of the amphibian pineal. *Am. Zool.* 10:201–16.

[6] Baringa, M. 1997. New jet-lag hormone does double duty in the brain. *Science* 277:480.

[7] Benitez-King, G., and F. Anton-Tay. 1993. Calmodulin mediates melatonin cytoskeletal effects. *Experientia* 49:635–41.

[8] Bronson, F. H. 2004. Are humans seasonally photoperiodic? *J. Biol. Rhythms* 19:180–92.

[9] Brzezinski, A., et al. 2005. Effects of exogenous melatonin on sleep: A meta-analysis. *Sleep Med. Rev.* 9(1):41–50.

[10] Carrillo-Vico, A., et al. 2005. A review of the multiple actions of melatonin on the immune system. *Endocrine* 27(2):189–200.

[11] Cavallo, A., and W. A. Ritschel. 1996. Pharmacokinetics of melatonin in human sexual maturation. *J. Clin. Endocrinol. Metab.* 81:1882–6.

[12] Chappell, P. E. 2005. Clocks and the black box: Circadian influences on gonadotropin-releasing hormone secretion. *J. Neuroendocrinol.* 17:119–30.

[13] Davis, F. C. 1997. Melatonin: role in development. *J. Biol. Rhythms* 12:498–508.

[14] de la Iglesia, H. O., and W. J. Schwartz. 2006. Minireview: Timely ovulation: Circadian regulation of the female hypothalamo-pituitary-gonadal axis. *Endocrinology* 147:1148–53.

[15] Ebisawa, T., et al. 1994. Expression cloning of a high-affinity melatonin receptor from *Xenopus* dermal melanophores. *Proc. Natl. Acad. Sci. USA* 91:6133–7.

[16] Fraschini, F., R. J. Reiter, and B. Stankov (eds.). 1995. *The pineal gland and its hormones: fundamentals and clinical perspectives.* New York: Plenum Press.

[17] Goldman, B. D. 2003. Pattern of melatonin secretion mediates transfer of photoperiod information from mother to fetus in mammals. *Sci STKE* 192:PE29.

[18] Heward, C. B., and M. E. Hadley. 1975. Structure-activity relationships of melatonin and related indoleamines. *Life Sci.* 17:1167–78.

[19] Horton, T. H., and Stetson, M. H. 1990. Modification of pubertal photoperiodic responses in rodents by factors acting during fetal development. *Prog. Clin. Biol. Res.* 342:639–47.

[20] Jin, X., et al. 2003. Targeted disruption of the mouse Mel(1b) melatonin receptor. *Mol. Cell. Biol.* 23:1054–60.

[21] Kitay, J. I., and D. Altschule. 1954. *The pineal gland.* Cambridge: Harvard University Press.

[22] Klein, D. C., et al. 1997. The melatonin rhythm-generating enzyme: Molecular regulation of serotonin N-acetyltransferase in the pineal gland. *Recent Prog. Horm. Res.* 52:307–58.

[23] Kolata, G. 1985. Finding biological clocks in fetuses. *Science* 230:929–30.

[24] Lincoln, G. A., Andersson, H., and Loudon, A. 2003. Clock genes in calendar cells as the basis of annual timekeeping in mammals—a unifying hypothesis. *J. Endocrinol.* 179(1):1–13.

[25] Liu, C., et al. 1997. Molecular dissection of two distinct actions of melatonin on the suprachiasmatic circadian clock. *Neuron* 19:91–102.

[26] Luboshitzky, R., et al. 1996. Abnormal melatonin secretion in male patients with hypogonadism. *J. Mol. Neurosci.* 7:91–8.

[27] Macchi, M. M., and J. N. Bruce. 2004. Human pineal physiology and functional significance of melatonin. *Front. Neuroendocrinol.* 25(3–4):177–95.

[28] McCord, C. P., and F. P. Allen. 1917. Evidence associating pineal gland function with alterations in pigmentation. *J. Exp. Zool.* 23:207–24.

[29] Middleton, B., J. Arendt, and B. M. Stone. 1997. Complex effects of melatonin on human circadian rhythms in constant dim light. *J. Biol. Rhythms* 12:467–77.

[30] Moore, R. Y. 1978. The innervation of the mammalian pineal gland. *Prog. Reprod. Biol.* 4:1–29.

[31] Morell, P. 1996. Setting the biological stopwatch. *Science* 271:905–6.

[32] Morell, V. 1995. A 24-hour circadian clock is found in the mammalian retina. *Science* 272:349.

[33] Panda, S., and J. B. Hogenesch. 2004. It's all in the timing: Many clocks, many outputs. *J. Biol. Rhythms* 19:374–87.

[34] Poeggeler, B. 2005. Melatonin, aging, and age-related diseases: Perspectives for prevention, intervention, and therapy. *Endocrine* 27:201–12.

[35] Pukkala, E., et al. 2006. Does incidence of breast cancer and prostate cancer decrease with increasing degree of visual impairment. *Cancer Causes Control* 17(4):573–6.

[36] Ralph, M. R., et al. 1990. Transplanted suprachiasmatic nucleus determines circadian period. *Science* 247:975–8.

[37] Reiter, R. J. 1991. Pineal melatonin: Cell biology of its synthesis and of its physiological interactions. *Endocr. Rev.* 12:151–80.

[38] Reiter, R. J. 1992. The ageing pineal gland and its physiological consequences. *BioEssays* 14:169–75.

[39] Reiter, R. J. 1993. The melatonin rhythm: Both a clock and a calendar. *Experientia* 49:654–64.

[40] Reiter, R. J., and A. Lerchel. 1993. Regulation of mammalian pineal melatonin production by the electromagnetic spectrum. In: H.-S. Yu, and R. J. Reiter, eds. *Melatonin: biosynthesis, physiological effects, and clinical applications.* Boca Raton: CRC Press, pp. 107–27.

[41] Reppert, S. M. 1997. Melatonin receptors: Molecular biology of a new family of G protein-coupled receptors. *J. Biol. Rhythms* 12:528–31.

[42] Reppert, S. M., D. R. Weaver, and C. Godson. 1996. Melatonin receptors step into the light: Cloning and classification of subtypes. *TiPS* 17:100–2.

[43] Reppert, S. M., and D. R. Weaver. 2002. Coordination of circadian timing in mammals. *Nature* 418(6901):935.

[44] Rosebloom, P. H., and D. C. Klein. 1995. Norepinephrine stimulation of pineal cyclic AMP response element-binding protein phosphorylation: Primary role of a β-adrenergic receptor/cyclic AMP mechanism. *Mol. Pharmacol.* 47:439–49.

[45] Roush, W. 1995. Can "resetting" hormonal rhythms treat illness. *Science* 269:1220–1.

[46] Sack, R. L., and A. J. Lewy. 1992. Human circadian rhythms: Lessons from the blind. *Ann. Med.* 25:303–5.

[47] Sack, R. et al. 1991. Melatonin administration to blind people: Phase advances and entrainment. *J. Biol. Rhythms* 6:249–61.

[48] Scheving, L. E., F. Halberg, and C. F. Ehret. 1987. *Chronobiotechnology and chronobiological engineering.* Dordrecht, The Netherlands: Martinus Nijhoff.

[49] Stehle, J. H. 1995. Pineal gene expression: Dawn of a dark matter. *J. Pineal Res.* 18:179–90.

[50] Stumpf, W. E. 1988. The endocrinology of sunlight and darkness: Complementary roles of vitamin D and pineal hormones. *Naturwissenschaften* 75:247–51.

[51] Takahashi, J. S. 2004. Finding new clock components: Past and future. *J. Biol. Rhythms* 19(5):339–47.

[52] Turek, F. W. 1997. Melatonin: A pathway from obscure molecule to international fame. *Persp. Biol. Med.* 41:8–20.

[53] Turek, F. W., and M. U. Gillette. 2004. Melatonin, sleep, and circadian rhythms: Rationale for development of specific melatonin agonists. *Sleep Medicine* 5(6):523–32.

[54] Weir, T. A., et al. 2001. A circadian signal of change of season in patients with seasonal affective disorder. *Arch. Gen. Psychiatry* 58:1108–14.

[55] Wurtman, R. J., J. Axelrod, and D. E. Kelly. 1968. *The pineal.* New York: Academic Press.

[56] Zweig, M., S. H. Snyder, and J. Axelrod. 1966. Evidence for a nonretinal pathway of light in the pineal gland of newborn rats. *Proc. Natl. Acad. Sci. USA* 56:515–20.

ANSWERS TO REVIEW EXERCISES

Chapter 1 Introduction to Endocrinology

Compare and Contrast each of the Following Terms. How are they Related? How do they Differ?

Baroreceptors/osmoreceptor: Baroreceptors are sensory nerve endings in the walls of auricles of the heart, aortic arch, vena cava, and carotid sinus that register stretching in the walls of these tissues, and convey signals to the CNS that trigger responses to reduce that stretching. *Osmoreceptors* are cells in the hypothalamus that are sensitive to changes in osmotic pressure of the blood, and convey signals to counteract deviations from normal. Activation of both result in altered vasopression secretion and compensatory changes in blood pressure and blood osmolarity.

Endocrine gland/exocrine gland: Endocrine glands are ductless and secrete hormones directly into the bloodstream, while *exocrine glands* secrete substances that reach external or internal body surfaces by ducts.

Intrinsic stimulus/extrinsic stimulus: Intrinsic stimuli are signals originating within the body, such as blood glucose or blood pressure, that affect physiological processes within an animal. *Extrinsic stimuli* are those that originate in the environment, such as changes in temperature, day length, or olfactory cues. Physiological systems can often integrate intrinsic and extrinsic stimuli to generate appropriate responses to prevailing conditions.

Inotropic/chronotropic: Inotropic refers to the regulation of the strength of contractility of muscular tissue, particularly cardiac muscle. *Chronotropic* refers to the regulation of the rate of rhythmic muscular contractions. Hormones such as epinephrine may regulate one or both of these characteristics of the heartbeat.

First messenger/second messenger: A *first messenger* is generally a hormone that binds to a receptor on the cell surface and thereby communicates with intracellular metabolic processes. A *second messenger* is an intermediary molecule that is produced as a consequence of the activation of a hormone receptor, e.g. adenosine 3′,5′-cyclic monophosphate, cyclic guanosine 3′,5′-cyclic monophosphate, calcium, and phosphoinositides. Thus, extracellular first messengers evoke the production of intracellular second messengers.

Estivation/hibernation: Both hibernation and estivation refer to a process of living in a quiescent, torpid state. *Hibernation* occurs with exposure to low temperatures, principally during winter seasons when there are lengthy periods of low environmental temperatures. Animals *estivate*, by contrast, when they are exposed to prolonged periods of drought or during hot, dry summers. Hibernation and estivation in animals are essentially indistinguishable, except for the nature of the environmental stimuli.

Homeotherm/poikilotherm: Homeotherms are "warm blooded" animals that maintain a relatively constant body temperature in the face of changing ambient temperatures. *Poikilotherms* are "cold-blooded" animals that vary in body temperature according to the environmental temperature.

Endocrinology/neuroendocrinology: Endocrinology is the broader science of the glands and hormonal secretions and their physiological and pathophysiological relationships. *Neuroendocrinology* is a sub-discipline of both endocrinology and neurobiology that is concerned with the functional relationships between the nervous and endocrine systems. Neuroendocrine studies generally address the regulation of hormone secretions by the brain, and the effects of peripheral hormones on brain function.

Negative feedback/positive feedback: In endocrinology, negative feedback usually refers to the inhibitory control of hormone secretion by a signal that is itself regulated by that hormone. Almost always, negative feedback is the major mechanism that maintains homeostatic control within an endocrine system, and is mediated by the metabolite or second hormone that is regulated by the first hormone. By contrast, positive feedback is the relatively rare control situation in which the consequence of hormone action exerts a stimulatory effect on secretion of that hormone, leading to uncontrolled amplification of the endocrine signal.

Define or Otherwise Characterize each of the Following Terms

Hypothalamus: The region of the diencephalon that is situated below the thalamus, anterior to the mammillary bodies, posterior to the septal regions, and lying dorsally to the pituitary gland. Its major functions include regulation of autonomic function, endocrine secretions by the anterior and posterior pituitary glands, and neural mechanisms underlying mood and motivated behaviors. Neurons that produce the hypophysiotropic hormones and the neurohypophysial hormones are located in certain hypothalamic nuclei.

Homeostasis: The state of equilibrium, or balance, between opposing internal or external pressures, in the body with regard to the various physiological functions and chemical compositions.

Oncogene: Any of a group of genes that are involved in the regulation of cell growth and development, and which may prompt malignancies when mutated or inappropriately activated.

Vagustuff: In 1921, Otto Loewi demonstrated the existence of an endogenous substance that is released by the Vagus nerve, and exerts inhibitory control over the heartbeat. He called the unknown chemical Vagustuff, which was later shown to be the neurochemical acetylcholine.

Diabetes mellitus: A chronic metabolic disorder that is characterized by an impairment of the utilization of carbohydrate and an enhancement of the utilization of lipid and protein. It results from a failure of insulin production (Type 1) or action (Type 2) and, depending upon the severity of the deficiency, it can lead to hyperglycemia, glycosuria, water and electrolyte loss, ketoacidosis, and even coma and death.

Hypophysiotropic factor: A neurohormone, usually produced in neurons of the hypothalamus, that exerts a stimulatory or inhibitory action on specific cells of the anterior pituitary gland (adenohypophysis).

Second messenger: An intracellular intermediary molecule that is induced by plasma membrane receptor activation, and functions to convey signals to downstream elements of one or more intracellular signal transduction pathways.

Chapter 2   The Vertebrate Endocrine System

Compare and Contrast each of the Following Terms

Mineralocorticoid/glucocorticoid: A *mineralocorticoid* is a steroid hormone produced by cells of the zona glomerulata of the adrenal cortex; they function as key regulators of electrolyte and water metabolism and balance. *Glucocorticoids* are steroid hormones produced by the zona fasciculata of the adrenal cortex that regulate intermediary metabolism and can be used clinically to reduce inflammation.

Androgen/estrogen: *Androgen* is the generic term for substances that stimulate the activity of the accessory male sex organs and can promote development of male secondary sex characteristics. Natural androgens include the steroids testosterone and dihydrotestosterone, which serve as endogenous hormones. *Estrogen* is the generic term for substances that have actions characteristic of the estrogenic steroid hormone 17β-estradiol, such as stimulation of secondary sex characteristics or regulation of menstrual cyclicity. Androgens and estrogens are both produced by the ovaries, placenta, testes, and adrenal cortex. Endogenous testosterone is a precursor in the formation of 17β-estradiol via aromatization.

Endocrine/neuroendocrine (delivery of a hormone): *Endocrine* secretions are generally those released from glands or tissues into the bloodstream; *neuroendocrine* secretions (neurosecretions) involve release of neurohormones from nerve terminals into either the systemic circulation (e.g. vasopressin, oxytocin) or into specialized vasculature, such as the hypophysial portal vessels (e.g., GnRH, CRH, TRH).

Translation/transcription: The synthesis of a protein hormone begins with the *transcription* of DNA to RNA, followed by the *translation* of mRNA to a preprohormone molecule. Translation is the process by which mRNA, tRNA, and ribosomes affect the production of proteins from amino acids, as per the sequences encoded by specific genes. Transcription is the process by which the base sequence of mRNA is synthesized on a template of complimentary DNA; this process is catalyzed by an RNA polymerase.

Endopeptidase/exopeptidase: An *endopeptidase* is an enzyme that catalyzes the hydrolysis of a peptide chain at points along the interior of the molecule, while an *exopeptidase* catalyzes hydrolysis of the terminal amino acid of a peptide chain.

Oxytocin/vasopressin: Both neurohypophysial hormones are produced in magnocellular neurons of the hypothalamus, in the supraoptic and paraventricular nuclei, and released from nerve terminals in the posterior pituitary gland. *Oxytocin* stimulates milk-ejection in the mammary glands of lactating females, and uterine contractility during pregnancy in advance of parturition. *Vasopressin* stimulates water resorption in the renal collecting ducts and contraction of smooth muscle in blood vessels.

Neurohormone/neuropeptide: *Neurohormone* refers to any endogenous substance that is produced in neurons and released into the bloodstream. *Neuropeptides* are small protein molecules that are produced in neurons and released into synaptic clefts as neurotransmitters, or from neurovascular endings as neurohormones, or both.

Adrenal chromaffin/adrenal steroid (tissue): *Adrenal chromaffin* cells comprise the medulla of the adrenal gland, and were originally identified because they give a brownish-yellow color when reacted with chromic salts. These are catecholaminergic cells that primarily produce and secrete epinephrine into the bloodstream. Cells of the *adrenal cortex* are steroidogenic, producing mineralocorticoids, glucocorticoids, and androgens.

Endorphin/opiate: *Opioid* peptides are endogenous neuropeptides that serve multiple functions, including the suppression of the perception of painful stimuli. They are so named for their opiate properties. *Endorphin* is one of the opioid peptides that is produced in high quantities in the hypothalamus.

Endocytosis/exocytosis: *Endocytosis* is the internalization of substances in the extracellular fluid by the formation of vesicles from the plasma membrane. *Exocytosis* is the release of substances from a cell, whereby the secretory granule or synaptic vesicle containing the substance fuses with the plasma membrane, allowing diffusion of the contents into the extracellular fluid. Exocytosis is the Ca^{++}-dependent process by which hormones and neurotransmitters are released in a regulated manner, a process called stimulus-secretion coupling.

Define or Otherwise Characterize each of the Following Terms

Hypovolemia: A decrease below normal in the amount of blood in the circulation.

Isohormone: Different forms of a given hormone occuring as a result of microheterogeneity, for example, in the degree of glycosylation or other post-translational modifications.

Arachidonic acid: An unsaturated fatty acid, and the biological precursor of the chemical messengers prostaglandins, thromboxanes, and leukotrienes, together known as the eicosanoids.

Adenohypophysis: The anterior pituitary gland, containing the hormone producing cells gonadotropes, somatotropes, lactotropes, and corticotropes. Hormone synthesis and secretion from these cells are controlled by their corresponding hypothalalmic hypophysiotropic hormones.

Pheromone: A type of hormone signal that is synthesized and released by one individual and then received and transduced by a second individual, usually of the same species.

Chemoreceptor: A neuron or other cell that senses a change in the chemical environment and changes its pattern of electrophysiological activity.

Autoinhibition: A negative feedback effect of a hormone on the cells in which it is synthesized.

Match the Glandular Tissues in Column A with the Hormone(s) That They Produce in Column B

Ovary: estrogen, progesterone, inhibin
Pancreas: Insulin, glucagon
Anterior pituitary gland: LH, FSH, GH, ACTH, PRL, TSH
Adrenal cortex: cortisol, aldosterone, testosterone
Heart: Atriopeptin
Posterior pituitary gland: vasopressin, oxytocin
Thyroid gland: T3, thyroxine
Testis: testosterone, inhibin
Hypothalamus: GnRH, TRH, SST, GHRH, DA, CRH
Parathyroid gland: calcitonin

Chapter 3   General Mechanisms of Hormone Action

Compare and Contrast each of the Following Terms. In What Way are they Related? How do they Differ?

Phosphorylation/dephosphorylation (and hormone action): Many hormones activate signal transduction pathways that involve intracellular signaling molecules that are activated upon *phosphorylation*. In the adenylyl cyclase –cAMP-PKA mediated intracellular signaling pathway, for example, PKA is a kinase that activates downstream targets by phosphorylation. *Dephosphorylation* deactivates these same messengers. In some signaling pathways, dephosphorylation may activate the molecule, and deactivation may be mediated by phosphorylation.

Regulatory/catalytic subunits: Several key protein kinases are comprised of complexed *regulatory* and *catalytic* subunits, and dissociation of the subunits leads to an activation of the catalytic subunit, which propagates signaling via phosphorylation of downstream targets. In the adenylyl cyclase –cAMP-PKA mediated signal transduction pathway, for example, cAMP binds to the regulatory subunit of PKA, causing dissociation of the complex and activation of the PKA catalytic unit.

Lipase/phospholipase: *Lipase* is the general term used for an enzyme with fat-splitting or lipolytic activity. *Phospholipase* is the more specific name for enzymes that catalyze the hydrolysis of phospholipids. Phospholipases function as important components of several signaling transduction cascades. For example, phospholipase C (PLC) is a G-protein activated membrane enzyme that catalyzes the splitting of the phosphodiester bond of phosphatidylinositol 4,5-biphosphate, providing the two messenger molecules Ins(1,4,5) and 1,2-diacylglycerol (Fig. 3.12) [10]. Eicosanoids are produced exclusively within the plasma membrane of cells and are derived mainly from arachidonic acid released from phospholipids by the action of PLA_2.

Adenylate/guanylate (cyclases): *Adenylate cyclase* is a membrane-bound enzyme that is activated by Gs and inhibited by Gi, and catalyzes the production of the second messenger cAMP from ATP. This cyclase is thus a crucial link in this ubiquitous cellular signaling pathway. *Guanylate cyclase* is analogous to adenylate cyclase, but it cyclizes guanosine 5'-triphosphate to guanosine 3'5'-cyclomonophosphate, and is generally activated by the enzyme nitric oxide.

Additive/synergistic (actions of hormones): Two hormones may exert *additive* effects on a cell by activating receptors that are both linked to the production of the same intracellular second messenger. *Synergistic* actions of hormones occur when different signal transduction pathways are activated by two different hormones via their respective receptors, and the net effect is larger than the simple sum of the independent actions of the two hormones.

Stimulus-contraction/stimulus-secretion/stimulus-response (coupling): In electrically excitable cells, the depolarization of the membrane is coupled to a cellular response that depends upon the functions of the cell. In general, this is referred to as *stimulus-response coupling*. In muscle cells, this is called *stimulus-contraction coupling*, as the depolarization of the membrane is coupled to the mobilization of intracellular Ca^{++} and the contraction of muscle fibers. In endocrine cells and neurons, the release of a hormone or neurotransmitter occurs in response to an electrical or metabolic stimulus, which is coupled to an elevation of intracellular Ca^{++} and Ca^{++}-dependent exocytosis of the hormone or neurotransmitter. This is called *stimulus-secretion coupling*.

G_s/G_i: These are intracellular membrane-associated GTP binding proteins that are activated by the GPCRs. They transduce receptor-activated signals into alterations in amplifying enzyme (e.g. adenylate cyclase, PLC) activity. G_s transduces stimulatory signals while G_i mediates inhibitory influences on adenylate cyclase and the generation of cAMP.

DAG/IP_3: Activation of GPCRs is often coupled via $G_{q/II}$ to the activation of phospholipase C, which mediates phosphoinositol hydrolysis and the production of both of these second messengers – *DAG* and IP_3. While DAG activates PKC, IP_3 acts to mobilize intracellular Ca^{++}.

G-protein-coupled receptor (GPCR)/nuclear receptor: The *GPCRs* are seven transmembrane domain-containing receptors that are bound by hormones or neurotransmitters, leading to activation of G-proteins, membrane cyclases, or phospholipases, and the production of second messengers. They commonly mediate the actions of most peptide, protein, or monoaminergic hormones and neurotransmitters. The *nuclear receptor* family of proteins are intracellular proteins that bind steroid, thyroid, and other hormones and primarily mediate their actions via the regulation of transcription of target genes.

Define or Characterize Each of the Following Terms

Receptor "crosstalk": This can occur because changes in concentration of one second messenger can lead to a change in the concentration of another. Thus, activation of a single or multiple receptor type may be able to activate G proteins of more than one family, and the effect of a particular G protein might be altered by the activation of another G protein.

Methylxanthine synergism: *Methylxanthines* inhibit degradation of cAMP by phosphodiesterase when used at low concentrations, may only slightly increase the basal activity of cells. Used at a low concentration, a hormone might also have a minimal effect. When used in combination, however, a hormone and a methylxanthine may produce a dramatic response. The synergism results from the combination of increased production and decreased degradation of cAMP.

Guanylate cyclase: Analogous to the actions of adenylate cyclase, *guanylate cyclase* cyclizes guanosine 5'-triphosphate to guanosine 3'5'-cyclomonophosphate. It is primarily activated by the enzyme nitric oxide.

Transacting zinc finger proteins: Steroid and steroid-like hormones mediate their actions via specific receptors that belong to a superfamily of transacting "zinc finger" proteins. After binding of the specific ligand, these ligand-induced transcription factors influence gene expression via association with specific DNA elements, known as hormone-responsive elements (HREs).

Protein kinase A (PKA): Cyclic AMP-dependent protein kinase (*PKA*) mediates many of the actions of cAMP on cellular function. The kinase is composed of two components a regulatory subunit and a catalytic subunit. Interaction of cAMP with the regulatory subunit results in the release of the catalytic unit. The catalytic unit is thus free to function as a *kinase*, that is, a phosphorylating enzyme that activates downstream targets which affect changes in cellular function.

Tyrosine kinase: This is an enzyme that phosphorylates tyrosyl residues on certain proteins. Many receptors for growth factors, e.g. insulin and insulin-like growth factor (IGF), are *tyrosine kinases* that convey signals via phosphorylation of intracellular signaling molecules on tyrosyl residues.

Synergism: This refers to the circumstances where the combined actions of two different hormones are greater than the sum of their individual actions.

Protein kinase C (PKC): This describes any of a number of cytoplasmic calcium-activated kinases that mediate a number of signaling functions in cells. *PKC* is a critical component of the phosphoinositol hydrolysis signal transduction pathway.

Chapter 4 Endocrine Methodologies

Compare and Contrast each of the Following Terms. How are they Related? How do they Differ?

Orchidectomy/ovariectomy: Orchidectomy is the removal of one or both testes, while *ovariectomy* is the removal of one or both ovaries. These can be used as experimental procedures to remove the source of most circulating androgens and estrogens, respectively.

Basophilic/acidophilic: Basophilic describes cells containing granules that stain specifically with basic dyes. *Acidophilic* cells have an affinity for acid dyes. Hormone-producing cells of the anterior pituitary gland have classically been distinguished on the basis of their relative affinity for these dyes.

Atrophy/hyperplasia: These terms describe the decrease and increase in cell size and/or number in a tissue, respectively. *Atrophy* in a hormone target organ can occur from the removal of a trophic hormone, while *hyperplasia* can result from an excess of trophic hormone.

Immunoassay/radioimmunoassay: These are assays that can be used for the measurement of hormones in body fluids or tissue

extracts. *Immunoassays* make use of specific antibodies that recognize and bind the hormone. *Radioimmunoassays* are a specific type of immunoassay that use a radiolabeled hormone in a competitive inhibition assay to quantitate hormone levels.

Northern blot/real-time PCR: Both of these methods are used to quantitate the levels of specific mRNAs in a tissue or group of cells. In *Northern blotting*, RNA is isolated from a group of cells, or a tissue electrophoretically fractionated by size in an agarose gel, and transferred to a nylon or nitrocellulose membrane. A radiolabeled cDNA probe corresponding to the mRNA of interest is then hybridized to the RNA on the blot, detected via exposure of apposed x-ray film, and quantified by densitographic analysis of the image. *In Real-time polymerase chain reaction (real-time PCR)* techniques, by contrast, RNA is first reverse-transcribed, and then the sequence of interest is amplified by PCR and detected in real time by the incorporation of a fluorescent indicator in the reaction.

Teleost/cartilaginous fishes: Teleosts are bony fishes while the *cartilaginous fishes* include sharks, rays, and skates. The bony fishes have been the subjects of a greater amount of endocrine research, perhaps due to the evolution of many interesting specialized functions of their endocrine systems.

Hypertrophy/hyperplastic: While *hypertrophy* is a general increase in bulk of a tissue or organ, *hyperplastic* refers to a tissue in which hyperplasia occurs, i.e. an increase in number of normal cells in a tissue. Hyperplasia can be the underlying reason for hypertrophy.

Unilateral/bilateral: In terms of the surgical removal of a tissue, *unilateral* describes the removal of one of a paired set of organs or tissues, while *bilateral* refers to the removal of both of the paired set.

Immunocytochemistry/in situ hybridization: Immunocytochemical techniques make use of specific antibodies that recognize and bind specifically to a protein of interest, and can thus be used to characterize the cell – and tissue-specific localization of a protein. *In situ hybridization* procedures utilize cDNA probes or riboprobes to hybridize to an mRNA of interest, and are thus used to characterize the cell- and tissue-specific localization of a mRNA.

Transgenesis/gene targeting: Both methods are used to alter gene expression in experimental animals. In *transgenesis*, a gene construct is introduced into the germ line in an animal, and transgene expression is characterized to assess the control systems that normally function to regulate a certain gene, or to permit identification of specific cell types by the expression of a reporter or marker gene. *Gene targeting* usually refers to the process of inactivating a certain gene, thereby creating a gene "knockout" animal. In some cases, a gene is replaced by an exogenous gene construct that is "knocked-in" to the genome.

Define or Characterize each of the Following Terms

Ectopic transplantation: Surgical removal of a tissue or organ and transplantation of it to an abnormal site in the body, particularly a location at which the tissue or organ can be quickly vascularized and can be sustained.

Axoplasmic transport: Many cellular proteins are conducted from neuronal cell bodies to axon terminals by means of *axoplasmic transport*. In peptidergic neurons, secretory granules containing the neuropeptide undergo axoplasmic transport prior to exocytotic release of the neuropeptide at synapses or neurovascular junctions. Some drugs (e.g. colchicine) can be used to block axoplasmic transport for experimental purposes, such as the enhancement of neuropeptide immunoreactivity in cell bodies. Radiolabeled amino acids can also be infused in proximity to cell bodies, and the rate of incorporation into newly synthesized neuropeptides, and their transport along neurosecretory axons can be estimated.

Atrophy: Wasting of tissues as a consequence of cell shrinkage and/or loss. This can occur as a consequence of the withdrawal of trophic hormone support.

Parabiosis: Surgical joining of the vascular systems of two organisms. This has been used to obtain evidence for the existence of certain hormones, such as leptin.

Immunosympathectomy: Antibodies have been used in certain studies to neutralize the actions of a specific hormone or growth factor. The consequences of immunoneutralization can reveal information about the normal functions of the substance. Injections of antibodies to nerve growth factor (NGF) cause a failure of the growth and development of the sympathetic nervous system, demonstrating the obligatory role of NGF in this process. The injected animals are effectively *immunosympathectomized.*

Reverse transcriptase PCR: This is a method for qualitatively, or in some cases quantitatively, assessing the expression of an mRNA in a particular tissue or cell population. Reverse transcriptase is used to produce cDNAs corresponding to the mRNAs in a sample. Polymerase chain reaction, an enzymatic method for the repeated copying of two strands of DNA containing a gene sequence, is then used to amplify the extremely small quantities of the cDNA corresponding to the RNA of interest.

Western blot: An analytical procedure in which proteins are electrophoretically separated in a polyacrylamide gel, transferred to a nylon or nitrocellulose membrane, and identified by complexing with specific antibodies that are pre- or post-tagged with a labeled secondary protein.

Reporter gene: A *reporter gene* is a recombinant DNA construct whose phenotypic expression can be easily monitored. These are commonly used to study promoter activity in different tissues or under different developmental circumstances. Recombinant DNA constructs are made which contain the reporter gene sequence fused to a promoter region of a gene of interest, and the constructs are transfected into a cell or an organism.

Conditional gene targeting: Conditional gene targeting, using, Crelox or related technology, permits a gene of interest to be knocked-out in only a subset of tissues or cells, or only at a particular time during development. In many cases, these conditional knockout procedures circumvent lethality that would otherwise occur in a complete gene knockout. Gene targeting can be controlled both spatially and temporally, and thus the function of a particular gene can be analyzed in a specific cell type and at a specific time point.

Binding protein: The general term *"binding protein"* can refer to a protein that binds to a circulating hormone, such as any one of the steroid binding globulins. It is also used to describe an intracellular protein that can be activated and thereby prompted to bind specific DNA response elements, thus regulating transcription of target genes.

Immunocytochemistry: Immunocytochemical techniques make use of specific antibodies that recognize and bind specifically to a protein of interest, and can thus be used to characterize the cell – and tissue-specific localization of a protein.

Glycoprotein: One of a number of proteins that contain covalently linked carbohydrate moieties. The anterior pituitary hormones LH, FSH, and TSH are *glycoproteins*, each being heavily glycosylated.

Hormone analog: A synthetic molecule that resembles the structure of a hormone. These can often be designed to activate hormone receptors with greater or reduced potency compared to the endogenous hormone ligand. Some *hormone analogs* are capable of acting as receptor antagonists, blocking the actions of the hormone while not itself activating the receptor.

Ion Channel: A protein, or complex of subunit proteins, that forms an aqueous pore in a lipid bilayer membrane and allows controlled cellular influx or efflux of specific inorganic ions. They are typically involved in maintaining or modulating the electrical potential across the membrane.

Immunohistofluorescence: A specific type of immunocytochemistry that employs a fluorescent dye to label the expression and location of specific protein in a tissue and/or group of cells.

Transfection: Any process by which DNA can be induced into cells, including electroporation, lipofection, and virally-mediated gene transfer.

Gene knockout animal: An animal in which the genome is altered by means of site-directed recombination, resulting in the deletion of a gene sequence.

Stem cells: Precursor cells, or daughter cells, that may differentiate into other cell types.

Chapter 5   Pituitary Hormones

Compare and Contrast each of the Following Terms. In What Way are they Related? How do they Differ?

Corticotroph/lactotroph: Both of these are endocrine cell types in the anterior pituitary gland. *Corticotrophs* produce adrenocorticotropic hormone (ACTH) and other peptides derived from the preprohormone POMC, while *lactotrophs* produce the hormone prolactin.

Follitropin/lutropin: Both of these are glycoprotein hormones of the anterior pituitary gland. *Follitropin, or follicle-stimulating hormone (FSH)*, supports gametogenesis in both sexes; *lutropin, or luteinizing hormone (LH)*, stimulates steroidogenesis in both sexes and a surge of this hormone triggers ovulation in female mammals. Synthesis and secretion of both gonadotropins are stimulated by the hypophysiotropic neurohomrone gonadotropin-releasing hormone (GnRH, or LHRH).

Somatocrinin/somatostatin: Somatocrinin, also called growth hormone-releasing hormone (GHRH), is a hypothalamic hypophysiotropic neurohormone that stimulates synthesis and secretion of growth hormone (GH). *Somatostatin* (SST) is a hypophysiotropic neurohormone that inhibits the secretion of GH.

Lactotroph/prolactin: Lactotrophs are endocrine cells of the anterior pituitary gland that produce and secrete the hormone *prolactin.*
ACTH/α-melanotropin: Both of these peptides are derived from the preprohormone POMC, and they share structural similarity. *ACTH* is the primary secretory product of the corticotrophs of the anterior pituitary gland.

Adenohypophysis/neurohypophysis: Both of these structures are contained within the hypophysis, or pituitary gland; the *adenohypophysis* is derived from oral ectoderm during embryonic development and consists of glandular cells that secrete the anterior pituitary hormones. The *neurohypophysis* is derived from neural ectoderm and primarily consists of axons of magnocellular neurons that secrete vasopressin and oxytocin.

Heterodimer/homodimer: As it applies to endocrinology, a dimer is defined as protein that is comprised of the combination of two subunits, often linked together via disulfide bonds. *Homodimers* consist of the combination of two identical subunits, while *heterodimers* consist of different subunits.

Pars distalis/pars nervosa: The *pars distalis*, along with the dorsal extensions of the anterior pituitary surrounding the pituitary stalk (pars tuberalis), comprise the anterior lobe of the pituitary gland. The *pars nervosa* is the neural lobe of the pituitary gland.

Gonadotropin/basophil: The anterior pituitary hormones, LH and FSH, are glycoproteins that regulate gonadal growth and function and are therefore called *gonadotropins*. Both gonadotropins, as well as the third major glycoprotein hormone TSH, share a common α-subunit, and each contains a unique β-subunit. The gonadotrophs are cells of the anterior pituitary gland that produce the gonadotropins; these cells are called *basophils* because of their affinity for basic histological stains.

Define or Characterize each of the Following Terms.

Anterior lobe: The anterior pituitary gland consisting of the pars distalis and pars tuberalis.

Chromophobe cells: Some cell types, such as the corticotrophs and cells of the pars intermedia, do not have an appreciable affinity for histological dyes, and are therefore referred to as *chromophobes*.

Corticotroph: The anterior pituitary cell type that produces and secretes ACTH.

Vasopressin: The neurohypophysial hormone that is produced in magnocellular neurons of the parvocellular and supraopic nuclei, is released into the circulation from nerve terminals in the posterior pituitary gland, and stimulates water reabsorption in the collecting ducts of the kidneys and contraction of arterial smooth muscle. It is also referred to as anti-diuretic hormone (ADH). *Vasopressin* also functions as a central neurotransmitter.

Ectopic secretion: Secretion of a hormone or other substance from tissue located at (often transplanted to) a site that the tissue does not normally occupy.

Myoepithelial cells: Contractile cells of the breast that are stimulated by the neurohypophysial hormone oxytocin.

Glycoprotein: Proteins that contain carbohydrate moieties, such as the anterior pituitary glycoprotein hormones LH, FSH, and TSH.

Rathke's pouch: An inward invagination of the oral ectoderm of the stomodeum (primitive mouth cavity) that gives rise to the adenohypophysis during development.

Describe the Etiological Bases (causes) for each of the Following Endocrinopathies.

Acromegaly: Excess GH secretion in adulthood.

Addison's disease: Deficit in cortisol secretion.

Goiter: Excess TSH secretion, usually as a compensatory response to deficits in T_3 and thyroxine production.

Cretinism: TSH and T_3/thyroxine deficiency in childhood.

Cushing's disease: Excess glucocorticoid secretion, in some cases due secondarily to excess ACTH secretion.

Galactorrhea: Excess prolactin secretion (hyperprolactinemia).

Hypopituitarigenic dwarfism: Deficits in pituitary GH secretion, in some cases due to developmental failure or tumor development, and in other cases due to altered GHRH or somatostatin neurosecretion.

Laron dwarfism: Failure of the liver to respond to GH with the production of somatomedins.

Panhypopituitarism: Complete lack of anterior pituitary hormone secretions due to the failure of the pituitary gland to develop normally, or as a result of injury to the gland.

Pituitarigenic gigantism: Excess GH secretion during childhood, due to the development of a pituitary tumor, or altered hypophysiotropin neurosecretion and regulation of somatotropes.

Chapter 6   The Endocrine Hypothalamus

Compare and Contrast each of the Following Terms. How are they Related? How do they Differ?

Hypertrophy/hyperplasia: While *hypertrophy* is a general increase in bulk of a tissue or organ, *hyperplastic* refers to a tissue in which *hyperplasia* occurs, i.e. an increase in number of normal cells in a tissue. Hyperplasia can be the underlying reason for hypertrophy.

Parvocellular/magnocellular (neurons): *Parvocellular* neurons are relatively small neurosecretory cells of the hypothalamus and pre-optic area that project axons to the median eminence, and release hypophysiotropic neurohormones into the hypophysial portal vasculature. *Magnocellular* neurons are relatively large neurosecretory cells whose axons terminate in the posterior pituitary gland, where they release vasopressin and oxytocin into the peripheral circulation.

Ectoderm/neuroectoderm: Ectoderm is the outer layer of cells in the embryo, after the development of the three primary germ layers (ectoderm, mesoderm, endoderm). *Neuroectoderm* is the central region of the early embryonic ectoderm that further develops into the brain and spinal cord.

Hypophysiotropin/hypophysiotropic   area: Hypophysiotropin refers to a neurohormone that stimulates the secretion of one of the anterior pituitary hormones; the *hypophysiotropic area* generally refers to the mediobasal hypothalamus, since this is the neural area that is capaple of maintaining the normal structure and function of pituitary grafts placed adjacent to it. This reflects the fact that hypophysiotropins are released from nerve terminals in the median eminence, which is contained within this tissue.

Hypogonadism/hypergonadism: Hypogonadism is a condition of inadequate gonadal function, manifested as reduced gametogenesis and/or steroidogenesis. *Hypergonadism,* by contrast, is the clinical condition that results from the excess secretion of gonadal hormones.

Primary/secondary (hypothyroidism): Primary hypothyroidism occurs as a result of an intrinsic defect in the ability of parafollicular cells of the thyroid to produce biologically active thyroid hormones. In *secondary hypothyroidism,* a deficit in the production and release of pituitary TSH is the cause of inadequate thyroid hormone synthesis and secretion.

Circadian/diurnal rhythms: Circadian rhythms are oscillations in physiological or behavioral processes that occur with a complete cycle of about 24 hour duration. A *diurnal rhythm* refers to the occurrence of a particular physiological or behavioral event once every 24 hours. A diurnal rhythm is not necessarily an oscillatory phenomenon.

Define or Otherwise Characterize each of the Following Terms (Then use each of the Terms in a Sentence):

Neurovascular hypothesis: This hypothesis, now uniformly accepted among neuroendocrinologists, holds that the hypothalamus contains neurosecretory neurons that release hypothalamic releasing and inhibiting factors into the hypophysial portal vasculature, which are conveyed to the anterior pituitary where they regulate synthesis and secretion of the anterior pituitary hormones.

Hyperprolactinemia: High levels of prolactin in peripheral serum, resulting from hypersecretion of prolactin from lactotropes.

Portal blood vessels, portal system: The hypothalamic-hypophysial *portal vessel system (portal blood vessels)* convey hypophysiotropins that are released from nerve terminals in the median eminence, to the anterior pituitary gland, where these stimulating and inhibiting factors regulate anterior pituitary hormone secretions.

Ectopic site: In anatomy, the position of a tissue at an abnormal location.

Median eminence: The neural tissue at the base of the hypothalamus where neurosecretion of hypophysiotropins into the portal vessel system occurs.

Match each Hypophysiotropin to its Corresponding Pituitary Hormone(s), Indicating (+) or (−) Control:

CRH: (+) ACTH
TRH: (+) TSH
GnRH: (+) LH, FSH
GHRH: (+) GH
SST: (−) GH
DA: (−) PRL

Chapter 7   Neurohypophysial Hormones

Compare and Contrast each of the Following Terms:

Baroreceptor/osmoreceptor: Baroreceptors are sensory nerve endings that are located in the walls of the heart, vena cava, aortic arch, and carotid sinus, that are sensitive to the stretching of the tissue wall, and secondary to changes in the pressure within the vessel/tissue. *Osmoreceptors* are cells in the central nervous system, most often in the preoptic area and hypothalamus, that respond to alterations in the osmotic pressure of the blood perfusing that tissue.

AVT/AVP: Arginine vasopression (AVP) is a nonapeptide neurohypophysial hormone that is structurally related to oxytocin and arginine vasotocin (AVT). It is a physiological regulator of water reabsorption in the collecting ducts of the renal tubules, and it also possesses vasoconstrictive properties. *Arginine vasotocin* is a nonapeptide that is present in the neurohyophysis of non-mammalian vertebrates. It contains an arginyl residue at position 8 and an isoleucyl residue at position 3.

Polydipsia/polyuria: Polydipsia is a condition of excessive and prolonged thirst, while *polyuria* is an excessive secretion of urine. Both are symptoms of AVP deficiency.

Paraventricular/supraoptic (nuclei): These two hypothalamic nuclei contain the magnocellular neurons that produce the neurohypophysial hormones, vasopressin and oxytocin.

Oviparous/viviparous: An *oviparous* animal is one that lays eggs, while *viviparous* animals give birth to live young.

Myometrium/myoepithelial cells: The *myometrium* is the muscular wall of the uterus, while *myoepithelial cells* are contractile, smooth muscle cells arranged around secretory alveoli of the mammary gland and sweat glands. Both are targets of the hormone oxytocin.

Neurogenic/nephrogenic: These terms indicate an origin in the nervous system or the kidneys, respectively. They describe two different types of diabetes insipidus, one due to the lack of AVP production or release from the neurohypophysis, and the other resulting from a lack of renal responsiveness to the hormone.

Uterotropic/nephrogenic/antidiuretic (actions of hormones): These refer to the action of hormones on the uterus (oxytocin) and kidneys (vasopressin), the latter action evoking an *antidiuretic* effect on the nephron, i.e. provoking reabsorption of water.

Pressophysin/oxyphysin: These are the neurophysins that are produced by the proteolytic processing of the preprovasopressin and prepro-oxytocin molecules, respectively. The neurophysins are proteins which are co-released with the neurohypophysial hormones into the circulation, and are of uncertain function.

Cysteine/cystine: Cystine is the disulfide product of the linking of two sulfhydryl groups to become a disulfide bridge between two *cysteine* amino acid residues in a protein.

Serosal/mucosal: In a renal tubule, the *serosal* side is the peritubular surface, and the *mucosal* side is the luminal surface.

Exocytosis/endocytosis: Exocytosis is the process by which a hormone or neurotransmitter is released from a cell; it involves a Ca^{++}-dependent fusion of the vesicular or granular membrane with the plasma membrane and diffusion of the contents into the extracellular fluid. *Endocytosis* is essentially the reverse process, in which substances in the extracellular fluid are internalized by the formation of vesicles in the plasma membrane.

Parvocellular/magnocellular: *Parvocellular* neurons are relatively small neurosecretory cells of the hypothalamus and preoptic area that project axons to the median eminence, and release hypophysiotropic neurohormones into the hypophysial portal vasculature. *Magnocellular* neurons are relatively large neurosecretory cells whose axons terminate in the posterior pituitary gland, where they release vasopressin and oxytocin into the peripheral circulation.

Urophysin/neurophysin: Urotensin I and II are peptides that are produced by a neurosecretory system in the spinal cord of many fish. *Urophysins* are by products of the production of urotensins, analogous to the *neurophysins* that are produced in the proteolytic processing of preprovasopressin and prepro-oxytocin.

Diabetes insipidus/diabetes mellitus: The term diabetes is used for any condition that includes the symptom of polyuria. Diabetes insipidus results from a vasopressin deficiency, and is characterized by polydipsia, polyuria, and hypotension, among other symptoms. Diabetes mellitus is caused by a defect in insulin production or action, producing sustained hyperglycemia.

Match the animal group(s) with its (their) neurohypophysial hormone(s):

1. Cartilaginous fishes: D, arginine vasotocin, G, valitocin, aspargtocin
2. Bony fishes: F, isotocin
3. Amphibians: D, arginine vasotocin, C, mesotocin
4. Reptiles: D, arginine vasotocin
5. Birds: D, arginine vasotocin
6. Mammals except domestic pigs and Macropodidae: A, arginine vasopressin, E, oxytocin
7. Domestic pigs and certain marsupials: B, lysine vasopressin

Chapter 8   Opiomelanocortins

Match the Hormone/Receptor/Cell with its Anatomical Location:

1. Melanocortin receptor MC1-R: E, melanocytes
2. α-Melanotropin: B, pituitary/hypothalamus
3. Melanocortin receptor MC2-R: D, adrenal cortex
4. Adrenocorticotropin: C, pars distalis
5. Chromatophores: E, dermis
6. Melanocortin receptor MC3-R: A, hypothalamus/limbic system
7. Melanin-concentrating hormone: F, pars intermedia/arcuate nucleus
8. β-Endorphin: B, pituitary, hypothalamus

Chapter 9   Hormonal Control of Calcium Homeostasis

Match the Disease/Defect with Its Primary Effect on Plasma Hormone Levels:

1. Hypoparathyroidism: A, lowered parathormone, C, lowered vitamin D
2. Paget's disease: B, elevated parathormone
3. Defective calcium sensing receptor: B, elevated parathormone
4. Parathyroid cancer (neoplasia or hyperplasia): B, elevated parathormone
5. Vitamin-D-responsive osteomalacia: C, lowered vitamin D
6. Secondary hyperparathyroidism: B, elevated parathormone, C, lowered vitamin D
7. Senile osteoporosis: A, lowered parathormone, C, lowered\ vitamin D

Chapter 10   Gastrointestinal Hormones

Match the GI Hormone with Its Cellular/Anatomic source:

1. GIP: C, K cells
2. CCK: E, I cells
3. Gastrin: D, G cells
4. Secretin: F, S cells
5. VIP: A, Meissner's and Auerbach's plexuses
6. Somatostatin: B, D cells

Chapter 11   Pancreatic Hormones and Metabolic Regulation

Match the Substrate with Its Metabolite:

1. Glucose: D, Glucose-6-phosphate
2. Glucose-1-phosphate: A, Glycogen
3. Phosphoenolpyruvate: B, pyruvate
4. Glucose-6-phosphate: F, glucose-1-phosphate
5. Fructose-6-phosphate: C, fructose-1,6-phosphate
6. Free fatty acids: E, ketones

Chapter 12   Growth Hormones

Match the Growth Factor with Receptor and/or Signaling Molecules:

	Receptor type (tyrosine kinase, serine/threonine kinase, cytokine receptor)	Intracellular signaling pathway (JAK-STAT, IRS/PI-3 kinase, Smads)
1. Prolactin	cytokine receptor	JAK-STAT
2. TGFβ	serine-threonine kinase	Smads
3. GH	cytokine receptor	JAK-STAT
4. insulin	tyrosine kinase	IRS/PI-3 kinase
5. EGF	tyrosine kinase	IRS/PI-3 kinase
6. IGF-1	tyrosine kinase	IRS/PI-3 kinase

Match the Stages of the Cell Cycle:

1. Apoptosis: F, a stage of programmed cell-death
2. G_0 stage: C, a resting stage
3. G_2 stage: D, a short growth stage
4. G_1 stage: A, a growth stage in preparation for DNA synthesis
5. S stage: E, the DNA synthesis stage
6. M stage: B, a cell division stage

Chapter 13   Thyroid Hormones

Match the Symptom to Its Cause:

1. Low basal metabolic rate: B, hypothyroidism
2. Cold intolerance: B, hypothyroidism
3. Rapid pulse: A, hyperthyroidism
4. Decreased T3-T4 levels: B, hypothyroidism
5. Elevated basal metabolic rate: A, hyperthyrioidism
6. Weight gain: B, Hypothyroidism

Chapter 14 Catecholamines and the Sympathoadrenal System

Match the Substrate with Its Enzyme:

1. Phenylalanine: C, phenylalanine hydroxylase
2. Dopa: E, L-aromatic amino acid decarboxylase
3. Tyrosine: A, tyrosine hydroxylase
4. Norepinephrine: D, phenylethanolamine- *N*-methyltransferase
5. Dopamine: B, dopamine β-hydroxylase
6. Epinephrine: F, monoamine oxidase

Fill in the blanks to complete the comparisons between the parasympathetic and sympathetic nervous systems:

Attributes	Parasympathetic nervous system	Sympathetic nervous system
Relative length of preganglionic fibers	long	short
Relative length of postganglionic fibers	short	long
Spinal cord regions giving rise to fibers	cranial, sacral	thoracic, lumbar
Preganglionic neurotransmitter	acetylcholine	acetylcholine
Postganglionic neurotransmitter	acetylcholine	norepinephrine
Active in resting state or stress	resting state	stress
Discrete or mass response	discrete	mass response

Chapter 15 Adrenal Steroid Hormones

Match the Steroid with Its General Classification:

1. Cortisol: B glucocorticoid
2. 11-Deoxycorticosterone: D, mineralocorticoid
3. Aldosterone: D, mineralocorticoid
4. Progesterone: A, progestin
5. Corticosterone: B, glucocorticoid
6. Dehydroepiandrosterone: C, androgen

Chapter 16 Endocrinology of Sex Differentiation and Development

Match the Steroid with Its Direct Steroid Precursor:

1. Pregnenolone: B, cholesterol
2. Progesterone: D, pregnenolone
3. 17α-OH-Progesterone: A, progesterone
4. Androstenedione: F, 17α-OH-Progesterone
5. Testosterone: C, Androstendione
6. Estradiol: E, testosterone

Chapter 17 Hormones and Male Reproductive Physiology

Match the Exons of the Androgen Receptor with their Function:

1. Exon A: C, transcriptional transactivation
2. Exon D: A, androgen-binding domain
3. Exon C: B, DNA-binding domain
4. Exon E: A, androgen-binding domain
5. Exon B: B, DNA binding domain
6. Exon F: A, androgen-binding domain
A. Androgen-binding domain
B. DNA-binding domain
C. Transcriptional transactivation

Match the Molecule with the Cell Type:

1. GnRH receptor: gonadotrope
2. LH receptor: Leydig cell
3. FSH receptor: Sertoli cell
4. inhibin receptor: gonadotrope
5. inhibin: Sertoli cells
6. LHβ subunit: gonadotrope
7. androgen binding protein: Sertoli cell
8. testosterone: Leydig cell
9. activin receptor: gonadotrope
10. androgen receptor: neurons in the SNB

Chapter 18 Hormones and Female Reproductive Physiology

Match the Terms:

1. Graafian follicle: B, mature follicle
2. Atretic follicle: D, expiring follicle
3. Primordial follicle: A, resting follicle
4. Egg: E, ovum
5. Interstitial tissue: F, theca folliculi
6. Epithelial tissue: C, granulosa cells

Chapter 19 Endocrinology of Pregnancy, Parturition, and Lactation

Match the Terms with their Description:

1. Zygote: E, the cell that results from fertilization
2. Morula: D, compact mass of cells
3. Blastocyst: B, a hollow sphere of cells
4. Ovum: A, unfertilized egg
5. Neonate: F, newly born offspring
6. Fetus: C, an embryo

Chapter 20 Endocrine Role of the Pineal Gland

Match the Manipulation with Its Effect on Plasma Melatonin Levels:

1. Decreased day length: A, increased melatonin
2. Increased day length: B, decreased melatonin
3. Pinealectomy: B, decreased melatonin
4. Blinding: A, increased melatonin
5. Inhibition of *N*-acetyltransferase: B, decreased melatonin.
6. Stimulation of the superior cervical ganglion: A, decreased melatonin

Books and Monographs

ADASHI, E. Y., J. A. ROOK, AND Z. ROSENWAKS (Eds.). 1996. *Reproductive endocrinology, surgery and technology.* Philadelphia: Lippincott-Raven.

BAXTER, J. D., S. MELMED, AND M. I. NEW (Eds.), L. MARTINI (Series ed.). 2002. *Genetics in endocrinology.* Philadelphia: Lippincott Williams & Wilkins.

BECKER, J. B., S. M. BREEDLOVE, D. CREWS, AND M. M. MCCARTHY. 2002. *Behavioral endocrinology,* 2nd edn. Boston, MA: MIT Press.

BENTLEY, P. J. 1998. *Comparative vertebrate endocrinology.* Cambridge, UK: Cambridge University Press.

BOLANDER, F. F. 2004. *Molecular endocrinology,* 3rd edn. San Diego, CA: Elsevier, Inc., Academic Press.

BRAVERMAN, L. E., AND R. D. UTIGER (Eds.). 1996. *Werner and Inghar's the thyroid, a fundamental and clinical text.* Philadelphia: Lippincott-Raven.

CONN, P. M., AND M. E. FREEMAN (Eds.). 2000. *Neuroendocrinology in physiology and medicine.* Totowa, NJ: Humana Press.

DEGROOT, L., AND J. L. JAMESON. 2005. *Endocrinology.* San Diego, CA: Elsevier Inc., Saunders.

FELIG, P., AND L. A. FROHMAN. 2001. *Endocrinology and metabolism.* New York, NY: McGraw-Hill.

GOODMAN, H. M. 2003. *Basic medical endocrinology,* 3rd edn. San Diego, CA: Academic Press.

GRIFFIN, E., AND S. R. OJEDA (Eds.). 2004. *Textbook of endocrine physiology,* 5th edn. New York: Oxford University Press.

HENRY, H. L., AND A. W. NORMAN (Eds.). 2003. *Encyclopedia of Hormones, Vol. 1–3.* San Diego, CA: Elsevier, Inc.

JONES, R. E., AND K. H. LOPEZ. 2006. *Human reproductive biology,* 3rd edn. San Diego: Academic Press.

LARSEN, P. R., H. M. KRONENBERG, S. MELMED, AND K. S. POLONSKY (Eds.). 2002. *Williams Textbook of endocrinology.* Philadelphia: W. B. Saunders.

LAUFER, H., AND R. G. H. DOWNER (Eds.). 1988. *Invertebrate endocrinology, Vol. 2: Endocrinology of selected invertebrate types.* New York: Alan R. Liss.

LEROITH, D., J. M. OLEFSKY, AND S. I. TAYLOR. 2003. *Diabetes mellitus: a fundamental and clinical text.* Philadelphia: Lippincott Williams and Williams.

NELSON, R. J. 2005. *An introduction to behavioral endocrinology,* 3rd edn. Sunderland, MA: Sinauer.

NORRIS, D. O. 1996. *Vertebrate endocrinology,* 3rd edn. Philadelphia: Lea & Febiger.

NORRIS, D. O., AND R. E. JONES (Eds.). 1987. *Hormones and reproduction in fishes, amphibians, and reptiles.* New York: Plenum Press.

PANG, P. K. T., M. P. SCHREIBMAN, AND A. GORBMAN (Eds.). 1986. *Vertebrate endocrinology, Vol 1: Morphological considerations.* San Diego: Academic Press.

PANG, P. K. T., AND M. P. SCHREIBMAN (Eds.). 1987. *Vertebrate endocrinology, Vol. 2: Regulation of water and electrolytes.* San Diego: Academic Press.

PANG, P. K. T., AND M. SCHREIBMAN (Eds.). 1987. *Vertebrate endocrinology, Vol 3: Regulation of calcium and phosphate.* San Diego: Academic Press.

PFAFF, D. W., A. P. ARNOLD, A. M. ETGEN, S. E. FAHRBACH, AND R. T. RUBIN. 2002. *Hormones, brain and behavior.* San Diego, CA: Elsevier, Inc.

RALPH, C. L. 1986. *Comparative endocrinology: Developments and directions.* New York: Alan R. Liss.

STRAUSS, J., AND R. BARBIERI 2004. *Yen and Jaffe's reproductive endocrinology: Physiology, pathophysiology, and clinical management.* San Diego, CA: Elsevier, Inc., Saunders.

Major Endocrinology Journals

Acta Endocrinologica (Acta Endocrinol.)
Advances in Cyclic Nucleotide Research (Advan. Cyclic Nucl. Res.)
Annales d'Endocrinologie (Ann. d'Endocrinol.)
Baillière's Clinical Endocrinology and Metabolism (Baillière's Clin. Endocr. Metab.)
Clinical Endocrinology (Clin. Endocrinol.)
Domestic Animal Endocrinology (Domest. Anim. Endocrinol.)
Endocrine

Endocrine Pathology (Endocr. Pathol.)
Endocrine Research (Endocr. Res.)
Endocrine Research Communications (Endocr. Res. Commun.)
Endocrine Reviews (Endocr. Rev.)
Endocrinologica Japonica (Endocrinol. Jpn.)
The Endocrinologist
Endocrinology
Endocrinology and Metabolism Clinics of North America (Endocrinol. Metab. Clin. North Am.)
European Journal of Endocrinology (Eur. J. Endocrinol.)
Experimental and Clinical Endocrinology (Exp. Clin. Endocrinol.)
Frontiers in Neuroendocrinology (Front. Neuroendocrinol.)
General and Comparative Endocrinology (Gen. Comp. Endocrinol.)
Growth Factors
Gynecological Endocrinology (Gynecol. Endocrinol.)
Hormone Research (Horm. Res.)
Hormones and Behavior (Horm. Behav.)
Hormone and Metabolism Research (Horm. Metab. Res.)
Journal of Clinical Endocrinology and Metabolism (J. Clin. Endocrinol. Metab.)
Journal of Endocrinology (J. Endocrinol.)
Journal of Endocrinological Investigation (J. Endocrinol. Invest.)
Journal of Molecular Endocrinology (J. Mol. Endocrinol.)
Journal of Neuroendocrinology (J. Neuroendocrinol.)
Journal of Pediatric Endocrinology and Metabolism (J. Pediatr. Endocrinol. Metab.)
Molecular and Cellular Endocrinology (Mol. Cell. Endocrinol.)
Molecular Endocrinology (Mol. Endocrinol.)
Neuroendocrinology
Pituitary
Psychoneuroendocrinology
Regulatory Peptides (Reg. Pept.)
Stress
Trends in Endocrinology and Metabolism (TEM)

Endocrinology-Related Journals

Acta Diabetologia (Acta Diabetol.)
Advances in Prostaglandin and Thromboxane Research
Advances in Steroid Biochemistry and Pharmacology
American Journal of Physiology (Am. J. Physiol.)
Biology of Reproduction (Biol. Reprod.)
Cell and Tissue Research (Cell Tissue Res.)
Clinical Investigation (Clin. Invest.)
Diabetes
Diabetologia
Federation Proceedings (Fed. Proc.)
Fertility and Sterility (Fertil. Steril.)
Human Reproduction (Hum. Reprod.)
Journal of the American Medical Association (JAMA)
Journal of Biological Chemistry (J. Biol. Chem.)
Journal of Clinical Investigation (J. Clin. Invest.)
Journal of Cyclic Nucleotide Research (J. Cyclic Nucl. Res.)
Journal of Experimental Zoology (J. Exp. Zool.)
Journal of General Physiology (J. Gen. Physiol.)
Journal of Neurophysiology (J. Neurophysiol.)
Journal of Neuroscience (J. Neurosci.)
Journal of Nutrition (J. Nutr.)
Journal of Physiology (J. Physiol.)
Journal of Pineal Research (J. Pineal Res.)
Journal of Receptor Research (J. Receptor Res.)
Journal of Steroid Biochemistry and Molecular Biology (J. Steroid Biochem. Mol. Biol.)
Laboratory Investigation (Lab. Invest.)
Life Sciences (Life Sci.)
Metabolism
New England Journal of Medicine (N. Engl. J. Med.)
News in Physiological Sciences (NIPS)
Obesity
Peptides
Physiology and Behavior (Physiol. Behav.)
Proceedings of the National Academy of Sciences USA (Proc. Natl. Acad. Sci. USA)
Regulatory Peptides (Regul. Pept.)
Thyroid

Serial Publications

Annual Review of Biochemistry (Annu. Rev. Biochem.)
Annual Review of Medicine (Annu. Rev. Med.)
Annual Review of Neuroscience (Annu. Rev. Neurosci.)
Annual Review of Pharmacology and Toxicology (Annu. Rev. Pharmacol. Toxicol.)
Annual Review of Physiology (Annu. Rev. Physiol.)
Contemporary Endocrinology (formerly The Year in Endocrinology)
Physiological Reviews (Physiol. Rev.)
Recent Progress in Hormone Research (Rec. Prog. Horm. Res.)
Vitamins and Hormones (Vit. Horm.)

INDEX

Some Common Endocrine Abbreviations and Terminology

ACTH	Adrenocorticotropic hormone (corticotropin)
ADH	Antidiuretic hormone
ANF	Atrial natriuretic factor (atriopeptin, atrial natriuretic peptide, ANP)
ANS	Autonomic nervous system
APUD	Amine precursor uptake and decarboxylation
AVP	Arginine vasopressin
AVT	Arginine vasotocin
cAMP	Cyclic adenosine monophosphate (cyclic AMP)
CaM	Calmodulin
CaBP	Calcium-binding protein
CBG	Corticosteroid-binding globulin, transcortin
CCK	Cholecystokinin
cGMP	Cyclic guanosine monophosphate (cyclic GMP)
CGRP	Calcitonin gene-related peptide
CNS	Central nervous system
COMT	Catechol-O-methyltransferase
CRH	Corticotropin-releasing hormone
CSF	Cerebrospinal fluid
DG	Diacylglycerol (or DAG)
DA	Dopamine
DBH	Dopamine β-hydroxylase
DHT	Dihydrotestosterone
DIT	Diiodotyrosine
DOPA	Dihydroxyphenylalanine
EGF	Epidermal growth factor
FGF	Fibroblast growth factor
FSH	Follicle-stimulating hormone (follitropin)
GH	Growth hormone (somatotropin, STH)
GHRH	Growth hormone releasing hormone (somatocrinin)
GIP	Gastric inhibitory peptide
GRP	Gastrin-releasing peptide
GLP-1	Glucagon-like peptide 1
GnRH	Gonadotropin-releasing hormone (LH/FSH-RH)
GPCR	G-protein-coupled receptor
GTP	Guanosine triphosphate
hCG	Human chorionic gonadotropin (choriogonadotropin)
HIOMT	Hydroxyindole-O-methyltransferase
hPL	Human placental lactogen
HRE	Hormone response element
5-HT	5-Hydroxytryptamine (serotonin)
IGFs	Insulin-like growth factors (I and II)